Concepts in HEALTH and WELLNESS

Concepts
in
HEALTH and
WELLNESS

James Robinson, III, EdD, FAAHE
Deborah J. McCormick, PhD

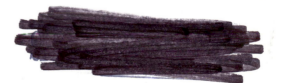

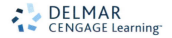
DELMAR
CENGAGE Learning™

Australia • Brazil • Japan • Korea • Mexico • Singapore • Spain • United Kingdom • United States

Concepts in Health and Wellness, 1st Edition
James Robinson, III, EdD, FAAHE,
Deborah J. McCormick, PhD

Vice President, Career and Professional
Editorial: Dave Garza

Director of Learning Solutions: Matt Kane

Acquisitions Editor: Matt Seeley

Managing Editor: Marah Bellegarde

Senior Product Manager: Juliet Steiner

Editorial Assistant: Samantha Zullo

Vice President, Career and Professional
Marketing: Jennifer Ann Baker

Marketing Director: Wendy Mapstone

Senior Marketing Manager: Kristin McNary

Marketing Coordinator: Erica Ropinsky

Production Director: Carolyn Miller

Production Manager: Andrew Crouth

Content Project Manager: Anne Sherman

Senior Art Director: Jack Pendleton

For product information and technology assistance, contact us at
Cengage Learning Customer & Sales Support, 1-800-354-9706

For permission to use material from this text or product,
submit all requests online at **www.cengage.com/permissions.**
Further permissions questions can be e-mailed to
permissionrequest@cengage.com

Library of Congress Control Number: 2009942712

ISBN-13: 978-1-4180-5541-7
ISBN-10: 1-4180-5541-7

Delmar
5 Maxwell Drive
Clifton Park, NY 12065-2919
USA

Cengage Learning is a leading provider of customized learning solutions with office locations around the globe, including Singapore, the United Kingdom, Australia, Mexico, Brazil, and Japan. Locate your local office at: **international .cengage.com/region**

Cengage Learning products are represented in Canada by
Nelson Education, Ltd.

To learn more about Delmar, visit **www.cengage.com/delmar**

Purchase any of our products at your local college store or at our preferred online store **www.ichapters.com**

NOTICE TO THE READER
Publisher does not warrant or guarantee any of the products described herein or perform any independent analysis in connection with any of the product information contained herein. Publisher does not assume, and expressly disclaims, any obligation to obtain and include information other than that provided to it by the manufacturer. The reader is expressly warned to consider and adopt all safety precautions that might be indicated by the activities described herein and to avoid all potential hazards. By following the instructions contained herein, the reader willingly assumes all risks in connection with such instructions. The publisher makes no representations or warranties of any kind, including but not limited to, the warranties of fitness for particular purpose or merchantability, nor are any such representations implied with respect to the material set forth herein, and the publisher takes no responsibility with respect to such material. The publisher shall not be liable for any special, consequential, or exemplary damages resulting, in whole or part, from the readers' use of, or reliance upon, this material.

Printed in the United States of America
1 2 3 4 5 6 7 12 11 10

CONTENTS

v

PREFACE

There is perhaps no other point in the history of our nation when we have been more concerned about the population's health, access to health care, and the cost of medical treatment. Our country's leadership is attempting to reform the entire health care system in an effort to improve the health status of all and make treatment more affordable. While all this is taking place, we must not forget that Americans have the personal power to affect their health status through the adoption of their own health behaviors. Health researchers have reported a number of important findings related to people who practice health-protective behaviors:

- People who practice good health behaviors are healthier than those people who do not practice such behaviors; thus, healthier people require less health care.

- When healthy people do require health care, they are less likely to require very expensive treatment.

- Healthy people recover from illness more rapidly when they do get ill.

In this regard, it is in everyone's best interest to engage in a personal lifestyle that encourages healthy behaviors. Developing healthy behaviors is easily accomplished if the individual possesses the motivation for developing behaviors and the knowledge and skills to develop and practice those health behaviors.

Concepts in Health and Wellness is an approachable, inviting, straightforward text that provides postsecondary students with the essential body of personal health information that they can use to develop a lifetime of wellness skills. The goal of this text is to help you enhance your motivation to develop the knowledge and skills necessary to ensure optimal wellness throughout adulthood. The purpose of this text is to provide you with meaningful literary support for class instruction but, more important, to empower you with the skills to access credible health and wellness information now and in the years to come. This text is meant to meet the diverse needs and interests of college and university students regardless of the academic setting. It is written in a style that is easily understood by learners at all levels.

Organization of Text

The text is composed of 17 chapters covering a wide range of contemporary personal health issues. This organizational structure allows the entire text to be used during what is typically a semester-long college health course. The instructional style is designed to encourage a personal wellness emphasis to include healthy behaviors. Health behavior theory was used to craft the narrative style throughout the text.

Knowledge that does not lead to behavior is not very useful. Philosophically, we believe what students *do about their health and wellness* is just as important, if not more so, as *the health knowledge they develop*. This text does more than present health information. The authors created the chapter components to provide opportunities for you to think critically about personal and community health issues and engage in problem-solving activities to address important health problems. Many of these activities give you the opportunity to do research, perform interviews, and write down personal information, all of which can be used or modified to suit health needs as necessary. It is recommended that you create a wellness journal where you can keep track of personal health information and resources developed during the course.

The many special features and activities included in each chapter are designed to make learning health and wellness concepts engaging, interesting, and entertaining. Our intention was to produce a student-friendly text that does the following:

- Promotes the adoption of a wellness lifestyle

- Encourages the development of health literacy skills so that you can access valid and reliable online and hard-copy materials to support your wellness program

- Includes wellness planning exercises that can be completed and archived for use at a later time

- Promotes a sense of personal advocacy so that you can serve as a health resource for family, friends, and community

Organized into the back of the textbook are wellness plan worksheets for each chapter. These worksheets provide opportunities for you to apply the knowledge and skills derived from the chapter activities. The prompts in the wellness plans invite you to apply chapter information to real-life situations. These perforated pages can be removed from the book and included in a personal wellness folio or journal for reference at a future time. These worksheets support the chapters, but they are useful tools for developing and maintaining a lifetime wellness plan.

Chapter Components

Chapter elements were developed to support the overall philosophy of the text. Each chapter includes a number of pedagogical elements to enhance your motivation and interest.

Chapter Opening

Each chapter begins with an introduction to the specific chapter topic. Each chapter also includes student-centered learning objectives, written to match the

academic skills of the postsecondary learner. These objectives will serve as instructional guidelines to help you attain mastery of the knowledge and skills emphasized in the chapter. You will find a list of key terms featured in the chapter. Within each chapter, all new terms are highlighted and described in the chapter margin on the same page where the term is introduced. These terms are also included in the comprehensive glossary at the back of the book. At the start of each chapter, you are presented with a personal assessment activity designed to measure your understanding of the chapter theme or to assess individual behaviors associated with the chapter's wellness message. Interpretations of personal assessment items are included for reference at the end of each chapter, but you will also find assessment-related information embedded within the chapter.

Chapter Features

Each chapter contains the special features described in the following sections. The features were designed to enhance your interest in the topics, present cutting-edge news related to key chapter topics, or present thought-provoking activities to challenge student knowledge or critical thinking:

- The *Did You Know…?* feature contains little-known facts intended to reinforce chapter topics in an entertaining manner. This feature is located in the margin near related textual material.

- *Web Links* include URL addresses for Web sites that add additional clarity/information on the particular chapter topics. The Web links have been researched for reliability, accuracy, and suitability and are annotated for easy student reference. All Web links were verified at the time of production, but, as we know, Web sites are subject to change. In that regard, each feature contains the search terms that can be used to find other sites using search engines.

- *What's News?* is a feature designed to deliver late-breaking research findings or other news items that will be of interest. Moreover, this feature teaches that health and wellness–related information is constantly evolving and that health literacy skills are important to your wellness plan.

- *What's Your View?* is designed to provide thought-provoking scenarios related to the chapter themes. Your can use the scenarios to make use of their health literacy and problem-solving skills. Many of the *What's Your View?* responses can be written down and included in your wellness plans.

- The *Talking It Over* feature provides discussion triggers linked to a central theme within the respective chapter. You can share the discussion triggers with family, friends, or class mates. Depending on the personal nature of the features, the instructor may want to have small groups of students discuss the feature topic and share with the class for a larger discussion on the topic.

- Each chapter concludes with *End-of-Chapter Activities* to reinforce learning. You can complete application exercises and discussion questions to enhance mastery of the chapter key concepts.

- Finally, at the back of this text, there is a worksheet for each chapter, labeled the *Personal Wellness Plan*. The wellness plan is a self-directed way for you to develop or enhance lifelong wellness skills as you moves through the text. You can develop their personal wellness folios during the course as you complete the wellness plan worksheets for each chapter.

Learning and Teaching Package

The complete supplements package for *Concepts in Health and Wellness* was developed to achieve two goals:

- To assist students in learning the information presented in the text

- To assist instructors in planning and implementing their course for the most efficient use of time and other resources

Instructor Resources

Instructor Resource to Accompany Concepts in Health and Wellness

ISBN-10: 1-4180-5542-5
ISBN-13: 978-1-41805-542-4
The Instructor's Resource CD-ROM has three components to assist the instructor and enhance classroom activities and discussion.

Instructor's Guide

An electronic Instructor's Guide provides excellent tools to help the instructor create a dynamic and engaging learning experience for the student. The Instructor's Guide

contains the tools listed here but can be downloaded and modified to meet individual instructional goals:

- **Teaching Strategies:** This section provides engaging ideas and tips for the instructor to use in conjunction with the chapter topics.

- **Strategies for Stimulating Class Discussion:** These excellent and provocative discussion topics can be used to challenge student critical thinking and to create an interactive classroom experience.

- **Additional Internet Activities, Writing Exercises, Role-Playing Activities, or Assignments:** These additional ready-to-use activities and assignments are provided to support the instructor with thoughtful activities directly supporting the individual chapters.

- **Answers to End of Chapter Questions:** Answers and intended outcomes for the end of chapter questions are provided to assist the instructor in grading and evaluation.

Computerized Testbank in ExamView™

- Includes 680 multiple-choice, short-answer, and matching questions that test students on retention and application of material in the text.

- All questions provide correct answers and rationales.

- Allows instructors to create custom tests by mixing questions from each of the 17 chapters of questions, modifying existing questions, and even adding additional questions to meet individual instructional needs.

Instructor Slides Created in PowerPoint

- A comprehensive offering of over 250 instructor slides created in PowerPoint outlines the concepts from the text to assist the instructor with lectures.

- Ideas presented to stimulate discussion and critical thinking.

Concepts in Health and Wellness Online Companion

The Online Companion gives you online access to a range of additional resources to support understanding of the material. On the password-protected instructor side, instructors will find all the components of the Instructor's Resource CD. To access the Online Companion Web site, simply point your browser to http://www.delmar.cengage.com/companions. Select the Health Education Discipline and then select Concepts in Health and Wellness.

Student Resources

Concepts in Health and Wellness WebTutor on Blackboard

ISBN-10: 1418055441
ISBN-13: 978-1-4180-5544-8

Concepts in Health and Wellness WebTutor on WebCT

ISBN-10: 1418055433
ISBN-13: 978-1-4180-5543-1

Our WebTutors are a complete online environment supplementing your course, provided in both Blackboard and WebCT format. Chapter resources including Chapter Objectives, Building your Wellness Plan, and Weblinks are provided, along with useful classroom management tools including chats and calendars. The complete contents of the Instructor Resource CD-ROM is provided, allowing for easy implementation of the extensive instructor package in these online course management environments.

ABOUT THE AUTHORS

James Robinson, III, EdD, FAAHE

James Robinson is currently professor and graduate coordinator in the Department of Public Health Sciences at New Mexico State University. Dr. Robinson received his BS in health and physical education and his MEd in health education from West Chester University and his EdD in health education from the University of Northern Colorado. He taught health education for nine years in the Downingtown Area School District, Downingtown, Pennsylvania. After his doctoral studies, he held faculty appointments at California State University, Northridge; the University of Northern Colorado; Texas A&M University; and Texas A&M Health Science Center. Dr. Robinson's health education consultations include school districts in California, Colorado, Texas, and Wyoming as well as the state health and education departments in Colorado and Texas. Dr. Robinson is author or coauthor of more than 25 professional publications and has delivered more than 75 professional presentations to local, state, and national audiences. He is lead author of *Essentials of Health and Wellness*, a health textbook for high school students, and is currently the executive editor of the *Journal of Drug Education: Substance Abuse Research and Prevention*. Dr. Robinson has served on numerous committees and boards of the American Association for Health Education and the American School Health Association. The American Association for Health Education honored him with fellow status in 1999 and with the association's Professional Service Award in 2003. In addition to his teaching, scholarly activity, and service, Dr. Robinson has generated approximately $2.5 million in grant support for his research and projects.

Deborah J. McCormick, PhD

Deborah McCormick is currently an associate clinical professor in the Department of Health Sciences in the College of Health and Human Services at Northern Arizona University in Flagstaff, Arizona. She received her BS in health and physical education from the University of Mary Hardin-Baylor, her MS in health and physical education from Baylor University, and her PhD in health education from Texas A&M University. Dr. McCormick has also held faculty appointments at Lamar University, University of Texas at San Antonio, and Texas State University. She has delivered more than 50 professional presentations to local, state, and national audiences on topics related to health promotion. She is coauthor of *Essentials of Health and Wellness*.

ACKNOWLEDGMENTS

A project such as this is not completed without the support from many individuals. The authors wish to thank the following professionals who contributed to the completion of this text:

Aisha Kudura, Health Content Consultant
Bianca Zamora, Health Content Consultant
Dierdra Bycura, EdD, Health Content Consultant
Kirsten Maanum, MPH, Health Content Consultant

The authors wish to express their appreciation to all those individuals who contributed to the completion of this book: all the students, parents, and others who served as photographic subjects and the many professionals who offered comments, suggestions, and professional insights following their review of the initial draft of this text; their time and effort are greatly appreciated.

Dr. Robinson and Dr. McCormick would like to express their heartfelt gratitude to all the teachers, professors, and colleagues who have contributed to the development of their academic abilities. Dr. Robinson would also like to dedicate this work to his late professional friend, Dr. Thomas Fleming, who was instrumental in starting Dr. Robinson on the path toward textbook publishing.

REVIEWERS

Diana E. Alagra, RN, AHI, CPT
Medical Assistant Program Director
Branford Hall Career Institute
Southington, CT

Tania Dickson-Humphries, BS, ACSM ES/HFI
Exercise Physiologist
Adjunct Faculty
Lake Tahoe Community College
South Lake Tahoe, CA

Susan S. Erue, RN, BSN, MS, PhDc
Professor
Division of Health and Natural Sciences
Nursing Program
Iowa Wesleyan College
Mount Pleasant, IA

Anne M. Loochtan, PhD
Assistant Dean, Health and Public Safety Division
Cincinatti State Technical and Community College
Cincinnati, OH

Kathleen Malachowski, MEd
Assistant Professor, Coordinator of Health and Human
Performance Department
Ocean County College
Toms River, NJ

Anita K. Reed, MSN, RN
Instructor of Nursing
St. Elizabeth School of Nursing
Lafayette, IN

Betty Kehl Richardson
Professor Emeritus
Austin Community College
Austin, TX

Deborah Ruh, RN, BSN, MSEd
Erie Community College
Wiliamsville, NY

Marcea Wiggins, ND
Director of Education
Health Career Institute at Pioneer Pacific College
Wilsonville, OR

Jeffrey W. Wimer, PhD, ATC
Associate Professor of Wellness and Sports Sciences
Millersville University
Millersville, PA

HOW TO USE THE WELLNESS PLANS

This text focuses purposefully on helping you understand how health information can be used to improve your life, health, and wellness. At the end of each chapter, you'll find a section called "Personal Wellness Plan." This section takes concepts and information presented in the chapter and shows how you can apply what you've read to "real life." This section asks you to reflect on your personal life choices. It challenges you to take what you've learned and apply it to the choices and decisions you make for yourself. Through this section, you may find that you already make positive choices for your health and wellness. Or you may learn that there are changes you can make that lead to improvement. These plans are personal; they belong to you and can be revisited after your course is over.

168 **Concepts in Health and Wellness**

BUILDING YOUR LIFETIME WELLNESS PLAN

In this chapter, you learned about the importance of building successful relationships within your family and with friends and romantic partners. All these relationships are part of being a healthy adult. Your wellness plan should include information and strategies to help you gain additional insights and strategies to support your contributions to your family, your friends, and your romantic partner. Because we exist in a social network, we cannot avoid relationships and conflicts. We can go through life ill prepared to interact in a value-creating manner, or we can do all we can to hone our wellness skills, such as the following:

- Recognizing that you may have a variety of types of friends and that each of those relationships can be rewarding and fulfilling

- Understanding the different stressors that can affect your relationships with others and developing ways that you can cope with these stressors while maintaining good relations

- Developing certain qualities and skills that will help you establish and maintain successful relationships

- Work on developing good communication skills, including becoming a good listener

- Understanding the three components of romantic relationships: passion, intimacy, and commitment

- Recognizing the warning signs of unhealthy relationships and knowing strategies to avoid or leave them

CHAPTER FIVE: RESOLVING CONFLICT
Personal Wellness Plan

1. Use your health literacy skills to search the Internet for personal assessments that assess one's personal and psychological qualities related to conflict. List the sites you found and their URL addresses in the table. You may want to enter some notes about the sites in the second row. One site you may want to visit is http://www.nvcc.edu/home/npeck/conflicthome/index.htm. Go to "Personal Conflict."

Site Name
1.
Comments
2.
Comments
3.
Comments

CHAPTER SIX: DEVELOPING HEALTHY RELATIONSHIPS
Personal Wellness Plan

1. Consider family relationships, friendships, and romantic relationships. What positive qualities do you have to contribute to these relationships?

_____
_____
_____
_____
_____

2. What qualities would you like to develop more fully?

_____
_____
_____
_____

3. What can you do *this week* to begin working toward improvement in these areas?

_____
_____
_____
_____
_____

4. What qualities would be important to you in making new friends or finding a new romantic partner?

_____
_____
_____
_____
_____

517

To help you organize your thoughts surrounding your Personal Wellness Plan, a special section called "Lifetime Wellness Plan" has been included at the back of the book. These perforated pages are meant to be removed from the book, written on, and kept with you after your course has concluded. The Lifetime Wellness Plan for each chapter is based on the health and wellness concepts covered in the chapter. However, the questions are personal, asking you to think about specific behaviors and attitudes. In taking the time to answer these questions thoughtfully, you are taking an important step toward creating a wellness plan that you can carry with you throughout your life. You may want to revisit these questions in the months and years to come to check in on your progress or readjust your wellness goals.

CHAPTER 1

Current Health Issues

CHAPTER OBJECTIVES

When you finish this chapter, you should be able to:

- Describe the current definition of health.
- Compare and contrast valid sources of health information.
- Discuss the significance of the four dimensions of health.
- Describe factors that contribute to longevity.
- Explain why health promotion should be important to one's life throughout the life span.
- Describe the characteristics of a health-literate person.
- List the seven skills that are practiced by a health-literate person.

KEY TERMS

chronic diseases	genes	longevity	risk factors
credentials	health literacy	metabolic rate	social support network
critical thinking	homeostasis	mind mapping	testimony
deductive reasoning	inductive reasoning	opinions	valid
diabetes	infectious diseases	optimal health	
feedback	life expectancy	osteoporosis	

●●● Introduction

Before you begin reading this chapter, take a few moments and reflect on the kind of life you want for yourself in the immediate and distant future. Among other things, your reflection may include the knowledge and skills you are gaining from your college education. You may see this training as something that increases the likelihood of obtaining a good job. You may be interested in this material because you are thinking about a good quality of life for you and your family. You may also have a personal interest in preparing for a healthy quality of life and health care as you get older. No doubt these factors may be why you are in college at this time. You expect to acquire the knowledge and skills necessary for your preparation as a competent and productive professional. You may see your transition from learner to professional and visualize the security you will gain from having a good job so you can achieve a good quality of life. While all these things are important, let's not lose sight of what is probably the most important aspect of a good quality of life: your good health. Without your health, all other things can come to a halt. Good health has many advantages. It can improve your ability with learning, it can prevent lost workdays and loss of income, and it can produce vitality and improve work performance and enjoyment of daily activities. In the long run, good health enhances your quality of life, while poor health reduces your ability to enjoy your life and may even affect how long you actually live.

Once a person leaves home and begins to live independently, health and health care become that individual's responsibility. As a young adult, statistically speaking, you are probably enjoying good health; childhood diseases are behind you, and the illnesses facing older adults are years away. If you happen to be someone who is beyond young adulthood, your risk for the health concerns of aging increases as the years go by. Regardless of your age, knowing and performing the behaviors that reduce health risks is in your best interest. It is less expensive to practice prevention than it is to pay health care costs for treatment. Adults have control over their health; in fact, they *must* take responsibility because it is not likely that they will have anyone else to take care of it for them.

The purpose of this course and the content in this text is to help you develop the knowledge and life skills to obtain and maintain optimal health (Figure 1-1). You may find some of the information useful to your friends or family members as well. It is hoped that the material this semester will provide you with the knowledge, skills, and motivation to take charge of your health. Taking advantage of these learning and skill-building opportunities, you will lay the foundation for a lifetime of health and wellness.

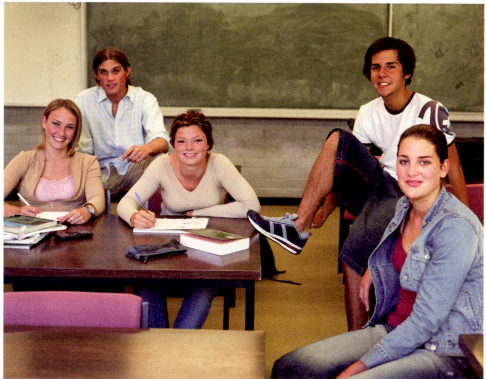

Courtesy of Photodisc

FIGURE 1-1 • Regardless of who you are or your motivations for attending college, this text and this course will help you develop life-long skills for obtaining and maintaining optimal health and personal wellness.

PERSONAL ASSESSMENT
Health Behavior Assessment

Think about the things you are doing or not doing that affect your health. Read each of the following statements and indicate whether the statement applies to you. Feedback is at the end of the chapter.

1. I currently have all the immunizations I am supposed to have.

2. I do not smoke cigarettes.

3. I make an effort to eat fruit and vegetables every day.

4. I choose not to use drugs.

5. I choose to consume alcoholic beverages seldom or not at all.

6. I use a safety belt every time I ride in an automobile.

7. I am able to deal with stressful situations without anger or urgency.

8. I have someone I can talk to when I need help solving problems.

9. I can communicate well with members of my family.

10. I understand the structure of the health care system and know how to use it.

11. I make decisions that are good for my health and act on them.

●●● Acquiring Health and Wellness Information

Before we embark on this journey to good health, we want to introduce you to some information to help you navigate through the chapters and gather useful information from outside reading. Our intention is to make this text as useful as possible—so much so that you want to keep the book and the materials you develop during the semester for future reference.

Making good decisions for your life requires having accurate and meaningful information. It is easy to find numerous sources of information in this electronic age, but determining whether the information is **valid** is not so simple. One should not take such information simply on face value. All too often, health facts seem to contradict each other or change as a result of new medical studies. How does someone know what to believe? The best way to obtain good information is to examine information to see if it is based on evidence supported by scientifically accurate data. For example, many "wonder diets" presented and advertised in the media have not been tested in a scientific manner. The diets are generally advertised using the **testimony** of pleased customers. The diets are seldom based on valid research, and they avoid including information about failures. So where can someone get accurate health information?

valid
based on evidence or supported by scientifically accurate data

testimony
a firsthand declaration of fact

Family and Friends

Friends and family members are often good sources of information, but how reliable and valid is their information? The truth is that their intentions may be good, but what they have to say may not be valid. Rather than act immediately on their information, take the time to confirm the accuracy of the information you get from them or anyone else. One good way to check the accuracy of information is to search for and find the same information in several sources. For example, if you hear something from a friend, read the same thing in your city's daily newspaper, and then locate the same information in a book, you are more likely to have validated what you heard originally. Validating information is important when it comes to health and wellness because following unsound information can result in wasting money or using products and practices that are actually harmful to your health.

Did You Know...?

Some health food companies publish their own newsletters and magazines. They print articles in their publications explaining why special health foods and products are needed for good health. If you read some of the articles in these publications, you will notice that the companies producing the literature also advertise their own brand of the products cited in the articles claiming better health results from using the products.

Printed Materials

You can read books, magazines, journals, and newspapers to gather information, but you need to be careful because not all printed material is accurate. The literature ranges from unbelievable and ridiculous articles, sometimes printed in tabloid newspapers sold at supermarket checkout stands, to reports of carefully conducted scientific studies, found in journals published by major universities or professional organizations. Here are some tips for determining the validity of written information:

- If a claim seems unbelievable, it almost certainly is. Follow your common sense.

- Locate more than one source and compare the information. If it is repeated in a number of reliable publications, the chances increase that the information is true.

- Check the **credentials** of the authors. They should have the proper education and experience to know the subject. Keep in mind that celebrities generally do not have the credentials to endorse books, products, and services. Name alone does not qualify one as an expert.

- Determine the purpose of the writing. If it is to sell a product or to promote its own viewpoints, question the "facts" carefully.

credentials
titles, education, or training that verify a person's intellectual or professional ability

The Internet

The Internet contains numerous sources of health information. There are a number of sites on the Internet specifically designed to help people find many forms of health information. Each of these sites contains identifying information for the wide array of Web pages connected to the Internet. These helpful sites are known as "search engines" (Table 1-1). There are some similarities among search engines, but they are not identical. Some sites have more stored pieces of information than others; thus, you may find links on one site that you won't come across on other sites. Using a good search engine, you can search almost any topic imaginable.

TABLE 1-1 • Top Web search engines for August 2009.

Search Engine	URL	Number of Searches
Google	http://www.google.com	6,986,580
Yahoo	http://www.yahoo.com	1,726,060
MSN	http://www.msn.com	1,156,415
America Online	http://www.aol.com	333,231
Ask.com	http://www.ask.com	186,270

Source: http://searchenginewatch.com.

To use a search engine, simply type in the topic you are researching in the search window and click "search," and the search engine will supply you with a list of Web sites containing information about the topic *according to the terms you entered.* The topic you enter is known as a "search term." You can post a search term as one word or as a series of words. If your topic has more than one word and you enter the words in the search window, the search engine will look for Internet sites having *any* of those words but not necessarily together or in the order you wanted. To acquire a more precise search, look for an "Advanced Search" button on the search page and use it to access a more advanced search menu. Enter your term in an "Exact Phrase" bar, and the engine will search for the terms in the *exact order* you presented them. Your entry can be a couple of words or even an entire sentence.

The location of the Web site will appear as an Internet address known as a URL (Uniform Resource Locator). Once you have found a site that looks interesting, how do you know if the information is accurate? The following tips will help you evaluate health Web sites (Figure 1-2):

- Check the credentials of the person who put the information on the site. Medical and advanced graduate degrees, such as MD and PhD, are often indications that the person is knowledgeable. If there is no author listed, look for the sponsoring organization. Universities, health agencies such as the American Diabetes Association, and federal and state health departments can be reliable sources of information.

- Determine the purpose of the site. Is it trying to sell you something? Be careful of Web sites promising that your life will be better if you buy what they are selling. If the purpose is only to provide information, there is a greater chance that the information is more credible than if the purpose of the site is to sell products.

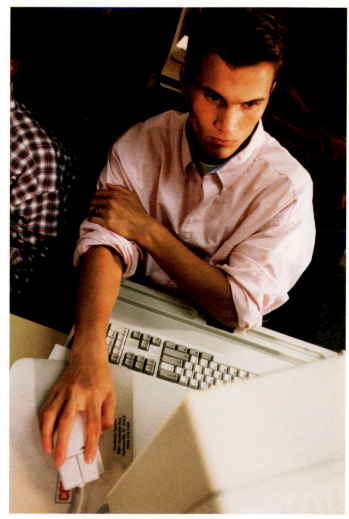

FIGURE 1-2 • The internet has a wealth of accurate and inaccurate health information. Using a reliable search engine and critical thinking skills will help you evaluate health Web sites.

- Seek the same the information on other Internet sites. See if they present the same facts. If so, you will be making a step toward validation of the information.

- Check the date of the material. This should be stated on the Web site, often at the bottom of the page. Dates are especially significant for health information because information may change as new discoveries are made.

- Evaluate how the information is presented. Watch for sweeping generalizations, forcible language, personal testimonies, and claims lacking scientific references.

Search engines are fine for general topics, and there are specific sites you could find via search engines, but you can access sites directly if you already have the URL addresses. For example, there are numerous reliable and stable health and medicine Web sites that you can trust for health information. The following are but a handful of excellent sites. They are all backed by scientific research studies from medicine and social science and are associated with credible medical and health facilities:

- Web M.D.—http://www.webmd.com

- InteliHealth—http://www.intelihealth.com

- U.S. Centers for Disease Control and Prevention—http://www.cdc.gov

- National Institute of Health's Medline Plus—http://www.nlm.nih.gov/medlineplus

- Mayo Clinic—http://www.mayoclinic.com

When using the Internet, remember that Web sites can come and go without notice. The most valid and permanent sites tend to be those supported by reputable organizations. Throughout this text, you will find feature boxes called "Web Links." Each feature will give you the name of a Web site and the URL address for the site. You will also find a description of the information that you will find at the Web site. We have made every effort to validate the existence of the Web site up to the time of printing. If the Web site is no longer up or if you want to find other sites to find information on your topic, the "Web Links" features also have a several usable search terms that will bring up a number of good sites.

●●● Current Health Issues

Tremendous progress has been made in medical research resulting in cures and treatments for many diseases and injuries. Health professionals currently understand more about how the human body works—and does not work—than at any time in history. Prior to the middle of the previous century, the major causes of death in the United States were **infectious diseases**, conditions over which people had little control. When we learned more about "germs" in the late 1800s, people and communities put in practices that prevented many illnesses. Until the development of vaccines and antibiotics, people had few opportunities to prevent or cure infections. Currently, we have many vaccines to prevent diseases and a wide range of antibiotics to treat infections. With medical advances and preventive health practices, the disease conditions of the past are not major areas of concern today in the United States. Look at the leading causes of death for 1900 and 2004 listed in Table 1-2. You will see that there are distinct differences among the top causes of death.

infectious diseases
diseases caused by organisms that can spread through water, food, air, or human contact

TABLE 1-2 • Causes of death in the United States, 1900 and 2004.

1900[1]	Rate*	2004[2]	Rate*
Pneumonia and influenza	202.2	Diseases of the heart	222.7
Tuberculosis	194.4	Cancer	187.4
Diarrhea, enteritis, and ulceration of colon	142.7	Stroke	51.1
Diseases of the heart	137.4	Chronic respiratory disease	42.2
Stroke	106.9	Accidents	37.0
Kidney disease	88.6	Diabetes	24.8
Accidents	72.3	Alzheimer's disease	22.4
Cancer	64.0	Influenza and pneumonia	20.9
Senility (Alzheimer's disease)	50.2	Kidney disease	14.6
Diphtheria	40.3	Septicemia	11.4

[1]National Office of Vital Statistics, December 1947.
[2]National Vital Statistics Reports, June 28, 2006.
*Number of deaths per 100,000 population.

Delmar/Cengage Learning

In 1900, people died from conditions such as pneumonia, flu, tuberculosis, and abdominal infections, all caused by infectious organisms such as bacteria and viruses. Today, the three leading causes of death are heart disease, cancer, and stroke, all of which are conditions related to lifestyle factors and environmental conditions, not infectious organisms. You may think that the leading causes of death and other serious diseases, such as **diabetes** and **osteoporosis**, are for older people to worry about. But there is ample evidence that many of the habits practiced during young adulthood and throughout the life span determine the condition of one's health in later adulthood. For example, research reported by the U.S. Department of Health and Human Services (2004) confirms that weight-bearing exercise such as walking, jogging, and floor aerobics along with a diet rich in calcium beginning in young adulthood can reduce the likelihood of osteoporosis later in life.

Of equal importance are health concerns that may not be listed specifically as causes of death but that still present numerous threats to the individual and/or society. Drug use is one of these concerns. Drug use per se is not listed as a reason for death on a death certificate, but involvement in drug abuse can be very unhealthy. There are health risks, such as overdose, infections, and psychological stress, but there are also associated risks, such as violence, crime, and legal consequences making drug use a risky and unhealthy behavior.

Think of health as a reflection of your body's state of **homeostasis**, the condition of your body at any given point in time. In that regard, your health is constantly changing, varying from day to day and even from hour to hour. Sometimes changes come suddenly; you wake up one morning with a fever and a headache. At other times, changes are not quite as obvious. As a person ages, his or her body may develop conditions leading to heart disease or cancer, and the person may not feel any symptoms at all. Because adults can have an illness without feeling symptoms, it is a good idea to obtain regular medical examinations in order to detect illnesses so that they can be treated in a timely fashion.

diabetes
disease in which the pancreas does not produce enough insulin, a hormone needed to properly convert sugar to energy

osteoporosis
a condition in which the bones lose their density and strength

homeostasis
a condition of the body's internal harmony as regulated by interaction of many body systems

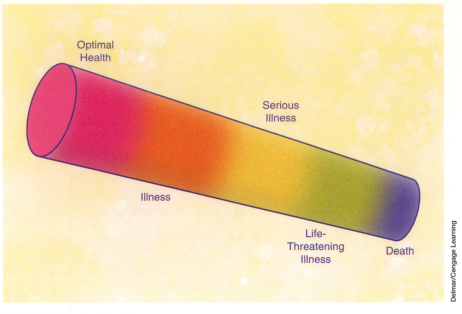

Delmar/Cengage Learning

FIGURE 1-3 • The health continuum.

The health continuum shown in Figure 1-3 illustrates fluctuations in health status. The image depicts how health can range from **optimal health**, the highest level of health a person can possibly have, to life-threatening illness.

Your health does not usually remain at its optimal level for long periods at a time. As a young adult, your level of health will often be close to the optimal end of the continuum; if you are an older adult, you are faced with the health effects of aging. When physical health problems do develop, homeostasis can be interrupted, and the body gets out of balance. We know that homeostasis is compromised when we develop fever, feel aches and pains, and lack energy for daily activities. When homeostasis is disrupted, the body works overtime to return to a balanced, steady state. What happens when you jump into a cold pool of water? The shock to your system causes many of your internal systems to work together: your heart rate goes up to circulate blood throughout the body in an effort to warm it back up, blood vessels near the surface of the skin constrict to keep heat in the body, and your breathing rate increases to deliver more oxygen to your bloodstream. If the struggle to overcome the cold temperature takes too long, shivering will occur to help warm the body's core. If the cold persists too long, the body temperature may drop low enough to cause unconsciousness and death. The more serious the assault on the body, the greater the struggle for homeostasis.

Did You Know…?

Normal body temperature is 98.6 degrees Fahrenheit. When the body temperature drops below 90 degrees, the exposure to cold becomes life threatening. Survival depends on the environmental temperature, length of exposure time, the individual's amount of body fat, and his or her adaptive processes.

●●● The Meaning of Health

How would you define *health*? Is it the way you feel? Does it mean not being sick? Most people think of health as a physical condition because they are taught from a young age to assess how they "feel." It is important to understand that health is a condition with more than one dimension. Health is a measure of how we feel physically, mentally, socially, and spiritually at any point in time. Are you surprised to see the words *mentally*, *socially*, and *spiritually* in a definition of health? The World Health Organization (WHO), an agency of the United Nations created to work on international health issues, expanded the definition of health in 1947 and later reaffirmed the definition at a world conference in 1978. Members of the WHO believed that they should be concerned about the total quality of a person's life. They believe that health is "a state of complete physical, mental and social well-being, and not merely the absence of disease or infirmity, is a fundamental human right, and that the attainment of the highest possible level of health is a most important world-wide social goal." Health-and-wellness experts think of health as a multidimensional concept with health having up to six dimensions. For the purpose of this discussion, we consider health as having four dimensions, each of which can contribute to explaining the quality of our lives (Figure 1-4):

1. Physical health

2. Mental and emotional health

3. Social health

4. Spiritual health

Physical Health

Physical health refers to the condition of your body structures and systems. It is the first of the health dimensions you learned as a child. Your parents taught you to describe "what hurt" when you did not feel well. You can sense, for example, when a cold is coming on because you get a sore throat and just don't feel well. When your physical health is affected, you experience signs or symptoms that may include pain and discomfort. Common examples are stomach pain, headaches, painful joints, or tiredness. Some people may have unhealthy physical conditions, such as leukemia or early HIV

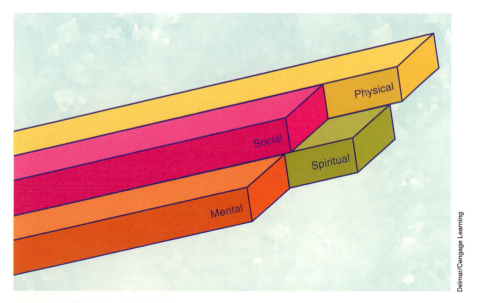

FIGURE 1-4 • The dimensions of health.

infection, but have no obvious physical symptoms. As adults, we learn to watch for specific physical symptoms that may indicate serious physical illness. For example, a change in a wart or mole or persistent skin sores, though not painful, could be an important sign of skin cancer. Can you think of other examples of illness signs or symptoms you have learned as an adult?

Mental and Emotional Health

Mental and emotional health is characterized by the condition of your mind and the capacity to balance your emotions. It includes how you respond to life situations around you. For example, a measure of a person's mental health is how he or she responds to stress and the problems of daily life. A person who has poor mental health may respond to normal situations with unusual or inappropriate behavior. Additionally, there may be individuals who are completely incapable of dealing with significant stress levels in healthy ways. How mentally healthy is an individual who physically assaults another person because that person "looked at them wrong"?

People often fail to recognize the symptoms of poor mental and emotional health. They may be unaware that their behavior is unusual. Lack of self-awareness can be one of the barriers to improving mental health; however, there are also many people who recognize that their mental health is not good but refuse to do anything to correct it. Many people don't spend time reflecting on their mental health until they have trouble dealing with daily life. Even then, it may take a friend or family member to encourage them to seek medical help.

Are you satisfied with your ability to handle stress? Would you feel comfortable seeking counseling or medical help if you had trouble coping with daily life? Would you encourage a friend or family member to seek help if it appeared to you that he or she was mentally or emotionally unhealthy? As an adult, these are important things to consider because stressful conditions are a part of everyday life, and having the skills to address these conditions can be helpful to you, your friends, and your family members.

social support network
people who are willing and able to provide emotional and physical resources to help you in time of need

Social Health

Social health refers to the quality of the relationships you have with other people (Figure 1-5). It is a measure of how you get along with all types of people, from family and close friends to people you do not know well or people of a different culture. The degree of tolerance and respect one has for others is part of social health. The ability to develop and maintain friendships that add value to your life is another measure of your social health. The depth and breadth of your social relationships will determine your **social support network**. People in your social support network are individuals who are willing and able to provide emotional and physical support when you need

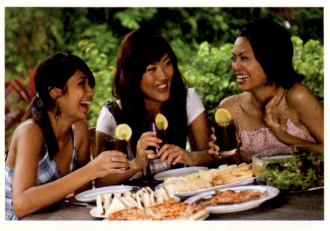

Courtesy of Shutterstock

FIGURE 1-5 • Social Health is a dimension of health that refers to the quality of one's relationships with other people.

help. For example, friends and acquaintances may be there to provide encouragement as you embark on an exercise program, or, knowing that you may be modifying your diet to prevent heart disease and/or lose weight, coworkers or friends will intentionally suggest that your group go to a restaurant where healthy food choices are included on the menu.

Spiritual Health

The spiritual health dimension is characterized by the values that direct your life. These values come from the forces that shaped your morals and the beliefs that guided your decisions about right and wrong. Spiritual health also means being able to seek out the meaning of human existence and the impact of nature on the health of populations.

Spiritual health does not necessarily refer to religious beliefs, although for many people a religious philosophy is the main component of their spiritual well-being. Spiritual health is the part of us that is beyond the physical and mental aspects of our existence. It also includes an inquiry into the meaning of life. Of all the dimensions of health, spiritual health is the most difficult to measure because it is not a tangible part of a person's life, nor is it something that can be assessed with medical tests. It may be that many people do not even recognize the spiritual aspects of their being. What are the factors in your life that contribute to your spiritual health? How might you know that you are having trouble with your spiritual health? To help answer these questions, think about what you do to lift your spirits and the spirits of others and consider the things that connect you to the environment. The answers you derive will help put your spiritual health in perspective. These are excellent issues to consider as you determine your overall personal health status.

⬤⬤⬤ The Total Picture of Health

As you consider your overall health status, evaluate all four of the health dimensions. The dimensions are not present in equal levels at any single point in time. The dimensions may appear as different levels of intensity. For example, a person with good physical health but very poor social health would not be described as having a high level of overall health. Consider the case of Jerry, a player on the college football team. Jerry is in great playing condition and an asset to the team, but he has a short temper, often gets into fights, and has been in trouble with the law. Lately, he has been trying to develop his spiritual self to overcome his social and mental health shortcomings. Although Jerry is physically strong and fit, his social health and emotional health are weak. It is important to remember that health is more than just feeling good or bad in a physical sense. It is in your best interest to be mindful of all four dimensions so that when you plan ways to achieve and maintain good health, you can attend to all of your health dimensions.

Interaction of the Four Dimensions

Have you ever known anyone who has become physically ill from stress? How about someone who became psychologically affected following an accidental injury? Health professionals have known for some time that the four dimensions of our health are interconnected. For example, medical researchers are discovering more about how emotional stress can contribute to physical symptoms. Some activities once considered to be only emotional or spiritual in nature appear to have an influence on physical health. Meditation, which simply means clearing the mind of thoughts, is one example. Meditation has been shown to influence physical health by lowering blood pressure and reducing the physical signs of stress. High blood pressure and high stress levels are contributing factors to stroke and heart disease.

●●● The Importance of Health

An ancient proverb states, "He who has health has hope, and he who has hope has everything." What is your reaction to this proverb? Many people believe that good health is more important than money or fame. In fact, good health increases the chances for achieving whatever it is you want in your life. Dealing with injuries and illnesses makes it difficult to participate fully in the activities that address your life goals. You can't perform well in a sport if you are injured or sick. It's difficult to do well in classes or a job if you are sick much of the time. Even being with friends is not enjoyable if you do not feel well. Being healthy not only makes life more enjoyable but also ensures that you will have the energy to do just about anything you want to do.

Good health also means having the stamina for study, work, and play. There are many demands on college learners these days. Maybe you participate in sports or other school activities or community programs or have a job in addition to your responsibilities at home. The more you do, want to do, or need to do, the more important it is to be healthy.

How would you rate your overall health? Do you feel well most of the time and have the energy you need? Think of your four dimensions of health. At this moment, is each of your four dimensions at its optimal level? If not, is there anything you could do to strengthen any that need improvement? In order to address any health dimension needing development, you need knowledge and a plan. As you progress through this text, you will find the tools to keep the dimensions of health in balance and performing at optimal levels.

Good Health Starts Now

Health behaviors you engage in now will influence health status in the future. Believe it! Healthy behaviors help reduce the risks of health threats almost immediately. Good health practices will have a cumulative effect because some of the things you do now will promote other healthy practices as you grow older. This statement is especially true for **chronic diseases**. Chronic disease is often caused by a lifetime of poor health choices that develop into serious problems later in life. In the same way, a lifetime of good choices can contribute to a healthy adulthood and old age.

chronic diseases
diseases that last for a long time with little change

An example of a healthy behavior that you could do right now might be choosing to eat well in order to maintain a healthy weight. Doing so makes it easier to keep a healthy weight throughout your lifetime because you become accustomed to eating well, and your body's need for extra calories is reduced. Maintaining weight in a healthy range diminishes one's risk of developing heart disease and/or diabetes. An example of a health-damaging behavior is choosing to smoke. Almost all adults who die from smoking-related diseases started smoking as teens. The cumulative effects of years of tobacco exposure can lead to tragic results. The choice is yours: good health behaviors now for good health later or bad health behaviors now for health risks as you age.

Your Life Expectancy

Would you like to live to be 100 years old? Living to that age was once considered rare, but more and more people are living for an entire century or even longer. The number of years a person might live is called **life expectancy**. The current life expectancy for Americans is almost 78 years. In Japan, the country with the highest life expectancy, it is over 81 years. Life expectancy is usually stated in terms of life expectancy at birth, but at any age the people in that age-group share a life expectancy for that group. The number of years given as one's life expectancy is the estimated years of life remaining. For example, a teen who has a life expectancy at age 16 of almost 62.5 years should live to be about 79 years old. A person who is 50 years old and has a life expectancy of about 26 years should live to be 76 years old. According to data on aging, an individual's life expectancy will end up being higher as he or she ages because the longer one survives in their later years, the remaining years are more additive. For example, a person who lives to be 90 may expect four to five more years of life compared to someone who is 50 and expects 28 more years.

Life expectancies are determined by health professionals and insurance company analysts when they examine death certificates for every age, race, and gender. An interesting point is that, at birth, females in the United States have a longer life expectancy than males. In fact, females can expect to live six years longer than their male counterparts (Figure 1-6). White Americans have a longer life expectancy than African Americans. In fact, white Americans live longer than members of all other minority groups. What do you think contributes to these differences? Life expectancy worldwide for all people is 64.3 years. Can you explain why this is so?

There are many people who outlive their life expectancy; there are others who die at birth before they have a chance to pursue their life expectancy. There is no way of telling which of these two outcomes await any individual, and there is no single factor explaining why some people live longer than others. The length of time a person actually lives is called **longevity**. We now have enough medical research data to suggest that longevity is influenced by four conditions:

- Heredity
- Environment
- Economics
- Personal health behaviors

life expectancy
a measure of how long a person has left to live based on data related to current causes of death

longevity
the length of a person's life

Did You Know...?

In 1776, a person's life expectancy at birth was 23 years of age. In 1900, a person's life expectancy at birth was about 48 years of age. In 2004, a person's life expectancy at birth was slightly more than 77 years of age. What do you think contributed to the increase?

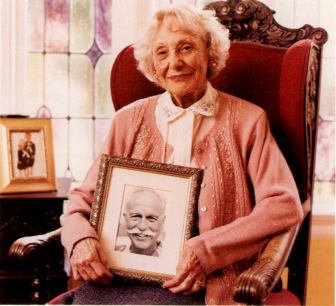

FIGURE 1-6 • In the United States, at birth, females have a life expectancy that is six years longer than their male counterparts.

Courtesy of Photodisc

Heredity

You inherit characteristics (traits) from each of your parents; some of those characteristics your parents inherited from their parents. Your inherited traits, such as eye color, come from your mother and father. Each parent contributed 50 percent of the characteristics that make up the unique person you are. Some traits, such as hair color, skin tone, and height, can be seen. Some traits, such as **metabolic rate** or an ability to process cholesterol, cannot be seen. These biological traits were passed to you from the **genes** you received from your parents' reproductive cells at the time you were conceived.

Some of the genes you inherit have an influence on your health. For example, your metabolic rate influences your ability to process the calories in food, which in turn has an impact on how easy it is for you to maintain your weight at a healthy level. Some health conditions, such as heart disease or diabetes, are more likely to occur in someone who has family members who had one of the diseases than in someone whose family members did not have either condition. This explains why your doctor may ask if any of your relatives have or had certain medical conditions. Knowing this information can allow you and your health care providers to safeguard your health.

Environment

There are many environmental events that are beyond your control. For example, in places where there is war, disease, famine, or natural disasters, people might not live as long as people in safer environments. Less dramatic examples of environmental factors affecting health include things like motor vehicle traffic and hazardous living conditions such as air pollution and toxic waste. Other things like overcrowding and poor living conditions can contribute to stressful living conditions, producing violence and drug abuse. In short, any adverse environmental condition can contribute to poor health status that, in turn, may have a negative impact on longevity.

Economics

People with more education and more financial resources tend to be healthier and live longer than people with less education and fewer financial resources. People with more financial resources can afford better food choices, they can afford time for leisure activity and exercise programs, and they can afford quality health care. When people cannot afford preventive care or medical attention, they may disregard early symptoms. They tend to wait until health problems become so serious that health care services are more comprehensive and costly. Health insurance is one way to pay for health care, but it can be too expensive for many people. Notice in Figure 1-7 the distribution of adults in the various age groups who are covered by health insurance. In no instance is there a group where 100 percent of the population is covered. In fact, the Centers for Disease Control and Prevention (CDC) reported that in 2000, there were 45 states where 10 to 20 percent of the adults did not have adequate health insurance. Data from surveys reported by the Kaiser Family Foundation indicate that approximately 43 percent of the nonelderly population of the United States is not covered by health insurance.

Individuals with limited income and no economic assets or resources may qualify for Medicaid, a program funded by state and federal governments and managed by the states. Created in 1965, Medicaid currently funds more than 50 million people each year. Individuals have to meet specific eligibility criteria established by individual states. A person must be a U.S. citizen to qualify, but under certain circumstances, lawfully admitted immigrants can receive Medicaid benefits. One of the primary criteria for Medicaid enrollment is the amount of personal income based on family size in relation

metabolic rate
the rate at which your body uses food and oxygen to carry out various body processes

genes
the small units of hereditary material found inside the nucleus of a cell

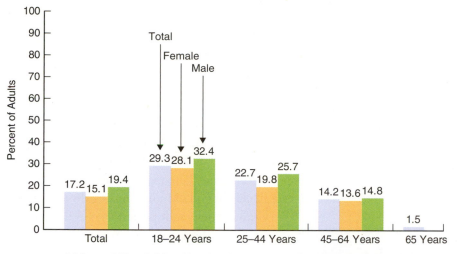

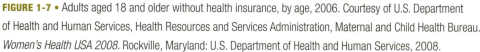

FIGURE 1-7 • Adults aged 18 and older without health insurance, by age, 2006. Courtesy of U.S. Department of Health and Human Services, Health Resources and Services Administration, Maternal and Child Health Bureau. *Women's Health USA 2008*. Rockville, Maryland: U.S. Department of Health and Human Services, 2008.

to poverty-level data. Poverty-level qualifications relate to two conditions: income related to the "percent of poverty" and the number of individuals in the family. As an example, in 2006, 100 percent of the poverty level for a family of four was $20,000. One of the serious problems affecting health care coverage for Americans is the matter of "near-poor" individuals in the population. These are people who earn too much to qualify for Medicaid and may be working in positions where their employers do not provide health insurance or who lack the finances to purchase their own insurance coverage. These near-poor people make up a group of individuals who must pay their own medical expenses.

Personal Health Behaviors

Many people are not aware that personal health behaviors and habits have more influence on how long and how well you live than do heredity, environment, or economics. It is not uncommon for individuals to rely on doctors and hospitals to keep them well, but evidence since the 1960s indicates that the greatest contribution to increasing life expectancy in the United States is practicing healthy behaviors. Medicine cannot cure every illness and repair every injury because there are many people who cannot afford to get the care. Personal actions have the most power in determining one's level of health. For example, the likelihood of injury in a car crash is reduced if a person drives safely, does not operate a vehicle under the influence of drugs or alcohol, and wears a safety belt. No matter how you look at it, it is less costly to prevent illness and injuries than it is to use medical care to treat them.

●●● Risks to Health

We are all exposed to conditions and have engaged in behaviors that can contribute to disease, death, or injury. We call these circumstances **risk factors** because exposure to them may result in a harmful outcome. Some risk factors are easier to recognize than other risk factors. For example, driving while under the influence of alcohol or without using a safety belt are obvious risk factors. Breathing secondhand cigarette smoke is not as obvious, but it is still a risk factor for poor health. Some risk factors are short term because they can result in immediate harm, like riding a bicycle without a helmet. Other

risk factors
identifiable conditions or behaviors that increase one's risk of getting ill or injured

risk factors do harm over a long period of time because their effects accumulate as a person continues to be exposed to the health risk. Teenagers don't get lung cancer when they begin smoking; the damaging effects of smoking appear after years of exposure.

There are also compounding effects of risk exposures. This means that the more risk factors for a particular health problem you are exposed to at one time, the greater the likelihood of a negative outcome. Take the skateboard example illustrated in Figure 1-8. At first glance, the rider is at risk for injury because he is performing a risky stunt, but there may be other unseen factors that could increase the likelihood of injury. Riding the skateboard without a helmet or protective gear is a risk factor. Using the skateboard in a busy traffic area would be another risk factor. If the rider is also under the influence of alcohol or drugs, that would be another. The possibility of an accident increases with each additional risk factor. Also note that among the risk factors mentioned previously, there are some conditions with a greater potential for harm than others. Thus, it is not just the number of risky behaviors; it is also the magnitude of those behaviors.

A Healthy Life

The quality of a person's life is not measured by his or her longevity; rather, it is measured by how long that person lives *well*. Although certain health conditions are to be expected with aging, the health goal is to have optimal health as long as possible. As an older adult, you'll want to feel well and have the energy and ability to do the things you enjoy. It's one thing to spend the last years of your life in and out of the health care system battling serious health

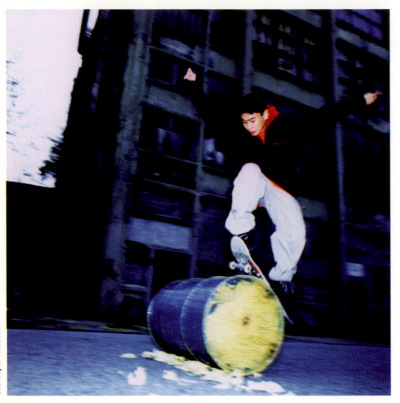

Courtesy of Photodisc

FIGURE 1-8 • The more health risk factors one is exposed to at one time, the greater the likelihood of a negative outcome.

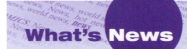

What's News

The CDC (Pan, et al., 2009) reported on a study that certain minority groups have much higher rates of obesity than whites. Blacks had 51 percent higher prevalence of obesity, and Hispanics had 21 percent higher obesity prevalence compared with whites. The study used data from the 2006–2008 Behavioral Risk Factor Surveillance System, an ongoing, state-based, random-digit-dialed telephone survey of the U.S. civilian, noninstitutionalized population aged 18 years and older.

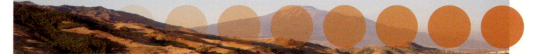

What's Your View?

Paying for Health Care

People who practice poor health habits tend to be sick more often than people who practice good health behaviors. For example, cigarette smoke is linked to numerous adverse health conditions. In that regard, cigarette smokers are likely to use more health care resources than nonsmokers. Some health professionals and insurance companies believe that individuals who practice poor health habits, such as smoking, should be required to pay more for their health care than nonsmokers. Should smokers be required to pay more for treatment of smoke-related illnesses? Is it fair to give nonsmokers discounts for their health and life insurance?

problems resulting from practicing health damaging behaviors; it's another thing to have the physical and mental capacity to do all the things you want to do with your life. Good health is not something that just happens. Part of being an adult, no matter what your age, is getting involved in making the right decisions and practicing the health-generating behaviors in order to ensure good health and minimize health risks. The first step toward health behaviors is to recognize that there are things you can do now to enhance *health and longevity*. The information in this book, class presentations, and class assignments will help you develop the knowledge and skills to meet your health goals.

Financial Benefits of Good Health

Good health can be financially beneficial. People who practice good health behaviors tend to miss fewer workdays; they have a high level of energy throughout the workday and are more productive. Individuals who take responsibility for their health also have lower health care expenses than do people with poor health habits. This factor alone is an important economic condition as a person enters his or her retirement years. Healthy people are not as sick when they enter the health care system; therefore, they require less treatment, heal faster, and are less likely to return for follow-up care. In the United States, we spend more than $1 trillion each year on health care. This means that the average cost for each person's health services is more than $4,000 annually. Notice in Figure 1-9 that health care costs per person keep going up each year. Furthermore, the increases each year are outpacing the rate of inflation.

If more people practiced good health habits, we would all save money. Because healthy people require fewer medical services than do unhealthy persons, the decreased need for services would reduce the amount of money insurance companies pay for health services. It is a matter of economics: increased reimbursements from the insurance companies result in increased premiums for health insurance. This is because the insurance companies are in business to make money. If they have to pay more claims, they eventually must raise rates to keep their profits. Understand also that many people living in the United States do not have health insurance, nor do they have the money to pay directly

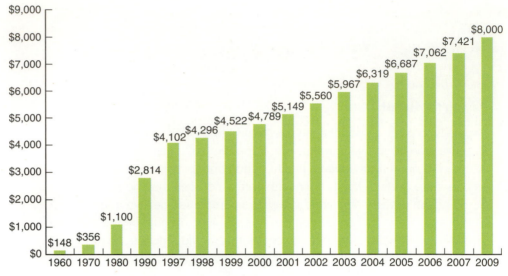

FIGURE 1-9 • Annual costs of health care per person in USA, 1960–2007 and 2009 (expected). Adapted from Centers for Medicare and Medicaid Services, Office of the Actuary, National Health Statistics Group, www.cms.hhs .gov/NationalHealthExpendData/02_NationalHealthAccountsHistorical.asp.

for health services. If those services are provided free or at low cost by the city, county, or federal government, the revenues to cover the services eventually come from tax dollars. Thus, we would all win if we practiced healthy behaviors; we would have more healthy people and fewer dollars spent on health care. With or without health insurance, health promotion is a good financial investment.

Health Role Model

When you practice health-generating behaviors, you may not be doing something just for yourself. You may also be presenting yourself as a role model for friends and family members. At some point, you may be a parent, if you are not one already. The family is the primary learning environment for children, and considerable research evidence demonstrates that children indeed emulate the behaviors of parents. If parents perform healthy behaviors, the children are likely to do so. Research studies have found that if parents drink and drive, use drugs, or smoke cigarettes, their children are likely to follow. Not only do children look up to and copy the behavior of their parents, but they may also try to be like older siblings. You may be surprised to know how much influence you may have on the people around you.

●●● Health Literacy

Being motivated to perform healthy behaviors is but one important aspect of being healthy. It is equally important for the individual to access and understand information useful for developing these behaviors. Unfortunately, not everyone is able to do this. Some people are unable to comprehend how important it is too seek out health information, others don't know how to access the information, and still others are unable to read and interpret the information once they acquire it. Education, occupation, and income are specific markers of good health. Education can lead to a better job, a better job can lead to higher income (and/or health insurance), and a better income results in better health status. People with good incomes are more likely to have access to health-promoting products and services and better health care. The education you are currently pursuing will serve you well in the future, but only a very small portion of that education will deal with health issues, so being able to locate information on your own is an important skill. If you have not mastered that skill, it is hoped that you will develop the ability to research reliable and valid health information on your own by the time you complete this course.

At the beginning of this chapter, the importance of being able to access information was presented. Do you feel capable of obtaining important health information when you need it? Do you know where to find reliable health information on the Internet or in the library? Can you take care of simple injuries, such as cuts or bruises? Can you read and interpret health care coverage policies and procedures? Are you capable of understanding inserts and labels for medications? The knowledge of these tasks and the ability to gather the information is a function of **health literacy**, the ability to obtain, interpret, understand, and use essential health information and services. Health-literate people can properly use the information and services to advance their health and the health of others. Here are more examples of health literacy skills:

health literacy
the ability to obtain, interpret, understand, and apply basic health information and services

- Interpreting a doctor's written instructions
- Reading and understanding guidelines for using health treatment devices
- Understanding a hospital's billing statement
- Using library resources to design a nutrition program
- Recognizing the symptoms of common diseases
- Locating valid health information on the Internet
- Understanding basic health and medical terms
- Knowing when to consult a doctor or access emergency care

Health literacy skills increase your chances of maintaining your health and the health of your family. It is estimated that 90 million adults in the United States have only limited health literacy skills (Kutner, Greenberg, Jin, & Paulsen, 2006).Unfortunately, this group also has more medical needs and requires more days of hospitalization than people with higher health literacy skills. Poor health literacy contributes to unnecessarily spending approximately $73 billion annually on health care to cover longer hospital stays, misuse of the emergency room, noncompliance with health care instructions, and so on (Kutner et al., 2006).

The Health-Literate Person

Health literacy starts with believing that health is important and wanting to learn how to care for your health and, to the extent possible, the health of your friends and family. Health-literate individuals share four common characteristics:

- Being a self-directed learner
- Being a critical thinker
- Being an effective communicator
- Being a responsible member of society

Self-Directed Learner

A self-directed learner is someone who doesn't limit learning to the educational setting or to what he or she learns from family members. The self-directed learner is a person who is motivated to learn more about health issues and uses the library, the Internet, and other sources to gather information about those issues. For this type of person, classroom learning merely serves as a starting point for lifelong learning.

Because health has an impact on the quality of your life now and in the future, health should be much more than a subject to study in college. As a self-directed learner, you will seek additional information to help you make good health choices. Medical science is changing so rapidly that some of what you are learning now may be revised in only a year or two, depending on the medical and social research. Scientists are continually learning more about disease processes and are discovering new treatments and drugs. There is also a need to know and understand information regarding the financial aspects of health care. A health-literate person will be able to seek out pertinent information about health services or products. For example, the federal government established Medicare Part D, a prescription drug program that became law in January 2006. The program took effect for Medicare enrollees later that year. This meant that everyone covered by Medicare had to learn about the prescription drug program. The plan contained numerous complexities that affected individual benefits under the program. As a health-literate individual, you should be able to locate information and learn how to use the Medicare system or any other health coverage program to ensure that you have access to appropriate coverage. It is possible that you may be faced with helping family members and/or relatives navigate this program and many like it in the not-too-distant future.

WEB LINK

Medicare

http://www.medicare.gov

One interesting feature of this Web site is being able to access information translated into foreign languages.

SEARCH TERMS: Medicare, Medicare benefits, health insurance

Critical Thinker

When you hear something presented as a fact, do you simply accept it, or do you look for ways to confirm that the information is accurate? Do you try to solve difficult problems by comparing several possible solutions before deciding what to do? **Critical thinking** is an important skill for everyone. You already use critical thinking skills to solve math problems, organize term papers, and judge the validity of advertising claims you see on television. Although critical thinking has been defined in many ways, it generally means that a person can do the following:

critical thinking
evaluating the worth, accuracy, or authenticity of issues and information, leading to a level of conclusion that can direct thoughts or actions

- Recognize problems: identify and understand their importance.

- Analyze: separate an idea into parts and examine in detail.

- Synthesize: put parts of ideas together in a meaningful way.

- Evaluate: judge or determine the worth or quality of something.

These skills require more than simply memorizing and recalling facts, such as the skills needed when taking true-or-false and multiple-choice tests.

deductive reasoning
reasoning that begins with the general and ends with the specific (arguments are based on laws, rules, and established principles, and conclusions are based on two or more premises)

Reasoning

Thinking critically often requires the use of reasoning, or drawing valid conclusions from facts or observations. There are two types of reasoning: deductive and inductive. **Deductive reasoning** begins with general statements and proceeds to a conclusion about something specific. *It is based on known laws or rules about the nature of things.* Two or more of these laws and rules, known as premises, are used to reach a conclusion. Here is an example of an argument using deductive reasoning:

Premise: All dogs have four legs.

Premise: Tipper is a dog.

Conclusion: Tipper has four legs.

Applying deductive reasoning to health concerns, it might look something like this:

Premise: Research indicates that health screenings save lives and reduce medical costs of treatment.

Premise: Mammography is a recommended screening for breast cancer and can detect breast cancer in early stages.

Conclusion: A mammogram can save one's life and reduce medical costs with early detection.

Inductive reasoning is based not on laws and rules but on using your experience and observation. *General conclusions are drawn from specific things that we know and see.* An argument based on inductive reasoning would be as follows:

Premise: Every time I pet a dog, I get bitten.

Premise: Your dog just bit me after I said that.

Conclusions: All dogs bite.

Some people apply inductive reasoning to justify unhealthy behaviors:

Premise: I have been smoking for seven years, and my health is fine.

Premise: My Aunt Ethel smoked all of her life and died in her sleep at age 75.

Conclusion: I will be like my Aunt Ethel—I won't die from smoking cigarettes.

You can see that inductive reasoning may be less valid than deductive reasoning because it lacks scientific validation. A person *can* use inductive reasoning to solve problems, but he or she must be able to validate observations to justify the conclusion. Taking the previously mentioned smoking example, what do you think would happen if the person using inductive reasoning sought scientific verification of the premises? To the best of your ability, you may want to arrive at critical decisions based on deductive reasoning. Critical thinkers listen, observe, and read carefully to gather information. They check the credibility of their sources and learn to distinguish between facts and opinions. They use the prior learning and the information they gather to form learned opinions and to solve problems.

Creativity

Creativity plays an important role in critical thinking because it enables you to see the world in a variety of ways. Not every problem has an easy solution, and many problems are quite complex. When faced with difficult or complex problems, we can use creativity to generate new solutions and then apply critical thinking and reasoning skills to see if any of the solutions might work.

inductive reasoning reasoning that moves from the specific to the general; reasoning in which arguments are based on experience or observations rather than on laws or proven facts

It's possible to score high on creativity but low on critical thinking and reasoning. The following laws, actually created by politicians to protect the public, illustrate why *all* these skills are needed:

- The Chico, California, City Council passed a ban on nuclear weapons, setting a $500 fine for anyone detonating one within city limits.

- In St. Louis, it's illegal to sit on the curb of any city street and drink beer from a bucket.

- In Denver, it is illegal for barbers to give massages to nude customers unless it is for instructional purposes (Koon & Powell, 2002).

You can use the search term "Dumb Laws" to find numerous other dumb and amusing laws related to health topics, past or present.

Thinking creatively has often been described as "thinking outside the box." This means seeing the world in many different ways, considering new ideas, and having the courage to be inventive. It starts with mentally walking around a problem and seeing it from various angles. It continues with proposing solutions that are different from "what we've always done" and trying to come up with something new and original. It means using known ideas and things in new ways. For example, have you ever used a screwdriver as a doorstop? This is an example of using a familiar object in a new, perhaps unexpected way.

Brainteasers. Brainteasers are like gymnastics for the mind. You can use them to sharpen your creative thinking skills. They are little puzzles that give you a chance to test your mental skills in a fun ways. Using your mental energies to work through the problems provides you with the opportunity to test your ability to solve problems. There are similarities between finding solutions to brainteasers and finding solutions to more complex problems in your life. You recognize and define the problem and think it through to a solution. Problem solving is a skill, and, as does any other skill, it improves with practice. Here is an example of a brain teaser: Daisy, Rose, and Lily each entered the county fair's flower competition. Coincidentally, the flowers they entered were a daisy, a rose, and a lily, but none of the women entered her namesake flower. If Daisy did *not* enter a rose, which flower did each woman enter? (answer at the end of the chapter)

Mind Mapping. **Mind mapping** is a technique that enables you to more freely use your brain (Buzan & Buzan, 1996). Scientists and psychologists recognize our brains have two separate sides. We use the left side of the brain for logical, structured thinking and the right side for artistic, creative thinking. In classroom settings, we are more likely to use the left side. For example, we are often encouraged to think and write in outline form, moving systematically from one level to the next. Mind mapping is a technique that allows you to think about topics in a less systematic way.

Mind mapping is a technique you can use to write down, organize, and illustrate your thoughts. A mind map represents a single major subject and consists of words, images, lines, and objects that are connected to the main subject and that have relationships to each other. You can be creative and color or illustrate a mind map any way you like. Essentially, a mind map has four major features:

1. A center image or circle that represents the major subject

2. Main themes that radiate off the center as branches

3. Minor themes that are linked to the main themes

4. No particular order required for adding themes

mind mapping
a technique that enables you to organize and illustrate your thoughts using both sides of your brain

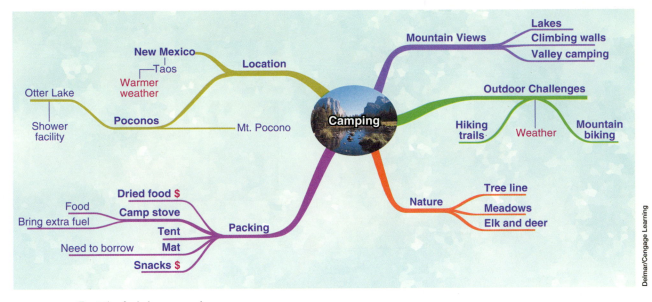

FIGURE 1-10 • Example of mind map: camping.

Figure 1-10 is an example of a mind map about camping. It provides a structure that could be used for preparing an oral report on camping. Can you imagine how this process could be used to take class notes? Try to create a similar map for yourself.

Many of the popular health fads in the media today, especially those advertising easy cures for difficult problems, generally are not based on scientific evidence. A critical thinker looks beyond the media proclamations, uses deductive reasoning, and forms valid **opinions** about products and services. As an example, consider the number of advertised devices, video programs, and other self-help gadgets intended to increase your fitness level. Have you ever wondered if they really work? Some of these products or services are more suitable than others. It is important to apply critical thinking skills to examine the claims and costs instead of just taking for granted the claims of products that are useless or even harmful. Imagine how important it would be to apply the same critical thinking skills to decide on your choice of medical treatment for a severe health problem.

opinion
a belief based on what seems to be true rather than on tested knowledge

Effective Communicator

Can you express yourself to others so that they understand what you mean? Do you listen attentively when others are speaking? Do you always comprehend everything a doctor tells you? A health-literate person is able to communicate and comprehend effectively. Let's take a quick look at the communication process to see how it works. People tend to view communication as simply a two-way interaction. One person talks while someone else listens, followed by a response from the second person. But communication research has demonstrated that communication is far more complex than that.

Observe the communication model depicted in Figure 1-11. Communication means formulating ideas before speaking or writing (ideation) and creating messages to be transmitted to others (encoding). It also means being able to decode information that is sent from others and to determine the intended meaning (ideation). This process is affected by outside forces known as interference. If two people are trying to talk and there is loud noise (interference) in the environment, they may not hear each other well. Sometimes even the slightest noises can interfere with communication. If someone in your class

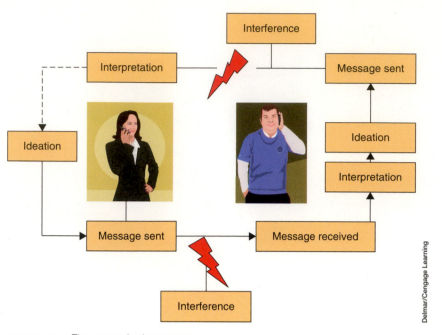

FIGURE 1-11 • The communication process.

is near you and talking to someone else, you may become distracted, not necessarily because they are loud but because the conversation occupies a space in your consciousness that prevents you from fully attending to the instructor.

Effective communicators are also good listeners. They check their own understanding of messages by asking questions of the sender and using **feedback**, restating the message back to the sender to validate understanding. Feedback results in exchanges that are helpful to both the receiver and the sender. An effective communicator is able to ask questions of caregivers in a medical encounter, and they can understand what they hear from health care personnel. Being an effective communicator does not mean that you have to be a great speaker. It simply means that you can formulate your thoughts so that you can express your position on issues and make the effort to give accurate and complete health information to others in a form they can understand and use.

Responsible Member of Society

You may ask yourself, "What is the connection between being a good citizen and being health literate?" Good citizens understand the importance of community health, know what their community health issues are, and become involved with keeping their neighborhoods and communities safe and well. Have you ever participated in community activities, such as food drives for the poor? Are you willing to volunteer for projects that make your community a safer place to live? Responsible members of society take an interest in the health and needs of others. They stay away from activities that threaten their own health or the health of others. Responsible citizens realize that their actions can make a positive difference in their community.

English as a Second Language

Health literacy is a problem for many Americans who lack the educational training to master literacy skills. The 2003 National Report on Health Literacy by the National Center for Educational Statistics reported that 14 percent of American adults had less

feedback
a way to check if you understand what someone has said (a common method is to restate in your own words what you heard and to ask the speaker if this is what he or she meant)

than basic health literacy skills. This accounts for approximately 11 million adults. These figures do not represent the many recent immigrants. Imagine the difficulty faced by recently immigrated persons trying to make their way through the health care system and/or developing a basic understanding of heath education materials. Studies demonstrate that the average Medicaid recipient reads at a fifth-grade level. Recently immigrated individuals may read at a level far below that. It is not uncommon for Hispanic immigrants to come to the United States being illiterate in *Spanish*, thus adding to their difficulty of developing health literacy in English.

Health Literacy Skills

How would you rate yourself today on health literacy? This textbook and the course activities will provide you with many learning opportunities to enhance your healthy literacy, such as understanding medical terms and health promotion principles, validating health information, and making good decisions to fulfill your potential for a healthy, happy life. You may or may not realize the importance of health literacy at this time. The extent to which you comprehend the significance of health literacy will depend greatly on your past experiences with the health care system. The significance of these skills may go beyond what you can do for yourself. As an adult, you may be placed in a position where you need to call on these skills to advocate on behalf of a family member. Read the learning objectives and skills in Box given below and assess the scope of your health literacy skills at this time. Make note of those you would like to improve during the semester.

WEB LINK
California Literacy Initiative
http://cahealthliteracy.org/index.html
The Web site is a project of California Literacy, Inc., and has numerous Web links to other sites containing easy-to-read health information. Of particular interest might be a section dealing with health issues of various cultural groups in numerous languages. On the home page, click to enter the resources center, and you can browse for pertinent pages.

SEARCH TERMS: health literacy, health literacy competencies, literacy and health

Health Literacy Objectives and Skills

1. Understanding health promotion and disease prevention

   - Knowing about the policies and programs organized by federal, state, and local governments and private agencies to promote good health
   - Promoting and participating in the activities sponsored by those organizations
     Examples: Raising funds for multiple sclerosis by participating in The Walk for Multiple Sclerosis
     Volunteering for community cleanup projects at public parks
     Doing your personal best to meet the nation's health objectives

2. Accessing valid health information and health-promoting products and services
   - Knowing where to gather reliable information about products and services
   - Investigating to see if the information is based on facts
     Examples: Researching and evaluating products promising quick and easy weight loss before purchasing them
     Helping a family member choose a physician
     Knowing your rights and responsibilities related to health insurance programs

3. Practicing health-enhancing behaviors
   - Learning about healthy behaviors
   - Incorporating health behaviors into daily activities

Examples: Committing to practice a sport or activity at least three times a week

Receiving regularly scheduled physical and dental examinations

Incorporating nutritionally sound eating behaviors into your daily life

4. Recognizing the influence of culture, media, technology, and other factors on health
   - Examining the validity of ideas you have always taken for granted
   - Examining your beliefs in view of what you learn about health
   - Learning to resist pressures to engage in unsafe behaviors

   Examples: Deciding to eat fewer fast foods after studying the basics of nutrition

   Turning down someone's offer of a cigarette at a party

   Being cautious of how loudly you use your MP3 player

5. Using communication skills to promote health
   - Listening attentively to information about health topics
   - Orally explaining your points of view in a clear manner

   Examples: Describing health concerns or problems to your physician

   Advocating concerns to a health care provider on behalf of a family member

   Communicating effectively with a representative of a health insurance carrier

6. Setting goals and making decisions
   - Making plans to achieve optimal health
   - Designing and following health improvement programs for yourself or family members
   - Gathering information and thinking about alternatives and consequences when making health decisions

   Examples: Creating an exercise program you can stick with

   Deciding whether to get a job on the weekends or to spend the time studying or partici-pating in outdoor activities

7. Advocating for personal, family, and community health
   - Being willing to state that health is important
   - Speaking out about health issues with friends and family

   Examples: Explaining to a friend the dangers of illegal drug use

   Sharing with family members what you've learned in your health class about nutrition

   Researching and providing valid information on health issues to family or friends

   Participating in the policy development process to protect the health of your community

Talking it Over

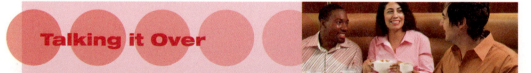

Use the information from the health literacy section and develop a short questionnaire to measure health literacy. Request family members and/or friends to take the questionnaire. Ask if they think more about their personal health now than they did a few years ago. Do they wish they had done any-thing differently back then to impact their health now? Are there habits they started as teenagers that were difficult to change? Write a summary of their responses and compare the summary with your own health literacy skills.

BUILDING YOUR LIFETIME WELLNESS PLAN

This chapter provided you with information about contemporary health issues and the different dimensions of health. By now, you probably understand that health is a physical and psychological condition that can be assessed at any point in time and is always changing. As an adult, you have more personal responsibility for your health and possibly the health of family members. Because optimal health is a lifelong challenge, you will need to hone your health literacy skills so that you can develop a lifestyle to prepare you for this challenge. The remaining portion of this book and the work you do during the course will focus on a new concept: *wellness*. In the next chapter, you will learn about wellness, its relationship to health, and the steps you can take toward developing a personal wellness plan. The intent of the wellness plan is to help you build health behavior and personal decision-making skills to ensure good health for a lifetime. Remember, it is not how long you live; it is how long you live *well*! Your wellness plan will become a health journal filled with information, resources, and strategies that you can take with you after the course, and you may use the materials as reference tools for years to come. You may want to create a personal folder, file, or binder to use as a wellness folio, which will be a place to store copies of your personal assessments, class assignments, chapter activities, and topic-specific wellness plans.

●●● End-of-Chapter Activities

Opportunities for Application

1. Carlos has been driving for about five years and thinks he is a pretty good driver. He doesn't usually wear his safety belt. He knows that state law requires everyone in the vehicle to wear their safety belts, but he thinks that this law doesn't really apply to him because he considers himself such a good driver. Besides, Carlos heard about people who died in accidents because they were wearing seat belts and got trapped in burning cars or drowned, so seat belts didn't sound so safe after all.

   Help Carlos with his health behaviors. Search the Web or a library and gather information related to the value of safety belts and prepare a paper for Carlos. Summarize this information in a manner that might influence Carlos to develop a habit of fastening his safety belt every time he gets into an automobile.

2. Imagine that you have grandparents (or parents) who are going to reach retirement age in the not-too-distant future. Go to the Medicare Web site and research what Medicare services are, the qualifications for coverage, and payment procedures. What does a person have to do to obtain a Medicare account? How does one sign up for Medicare? Where can one go to get services? Do a search for "Medigap" insurance and find out what Medigap covers. Using the information you gathered, produce a three-page summary of Medicare benefits and what the retiree needs to do to obtain Medicare services.

Key Concepts

1. Draw the four dimensions of health to illustrate your health status for this week. Are all dimensions equal in strength? If any dimension is lower, explain why. Do you think you can do anything to enhance any of your dimensions to strengthen your health status?

2. Explain why personal behaviors are important to health.

3. Describe the components of health literacy.

4. List the top 10 causes of death in the United States at this time. Explain the difference between the top 10 causes of death now and the top 10 causes of death in 1900.

Answers to Personal Assessment Quiz

Personal Assessment: Health Behavior Assessment

1. I currently have all the immunizations I am supposed to have.

2. I do not smoke cigarettes.

3. I make an effort to eat fruit and vegetables every day.

4. I choose not to use drugs.

5. I choose to consume alcoholic beverages seldom or not at all.

6. I use a safety belt every time I ride in an automobile.

7. I am able to deal with stressful situations without anger or urgency.

8. I have someone I can talk to when I need help solving problems.

9. I can communicate well with members of my family.

10. I understand the structure of the health care system and know how to use it.

11. I make decisions that are good for my health and act on them.

These 11 items are important elements of a wellness life-style. It is hoped that you can respond in the affirmative for all 11 items. If not, consider how important that item might be to your health. You are likely to uncover other behaviors during the course that will help you shape your course for health and wellness.

Answer to Brainteaser on page 22

Daisy entered a lily, Rose entered a daisy, and Lily entered a rose.

References

Buzan, T., & Buzan, B. (1996). *The Mind Map Book.* New York, NY: Plume.

Carter, R. (2000). *Mapping the Mind.* Berkeley, CA: University of California Press.

Centers for Disease Control and Prevention. (2006). *Behavioral Risk Factor Surveillance System* [Web Page]. URL http://www.cdc.gov/brfss/about.htm [2006, October].

DeNavas-Walt, C., Proctor, B. D., & Lee, C. H. (2006). *Income, Poverty, and Health Insurance Coverage in the United States: 2005.* Washington, D.C.: U.S. Government Printing Office.

Devine, C. M., Sobal, J., Bisogni, C. A., & Connors, M. (1999). Food Choices in Three Ethnic Groups: Interactions of Ideals, Identities, and Roles. *Journal of Nutrition Education, 31,* 86–93.

Koon, J., & Powell, A. (2002). *You may not tie an alligator to a fire hydrant: 101 real dumb laws.* New York, NY: The Free Press.

Kutner, M., Greenberg, E., Jin, Y., & Paulsen, C. (2006). *Health literacy of America's adults: Results from the 2003 National Survey of Adult Literacy (NCES 2006–483).* U.S. Department of Education. Washington, DC: National Center for Education Statistics.

Pan, L. et al. (2009). Differences in prevalence of obesity among Black, White, and Hispanic adults—United States, 2006–2008. *MMWR Weekly, 58*(27), 740–744.

U.S. Department of Health and Human Services. (2004). *Bone health and osteoporosis: A report to the surgeon general.* Rockville, MD: Public Health Services.

CHAPTER 2

Building Wellness Skills

CHAPTER OBJECTIVES

When you finish this chapter, you should be able to:

- Explain the relationship between health and wellness.
- Describe several wellness behaviors that protect and promote health.
- Describe the significance of the U.S. Public Health Service's Leading Health Indicators.
- Describe the various forms of wellness.
- Explain how to develop a personal wellness plan.
- Describe the psychological elements that form health motives.
- Discuss models that help explain the development of wellness behaviors.

KEY TERMS

ecosystem

health promotion

health risk appraisal

public health

social psychology

social support

surgeon general

wellness

wellness motives

●●● Introduction

If someone asked you right now, "How are you doing?," you would quickly do a mental check of yourself and probably answer with something like the following: "I've never been better!" or "Fine, except for my headache" or perhaps "Well, right now I'm upset because I didn't get the job I wanted." Whatever your response, it would be based on a quick but complete assessment of yourself, especially all of your health dimensions. Describing how you *are at that moment* takes into account each of your health dimensions.

Obviously, life is much more enjoyable when you have good health than when you are sick, injured, or emotionally upset. Health is a measure of your physical, social, mental, and spiritual conditions at any point in time. Recall from the previous chapter that all our health dimensions are rarely at optimal levels simultaneously. All the dimensions need not be at peak levels at the same time in order to achieve optimal health. Nonetheless, we should strive to maintain the dimensions at as high a level as possible. Doing so ensures optimal health. Just about everyone will agree that optimal health is a significant

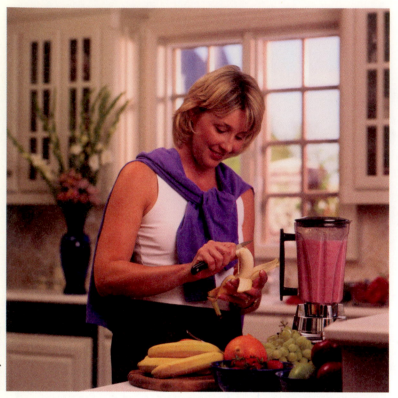

Courtesy of Photodisc

FIGURE 2-1 • Wellness represents the collective behaviors and habits that have a positive influence on health.

personal achievement. The process of developing a personal lifestyle that includes the decisions and behaviors to achieve your health goals is a process called wellness (Figure 2-1). In this chapter, you will learn about practicing wellness to attain your health goals. Your knowledge of wellness behaviors and accepting the importance of including them in your daily life can lead to a lifestyle resulting in good health now and in the future.

A classic study of almost 7,000 adults in Alameda County, California, was conducted by researchers Nedra Belloc and Lester Breslow (1972). The researchers categorized the subjects according to health status and collected information on seven basic health practices over almost 10 years. Those seven health practices are included in the previously mentioned assessment. The study revealed that the more health practices the subjects reported, the better their physical health status. In fact, the researchers reported that the behaviors were cumulative, meaning that people who reported performing all or most of the behaviors were healthier than *younger* subjects who reported following fewer habits. You will read more about this study later in the chapter.

PERSONAL ASSESSMENT
Current Health Behaviors

Write down your answers to each of the following questions. Feedback is at the end of the chapter. You can also read further in this chapter to see how these behaviors impact health.

1. Do you avoid the use of tobacco?

2. Do you exercise regularly?

3. Do you keep your weight within the normal range for your height and age?

4. Do you avoid eating between meals?

5. Do you eat breakfast every day?

6. Do you sleep seven to eight hours each night?

7. Do you consume no more than one to two alcoholic drinks, three or less times per week?

●●● Health and Wellness

As discussed in chapter 1, health is a measure of how you feel physically, socially, mentally, and spiritually at any point in time. **Wellness** is the process of incorporating behaviors into your daily life to positively impact your health. Wellness is a lifestyle that gives you personal power over your health. The goal of wellness is to develop a way of life that is health enhancing. You can see in Figure 2-2 that education is a key component in developing wellness knowledge, attitudes, and skills. You can be exposed to and seek out abundant amounts of information. As mentioned previously, it is important to validate the information you receive and the source from which it came. Knowledge, attitudes, and skills have an effect on your motivation to engage in wellness behaviors. Motivation is the prime mover toward wellness. Motivation means that you *have a desire* to practice it. Education in and of itself doesn't necessarily lead to behavior. People may *know* about health risks such as smoking, yet some people choose to engage in risky behaviors. Wellness cannot occur unless the individual is motivated to practice it. One's education can contribute to the formation of health-generating motives, but keep in mind that engaging in wellness behaviors can result in feedback that reinforces your attitudes toward the behavior and support the knowledge that you are doing something good for your life. The reinforcement also leads to the likelihood that you will seek out additional information on the health issue or seek information about other topics.

Wellness can be practiced by anyone regardless of their health condition. Take the example of two young women leaving a hospital at the same time after recovering from serious accidents. Both suffered spinal cord injuries, and neither is expected to walk

wellness
behaviors and habits that have a positive influence on health

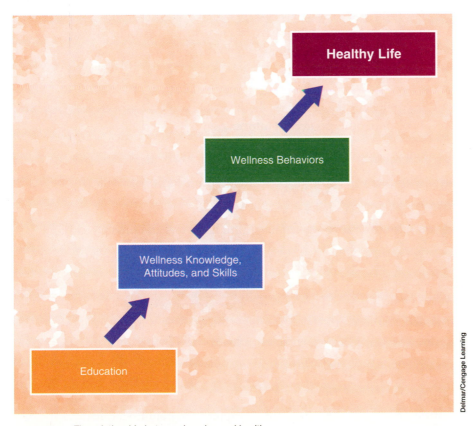

FIGURE 2-2 • The relationship between learning and health.

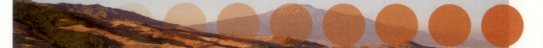

What's Your View?

People with spinal cord injuries can be paraplegic (paralysis in both legs) or quadriplegic (paralysis in all four extremities). Do you think that individuals with spinal cord injuries can achieve optimal wellness? Is there a greater likelihood that paraplegics can achieve better health status than quadriplegics? Explain what you think health would be like for individuals with these two types of injuries.

again. One of the patients, Kathy, feels miserable about her injuries and her loss of mobility and refuses to see her friends. She spends much of her time feeling angry and sad. Marta, the other patient, is grateful for visits from her friends and family. She looks forward to their continued support and hopes to make the best of her condition. Marta recalls learning about the Wheelchair Olympics in one of her classes and wants to learn how to play wheelchair basketball. Both young women may be low on the physical health dimension, but Marta is practicing wellness behaviors and, as a result, is much healthier overall than Kathy.

Wellness can be an invigorating component of your lifestyle because it allows you to exercise personal control over your life for the rest of your life. This control and the independence you have as an adult can assist you in making decisions about your health and creating your own wellness lifestyle. But it may not be easy. If you are not already motivated to practice wellness, you will have to redirect your attitudes. If you do adopt wellness motives, you will have opportunities to do the following:

- Take responsibility for your health and how you feel

- Use your health literacy skills to learn about wellness behaviors from class presentations, this book, and other sources of information

- Become an informed consumer of health products and services

- Make decisions that will affect the present and future health of you and/or your family

- Protect yourself and your family from harmful behaviors and unsafe conditions

- Reduce or delay the need for health care, thus improving the quality of your life

You may recall reading the information on health risk in chapter 1. Information from studies conducted by medical records, insurance companies, and health researchers opened up the science of **health risk appraisal** (HRA), sometimes referred to as health risk assessment. The HRA begins when an individual enters personal information on a questionnaire. The information consists of physical assessment values, such as blood pressure, cholesterol, height/weight, family history, health behaviors, and so on. The questionnaire data are entered into a computer and analyzed in comparison with the numerous entries in the HRA database. The computer program then calculates the person's health risk factors and computes that person's "health age." Ideally, the individual

health risk appraisal
a computerized assessment of an individual's health age in relation to his or her actual age

should achieve a health age that is much younger than his or her actual age. It would look good, for example, if a 45-year-old person scored a health age of a 38-year-old; on the other hand, if the 45-year-old had a health age of a 50-year-old, that would not be a good sign. A young health age indicates that the individual has behaviors that are health enhancing, a family history that may be health protective, and physical markers indicating an absence of negative health conditions.

Wellness Behaviors

In the personal assessment at the beginning of the chapter, how many questions did you answer with a "yes"? Each of the questions corresponds to the wellness behaviors examined in Belloc and Breslow's Alameda County study (1972) as producing a positive impact on health. The 12-year Alameda County study of 6,928 people revealed that people who practiced the seven behaviors listed in the personal assessment enjoyed better health and had a longer life expectancy than people who did not practice the behaviors. More important, it was not just the individual behaviors that made a difference; it was also the magnitude of the behaviors. For example, people who slept seven to eight hours a night were more healthy than those who slept more than eight hours (those people were more likely to be depressed) or fewer than seven hours (those people were more likely to be under great stress). Here are some interesting facts from the study:

- People who practiced six or more of the behaviors lived longer than people who practiced fewer than six of the behaviors.

- Men who practiced two or fewer of the behaviors were three times more likely to die prematurely than were men who practiced four or five of the behaviors.

- Women who practiced two or fewer of the behaviors were almost three and a half times more likely to die prematurely than were women who practiced four or more of the behaviors.

- People who did not eat breakfast had a 50 percent higher risk of premature death than did people who did eat breakfast.

Medical and social science research such as the Alameda County study has confirmed specific connections between personal habits and a person's risk of developing illness. As an example, consider heart disease or cancer. These two diseases account for almost two-thirds of American deaths each year. Knowing the connections between personal habits and these two diseases gives individuals some control over preventing the diseases from occurring or at least delaying their onset. Simply stated, there are five behaviors that people can perform to reduce their personal risks of heart disease and cancer:

1. Stay away from all tobacco use.

2. Engage in regular physical activity.

3. Follow good nutritional practices.

4. Consume alcohol in moderation, if at all.

5. Engage in known prevention practices, such as recommended physical examinations and medical screenings.

Take another look at your answers to the personal assessment. Are you on the road to optimal health and longevity? Are there behaviors you'd like to develop or habits you want to change? No matter what your age, you can develop a wellness lifestyle that can make a difference in your life. As you can see from the Alameda County study, there is much to be derived from very simple practices. By the way, research confirms that you benefit from practicing health-generating behaviors no matter how old you are when you start performing them. Remember, the quality of your life is not to be measured by how long you might live; rather, it will show in the *quality* of your life for as long as you live. The knowledge and skills you gain from this text and the additional learning you obtain from presentations, library readings, and the Internet will give you what you need to develop a *personal wellness plan* that will serve you well now but will likely evolve as you use your health literacy skills for the rest of your life.

Nation's Health Objectives

About 30 years ago, the U.S. Public Health Service took an active role in promoting wellness. Before then, the health care system focused mainly on what is now referred to as the "medical model" of health. The medical model is physician centered (Figure 2-3). The model is based on an ill person going to the doctor or hospital *after* he or she gets sick. The physician is responsible for the diagnosis and treatment. The patient is responsible for

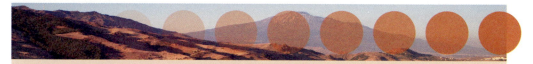

What's Your View?

Is Health Care a Right or a Privilege?

The United States has one of the finest health care systems in the world, but sadly a very large segment of the population lacks access to this system. Some people cannot afford health care, lacking insurance or the ability to pay out of pocket. Some live in rural areas where medical resources might be many miles away. The increased cost or the lack of health care has motivated some people to actively engage in health promotion. Others believe that health care is a right and that everyone should have access to medical treatment. This has become a source of social and political debate: personal responsibility versus medical treatment for disease and disability. What do you think? Should people be more responsible for maintaining their own health, or should they depend on a health care system to keep them well?

following the physician's recommendations. Unfortunately, the medical model does not focus on disease prevention. In many cases, patients go for care after their illness is very advanced and receive treatment too late to improve their health status or to save their lives. Moreover, they enter the health care system at a point when their treatment is complex and costly. For example, in its early stages, cancer of the lung does not cause a great deal of discomfort, so by the time the cigarette smoker feels the symptoms of lung cancer, it is usually too late to save his or her life, even after heroic and costly treatments.

A U.S. Public Health Service initiative in 1979 changed the way physicians and the public looked at health. That initiative was the release of *Healthy People—The Surgeon General's Report on Health Promotion and Disease Prevention*. The **surgeon general** is the highest-ranking U.S. government medical official in the country, and the 1979 report focused on using the **public health** system to prevent disease instead of simply trying to cure it. This report identified five major goals aimed at improving the health and quality of life for all Americans, and it included 225 specific objectives to support the achievement of the goals.

In 1980, the report was revised, and a new list of goals was presented in *Promoting Health/Preventing Disease: Objectives for the Nation*, such as to reduce smoking by adults to less than 25 percent by 1990. You can see from the title of the report that emphasis was on helping Americans achieve better health. The belief was that if businesses, communities, and individuals worked together to achieve the objectives, the need for costly medical care could be reduced and there would be more productivity within the workforce.

Health officials in the United States evaluated the outcomes of *Objectives for the Nation* and concluded that the emphasis on prevention was working well. Meeting with health professionals and citizens at conferences across the nation, officials used the information to develop objectives for the 1990s. The result was a report called *Healthy People 2000*, published in 1990. The current version, *Healthy People 2010*, published in 2000, is being used to guide the development of health behaviors, health programs, and medical interventions for continued improvement of the nation's health through 2010. *Healthy People 2010* is organized into 28 focus areas with 467 public health objectives. These objectives, developed and selected through consultation with a broad range of organizations, professional groups, and individuals, provide a framework for monitoring and measuring improvements in the health status of the American population over the 10-year period from 2000 to 2010. (*Healthy People 2020* is expected to be released in the fall of 2010). Sample objectives for *Healthy People 2010* are presented in Table 2-1.

Recommendations published in *Healthy People 2010* include more personal responsibility and behaviors than did the previous reports. It also contains a section titled "Leading Health Indicators." These indicators make up the 10 most important public health issues facing Americans at this time; they are listed in Table 2-2. Most of the indicators

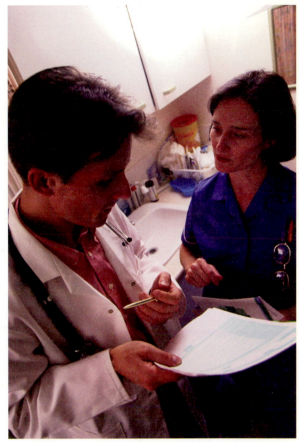

FIGURE 2-3 • The medical model of health care delivery is physician centered.

Courtesy of Photodisc

surgeon general
highest-ranking medical officer in the United States

public health
sum of federal, state, and local health agencies and organizations working together to promote health and prevent disease for the community as a whole

TABLE 2-1 • Sample health objectives, *Healthy People 2010.*

Focus Area	Objective	Baseline Measure
3 Cancer	3-2 Reduce the lung cancer death rate to 44.9 deaths per 100,000 population	57.6 lung cancer deaths per 100,000 population
5 Diabetes	5-1 Increase to 60 percent the proportion of people with diabetes who receive formal diabetes education	45 percent of persons with diabetes received formal diabetes education in 1998
11 Communication	11-1 Increase to 80 percent the proportion of households with internet access	26 percent of households had access to the Internet at home in 1998
12 Heart disease and stroke	12-10 Increase to 50 percent the proportion of adults with high blood pressure whose blood pressure is under control	18 percent of adults aged 18 years and older had it under control
17 Maternal, infant, child	17-6 Increase the proportion of persons who donate blood to 8 percent and in so doing ensure an adequate supply of safe blood	5 percent of the total population donated blood in 1994
27 Tobacco use	27-9 Reduce to 10 percent the proportion of children who are regularly exposed to tobacco smoke at home	27 percent of children aged six years and under lived in a household where someone smoked inside the house at least four days per week

Delmar/Cengage Learning

TABLE 2-2 • Leading health indicators, *Healthy People 2010.*

Indicator	Reason for Including
1. Physical activity	There are numerous benefits from regular exercise, including a healthy body, reduced stress, and prevention of premature death. Yet only 75 percent of teens and 15 percent of adults exercise at least three times a week.
2. Overweight and obesity	Overweight and obesity are major contributors to many causes of preventable death and disability. More than 32 percent of adults between the ages of 20 and 74 are obese.
3. Tobacco use	This is currently the most preventable cause of disease and death in the United States. Almost 25 percent of adults are smokers, and in 1999, 35 percent of teens surveyed reported that they had tried at least one cigarette in the past 30 days.
4. Substance abuse	Alcohol and illicit drug use are related to many of America's most serious problems, including violence, injury, and HIV infection. In 1995, the costs of dealing with drug abuse were estimated at $110 billion.
5. Responsible sexual behavior	Unintended pregnancy and sexually transmitted diseases, including HIV infections, can result from unprotected sexual behaviors. Abstinence is the only behavior that can completely prevent these conditions.
6. Mental health	Approximately 20 percent of the U.S. population is affected by mental illness each year. Depression is a real threat to both adults and teens.
7. Injury and violence	More than 400 Americans die each day from car crashes, murder, poisoning, drowning, and falls. These deaths are preventable.
8. Environmental quality	It is estimated that 25 percent of all preventable illnesses worldwide are related to environmental conditions. In the United States, it is believed that 50,000 premature deaths are related to poor air quality each year.
9. Immunization	Among the most important advances of the twentieth century, immunizations prevent numerous diseases, yet 28 percent of the nation's children are not immunized.
10. Access to health care	Not everyone has access to quality health care because they lack financial resources and education. Approximately 20 percent or more of the 50 million people under the age 65 have no health insurance.

Delmar/Cengage Learning

represent areas that we as individuals can control by our choices and behavior (Figure 2-4). A major purpose of the indicators is to motivate the public to accept responsibility for their health and encourage health promotion activities for health improvement.

As you gain interest in your health and practice wellness behaviors, you may want to join planned health promotion activities at your university, workplace, or community. Imagine: in addition to improving your quality of life, you will be helping to meet the nation's health objectives.

Planning for Wellness

The first step toward a wellness lifestyle is to know and appreciate the importance of wellness; the next step is to put wellness into action. When you were a child, your family was instrumental in caring for your health; now, as an

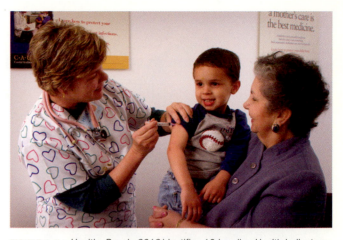

FIGURE 2-4 • *Healthy People 2010* identifies 10 Leading Health Indicators, including immunizations, as areas where individuals can take responsibility for their own health and the health of others. Photo courtesy of CDC; photo taken by James Gathany.

adult, you are personally responsible for your well-being and perhaps for family members as well (Figure 2-5). In that regard, it is up to you to determine what your wellness lifestyle will be and what information you can gather to help you and your family. To bring wellness into your life, you first need to set goals and develop a plan. Just as you would want to develop a financial plan that prepares you for and sustains your retirement years, your wellness plan will position you for health and vitality for the rest of your life. This section will help you develop wellness goals and make that plan. Be sure that your wellness plan is something you will enjoy. Practicing wellness is something you will do for a lifetime; you should enjoy it!

Wellness Domains

Wellness means doing those things that ensure not only your good health but also the health of the people around you. Wellness is a complex process; while it includes the personal elements, it also implies the interaction of the individual with the social and physical environments. As such, wellness extends beyond you as an individual to affect your friends, family, and the environment. Just as there are four dimensions of health, there are several wellness domains that interact with one another while they influence

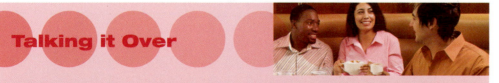

Talking it Over

Prepare a list of the 10 Leading Health Indicators and discuss the list with family or friends. Share information you have about selected indicators and see what they know about the indicators. Talk about the health practices and attitudes that relate to each of the 10 indicators. You can use the information to encourage family members or friends to examine their wellness behaviors and see if there are some they might like to put into practice or strengthen.

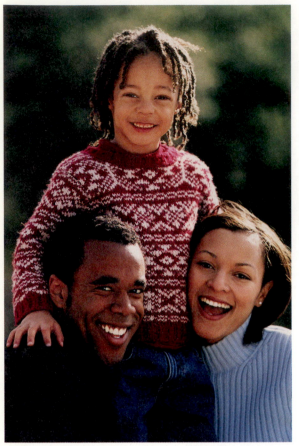

Courtesy of Photodisc

FIGURE 2-5 • Children rely on their parents to care for their health. Adults are responsible not only for their own health but for the health and well-being of their family as well.

all dimensions of health (Figure 2-6). The common wellness domains include the following:

1. Personal wellness
2. Social wellness
3. Emotional wellness
4. Intellectual wellness
5. Environmental wellness
6. Cultural wellness
7. Spiritual wellness
8. Community wellness

Although the importance of each domain may vary from person to person, it is a good idea to include all domains when developing a personal wellness plan. An understanding of all the wellness domains can facilitate your involvement in the wellness process and your ability to help friends and family with their health concerns.

Personal Wellness

Personal wellness implies accepting responsibility for utilizing your health-related knowledge and skills as you strive toward optimal health. Wellness includes developing positive attitudes about you and about planning, implementing, and maintaining

Wellness Domains

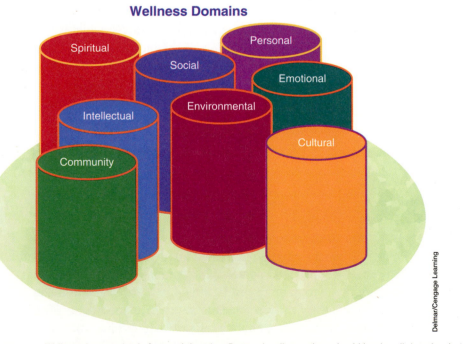

Delmar/Cengage Learning

FIGURE 2-6 • Wellness is comprised of several domains. Personal wellness plans should involve all domains, but the importance of each individual domain can vary from person to person.

a healthy lifestyle. Personal wellness also means gathering the information necessary to make good health decisions. People practice personal wellness if they do things such as the following:

- Knowing how to eat well and doing so

- Avoiding risky behaviors, such as drinking and driving, engaging in unprotected sexual activity, and/or consuming a high-fat diet

- Practicing personal health habits, such as twice-daily dental care, getting plenty of exercise, and getting necessary immunizations

- Practicing personal wellness, which requires a conscious commitment to setting and working toward your goals and encouraging personal wellness among family members

WEB LINK
iVillage

http://www.ivillage.com

This Web site is designed especially for women, but it may be a good site for husbands and significant others to visit as well because there are numerous pages related to wellness topics that are of mututal interest to men and women, such as pregnancy and parenting.

SEARCH TERMS: women's health, family health, health and well-being

Social Wellness

Social wellness means forming positive relationships with other people. It is developing the interpersonal skills needed to interact effectively with others. Social wellness enables you to be comfortable with people at home, at school, and at work. It includes getting along with others even if sometimes you don't particularly like them. Perhaps you can recognize some social wellness characteristics:

- Send thank-you notes to friends and family members when they do something nice for you.

- Remember birthdays and anniversaries and act on them.

- When you are in a conversation with someone, listen and learn something from them.

- Accept and give compliments.

- Think before you speak.

- Attend social events.

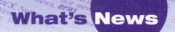

What's News

Even with the proven benefits of physical activity, more than 50 percent of U.S. adults do not get enough physical activity to provide health benefits; 24 percent are not active at all in their leisure time. Activity decreases with age, and sufficient activity is less common among women than men and among those with lower incomes and less education.

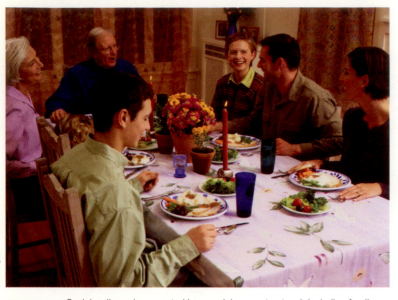

Courtesy of Photodisc

FIGURE 2-7 • Social wellness is supported by a social support network including family members and friends.

social support
real or perceived emotional and physical support received by family, friends, neighbors, and coworkers

Social Support

An important aspect of social wellness is developing a **social support** network that includes family members and friends (Figure 2-7). There is a considerable amount of research confirming the value of social support. Increased levels of social support have been responsible for reduced risk of disease, mental illness, and mortality. For example, Dr. Corey Keyes and his associates (Keyes, Michalec, & Kobau, 2005) studied more than 3,000 older adults and found that subjects who reported seldom visiting relatives or friends had almost four times the number of mentally unhealthy days than those who had visited relatives or friends. Persons who reported having no close friends for emotional support during the 30 days prior to the study reported more physically unhealthy days (8.1 vs. 5.5 for those with three or more friends). There is no doubt that social support is good for one's health.

What can one do to ensure that one has a strong social support network? There is no absolute answer to this question. The strength of a person's social support network depends on a number of factors. It may be nice to have a large number of people in your social support network, but if those individuals cannot be counted on to provide support when you need it, the sheer number is of little value. On the other hand, fewer network members who are truly there for you in many respects will contribute more to your well-being. To develop a good social support network, do the things mentioned previously that contribute to social wellness. You need to develop your circle of friends. This includes *being a good friend*. Make sure you are someone who is available to provide social support for the people close to you. Just be careful not to overdo it. Be there for people when they need the support, but be aware that people will demonstrate a need for support in a variety of ways, and sometimes they may prefer to handle things on their own. A good rule of thumb is to let your friends and family know that you care about them, to let them know that you are available to help when they need it, and to let them come to you.

Did You Know…?

Marriage is good for your health. Almost 30 years of research has demonstrated that married couples are healthier and that they live longer than people who are unmarried.

Emotional Wellness

An emotionally well person can effectively deal with the disturbing and sometimes challenging situations that are part of everyday life. We all experience setbacks in life, such as performing poorly on a test, not getting the new job we applied for, or losing someone we love. It is natural to feel uncomfortable, even angry, when we face these kinds of difficulties. The feelings aren't unhealthy; what is unhealthy is expressing our hurt or disappointment in unproductive, even damaging ways, such as angry outbursts, yelling at someone, or turning to alcohol or other drugs for comfort and escape. The emotionally well person finds constructive ways to deal with life's problems. This may mean turning to your social support network to seek someone to talk to and to get emotional support for the disappointment. Other tips you might want to consider are the following:

- Don't make big worries out of small problems.
- Reduce the level of drama in your life; don't get uptight about every little thing.
- Look for humor in the things that go wrong in your life.
- Open up to people and talk about the hurt you are experiencing.
- Seek professional help if you feel you need it.

Intellectual Wellness

Intellectual wellness means enjoying learning and pursuing knowledge beyond the classroom. It involves exploring new topics, learning new skills, and developing the ability to solve problems and to think critically. There are many ways to learn, such as reading, visiting museums and cultural events, using the Internet, and talking with friends and family members about topics of interest. People who exhibit intellectual wellness use a variety of methods to increase their knowledge and skills:

- Read things that entertain you in addition to reading for academic purposes.
- Set aside specific time for studying and library work and put it on your calendar.
- When you have a lot of homework, do the most challenging work first.
- Eat well (protein helps learning).

Environmental Wellness

Environmental wellness means understanding and caring for the environment. Similar to all other organisms, we live in an **ecosystem**. We share our environment with our friends, neighbors, and other living things. Our ecosystem is a fragile environment, so we must do our part to use resources respectfully and efficiently. Living in a culture where it is easy to overuse resources and to ignore the environment leads to an altered ecosystem for future generations. Each of us needs to practice conservation and environmental protection in our own way. It is wise to remember the Amish proverb, "We do not own the earth, we are borrowing it from our children." What we do or do not do will affect the condition of the environment for future generations. Doing your part to care for the environment could include things like the following:

ecosystem
a complex collection of living things that share a specific environment

- Recycling materials to reduce the amount of waste in the environment.
- Driving less in order to reduce the consumption of fossil fuel.
- Keeping your residence clean and neat.
- Looking for ways to conserve resources, like walking to the store rather than driving and turning out lights when not at home. Imagine if everyone used just one paper towel to dry their hands.

Cultural Wellness

Cultural wellness is being aware of and celebrating your own cultural background as well as understanding and respecting the diversity and richness of other cultures. It involves interacting well with others, regardless of their gender, sexual preference and identity, race, talents, ethnic backgrounds, ages, and so on. Cultural wellness also means passing on the traditions of your family while blending them with the traditions of new family members. Practicing cultural wellness could include things like the following:

- Recognize that everyone you meet knows something that you don't. Take the time to learn from them.

- Most likely, your ancestry is a blend of cultures. Learn as much as you can about your ancestors and find out what cultural factors have blended into your immediate family.

- Visit cultural fairs and celebrations and buy something you can use in your home.

Spiritual Wellness

Spiritual wellness means looking within yourself and getting in touch with your spiritual nature. This might mean reading a holy book, attending a religious service, practicing relaxation, or simply sitting in a quiet place to think about the world. Spiritual wellness may or may not include any particular religion or belief in a higher power. It does include setting aside quiet time for yourself to think about who you are and what you stand for, to reflect on your life's purpose and goals, and to mentally explore possible solutions to important problems (Figure 2-8). Good places to seek quiet time include your home, a park, a beach, a forest, or a place of worship. Some characteristics of spiritual wellness include the following:

- Being able to sit quietly and contemplate your self and getting in touch with the inner you

- Respecting your thoughts, feelings, and emotions

- Being able to embrace the beauty of the environment

- Observe the interconnectedness of environmental elements

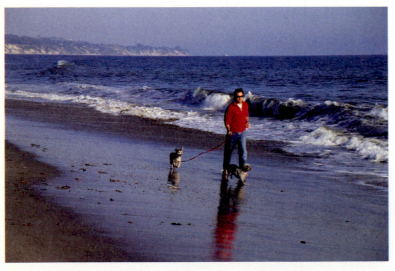

Courtesy of Photodisc

FIGURE 2-8 • Spiritual wellness involves setting aside quiet time to think about your purpose and goals, to reflect on life, and to contemplate the world around.

Community Wellness

Community wellness is engaging in activities to protect the health of the community. The health of a community depends on all the individuals who live in it. Even if your community is very large, your individual behavior can have an impact, especially when you can influence others to participate in developing the community. Community health is enhanced through personal actions, volunteer programs, and environmental protection. Your actions can set an example for others. Having an impact on community wellness includes such things as the following:

- Encouraging tolerance and respect for all members of the community

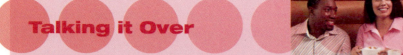

Talking it Over

Talk with your family members or friends about their health beliefs. Find out how they feel about things such as eating habits, the causes of illness, how to treat simple ailments such as colds and injuries, the importance of medical checkups, and so on. If you speak with grandparents, you may get a different perspective than that of your parents, siblings, or friends. List your family members' health beliefs and wellness behaviors and see how many of them have been passed down from generation to generation. Discuss whether these beliefs and behaviors agree with recent scientific information:

• Where do you think these health beliefs originated?
• Do you think the health beliefs are medically valid?

• Developing programs with the help of all constituents that benefit all of the community, not just specific neighborhoods

• Volunteering for community programs, such as "fun runs," Habitat for Humanity, "Toys for Tots," or Meals on Wheels

• Getting involved in community service organizations, seeking election to or supporting candidates for city council, or serving on local government committees

Creating Wellness

As important as wellness is to maintaining optimal health, it is not a way of life that comes naturally to every person. This is especially true in light of the fact wellness is something that has not been institutionalized into the American family's way of life. On the contrary, our culture tends to support unhealthy behaviors with fast foods, high-fat diets, stressful lifestyles, acceptance of obesity, lack of meaningful physical activity, and so on. But there are many individuals who are motivated to practice wellness behaviors. Let's examine some of the factors that play a role in influencing the adoption of wellness behaviors.

Psychological Factors

For almost 50 years, social scientists have been studying human populations to explain why some people protect their health and others don't. The data from these studies not only help explain these behaviors but also help health professionals develop theoretically sound programs encouraging people to develop health-generating behaviors. Much of this information has come from the field of **social psychology**. Social psychologists seek to explain the social-environmental influences on people's attitudes and behaviors. It is from social-psychological research that we learned about things like peer pressure, principles of persuasive communication, and attitude change. But, after all this research, there are no absolute explanations as to why people think and act the way they do. Human beings have free will and varied personalities. Not every person responds the

social psychology
the study of how people's thoughts, emotions, and behaviors are influenced by the actual, imagined, or implied presence of others

same way to every life circumstance. Studies of the psychological responses to events are ongoing in an effort to gather greater understanding about the human response to health and self-preservation. Researchers someday may be able to explain why some people defy logic and engage in health-damaging behavior, such as avoiding safety belt use when they ride in a car. Human motivation is a complex phenomenon. Researchers someday may come up with "recipes" for strategies to encourage wellness practices.

Knowledge, Beliefs, and Attitudes

Our responses to health threats and the behaviors we choose or refuse to perform depend on a number of psychological factors that guide our decision making and behaviors. *Knowledge* is a necessary foundation for making such a decision. What you *know* can have an important influence on how you act. For example, you are not likely to purchase a new product unless you know about it. Moreover, as you learn more about the attributes of the product, you will have more information on which to base your decision. Once you trust the information received, your knowledge is reinforced, and you establish *beliefs* about the product. A belief is an unconfirmed conviction that something you know, you believe to be true. In this sense, the information can actually be true. Sometimes people rely on invalid information to form beliefs. You may gain more information on the product, sort through the number of attributes, and derive information that causes you to think positively or negatively toward the product. The positive or negative response toward the product would be your *attitude* toward the product. If you talk to someone or complete a questionnaire to state an attitude about the product, you are giving an *opinion*.

Attitudes are very important to health and wellness. Attitudes are derived from our knowledge, beliefs, and experiences, and they form the bases for our behaviors. If you hold positive attitudes toward eating fruit and vegetables, you are more likely eat fruit and vegetables. If you have negative attitudes toward smoking cigarettes, you will not smoke cigarettes. The point of all this is that if you have favorable attitudes toward protecting your health and reducing health care costs by practicing wellness, you will practice wellness.

Perception

Another factor that brings information into our psychological framework is perception. Perception is taking sensory information (what we hear, see, feel, and so on) and formulating interpretations of the information. Look at Figure 2-9. What do you see in each figure? Illustration A appears as a cube, but where you see the "opening" to the cube can be just about any of the eight sides. See how many you perceive, ordering them from most obvious to hardest to detect. Share the image with a friend and ask him or her to do the same thing. Was your friend's first choice the same as yours? If not, who is correct? The answer is "neither of you." Perception is an individualistic process. There is no right or wrong—it just is what it is to the individual. By the way, illustration B can be either a vase or the profiles of two people facing one another. You might imagine how our perceptions of the world around us influence our attitudes and behaviors. When you were a child, did you look at something new that was prepared for dinner and, just by appearance, think, "I am not going to like this." Someone may have said to you, "Try it; you'll like it." Maybe you tried it, and you *did* like it. Your taste receptors had a more positive effect on your perceptions than your visual receptors.

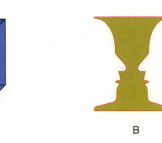

FIGURE 2-9 • Perceptual ambiguity.

A

B

Delmar/Cengage Learning

Perception is an important factor in health and wellness because of the role that perception plays in evaluating our internal and external environments. As a child, you learned from your family how to identify signs and symptoms of illness. Did you ever have a family member or doctor say, "Tell me where it hurts," "Tell me how it feels," or "Describe the pain"? These personal assessments depend on your perception. Hospitals now have "pain charts" asking patients to describe the pain level they are experiencing at the time by selecting the level from the chart. Now that you are older, you are able to make more interpretations, maybe to the point of diagnosis. You may sense, for example, that you are getting sick because you "just don't feel right." Perception of our external environment is significant because we observe behaviors of others and assess things in our environment posing threats to our well-being. A young person living in a neighborhood where there is a lot of gang activity may, over time, develop the perception that people in gangs are subject to violence, serve jail time, and have a shorter life expectancy. These perceptions may encourage this person to take protective action.

Perceptions and the Health Belief Model

In the early 1950s, health psychologist Godfrey Hochbaum was working for the U.S. Public Health Service. Tuberculosis was a major public health threat at the time. Despite the fact that the Public Health Service was offering free X-rays for early detection of tuberculosis, people were not responding to the offer. Dr. Hochbaum wanted to find out why, so he collected data from about 1,500 people to find out why some took advantage of free screening and why some did not. The subjects were asked if they perceived tuberculosis as a serious health condition and if they perceived themselves susceptible to getting tuberculosis. The results of the study indicated those who considered tuberculosis a serious threat were more likely to get the X-ray than those who did not consider tuberculosis a serious threat. In fact, those *most* likely to get screened were those individuals who perceived threat and susceptibility. This work became the basis for what is now the Health Belief Model (HBM). The HBM has been widely used and modified since Hochbaum's original work. The current model is illustrated in Figure 2-10. Notice the role that perception plays in the model. It appears that people will take action if they *perceive*

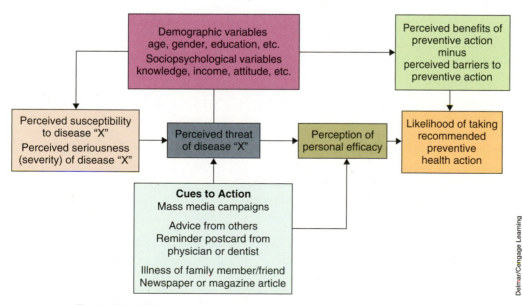

Delmar/Cengage Learning

FIGURE 2-10 • The Health Belief Model.

that a threat is imminent, in some cases even if the threat doesn't really exist. In 1976, U.S. health officials felt that an epidemic of swine flu was going to sweep the country. In response to that suspected threat, there was a plan to immunize every person in the United States. The government appropriated $135 million for the program, and people lined up to get their immunizations. They perceived that an epidemic *was coming*. The problem was that the epidemic never did come. There was only one death associated with the flu, but there were many more deaths among elderly citizens who died from the stress of receiving the injection and some who developed Guillain-Barre syndrome, a neurological condition associated with the vaccine itself. As a result, more than 40 million people were immunized for an epidemic that never occurred.

The HBM is perhaps the most widely used model to explain why people take action to prevent a health threat. The model has been used as a framework for research projects designed to test interventions intended to encourage preventive health behavior. Consider applying the HBM to your wellness program. If you obtain some information on something that poses a threat to your health, apply information about the threat to your own understanding of the HBM. Do you think the threat is serious? Do you perceive yourself susceptible to the ill effects of the threat? Is there anything in your family history that might enhance your susceptibility to the threat (or that protects you from the threat)? Do you have the personal efficacy to take action to reduce or eliminate the threat? Can you identify more benefits than barriers to preventive action?

WEB LINK

Health E-Notes.com

http://health.enotes.com

At this Web site, you can review more information on the HBM and many other health and wellness principles. Enter "Health Belief Model" in the search bar on the home page of the Web site.

SEARCH TERMS: health belief model, health planning models, health promotion theories

Theory of Planned Behavior

One other model that helps explain the adoption of healthy behaviors is the Theory of Planned Behavior (Ajzen, 1991). The model assumes *behavioral intention* as the most important determinant of behavior. The major components of the Theory of Planned Behavior are illustrated in Table 2-3. According to the theory, behavioral intention is

TABLE 2-3 • Theory of Planned Behavior.

Concept	Definition	Description
Attitude	Your personal evaluation of the behavior.	Is the behavior important enough for you to perform it?
Behavioral intention	The perceived likelihood that you will perform the behavior.	Are attitudes strong enough to cause you to take action?
Subjective norms	Beliefs about whether important people around you approve or disapprove of the behavior. Motive to behave to gain approval. Perception of norms will increase likelihood of behavioral intention.	Do you feel that most people will agree or disagree with the behavior?
Perceived behavioral control	The belief that one has the skills and resources to perform the behavior.	Do you feel that you have the ability to adopt the behavior? If not, what do you need?

Source: Adapted from National Cancer Institute (2005).

influenced by a person's attitudes toward the behavior and the degree to which the person perceives that important people approve or disapprove of the behavior (subjective norm). Reaction to perceived norms is an authentic part of social psychology. People want to be liked and admired, so it is not uncommon for them to adopt behaviors that are exhibited by people they know and admire. In particular, we see actions like this among adolescents. Young people will engage in risky behaviors such as drug use, smoking, and unprotected sexual activity if they *think* their peers are involved in the same behaviors. In truth, it may be just the opposite—*most* of their peers may not be engaging in the behavior.

An important construct within the theory is the aspect of *perceived behavioral control.* Researchers who developed the theory added this element to the model because they felt that people would try harder to perform a behavior if they perceived that they had the ability to perform the behavior. Notice that this concept was also part of the HBM. Although these two models were approached in different ways, they share some common themes. Their theoretical frameworks include (1) a response to a health threat that is influenced by perceptions and (2) attitudes to address the threat with healthy behavior as long as the individual perceives that he or she has the skill and resources to perform the behavior.

Health Promotion

Health promotion is a combination of policies and activities designed to help people achieve wellness. Health education and risk reduction programs may be conducted in communities, workplaces, and schools to help prevent or solve common health problems. It is not uncommon for these programs to be built on theoretical frameworks like those described previously. Examples of health promotion programs would include a hospital delivering nutrition education to pregnant women attending birthing classes, a community health center providing free or low-cost immunizations, a major corporation offering smoking cessation classes for employees, and an after-school walking program for school employees and learners. Health promotion programs may be sponsored by both public and private organizations. Whether the programs are intended for small groups or the entire community, the programs stress the prevention of illness and injury

health promotion
policies and activities designed to encourage wellness

and the promotion of wellness behaviors. Providing free infant-restraint car seats to low-income families would be a health promotion activity, but it is a cost-effective risk reduction program that would reduce medical costs to the community. Numerous corporations realize that healthy employees are more productive and profitable to the company than unhealthy employees (Figure 2-11), so employees are offered wellness programs such as exercise classes, nutrition education workshops, smoking cessation classes, and stress management workshops. Some companies even offer child care programs for employees, thus removing the stress of finding home-based child care. These companies would not sponsor these kinds of programs without first measuring the value of the activities against the expense of running

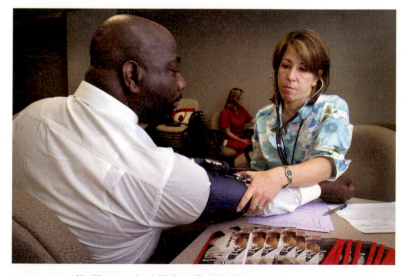

FIGURE 2-11 • Health promotion initiatives, like this blood pressure screening, can be conducted in communities, workplaces, and schools to help prevent or solve common health problems. Courtesy of CDC; photo taken by James Gathany.

them. Remember that companies save money when employees are working and not absent, when companies spend less money on health insurance because of fewer health care claims, when there is less employee turnover, and when morale and productivity go up. Health promotion contributes to beneficial outcomes.

Here is a sampling of companies and the savings derived from their health promotion programs:

- DuPont evaluated its work site health promotion program over a two-year period and found that, on reduced absenteeism alone, DuPont recovered $1.42 for every dollar invested in the program.

- Johnson and Johnson cut its hospitalization costs 34 percent after three years.

- Honeywell, Inc., reported returns estimated at 70 to 150 percent.

There are lessons to be learned from work site health promotion. If corporations are able to demonstrate that health promotion saves *corporations* money, it follows that health promotion can benefit everyone. Many universities offer health promotion programs to learners, faculty, and staff, generally under the sponsorship of the campus health center. The models vary from campus to campus depending on staffing and funding. The programs may include outreach workshops and training sessions, health fairs, sponsored exercise programs like fun runs, and health care planning seminars. Do you know how to access health promotion activities on your campus?

Recognizing Your Personal Value

Individuals have total control of their wellness behaviors. For example, as an adult, you make choices about what you eat, how much you exercise, and whether you use substances proven to be harmful to your health. At this stage of your life, you are making your own life decisions. This being the case, you now rely more on your personal decision-making skills to guide your wellness decisions now and as you get older. The importance of valuing this privilege and being able to act on it cannot be overstated.

A first step toward wellness is developing a positive attitude about yourself and a concern for your well-being. This means forming positive attitudes such as the following:

- "I am a good person, and I have value to others."

- "My health is important to me, and I am willing to dedicate myself to protect it."

- "I want to live a long, healthy, satisfying life."

- "I want to set a good example for my family."

- "I am willing to take responsibility to practice wellness."

Positive attitudes can help motivate you to plan for and reach your wellness goals. Having good **wellness motives** is important because some behaviors require self-discipline. This is especially true if you are trying to add a new health behavior to your way of life or if you want to give up some behavior that is not good for you. Have you ever started something like an exercise program and then quit because it just seemed like too much

---

WEB LINK

Go Ask Alice

http://www.health.columbia.edu

Go Ask Alice is a searchable Internet-based question-and-answer site at the Columbia University Health Services program. It is a Web site developed in 1993 where students can post questions and get answers about any health topic. The questions and answers are archived for quick retrieval. When you arrive at the Health Services Web site, go through the **Alice! Health Promotion Program** link.

SEARCH TERMS: campus wellness, campus health promotion

---

wellness motives
the sum of knowledge, beliefs, attitudes, and values that contribute to forming reasons for practicing wellness behaviors

trouble? When you feel like you can't stick with your program, there are some strategies you can use to keep yourself motivated:

- Remind yourself why you wanted to practice the new behavior in the first place. What are the financial, social, or physical benefits of the new behavior?

- Keep the end result in mind. Concentrate on how fit you will feel when you reach your goal and how much energy you will have.

- Look for additional rewards. If you are exercising, for example, think about how you are protecting your heart, managing your weight, or reducing your stress.

- Challenge yourself to have fun. Look for healthy foods and recipes that taste good. Find a physical activity or sport you enjoy.

- Look for an exercise partner. Putting exercise into a social context helps eliminate boredom.

- Enjoy your success. Plan rewards as you achieve your wellness goals. Give yourself credit for sticking with a wellness program. Permit yourself to feel good about what you have accomplished.

Did You Know...?

The increase in life expectancy that Americans now enjoy is the result of people's use of health information and health education to create improved health behaviors, not medical care. Practicing healthy behaviors has done more for improving health than has the advancement of medical procedures.

Setting Wellness Goals

Goals are important because they give direction to your life. They provide you with a kind of compass to help you stay on course. If you think about it, all the things around you—electronic and mechanical devices, sound equipment, transportation, and so on—are the result of goals someone set for themselves. Take Thomas Edison, inventor of the common lightbulb, for example. Developing a way to produce light from electricity was Edison's goal. He stayed with it even though he produced hundreds of bulbs that didn't work. When asked about the hundreds of failures, Edison remarked, "I have not failed almost 700 times. I have not failed once. I have succeeded in proving that those previous 700 versions will not work."

Goals keep you focused on solving problems. Here are some suggestions for setting good goals:

1. Be sure you have a clear assessment of your current health behaviors and health status.

2. Your goals should be something you really want to achieve.

3. Be clear about exactly what it is you want. A goal of "to be healthy" is not specific enough. You need a specific target, such as "I will engage in an exercise program that is healthy and fun," "I will create a walking program to help manage the stress in my life," or "I will become active in activities that protect the environmental condition of my community."

4. Set a reasonable number of goals so that you will not get frustrated trying to achieve them all.

5. Make sure your goals are attainable.

6. State goals in the positive rather than the negative. For example, "wanting to be smoke free" is better than "wanting to not smoke."

7. Write them out. The act of writing your goals helps reinforce them and increases the chance you will achieve them.

8. Identify the barriers that may prevent you from reaching each goal. Then think about ways you can eliminate the barriers.

9. Identify the resources such as people, information, materials, and money that can help you reach your goals.

10. Develop a plan for reaching each goal. Write out the plan.

Once you have planned and written out your goals, use the following strategies to increase your success rate:

- Keep your goal list posted where you will see it often.

- Make a commitment with yourself to achieve your goals.

- Keep a mental picture of the goals and their outcomes. Post a list of strategies you will use to reach the goal.

- When faced with obstacles, use your resources, that is, friends, family, and health literature, to overcome them.

- Repeat methods that *do* work.

- Do something to move toward your goals *every* day.

- Have someone close to you provide social support to help reach your goals.

- Evaluate your progress regularly and reward yourself for your accomplishments.

- Be persistent. This is the main ingredient in achieving goals: *persistence*.

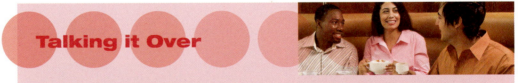

Talking it Over

Use the information from the health literacy section to construct a short questionnaire to measure health literacy. Ask each of your family members, roommates, or friends to answer the questionnaire. Ask if they currently think more about their personal health than they did when they were younger. Do they demonstrate health literacy; that is, do they seek health information? Are there unhealthy habits they started as teenagers that they have found difficult to change? Write a summary of their responses and compare the summary with your own health literacy skills and behaviors at this point in time.

BUILDING YOUR LIFETIME WELLNESS PLAN

Your wellness plan is likely to include some behaviors you already do, but your plan may also include some behaviors you want to eliminate, add, or modify. Let's say you currently spend a lot of time on the sofa watching television or just surfing the Internet or participating in chat rooms or having to work many hours in addition to school. You decide that exercise is to be part of your wellness plan. You will be more successful carrying out your plan if your goal is stated in terms of what you plan *to do* rather than what you plan *not to do*. You will increase your chances of success if you say "I will exercise for no less than 30 minutes at least four times a week" instead of "I will quit watching so much TV." Research tells us that people are more successful adopting new, improved behaviors than they are at quitting unwanted behaviors. Replace the time you spend watching television with exercise, and you will be substituting a new, positive behavior rather than struggling to eliminate an old one.

● ● ● End-of-Chapter Activities

Opportunities for Application

1. Conduct an Internet search for the topic of wellness and list the key things you learned from the sites you visited that have meaning to the development of your wellness lifestyle or wellness plan.

2. Pick one of the topical areas from the table of Leading Health Indicators and conduct a literature search on the National Institutes of Health Web site.
   a. Summarize the most important pieces of information you found.
   b. See if you can find information on the Web site describing the progress the country is making to some of the specific objectives for your chosen topical area.

3. Using the information for the topic you chose in item 1, try your hand at creating a mind map for the topical area. Include what you know and what you might like to know about the topic.

Key Concepts

1. Compare and contrast the relationship between health and wellness.

2. List and briefly describe the eight domains of wellness.

3 Write a letter to a family member or friend encouraging him or her to make a behavioral change that would improve his or her level of wellness. Be sure to include information from the text and other sources.

4. Draw the Health Belief Model and leave space in each of the boxes in the model to include information for each of the components in the model. Select a health threat that can affect you, a family member, or a friend and include information in the spaces provided. Look at the information you included and prepare a report that highlights the prospect of the person adopting the health behavior in question.

Personal Assessment: Current Health Behaviors

This assessment will give you a measure of the quality of essential healthful behaviors. These are the questions asked of the 6,928 people mentioned in the Alameda County study.

1. Do you avoid the use of tobacco?

2. Do you exercise regularly?

3. Do you believe you maintain a normal weight?

4. Do you restrict your eating between meals?

5. Do you eat breakfast every day?

6. Do you sleep seven to eight hours each night?

7. Do you consume no more than one to two alcoholic drinks, three or less times per week?

The following is based on research information:

1. Tobacco use, specifically cigarette smoking, is a major health risk. Each cigarette a person smokes will shorten his or her life by 14 minutes.

2. Regular exercise is health protective. Exercise can reduce risks for heart disease, cancer, obesity, and diabetes and can help relieve stress.

3. Normal weight is health protective. Overweight contributes to diabetes, cancer, and heart disease. Severe underweight can be a sign of serious mental problems and can be life threatening.

4. People who eat between meals are not as healthy as people who do not. If you do eat between meals, eat only healthy snacks.

5. People who do not eat breakfast are ill more often than are those who do.

6. The healthiest people sleep between seven and eight hours each night.

7. Use of alcohol can lead to health problems, especially if it is used to excess. Alcohol also increases one's risk of auto accidents.

References

Ajzen, I. (1991). The theory of planned behavior. *Organizational Behavior and Human Decision Processes, 50*, 179–211.

Belloc, N. B., and L. Breslow. (1972). Relationship of physical health status and health practices. *Preventive Medicine 1*, 409–421.

Keyes, C. L., Michalec, B., & Kobau, R. (2005). Social support and health-related quality of life among older adults—Missouri, 2000. *Morbidity and Mortality Weekly Report, 54*(17), 433–437.

National Cancer Institute. (2005). *Theory at a glance: A guide for health promotion practice* (2nd ed.). Washington, DC: U.S. Department of Health and Human Services. Retrieved May 4, 2010 from http://www.cancer.gov/PDF/481f5d53-63df-41bc-bfaf-5aa48ee1da4d/TAAG3.pdf

CHAPTER 3

Managing Stress

CHAPTER OBJECTIVES

When you finish this chapter, you should be able to:

- Explain the terms *stress*, *stressors*, *eustress*, *distress*, and *stress response*.

- Describe how stress affects your body and your immune system.

- Explain the health risks associated with long-term stress.

- List and describe the most common categories of stressors.

- List and describe healthy techniques and strategies for managing stress.

- Create a personal plan for successfully managing stress.

KEY TERMS

autonomic nervous system

cortisol

distress

endocrine system

eustress

fight-or-flight response

general adaptation syndrome (GAS)

homeostasis

hormones

job stress

parasympathetic nervous system

posttraumatic stress disorder

psychoneuroimmunology (PNI)

stress

stress hardiness

stressors

stress response

sympathetic nervous system

●●● Introduction

If you are a traditional college-age student, you have probably heard these words: "College is the best time of your life!" "You're on your own now—you get to manage life on your own!" "You'll never have this much freedom of choice and so little responsibility again. Enjoy it!" Some days you probably agree with these statements. Other days, you certainly don't feel very independent. In fact, you may feel just the opposite; you may sense pressure to perform well at school in order to graduate or assure that you qualify for a particular job. You may have to juggle work and classes in order to afford the costs of going to college and supporting yourself. Or perhaps you realize you've been spending too much time having "fun" and now the resulting stress of your choices is negatively affecting your performance.

Perhaps you are a non–traditional-age student returning to college after an extended absence. You may share some of the feelings mentioned previously, or you may have an entirely different set of concerns. You may be balancing your academic activities with a full-time job and perhaps with significant family responsibilities for children or aging parents (Figure 3-1). Finding the time and energy to handle all your other needs and interests while still finding time for schoolwork can be quite stressful.

In an age where life choices and opportunities have increased dramatically, we find ourselves wanting to "have it all" and "do it all." These desires to "have it all" can create high, unrealistic expectations that are difficult or even impossible to fulfill. Learning to balance your desires for achievement with your personal and social requirements can be quite a challenge.

You may realize that adult lives are packed with responsibilities, many of which revolve around the relationships we have with family, friends, classmates, and coworkers. As a college student, you are probably living away from your family support system—or you may have a family of your own to manage. You likely will find yourself facing new challenges and decisions that you are making for the first time. The feelings associated with managing all these responsibilities are probably often like a roller-coaster ride. Life can be fun and stimulating one day and miserable the next day. Moreover, it is impossible to anticipate what's going to happen from one day to the next. Life is exciting, but at the same time, it can also feel very stressful.

You may wonder at times if there's something wrong because you feel "stressed out" about things. It may appear that people around you seem to handle life's challenges without getting upset. But you may find yourself having a hard time facing adversity when things pile up against you. Although learning to manage the multiple challenges of life is a normal part of adulthood, at times it can be very confusing and frustrating. The anxiety of addressing obligations and responsibilities of adult life can threaten to overwhelm you. In this chapter, you'll learn what contributes to stress, how stress affects one's body and health, and how you can arm yourself with wellness skills to help manage stress so that you can enjoy your life.

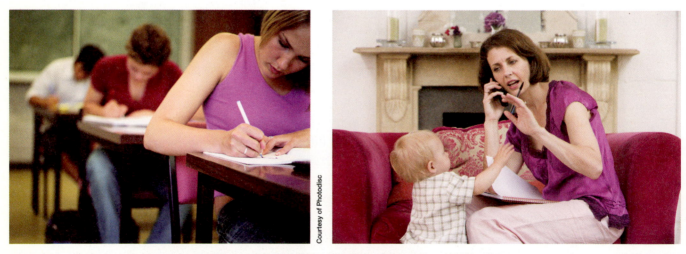

Courtesy of Photodisc

Image Copyright Monkey Business Images, 2009. Use under license from Shutterstock.com

FIGURE 3-1 • Whether you are (a) a traditional student or (b) a nontraditional student, college can be a stressful time.

PERSONAL ASSESSMENT
Stress Management Quiz

Before reading this chapter, see how much you already know about stress and managing stress. Read the questions below and answer True or False in the space provided. The answers are located at the end of the chapter.

1. We would be healthier if we could avoid all types of stress.

2. Even something positive, such as being selected for an award, can be stressful.

3. The amount of stress you feel depends on how you perceive (view and interpret) a situation, not just on the situation itself.

4. Your body responds differently to an imagined stressful situation than it does to an actual stressful situation.

5. The endocrine system controls breathing, heart rate, and blood pressure.

6. Stress hormones that circulate in your bloodstream over an extended period of time can damage the body.

7. At least two-thirds of all visits to health care providers may be for stress-related illnesses.

8. Feeling depressed, anxious, or upset causes immune system function to become stronger.

9. High levels of stress hormones in the body can increase learning and memory.

10. Getting plenty of sleep, eating a healthy diet, and exercising regularly can help you manage stress.

What Is Stress?

We hear about stress all the time. Chances are, you can't go through a day without hearing someone complain about stress, such as "I have so much pressure at work (school)" or "I'm just stressed out!" Perhaps you find yourself saying or thinking these words more often than you'd like.

What do we really mean when we say we're "stressed"? Are we worried? Fearful? Nervous? **Stress** refers to the physical and emotional states that we experience as a result of changes and challenges in our lives. These changes and challenges, which trigger a response in us, are called **stressors**. The effects of stress can be physical, emotional, or mental. It can cause physical symptoms such as headaches, stomachaches, and poor sleep patterns. It can also disrupt mental functions, making it more likely that we will forget things or have difficulty concentrating. The bottom line is that stress is a part of life. To be without stress is to be without life. Worry can be stressful, cold is stressful, heat is stressful, overcrowding is stressful, hunger can be stressful, and the list goes on. There can be degrees of stress. For example, cold can be a stressor at 60 degrees Fahrenheit, but at 15 degrees, the stressor is much more intense.

stress
the physical and emotional states experienced as a result of changes and challenges in our lives

stressors
situations that trigger physical and emotional reactions in our bodies

Stress can also affect emotions. When you're feeling stressed, you may become more moody or become upset more easily than usual. Prolonged stress can lead to apathy or lethargy toward life in general. In some people, prolonged stress can lead to depression. Stress, if not managed appropriately, can have a negative effect on all or most of your health dimensions.

We usually think of stress as occurring only in response to negative situations, such as getting a low grade on a test, receiving an overdue bill, or having an argument with a family member, friend, or coworker. These are stressors that are short term or limited in duration. Negative stressors can also be more long term, like the mounting pressure of an end-of-semester project or the prolonged illness of a family member. Negative forms of stress are called **distress**. Distress can be caused by something that's not very important, such as losing your sunglasses when you're in a hurry, or it can be a result of something major, such as the death of a parent or grandparent or being fired from your job or arrested.

The same physical response that happens to us during negative events can also happen to us when something good happens. This type of stress has a special name: **eustress**. Eustress can occur when receiving an award, presenting a project you are proud of at a business meeting, going to a big concert with friends, or going on a date with someone new. You can probably think of times when you have felt excited and had "butterflies" in your stomach, such as having to give an important presentation. This is an example of experiencing eustress. Eustress can also be long term, like the planning and preparation for a vacation or studying abroad in another country. Regardless of the type of stress, our bodies have physiological responses in place to deal with the stressors we encounter. The body responds the same way physically to both eustress and distress.

The Stress Response

The pioneer of stress research was Hans Selye (1976), a Canadian endocrinologist. His experiments with animals suggested that the body's response to a stressor was predictable. He postulated the definition of stress as "nonspecific response of the body to any demand imposed upon it." This meant that the stress response was not specific to each particular stressor; the response was the same regardless of the stressor. The stress response occurs in three phases. He called this response sequence the **general adaptation syndrome (GAS)**, shown in Figure 3-2. The three phases are the following:

1. *Alarm.* The brain alerts the body that extra resources are needed to deal with a challenge to the body's condition of homeostasis. Various body systems respond quickly to provide the needed resources. If the stressful situation doesn't last long, the body returns to homeostasis. During this phase of the GAS, the body prepares for a **fight-or-flight response**. This response was the kind exhibited by our ancient ancestors when they faced threats to their survival, such as animal attacks or battles. We may no longer face wild animals, but our biological response to stress is essentially the same as it was thousands of years ago. Our modern stressors don't always allow us to follow the fight-or-flight response. If a colleague raises our stress level, it is not socially acceptable to run away, nor is it appropriate to beat him or her up.

2. *Resistance.* If the stressful situation continues, the body would like to return to homeostasis, so it must first respond to the threat. Physiological changes in the

distress
a negative form of stress that occurs in reaction to something we perceive as bad

eustress
a form of stress that occurs in reaction to something we perceive as good but exciting

general adaptation syndrome (GAS)
the body's physiological response to continuous stress; it includes three phases: alarm, resistance, and exhaustion

fight-or-flight response
the response of the nervous and endocrine systems to supply the body with energy to fight back or escape from a stressor

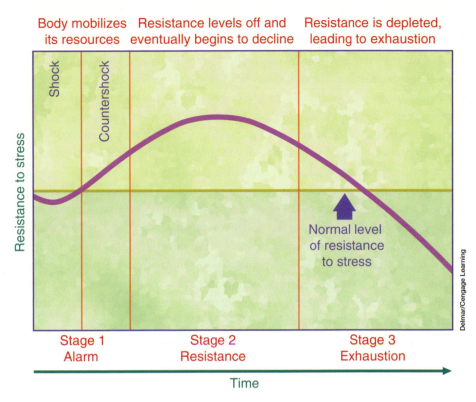

Body mobilizes its resources

Resistance levels off and eventually begins to decline

Resistance is depleted, leading to exhaustion

Shock

Countershock

Resistance to stress

Normal level of resistance to stress

Stage 1
Alarm

Stage 2
Resistance

Stage 3
Exhaustion

Time

Delmar/Cengage Learning

FIGURE 3-2 • *The general adaptation syndrome.*

body take place to allow the body to continue responding to the stressor. The body is remarkable in its ability to cope with extended stress, but it can't continue to produce enough resources to meet extra demands indefinitely.

3. *Exhaustion.* The body gradually becomes exhausted from trying to keep up with the increased demands, and it eventually breaks down. How long it takes for this breakdown to occur and what specific form it takes varies from individual to individual. All individuals, however, experience a decline of immune system function. This is serious because an individual with an impaired immune system is less capable of resisting disease.

Stressors

What makes something a stressor? Although it may be related to a situation, it is one's *perception*—the attitude and a picture created in one's mind about a situation—that determines whether something is a stressor. In fact, we learn to label situations as being "stressful." A young child, for example, is not afraid of an animal unless he or she has a negative encounter with the animal. Perceptions vary from one individual to another. How we perceive stress can be determined by our personalities, the environment in which we were raised, or the interactions with other people with whom we live and work. Some people can thrive on stress, while others may attempt to avoid it at all cost. Some people perform better under stress; some people have personalities that enjoy a lot of stimulation and may overschedule and overcommit, causing undue stress on themselves (and on others). People who have personalities that thrive on quiet, focused interaction are stressed by noise and what they consider chaotic activity. If you were raised in a free-flowing, high-activity environment, such as a large family, you might handle many things going on at once very well. If your family was quiet and controlled, however, any free-flowing activity may actually seem stressful to you.

You may perceive something as being stressful if you know that the people around you view it differently from the way you view it. Imagine telling your boss that you need the day off to take your child to the doctor when you know that the supervisor "blows up" whenever someone asks for time off. In this situation, just knowing that you have to confront this kind of boss about the need for time off may cause you significant stress. On the other hand, if your boss was more tolerant about taking leave time, you might not feel much stress at all about asking for the time off.

The same event can be considered eustressful by one person and distressful by someone else. Here's an example of how two people might perceive the same situation differently. Terry is the pitcher for his college baseball team. The bases are loaded, and there are two outs. Terry wants to strike out the next batter, Jason, to win the game. Both Terry and Jason are likely to be experiencing high levels of stress. Each may see the situation as either positive or negative—as an opportunity to win the game or to lose it. Depending on the outcome of the next pitch, one of them is likely to experience eustress while the other will probably experience distress (Figure 3-3).

Learners face many events in college that can cause a variety of emotional responses. Suppose there is a final exam in chemistry. Each learner in the class will have a different view of this situation. Some learners will feel completely prepared and experience little stress about the exam. Others will feel unprepared and very anxious. A few learners will think that they know the material well but will be afraid they'll forget everything when the test starts. A small number of learners will be completely unprepared but will recognize that there is nothing they can do about it now, so they might decide to relax and not worry about the exam. The situation is exactly the same for all learners: there is an important exam in chemistry. But each learner reacts according to his or her own individual perception of the circumstances and his or her personal motives. It is interesting to note that many times we become overly concerned prior to an event only to find out that it was not nearly as bad as we had envisioned in our minds. Sometimes we are our own worst enemies when it comes to being stressed out. Some people get stressed just wondering if stress will occur.

There are other factors that can influence how we experience a possible stressor. These factors include our past experiences with similar situations, how we are feeling physically and emotionally, and even the timing of the situation. For example, a red light is not usually a major stressor for most people. But if you are late for work or an important appointment, the red light that delays you suddenly becomes a stressor.

Other important factors that influence one's intensity of stress might be one's level of self-confidence and how prepared they are to handle life's events. The effects of stress are greatly reduced when the necessary resources, such as information, social support, coping mechanisms, and so on, are available to prevent stressors from being overwhelming. Suppose it comes time to pay your rent or car insurance. If you have enough money to pay the bill when it's due, you can take care of it without a second thought. If you don't have the money, however, the presence of the bill will become a stressor. Your ability to

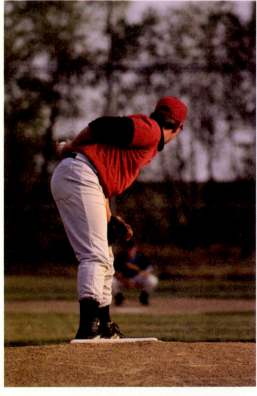

Courtesy of Photodisc

FIGURE 3-3 • Examples of eustress and distress can be vividly illustrated when thinking about sports.

handle life's events can be greatly enhanced by developing a resource "toolbox" to deal with the major categories of stressors. The toolbox can include those strategies that help you respond to stress or call on social support from those around you to help you get through stressful times.

Major Categories of Stressors

Many life events can be stressors (see the Holmes-Rahe Social Readjustment Scale in chapter 17). The stressors may come at any given time, and we don't necessarily experience all types, but it is good to know about them so that we can recognize them and deal with them when they do appear. We can categorize these events into three main categories of stressors: (1) personal, (2) interpersonal, and (3) environmental/societal.

Personal Stressors

Our lives are filled with events that sometimes are part of life, sometimes relate to achieving our goals, sometimes involve interacting with friends and family, and so on. Some of these stressors are listed in Table 3-1; perhaps you can identify more of your own. There are many personal circumstances that people might label as stressful. Being aware of potentially stressful circumstances can help you prepare a response to them by including toolbox strategies in your wellness lifestyle.

Physical, Emotional, and Social Changes

College is usually a time of change and adjustment—mentally, physically, emotionally, and socially. Regardless of your age, you will be challenged during all your college years to balance the demands of school, family, relationships, and your personal well-being. Emotionally and socially, you may be faced with challenges and new situations that you have not experienced before. Sometimes these changes occur so rapidly that you feel as if you're a stranger in your own body. Having it all together one day and then disaster the next as a result of your challenges can leave you feeling anxious and stressed.

TABLE 3-1 • Examples of personal stressors.

Personal Stressors	Examples
Physical and emotional challenges	Illness, injury, adjustment to new surroundings, separation from home, concern about family members
Academic pressures	Competition for grades, struggles with difficult subjects, career planning, adjusting to roommates, new academic skills
Financial stressors	College tuition, changing work environments, living costs, personal expenses
Relationships	Romantic relationships, spousal stressors, work relationships, classmates
Time	Demands of class attendance, work schedules, study time, project demands, desire for personal time

Delmar/Cengage Learning

If you are a non–traditional-age learner returning to school after being out for a while, you may find yourself wondering whether you "have what it takes" to succeed in today's academic environment. The people who are in your classes may seem very different from you, and you may have concerns about fitting in socially and keeping up academically. Some days you probably feel like your life experiences have prepared you well for the challenges that you face, while other days you may feel like a "fish out of water." Be confident in the fact that you bring a wealth of life's experiences to your classmates and your program of study.

Academic Pressures and Demands

The academic expectations in college will likely be higher than they were in high school. Because you have chosen to go to college, you expect to be taught well and challenged to perform well. As a result, it may not be uncommon to feel a great deal of pressure to perform academically. This is true whether you're a learner at the top of your class trying to do your best every time, a learner near the bottom of the class just struggling to keep moving on, or somewhere in between. You may feel challenged to complete class assignments, homework, and tests while trying to obtain good grades. There are constant pressures, such as meeting assignment deadlines and needing to perform well in class and for exams. On top of all these academic pressures, you may have work responsibilities and/or family obligations.

Like many college learners, you may be faced with the stress of working to pay for your education or living expenses and wanting to be sure that you get their money's worth from the experience. You may also be experiencing the stress of knowing that what you do now can affect your future opportunities and career choices. You may be concerned that you won't do well enough to get the job you want or to get into the graduate school program you want.

Negatives Feelings

Our reactions to stressors can include feelings of anxiety, insecurity, depression, or worry. These emotions can sometimes be very unpredictable. One moment you're on top of the world, and the next you're down in the dumps. You may feel insecure about your age, the way your body looks, your academic performance, and so on. You may feel depressed or anxious about your social relationships. You may be worried that you will disappoint important people in your life or that you won't be able to succeed at all the tasks that you must complete. All these feelings are normal, but the resulting stress can impact your level of wellness.

job stress
the harmful physical and emotional responses that occur when the requirements of the job do not match the capabilities, resources, or needs of the worker

Did You Know...?

According to labor reports in 2000, Americans put in what would be equivalent to an additional 40-hour work-week per calendar year as compared to 10 years previously.

Job Stress

Job stress can be described as the harmful physical and emotional responses that occur when the requirements of the job do not match the capabilities, resources, or needs of the worker. Stress related to and around issues involving people's employment has escalated in the past 20 years. The results of job stress include increased direct medical, legal and insurance costs, higher absenteeism, and employee turnover. Sources of job stress are things like longer work hours, workplace violence, job insecurity, economic downturn, and corporate restructuring.

Corporation outsourcing, downsizing, and bankruptcies have employees concerned about retaining their jobs. Just wanting to do one's job well can contribute to stress. Employees are constantly under pressure to do more in less time and with fewer resources in order to keep their jobs secure and to help keep the business stable. Additionally, there are certain job conditions that may lead to stress, such as interpersonal relationships, ambiguous work roles, management style, the design of tasks, and environmental conditions.

Many corporations are aware of the negative effects of job stress, which often results in low employee morale and poor health, which in turn lead to employee turnover. Many companies are taking steps toward rectifying poor working conditions and unpleasant work relationships and are trying to find ways to support their employees with personal concerns. Human resource departments are placing greater importance on job matching to make sure that the demands and nature of the job align more closely with the applicant's skill set. Some companies provide family day care, health benefits, comp time incentives, and salary bonuses to encourage employees to perform well and stay with the company.

Although it is relatively rare, another job-related stressor is the possibility of workplace violence. Approximately 1 million violent crimes, including sexual and physical assaults, take place each year during the workday. In addition to the injured party, many workplace violence incidents involve other employees who are working with that person. Workplace violence incidents can be triggered by numerous causes. Some employees bring the effects of their domestic disputes to the workplace. Occasionally, disgruntled employees or ex-employees take out their frustrations on others in the company.

Financial Stress

Worry and anxiety over finances can have a negative effect on your health. It can also occur the other way; poor health can negatively affect your financial situation. A 2005 study of 3,121 subjects identified health effects that resulted from financial problems. Over 42 percent of the respondents stated that their health was affected by their financial problems. Stress was the leading health concern, reported by over 46 percent of the subjects; depression was reported by 10 percent; high blood pressure by 7.2 percent (O'Neill, Sohaindo, Xiao, and Garman).

Funding a college education is not easy. More and more college learners are graduating from college with significant amounts of debt. If debt is a concern of yours, taking a short course in personal finance or spending time with a financial manager are two ways to help you understand and cope with your financial situation. Education about debt and spending are good first steps toward planning and feeling in control of your finances. This can help alleviate stress and undue worry over finances. As with other stressors, your financial stressors are determined by your perception of your financial situation and your ability to handle it, not by how much money you actually have. Stress occurs when your expectations are out of balance with your resources.

WEB LINK
The Centers for Disease Control

http://www.cdc.gov/index.htm

http://www.cdc.gov/niosh/homepage.html

Work site stress information can be found at these Web sites. From each of the home pages, you can search for excellent material, research, and resources to help with job stress.

SEARCH TERMS: job stress, work stress, workplace stress

WEB LINK
Debtors Anonymous

http://www.debtorsanonymous.org

At this Web site, you can find practical help for resolving financial stress, even if you don't consider your finances to be unmanageable. There is also a quiz to help you determine if you have a problem with compulsively acquiring debt.

SEARCH TERMS: debt management, financial planning, financial stress

Overscheduling or Too Much to Do

Effective time management is one of the most important skills for controlling stress. If you are not careful how you manage your time, things begin to pile up, and those anxious feelings reported earlier begin to emerge. As important as time management is, it is also one of the most difficult skills to consistently put into practice. Being overscheduled is one of the most common causes of long-term stress. Learning when enough is enough and maintaining a balanced lifestyle will help you control your stress levels and contribute to your overall wellness. Being able to manage your time requires planning, organization, and the ability to communicate your own needs.

WEB LINK
Time Management
http://www.timemanagementhelp.com

At this Web site, you can find numerous time management strategies related to your personal life as well as strategies for managing time in your workplace and college activities.

SEARCH TERMS: time management, time stressors, time management strategies

Interpersonal Stressors

The most common interpersonal stressors are related to family, friends, colleagues, and romantic partners. Conflicts with the people around you, especially with those who are important to you, can create lots of stress. Certainly, the conflicts are a part of life, unavoidable, and healthy if handled correctly.

An important part of most college experiences is learning to take more responsibility for your own life and becoming more independent. Increased independence requires changes in relationships with family. Moving toward independence can be threatening for all involved. Parents still want to help and yet have difficulty giving up control, while young adults need to make decisions and continue the process of managing things on their own. As a young college student, you probably find yourself wanting to spend less time with your family. As a nontraditional learner, you may be facing entirely different stressors. You may be under stress as your family is challenged to coping with your absence, or you find yourself balancing your studies with home responsibilities. You may find that you wish you had more time to spend with your family. You may also have children, experiencing the stress of college themselves, turning to you for support! A college education is challenging for the learner and the family.

As a learner, you may be developing new friends and groups of people who act as a support system for you. You may be involved in a romantic relationship. You may have responsibilities to children or aging parents. Balancing new and changing relationships in your life can be demanding. Learning and using good communication techniques and conflict resolution strategies (discussed more fully in later chapters) can help decrease the stress associated with relationships.

Another source of interpersonal stress is feeling lonely and isolated from other people (Figure 3-4). Sometimes it may seem as if you don't really fit well in the college environment. These feelings are more likely to occur if you are not engaged in campus activities or if you are a commuter who comes to campus for classes but may not stay to socialize with others. Humans are social beings. Feeling connected to the people around us is important for our emotional wellness. Developing the necessary emotional and social skills to make good connections with others is an important task of successful adulthood.

Environmental and Societal Stressors

Some of the stressors we encounter are not directly related to us as individuals. These stressors affect everyone. Examples of environmental stressors include heat, cold, storms, air pollution, overcrowded spaces, and noise. These factors exist in the background of our lives. We may not even notice them most of the time, but they can develop into major stressors. Think about what happens when the weather gets hot and humid. People tend to become more irritable, and tempers flare up more easily. Have you ever noticed how people act when there is overcrowding, such as in a bus or subway at rush hour? Or maybe you've been in a very noisy restaurant and don't notice how stressful that seems until you walk out onto a quiet street. As a learner, you may have been inconvenienced by weather so bad that you worried about getting to classes safely. Think about the kinds of environmental stressors that you personally experience and how perception influences your levels of stress.

In 2005, a very powerful hurricane, Katrina, came ashore along the Gulf Coast near Louisiana and Mississippi. The city of New Orleans was very vulnerable to damage and flooding, and Katrina was devastating. Low-income citizens who lived in the lower east side of the city did not have transportation to leave the city, so they fled to the New Orleans Superdome for shelter (Figure 3-5). Imagine the stress associated with the approach and arrival of the hurricane and being crowded into a sports arena with no power, no running water, and only the basics of medical care for a number of weeks.

Living among other people means that we're also exposed to societal stressors. One major societal stressor is discrimination. Being a target of discrimination can be very stressful because it affects many aspects of an individual's life. Discrimination can be based on race, religion, age, sexual orientation, or even the way someone looks or dresses. Often, people make judgments about other people on the basis of what they see or think about them without ever getting to know them. People who are discriminated against in this manner may experience a number of negative emotions. They may even feel irritated and angry that they are being unfairly judged.

Violence is another major societal stressor. Even if one is not personally a victim of violence, the constant news containing local and world reports about violence on the radio and television and in magazines and newspapers can create a low level of constant anxiety. Sometimes it seems as if the news is nothing but a steady stream of wars, murders, kidnappings, floods, fires, and children who have been neglected or abused. Even when you don't know the people who experience these events, you may be affected by the news reports. It's natural to begin to wonder if the same terrible things might happen to you or the people you care about. Threats of terrorist attacks or war add to our stress levels, even if they never affect us directly. It seems prudent that limiting your

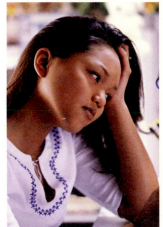

FIGURE 3-4 • Feelings of loneliness and isolation can be a source of interpersonal stress. Feeling connected to others is important for emotional wellness.

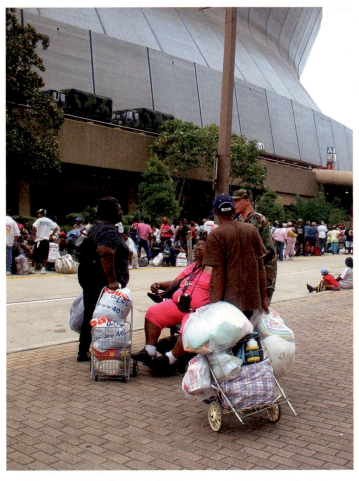

FIGURE 3-5 • Devastating environmental events such as Hurricane Katrina create significant stress. Courtesy of FEMA/Mary Bahamonde.

posttraumatic stress disorder
a mental disturbance that results from experiencing or witnessing a traumatic event that is replayed over and over in the mind after the event is over

homeostasis
the state of the body during relaxation when the body is functioning normally in a stable, balanced state

stress response
the physiological reactions that occur in the body when a stressor is experienced

exposure to reports about distressing events that you can't do anything about is a healthy way to decrease stress. It's important to be informed about current events, but it's also important to take care of yourself and minimize exposure to events that drive your stress level.

Personally experiencing a traumatic event can result in **posttraumatic stress disorder**. When this occurs, memories of the original event are played over and over in the mind. It is as if the person relives the event again each time it is remembered. The traumatic event may have happened to the person directly or may have been witnessed by the person. The event can even be a natural disaster that happens to an entire community, such as a tornado or hurricane, or a violent act, such as a shooting.

How Stress Affects Your Body

When your body is at rest and there are no special challenges, difficulties, or exciting events to deal with, it is in **homeostasis**. During homeostasis, the body has plenty of resources to maintain normal body functions and responses. But when you experience a stressor or a threat, a chain of reactions begins to take place in your body. This is known as the **stress response**. This response has been with humankind for perhaps millions of years. This response is designed to prepare the body for fight or flight, meaning that we could defend ourselves in the face of a threat, such as war, an attack from a wild animal, and so on. The physical responses meant to protect humans throughout history will occur whenever we are stressed, regardless of the reason.

Two major systems influence the physiological reactions of the body under stress: the nervous system and the endocrine system. Together, they prepare you for whatever action is needed to face a stressor. An important fact to remember is that stressors cause the

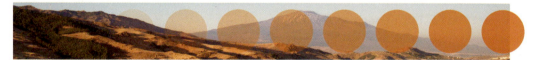

What's Your View?

Societal Stressors

How do you think societal stressors like discrimination and threats of violence affect us? Listening to the nightly news can cause concern about what's happening in our communities and in our world. It's difficult to hear the negative things that go on and realize that these may affect only a very small percentage of the population or may have a low chance of occurrence. Think about it—if it were common, it probably would not be on the news. How do you think we should balance our concerns about safety within families and community with the realities of our daily lives?

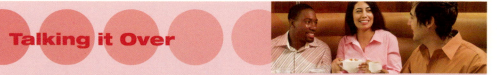

Talking it Over

What's Stressing Who?

Interview friends, workplace colleagues, or members of your family about what they consider their most common stressors. Into what categories do their stressors fall? Is there a difference between the type of stressors experienced by different individuals? How do these compare with the stressors that you experience? What can be done to help reduce the stressors or manage them to reduce their effects?

same physiological response in the body whether they are real or imagined and whether they are stress or eustress. This is why constant worry and negative thoughts can be just as unhealthy as real events.

The Nervous System

The brain acts as the signal caller for the rest of the body. It interprets every situation a human encounters and decides how the body should respond. If an emergency response is needed, the brain immediately alerts the rest of the body that special action is required. The nervous system relays these messages from the brain to the various parts of the body.

The **autonomic nervous system** plays an important role in stress responses. This part of the nervous system controls basic functions such as breathing, heartbeat, blood pressure, and digestion. These are involuntary actions, actions that happen automatically without our thinking about them.

The autonomic nervous system has two main branches, the **sympathetic nervous system** (Figure 3-6) and the **parasympathetic nervous system** (Figure 3-7). The role of the sympathetic nervous system is to "rev up" the systems and organs of the body, preparing them to respond to the challenges of stressors. For example, in the face of a real or imaginary threat, the heart will begin beating faster, breathing increases, and the blood pools to the body core. When the sympathetic nervous system is activated, all the energy resources of the body are put on alert and prepared to respond.

The role of the other branch, the parasympathetic nervous system, comes into play after the stress response has passed and helps "cool down" the body (i.e., shut down the responses of the sympathetic division) and bring it back to normal function. This system is in control when our bodies are in a relaxed state of normal functioning.

The Endocrine System

The **endocrine system** consists of glands, tissues, and cells that produce hormones. **Hormones** are chemical messengers that help regulate bodily processes. When the sympathetic nervous system responds to a stress alert, it triggers actions in the endocrine system. Certain hormones are associated with the stress response. These hormones target

autonomic nervous system
the division of the nervous system that controls basic body processes that are largely involuntary, such as breathing, heartbeat, blood pressure, and digestion

sympathetic nervous system
the branch of the autonomic nervous system that responds to a stressor by accelerating body processes

parasympathetic nervous system
the branch of the autonomic nervous system that slows down body processes and returns the body to homeostasis after a stressful situation has passed

endocrine system
a system of glands, tissues, and cells that produce hormones to help regulate bodily processes

hormones
chemical messengers produced by the endocrine system to help regulate bodily processes

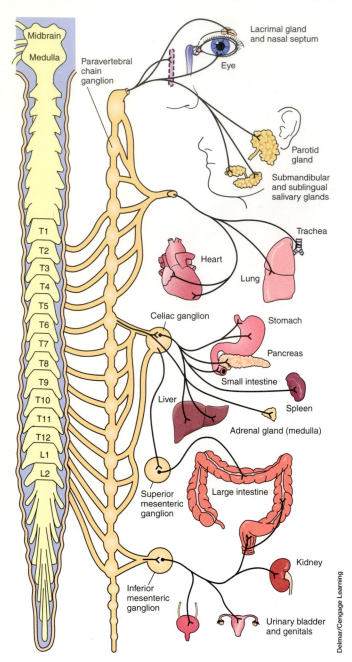

FIGURE 3-6 • The nerve pathways of the sympathetic division of the autonomic nervous system.

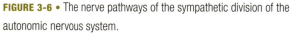

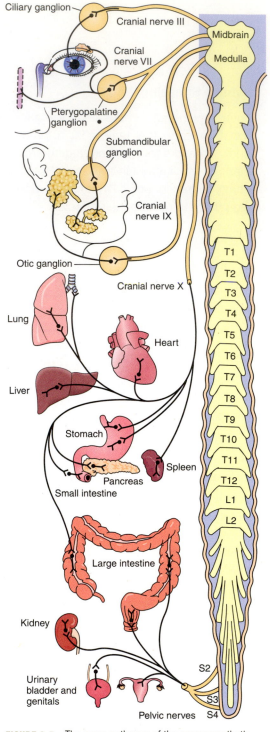

FIGURE 3-7 • The nerve pathways of the parasympathetic division of the autonomic nervous system.

specific cells in the body and provide them with "instructions" for the necessary response. The pituitary, thyroid, and adrenal glands, with the assistance of other parts of the endocrine system, produce most of the so-called stress hormones. When we are confronted with a stressor, these hormones, driven by the sympathetic nervous system, cause a number of changes in the body:

- Increased heartbeat

- Increased rate of breathing

- Narrower blood vessels

- Slower digestion

- Tensed muscles

These physical changes are preparing the body to fight or run. Figure 3-8 illustrates how the body responds in a fight-or-flight situation. You have probably heard of adrenaline. This is one of the stress hormones that enable people to do amazing things in an emergency, such as lift a heavy object off a loved one or run a long distance for help.

●●● How Stress Affects Your Health

The stressors our ancestors faced may have threatened their survival, but they were resolved rather quickly. Today our stressors are different. Although they may not threaten our immediate survival, many are long term in duration. In fact, these long-term stressors are so much a part of our daily lives that we barely even notice the toll they are taking on us. And it is these long-term, continuous stressors that are most likely to affect our health. Recall the General Adaptation Syndrome and the fact that being exposed to a stressor for a long period of time can result in exhaustion, meaning that the organism may die. The paradigm holds true for those stressors that compound their effects with continual stimulation of the autonomic nervous system. This results in overproduction of the hormones associated with the stress response.

The hormones the body produces in the presence of stressors are designed to help us respond quickly to short-term stressors. But these same hormones can do serious damage to the organs and systems if they stay in the body too long. One of the systems most affected by stress is the immune system. Stress hormones in excess, particularly **cortisol**, suppress immune system function, making an individual more susceptible to infection and disease. A weak immune system can make existing health problems worse, increase the likelihood of catching the common cold, and even increase the risk of a heart attack or cancer.

cortisol
a significant hormone produced by the adrenal glands and involved in a number of body functions such as regulation of sugar metabolism and blood pressure

What's News

Research suggests that high levels of stress hormones seem to interfere with memory. Normal memory function returns when the levels of stress hormones return to normal. This may be one explanation for test anxiety. The rise in stress hormones causes learners to temporarily forget information they actually know. Practicing techniques to relax and stay calm might be good ways to "study" for a test!

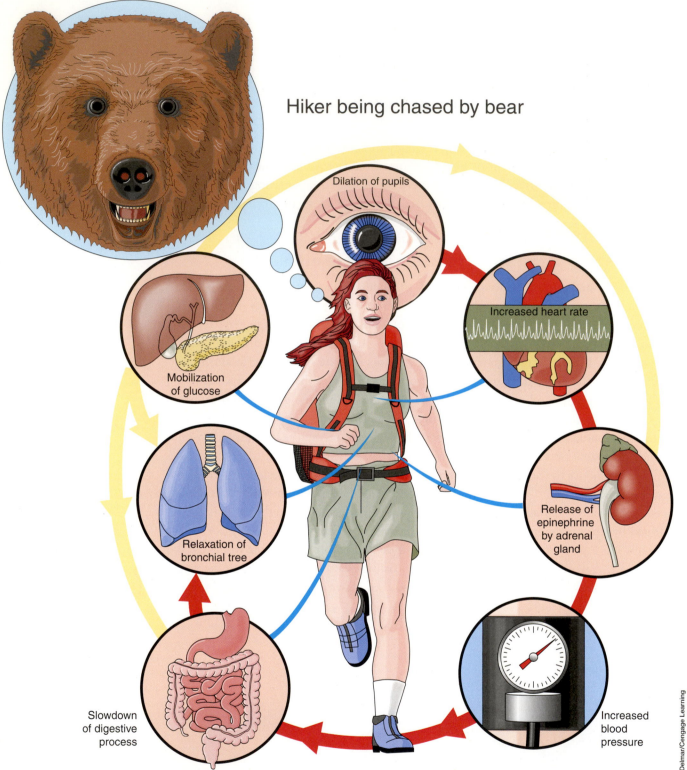

Hiker being chased by bear

Dilation of pupils

Increased heart rate

Mobilization of glucose

Release of epinephrine by adrenal gland

Relaxation of bronchial tree

Slowdown of digestive process

Increased blood pressure

Delmar/Cengage Learning

FIGURE 3-8 • The fight-or-flight response.

Stress as a Medical Problem

Stress has become a major medical problem in the United States. It is a leading contributor, either directly or indirectly, to the major causes of death and to many illnesses and diseases. Effective stress management could play a big role in decreasing medical costs, increasing work productivity, and improving the quality of life for millions of Americans.

We must keep in mind that not only major stressors—such as the death of a close personal friend or relative, personal illness, or severe financial difficulties—cause health problems. The accumulation of small life event stressors, such as rushing to be on time, being stuck in traffic, or having an argument with a co-worker, can also contribute to health problems. You can learn more about the effects of life events in chapter 17. The small hassles of daily living can also result in stress-related problems. A series of small stressors can add up until something quite insignificant makes the load seem more than a person can handle.

Evidence indicates there are numerous illnesses that have been associated with excessive and continued stress, including but not limited to diabetes, heart disease, obesity, ulcers, tooth and gum disease, ulcers, and possibly certain cancers.

●●● Protecting Yourself from the Effects of Stress

It is impossible to avoid stress completely. In fact, we wouldn't want to, even if it were possible. A certain amount of stress keeps life interesting, challenging, and fulfilling. If we never experienced stressful situations, we would almost certainly be bored and would miss opportunities to learn and grow as individuals.

The optimal amount of stress varies from person to person. The question is, How much stress is right for you? What level of stress allows you to function at your best? We know that too much stress over a long period of time can seriously damage our bodies. It can also result in feeling annoyed, frustrated, irritable, and unhappy. Finding the optimal amount of stress means balancing life's challenges with the resources you have to meet those challenges.

There are certain resources that can protect you from experiencing more stress than you can handle. These resources don't help you avoid stressors, but they can help you cope with them when stress does occur. Three of the most important protective factors are social support, specific personality traits, and a set of characteristics known as stress hardiness.

Social Support

Social support is one of the best protections against feeling overwhelmed by stressful circumstances. Having good social support means having a network of family, friends, and acquaintances who care about you and will provide assistance if you need it. You don't have to face stressful events alone. And, through other people, you have access to more resources. Good social support appears to reduce the likelihood that reactions to stressful events will result in illness. People who have good social support seem to have better health and well-being, whether or not they experience much stress, than do people without much social support.

Did You Know . . .?

It is estimated that between two-thirds and three-quarters of all visits to primary care physicians in the United States are due to an illness related to stress. Some medical experts say that the actual number might be closer to 90 percent! It is estimated that the medical costs of treating stress-related illnesses in the United States are more than $1 billion per year. This estimate doesn't even include job-related costs, such as high absenteeism, stress-related work injuries, and reduced productivity on the job. It also doesn't include the personal and emotional costs to the people who experience the problems and to those close to them.

WEB LINK
Effects of Daily Hassles

http://www.realage.com

Go to this Web site and enter the search term "daily hassles." The site will take you to a section that explains the significance of daily hassles on stress, and provide a number of links within the Web site to help you. Search within the site and you will have an opportunity to complete the Daily Life Equilibrium Calculator for an assessment of daily hassle influences on your life.

SEARCH TERMS: daily hassles, hassle assessment, stress assessment

psychoneuroimmunology (PNI)
the study of the interrelationships among the emotions, brain, nervous system, and immune system

An exciting field called **psychoneuroimmunology (PNI)** studies the interrelationships among the emotions, the brain and nervous system, and the immune system. PNI is still an emerging field of study, but through research in this area, we are learning about the direct connections between the brain, the emotions, and the immune system. According to Candace Pert, one of the leading researchers, chemical messengers called peptides communicate with cells throughout the body as a result of feeling an emotion. Your body systems actually talk among themselves in response to your emotions! Early indications are that stress associated with negative emotions interferes with proper immune system function. The good news is that experiencing positive emotions may improve immune system function.

Getting Connected

Sociologists and health experts are concerned about the state of social connectedness in the United States. Compared with previous generations, Americans today are more likely to live alone and less likely to have close family ties, be married, or belong to a social organization. People in countries that have close family ties and strong social connections, such as Greece, Spain, and Italy, have higher life expectancies than people in the United States. This difference in life expectancies occurs despite the fact that in the United States we spend far more money per person on health care than any other country in the world.

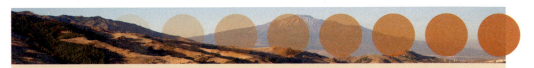

What's Your View: Are We Connected?

In our "wired world," we have more opportunities than ever to stay connected to others around us. Cell phones, texting, e-mail, and instant messaging allow us to stay in almost constant communication with others (Figure 3-9). Yet many people report feeling more disconnected than ever before.

- Do you think it's possible that having good social support and feeling a sense of connection and belonging is the best health insurance we can have?

- Do you believe there is a lack of social connectedness in the United States?

- How does the use of electronic technology affect social connectedness?

- Do you think connectedness affects physical health? If you do, what could you do to help build stronger connections with your family, friends, and community?

Personality Traits

Certain personality traits are believed to put people at increased risk for stress-related problems, yet there are some people who possess other traits offering protection against stress-related problems. Falling into the first group are people who possess what are known as type A personality traits. These traits include being results oriented, a perfectionist, and strongly motivated by the need to succeed. People with type A personalities are characterized by being ambitious, hurried, time conscious, and driven. They are usually very competitive and may exhibit impatience, anger, and hostility, especially if they don't get their way or are hampered in their efforts to achieve.

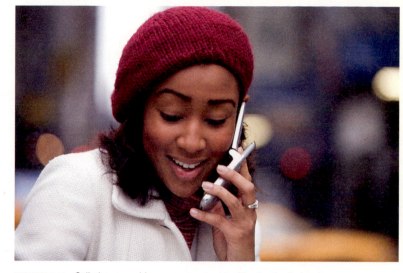

FIGURE 3-9 • Cell phone provide numerous opportunities to stay in touch.

In contrast, people possessing type B personality traits have a more relaxed attitude about life. They usually work and play at their own pace and don't feel an overwhelming need to always win when they compete with others. They tend to take life as it comes and "go with the flow." It isn't surprising that, given similar situations, a type A personality is more likely to produce a stress response, while a type B hardly notices it.

Research indicates that the type A personality traits of anger, cynicism, and hostility are linked to an increased risk of heart disease (Sprafka, et al., 1990). Personality traits are at least partly a result of experiences and learned behaviors. Consequently, individuals can learn to reduce their type A personality traits and become better at handling stress. Even if they can't change their basic personality type, they can make an effort to adopt behaviors to decrease stress in their daily lives.

WEB LINK
Discovery Health
http://discoveryhealth.queendom.com

At this Web site, you can take personality quizzes to determine how you normally respond to situations. For example, click on "Type A Personality Test."

SEARCH TERMS: personality traits, type A personality, type B personality, personality quizzes

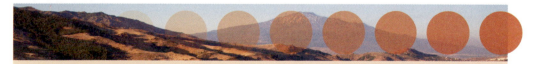

What's Your View?

It is likely that some aspects of our personalities are genetic and others are learned behaviors. Talk to members of your extended family about whether they consider themselves to have mostly type A or type B personality traits. Is there any pattern among their responses? Do you see any relationship between your personality traits and those of family members? Do you think the similarities, if any, are the result of genetics or learned behaviors? What evidence can you give to support your conclusion? Do you think you can change your personality?

Hardiness

Psychologist Suzanne Kobasa (1979) was interested in explaining why business executives exhibited various levels of illness given that they all functioned in similar stress-filled environments. She conducted a long-term study and found that, over time, some executives had symptomatic illness, while others had none and actually seemed to be thriving on stress. As a result of her research, she was able to identify certain attitudes and beliefs that protected some executives from the negative consequences of stressful situations. She proposed the term **stress hardiness** to describe the resilience or "bounce-back" quality that some people displayed in the face of stressors. In fact, the stress-hardy executives in her study exhibited 50 percent less illness than the executives who did not exhibit the characteristic. Kobasa's data revealed three key characteristics of these individuals, which can be remembered as the three Cs:

> **stress hardiness**
> resilience when confronted with stressors, as identified by the characteristics of challenge, control, and commitment

1. *Challenge.* Stress-hardy individuals don't feel overwhelmed by potentially stressful situations. Instead, they view these situations as challenges they can handle. Sometimes they even look forward to testing their skills in a challenging situation.

2. *Control.* Stress-hardy individuals believe that they have some control over situations. They don't feel helpless in the face of a stress. They accept responsibility for their own behavior and believe that they can make a difference with their own actions.

3. *Commitment.* Stress-hardy individuals are committed to something outside themselves. This might be a person, religion, community group, or cause that's important to them. They believe that their lives have meaning and purpose.

The significance of Kobasa's research is that stress in and of itself is not bad. It is our reaction to the life events that can bring the stress response. It is important to understand that it is okay to feel stress, but you can't let it bring you down. Rather than "suffer" with the stress, use it to your advantage. Actors, musicians, athletes, and coaches feel "butterflies" before performances. This feeling is the stress response. These individuals take the response and turn it into productive energy, much like you can do with your next big examination.

●●● Managing Stress

When you encounter a situation that seems stressful to you, there are several ways you can respond. Start by asking yourself these questions:

- Is it possible to reduce or eliminate my exposure to the stressor?

- What do I have control over?

- What must I accept?

- Is there anything I can do to change the situation?

- Can I change my perception of the situation?

- What coping mechanisms and resources do I have available to deal with the situation?

- With my available coping mechanisms and resources, what action can I take?

You can prepare yourself to handle unavoidable stressors by having a variety of coping strategies available. Coping strategies are habits and behaviors that help you manage stress and make the best of any situation. You might think of these strategies as tools you store in a stress reduction toolbox. When faced with a stressor, select the best tool to deal with the situation. All the strategies discussed in the next sections are simple and inexpensive and could be good additions for your stress reduction toolbox.

Practice Good Self-Care

Practicing good self-care reduces the chance that you will perceive situations as stressors. It also helps your immune system function at its best when faced with stressors. Three of the most important self-care activities are getting enough sleep, eating nutritiously, and participating in regular physical activity.

Sleep

Statistics indicate that at any given point in time approximately 40 percent of Americans are sleep deprived (American Sleep Foundation, 2002). The figure would be higher if only college students were studied. It is important to get adequate sleep in order for our bodies to function well. How much sleep each person needs for mental and physical rejuvenation varies, although the general rule of thumb is eight hours a night. Recall the information from the Alameda County study in chapter 1. The study revealed the health benefits of getting the appropriate amount of sleep. Napping is also good for the brain and can help alleviate stress. Some employers even advocate "power napping" for their employees, permitting them to take a 10- to 20-minute nap each day to clear their heads and increase their productivity in the afternoon. If you choose to nap, it is recommended that you do so between the hours of noon and 2:00 p.m. This allows for a mental break at midday yet does not interrupt your regular sleep patterns. If naps are taken too late in the day (after 3:00 p.m.), they can alter your nighttime sleep habits; this can be counterproductive to trying to get the rest you need. It's amazing how much better you'll feel, both emotionally and physically, when you get enough sleep.

Healthy Eating Habits

When you're busy and feeling stressed, you may eat too much without thinking, or you may even forget to eat. It's easy to grab whatever food is available and not pay much attention to what you're putting in your body. Sometimes eating without thinking or eating on the run results in overeating, thus increasing the workload on your gastrointestinal tract. This can lead to stomachaches, cramps, and discomfort in times of stress. Since food provides the fuel your body needs to function effectively, by eating healthy foods, in proper amounts throughout the day, you give your body high-performance fuel to get you through your daily activities. It is advisable to monitor the amount of caffeine you consume; too much during the day can increase your stress response.

Physical Activity

Putting your body in motion is a good way to release stress. Physical activity gives you time to unwind and relax while physically benefiting your body. Try taking a 10- to 20-minute walk whenever you find yourself beginning to feel stressed. Allowing a physical outlet for your stress by elevating your heart rate and opening up your capillaries increases blood flow and helps utilize stored-up energy that can be a result of stress, and it offsets the effects of excessive cortisol. In addition to releasing stress, exercise gives you a "time-out" so that you can reframe a stressful situation in a more positive light and develop an effective response. Even if you don't have much time, just taking a short break for a few minutes to get up and walk around a bit can help you refocus. You may find that this helps even more if you are able to go outside and get some fresh air at the same time.

Learn to Relax

When we are faced with stressors, it is a certainty that the stress response will kick in. Sometimes when you feel tension, a racing heartbeat, rapid breathing, and anxiety, you can minimize the stress effects if you just take the time to focus on relaxation. There are a number of activities you can employ to help you relax. Some methods require physical actions; others require you to focus on your mental and emotional state.

Deep Breathing

One of the simplest stress management tools is to pay attention to your breathing. Taking slow, deep breaths while concentrating on slowly inhaling and exhaling can produce a calming effect in your entire body. Many of us are in the habit of breathing shallowly and have to retrain ourselves to breathe deeply. You can tell if you are taking a deep breath by placing your hand on your abdomen. Does it rise and fall with each breath? If it doesn't, your breathing is too shallow. Taking 10 to 20 deep breaths can reduce the stress response and increase your ability to cope with a stressful situation.

Progressive Relaxation

Progressive relaxation requires a bit of practice, but it is quite simple to learn. It involves tightening and then relaxing the various muscle groups in the body. The following paragraph describes the basics of the technique. You may want to record the procedure in a quiet, calm voice so that you don't have to read it. To perform this technique, begin by sitting in a comfortable chair, closing your eyes, and taking a few slow deep breaths. Then take your legs and stretch them out, hold, and then relax; pull your toes toward you, hold, then relax; and then point your toes, hold, then relax. (Be sure to breathe slowly and keep your eyes closed.) Tighten your calves, hold, and release. Tighten your thighs, hold, and release. Allow your legs to return to the starting position. Stretch out your arms, make fists and tighten, hold, and relax and let your arms relax, allowing them to feel completely relaxed and sitting "heavy." Stretch your arms and contract the muscles in your forearms, hold, and relax. Let your arms drop relaxed once more. Now arch your back and hold, then relax. Tighten the muscles in your chest, abdomen, and back, hold, and relax. When you relax, feel all the tension go as you breathe quietly. Finally, tighten and relax the muscles in your neck, chin, and forehead. Finish the exercise with slow, relaxed breaths and let all the tension and energy leave your body.

Visualization and Guided Imagery

Visualization is the creation of a mental picture you can use as a focal point as you relax. Picture yourself in a pleasant environment or succeeding at something important to you. Visualization is something you can control. A technique similar to visualization is guided imagery. In guided imagery, you visualize a mental picture as it is described aloud or "guided" by someone else. Athletes often use visualization and guided imagery to improve their performance. Suppose you are a tennis player who gets really stressed during a match. You could use visualization to see yourself moving through the match successfully and easily. Or your coach could lead you through a guided imagery to help you focus and concentrate on maintaining good form during each stroke.

Meditation

The goal of meditation is to produce a state of relaxation, inner peace, and harmony. There are many different types of meditation practices. One type of meditation practice involves sitting quietly and focusing on a word or image of your own choosing while taking slow, deep breaths. Other meditative practices involve concentrating on relaxed breathing combined with a physical action repeated in a specific way, such as the practice of yoga or tai chi.

Enjoy Life

You may have seen a bumper sticker or button with the slogan, "Enjoy life. This is not a dress rehearsal." We often rush through life as if simply getting to the end of the day is our only goal. Someone once commented that "99 percent of people go through life like rats in a maze. The other 1 percent go through life amazed." We can enjoy our lives much more fully and reduce our stress levels at the same time if we choose to be among the 1 percent who go through life amazed. Try the following techniques to help you enjoy life more (Figure 3-10).

Mindful Awareness

Have you ever noticed how you can go through a good part of the day without ever really noticing your surroundings? Mindful awareness is really paying attention to each thing you experience and being fully aware of the present moment. For example, when you're eating, give your full attention to the food. When you're talking to a friend, pay careful attention to what your friend is saying. When you are outside, notice the sights, smells, and sounds around you. Practicing mindful awareness helps you reduce stress and experience life more fully.

Time Management

Good time management is a key factor in avoiding stress. Start by identifying your priorities. What is most important to you? Arrange your schedule so that you spend time on the things most important to you and still allow yourself some free time, as shown in Figure 3-11. You may discover that you prefer spending more time with family and friends and less time watching television and playing video games. When the way you spend your time is in balance with your priorities, you will feel less stressed.

Sometimes we all just need a time-out. This is a time when you can take a break from your responsibilities, work, and stressors so that you can come back more relaxed, refreshed, and

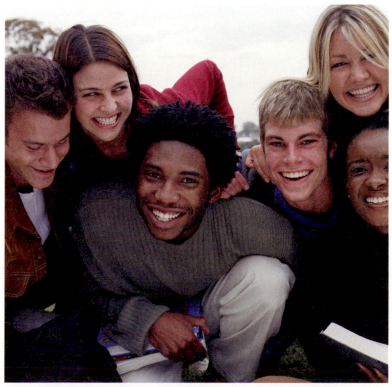

FIGURE 3-10 • Enjoying life is an important component for everyone's personal wellness.

Courtesy of Photodisc

Friday		Saturday	
8 am	Class	8 am	
9 am		9 am	Workout with Sarah
10 am	Biology test	10 am	
11 am		11 am	Laundry
12 pm		12 pm	
1 pm	Meet w/ advisor	1 pm	Library with Rob to work on report
2 pm		2 pm	
3 pm	Workout with Sarah	3 pm	Sociology research
4 pm		4 pm	
5 pm	Dinner with Mom	5 pm	
6 pm	Work	6 pm	RELAX!
7 pm		7 pm	
8 pm		8 pm	
9 pm		9 pm	

Delmar/Cengage Learning

FIGURE 3-11 • Managing your time effectively and scheduling time to relax may take a little extra work, but it can help reduce stress.

ready to cope more effectively. Every day, you should try to spend one hour for *yourself*—exercise, casual reading, shopping, fun with family, and so on. Do an activity you enjoy just for the pleasure of it. Even breaks as short as five minutes can make a major difference in your attitude and increase your enjoyment of life. The breaks give you a chance to relax and return refreshed and ready to face new challenges.

Humor and Laughter

Many studies have shown that laughter increases the efficiency of the immune system and lowers the levels of stress hormones. Laughter is even good exercise for your heart, lungs, and muscles. Try this activity. Pair up with a friend and just start laughing. It doesn't matter what you're laughing about, just concentrate on each other's faces and laugh for at least one full minute. Then notice how you feel when you finish. Chances are, you're feeling less stressed. You can also go to the video store and rent something from the comedy section. Perhaps you can find a movie that you have seen already but know that it is really funny or be venturesome and pick out something new.

BUILDING YOUR LIFETIME WELLNESS PLAN

From the information you learned in this chapter, you can see that stress has a major effect on your health. Stressors will always be a part of life. Learning and practicing techniques to manage stress effectively is one of the most beneficial things you can do to improve your health both now and in the future.

When stress is reduced or managed effectively, you are more productive, and life is more enjoyable. You can use the information in this chapter to develop your own personal stress management plan. This can be modified and used throughout your life whenever you encounter stressful situations.

●●● End-of-Chapter Activities

Opportunities for Application

1. Select a situation you currently find stressful. Focus on only one situation. Using the information you have learned in this chapter, describe some stress management activities you could employ to manage the stress associated with that situation.

2. Imagine that one of your family members or a friend comments on the amount of stress in his or her life. Given the information obtained from this chapter, what advice would you give that person to help him or her, and how would you present the information?

3. Think about your level of "stress hardiness." On a scale of 1 to 10, with 10 being the most hardy, rate your level of stress hardiness. Describe the characteristics you possess that make you stress hardy. If you feel your score is low, can you think of any things you could do to improve your hardiness scale?

Key Concepts

1. Distinguish among stress, distress, and eustress.

2. Describe the stages of the General Adaptation Syndrome.

3. List and describe some things you can do for yourself to increase your stress resistance.

Answers to Personal Assessment: Stress Management Quiz

1. False. Stress is a part of life and can actually be a productive force.

2. True

3. True

4. False. The stress response is the same no matter what the trigger happens to be.

5. False. It is the nervous system.

6. True

7. True

8. False. Actually, these feeling will stress the immune system.

9. False. Mild levels of stress can enhance learning and memory, but at high levels it can be counterproductive.

10. True

●●● References

Kobasa, S. C. (1979). Stressful life events, personality, and health: An inquiry into hardiness. *Journal of Personality and Social Psychology, 37*(1), 1–11.

Selye, H. (1976). *The Stress of Life, 2nd edition.* New York, NY: McGraw Hill.

O'Neill, B., Sorhaindo, B., Ziao, J. J., Garman, E. T. (2005). Negative health effects of financial stress. *Consumer Interests Annual, 51.* Retrieved April 30, 2010 from: http://www.personalfinancefoundation.org/research/efd/Negative-Health-Effects-of-Financial-Stress.pdf

Wolf, O. T. (2009). Stress and memory in humans: Twelve years of progress? *Brain Research, 1293,* 142–154.

Elzinga, B. A., Bakker, A., Bremmer, J. D. (2005). Stress-induced cortisol levels are associated with impaired delayed, but not immediate recall. *Psychiatry Research, 134*(3), 211–223.

National Sleep Foundation. (2002). *2002 Sleep in America Poll.* Retrieved May 7, 2010 from: http://www.sleepfoundation.org/article/sleep-america-polls/2002-adult-sleep-habits

Sprafka, J. M., Folsom, A. R., Burke, G. L., Hahn, L. P., Pirie, P. (1990). Type A behavior and its association with cardiovascular disease prevalence in Blacks and Whites: The Minnesota heart survey. *Behavioral Science, 13*(1), 1–13.

CHAPTER 4

Mental and Emotional Health

CHAPTER OBJECTIVES

When you finish this chapter, you should be able to:

- Define mental and emotional health.
- Identify several factors that affect mental and emotional health.
- Describe the characteristics of mentally and emotionally healthy individuals.
- Create a list of ways you can improve your mental and emotional health.
- Understand mental disorders as a form of illness.
- List and describe the factors that contribute to suicide.
- List and describe the warning signs for suicide.
- Describe what individuals, families, schools, and communities can do to prevent suicide.
- Discuss ways you can help people you care about who have mental health disorders.

KEY TERMS

cognitive-behavioral therapy
completed suicide
compulsions
defense mechanisms
emotionally healthy

manic
Maslow's hierarchy of needs
neurons
neurotransmitters
obsessions

phobias
psychiatrists
psychotherapists
psychotic
receptors
resiliency

schizophrenia
self-actualization
stigma

●●● Introduction

If you ask a group of college students what they want most in life, a common answer might be, "I just want to be happy." If you ask a group of parents what they want most for their children, they are likely to answer, "I just want them to be healthy and happy." But what does this actually mean? How can you take charge of your life and do those things that will lead to personal happiness? As a parent, how can you ensure that your children grow up happy and physically and mentally well?

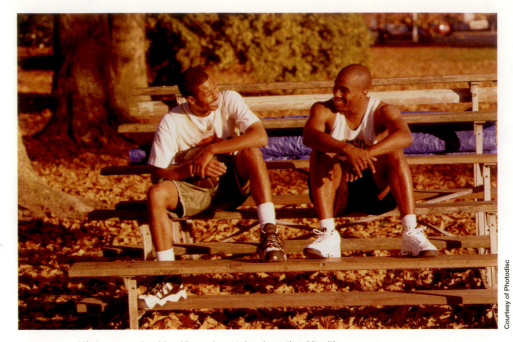

Courtesy of Photodisc

FIGURE 4-1 • Life is more enjoyable with good mental and emotional health.

Happiness means different things to different people. We might say that happiness comes from living life in ways that are meaningful and satisfying. For some people, happiness may be defined as "not being depressed." We often discover happiness when we are least focused on finding it. We know that our mental and emotional health have a lot to do with how much pleasure and enjoyment we get from our daily lives. Everything is just much more fun when we're mentally active and alert, when we feel good about ourselves, and when our relationships with other people are going smoothly. And good mental and emotional health can have a major positive effect on our physical health as well (Figure 4-1).

But for many, good mental and emotional health is difficult to achieve or maintain. According to the National Institute of Mental Health (2007), an estimated 26.2 percent of Americans ages 18 and older, about one in four adults, suffer from a diagnosable mental disorder in a given year. Applying this figure to the 2004 U.S. Census population estimate for ages 18 and older indicates that 57.7 million people have some form of mental disorder. Even though mental disorders are widespread in the population, the main burden of illness is concentrated in a much smaller proportion—about 6 percent, or 1 in 17—who suffer from a serious mental illness. In addition, mental disorders are the leading cause of disability in the United States and Canada for ages 15 to 44.

What does it mean to be mentally and emotionally healthy? It's often much easier to determine when people are *not* mentally or emotionally healthy than it is to determine when they *are* healthy. In addition to discussing positive mental and emotional health, this chapter includes information to help explain the conditions when things go wrong mentally and emotionally. Serious mental disorders and suicide are also presented in this chapter.

●●● Explaining Mental and Emotional Health

Mental illness has always been part of human existence. Historically, mental illness has been viewed as less acceptable than physical illness. In fact, as recent as the 1700s, mental illness was believed to be caused by devil worship and/or immoral practices. The mentally

PERSONAL ASSESSMENT
Mental and Emotional Health Quiz

Before reading this chapter, respond to the statements below according to the following scale: Strongly Agree, Agree, Disagree, or Strongly Disagree. See the interpretation of results at the end of the chapter.

1. Being realistic is associated with positive mental health.

2. Making decisions about people on their own merits, instead of by their race, religion, or style of dress, is an indicator of positive mental health.

3. Feeling lonely is an indicator of poor mental health.

4. Once you form a personal identity, that identity remains mostly the same throughout your life.

5. You can treat mental illness yourself if you just work through the problem.

6. People with mental health problems are usually violent.

7. If someone tries to talk to you about suicide, you should change the subject. Talking about suicide makes it more likely the person will attempt suicide.

8. Everyone who attempts suicide can be considered mentally ill, even if only temporarily.

9. Having easy availability to a method of suicide, such as a gun or pills, does not increase the risk of suicide.

10. If someone really wants to commit suicide, there is no way to keep that person from doing it.

---

ill were confined to institutions called asylums. Their confinement was designed not to cure them but to separate them from those who were not mentally ill. The conditions in asylums were very poor, with some "patients" being chained to the walls. Others lived in cells in which three or four people shared a bed.

During the mid-1800s, interest developed in providing more humane treatment for the mentally ill. Following World War I, mental illness began to be considered a health problem with medical causes. We now have a better picture of what mental illness is, although we still don't clearly understand what causes mental illness.

Can you distinguish between the terms *mental health* and *emotional health*? At first, the two terms seem very similar, but there is an important distinction. A person who is **mentally healthy** perceives reality in terms of facts and can respond appropriately to the challenges life presents to them. Being mentally healthy involves being able to evaluate a situation and interpret its meaning. Mentally healthy people can solve most of the problems of everyday life. People who are emotionally healthy are in touch with their entire range of feelings. They can express those feelings appropriately even when they are upset. Their feelings don't interfere with their ability to think clearly. Although being mentally healthy and emotionally healthy are not exactly the same, the terms are often used interchangeably when describing individuals who are usually successful in coping well with the mental and emotional challenges that life presents.

mentally healthy refers to a person who has the ability to perceive reality in terms of facts and can respond appropriately to a person who is in touch with his or her entire range of feelings and can express those feelings in an appropriate way

Being mentally and emotionally healthy does *not* mean that people never feel angry, sad, depressed, lonely, or frustrated. And it doesn't mean that they never need help and support from other people. We all have times when we feel overwhelmed by the demands of life. We may be faced with a difficult situation we've never encountered before. Sometimes our emotions are unpredictable. Experiencing a wide range of feelings, including negative ones, is normal for everyone. Having negative feelings does not mean that a person lacks emotional health or is not practicing emotional wellness. What is really important is being able to manage feelings so that they don't interfere with problem solving, decision making, and the ability to enjoy life most of the time.

Both internal and external factors contributed to creating the physical and mental person you are today. Internal factors include your genetics, personality, and physical health. External factors are the experiences that you've had as you've progressed on your life journey. Some factors are within your control (e.g., friends you choose, your choice of hobbies, and your education); others are not (e.g., the neighborhood you grew up in, your family's financial status, and how you were treated by peers). You may have grown up in a situation in which you were safe and well cared for by the adults in your life. Unfortunately, not everyone experiences this ideal environment.

Regardless of your past experiences or current situation, you can still practice mental and emotional wellness because many of the characteristics of mental and emotional wellness can be learned. Researchers have been studying a characteristic they call resiliency. **Resiliency** is the ability to bounce back from or deal effectively with distressing or traumatic events. Resilient individuals are able to trust and to form caring relationships, have good problem-solving skills, are independent and persistent, and believe that their lives have meaning and purpose. Experts believe that each of us has a natural capacity for resiliency that can be strengthened with training.

Mental Health Needs

Human beings have various needs that must be met in order for them to enjoy physical and mental well-being. Psychologist Abraham Maslow researched these needs and ranked them in order of importance for survival and well-being. These needs are organized in the shape of a pyramid called **Maslow's hierarchy of needs**, as shown in Figure 4-2. Maslow believed that people must satisfy their most basic physical needs before they can fully satisfy higher-level needs. Basic physical needs—such as food, water, and shelter—form the base of the pyramid and are believed to be our primary physical and psychological needs. Once those needs are satisfied, an individual can focus on developing a sense of safety and security, a sense of love and belonging, and good self-esteem. At the top of the pyramid is a quality Maslow called **self-actualization**. He defined this as functioning at or near one's optimal level of mental and emotional health.

Have you ever thought about what it would be like to be homeless? You would probably spend a lot of time trying to meet your basic needs for food, water, and shelter. Where would you get your next meal? Could you easily find shelter? What about sanitation and cleaning facilities? Most of us take fulfillment of our basic needs for granted. But in many places around the world and even in this country, there are people who face these problems every day. People have little interest in becoming self-actualized if they aren't sheltered from the elements and can't get food.

As with many other wellness tasks, growth includes assuming increased responsibility for meeting the needs that Maslow described. Adults should be able to provide for

resiliency
the ability to bounce back after experiencing distressing or traumatic events

Maslow's hierarchy of needs
a well-known representation of human needs progressing from most to least urgent; these needs include physical needs, safety and security, love and belonging, self-esteem, and self-actualization

self-actualization
the highest level in Maslow's hierarchy of needs, representing an optimal level of mental and emotional function

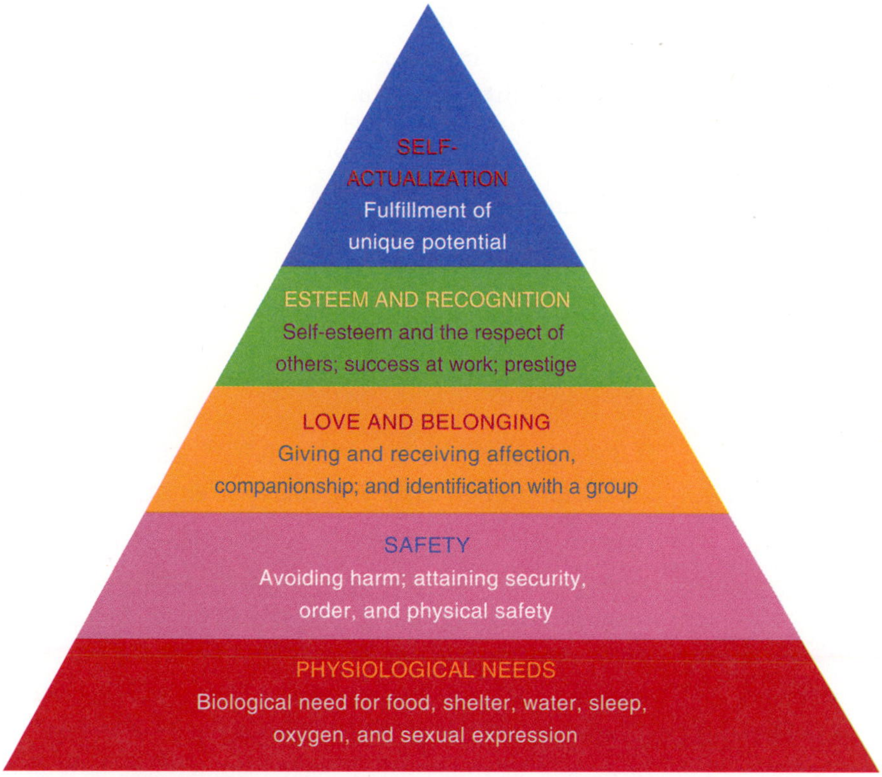

FIGURE 4-2 • Maslow's hierarchy of needs.

their own survival needs. They must also find ways to ensure their own safety and security. Independence from family support means that adults are on their own to establish meaningful relationships to satisfy needs for love and belonging. Moreover, adults may be a in a position to play a significant role in helping to satisfy the needs of others, such as their children or aging parents. One's self-esteem will be related to success in taking care of personal needs while doing things that contribute to the needs of others. Self-actualization is the most advanced of all the needs. As adults move closer to optimal levels of mental and emotional health, they are well on their way to achieving self-actualization. This process, indeed, is the work of a lifetime.

Developing Your Identity

Identity refers to all of the characteristics that make up who you are as an individual. The inherited genetic makeup you received from your parents provides the foundation for your individuality (Figure 4-3). Building on this foundation, your early identity was influenced by family members and other people who played significant roles in your life, such as extended family members, teachers, clergy, neighbors, and so on. These people served as models for your thoughts, values, attitudes, and behaviors. As a result, your identity as a child was probably largely a reflection of how other people related and responded to you. It was also shaped by personal experiences and the physical and social environment in which you lived.

As you grew older, you had more control over the continuing development of your identity. You began to shape your own attitudes, beliefs, and values along with determining your purpose for living. Your identity continues to develop throughout adulthood. This identity reflects your past experiences and the choices you made. A strong, healthy

identity
the recognition and expression of your uniqueness as a person, including your attitudes, beliefs, and behaviors

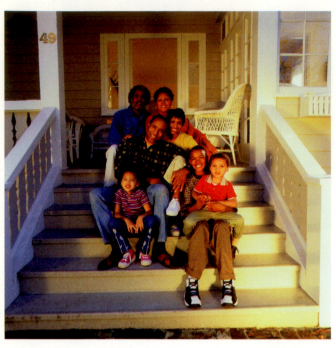

Courtesy of Photodisc

FIGURE 4-3 • Identity is influenced by genetic factors, relationships with family and community members, and the physical and social environment an individual grows up in.

identity plays an important role in mental and emotional health. Some of the most important tasks involved in creating a healthy identity include the following:

- Recognizing your personal uniqueness
- Identifying your strengths and weaknesses
- Defining your personal role in society
- Learning to form relationships with others without losing your self-identity

Characteristics of the Mentally and Emotionally Healthy Person

Maslow and other psychological researchers have identified characteristics of people who are mentally and emotionally healthy. Think of people you know who appear to be mentally and emotionally healthy, and as you read through the next sections, think about whether those people possess the qualities listed in Figure 4-4. Take an inventory of your own characteristics and see how well you compare to the checklist.

Realistic

People who are realistic see the world in terms of facts and actual events. They understand what things they can change and what things they must accept as they are. Suppose you were badly injured in a car accident. You were fortunate to survive, but now you walk

	Realistic
	Accepting
	Autonomous
	Authentic
	Capable of intimacy
	Creative
	Good self-esteem
	Value and purpose for living
	Optimistic
	Comfortable being alone

Delmar/Cengage Learning

FIGURE 4-4 • Checklist of characteristics among mentally and emotionally healthy people.

with a limp. The fact that you walk with a limp is a condition you may not be able to change. It's something you must accept. People sometimes stare at you, but you have learned to remind yourself how fortunate you are to be able to walk at all. You have decided not to let the actions or opinions of others spoil your outlook on life.

Accepting

Accepting refers to having positive but realistic feelings about yourself and others. People who are accepting don't demand perfection in themselves or in others. Using the previously mentioned example, they would have a compassionate understanding of the other person's defect. They understand that not everything in life will be to their liking, and they can handle it when things don't go their way. Imagine that a group of your friends wants to go to an outdoor concert, but you really want to go see a movie. You can accept the fact that not everyone in the group wants to do the same thing at the same time. You feel free to choose between going with your friends to the concert or going to the movie yourself. Either way, you aren't upset about the situation. People who are accepting also respect differences and value diversity among people. Their opinions about people are based on individual characteristics, not on group stereotypes.

Autonomous

Autonomous means being inner directed and not being controlled by the desires or wishes of other people. It is making choices on the basis of your own values and beliefs rather than following the crowd or trying to please other people. We all make choices about our future. You might decide to continue or postpone college. Or you might choose to work full-time. You might even decide to move to another state or country to pursue a dream that's important to you. You can take advice from others, but the choice will ultimately be yours. Making good decisions for yourself in such situations will depend on your ability to develop a strong inner compass that you trust.

Authentic

Authentic people are not afraid to be themselves. They are genuine and able to express their thoughts and feelings honestly. We might describe them by the phrase "What you see is what you get." Being authentic means being "real" and not pretending to be someone you aren't just to gain approval from others. Although it is normal for young adults to be somewhat self-conscious, people who are authentic don't spend much time worrying

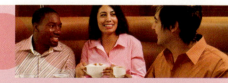

Talking it Over

Do you know someone who seems to be very happy and satisfied with life? Spend some time talking with this person. Ask for permission to conduct an informal interview and find out what qualities he or she believes are most important for happiness and mental and emotional health. What can you learn from this person? How is this person's perspective on what contributes to happiness similar or different from yours?

about what other people think of them. A wise person once said, "We would spend less time worrying about what other people think about us if we knew how seldom they think about us!" Although it may seem as if everyone is focused on you and forming judgments about you, they probably aren't. In fact, people are often most focused on themselves and their own concerns.

Intimate

People who are comfortable with themselves are capable of establishing appropriate physical and emotional intimacy (closeness) with other people (Figure 4-5). They have something to offer a relationship. They are able to express their feelings and are willing to take the risks necessary to create a relationship. They respect both themselves and others. Because establishing emotional intimacy can be quite threatening and challenging, some people are more comfortable with physical intimacy than with emotional intimacy. But physical intimacy without emotional intimacy can lead to shallow relationships that are not respectful of the individuals involved.

For many people, intimacy is described only as sexual contact. Actually, true intimacy is developed while communicating and sharing feelings with a significant person. Often, abstinence from sexual activity in a new relationship provides time for a couple to develop their level of intimacy. A sexual encounter that results in a pregnancy or the transmission of a sexually transmitted infection can actually have a harmful effect on intimacy, not to mention a person's emotional health.

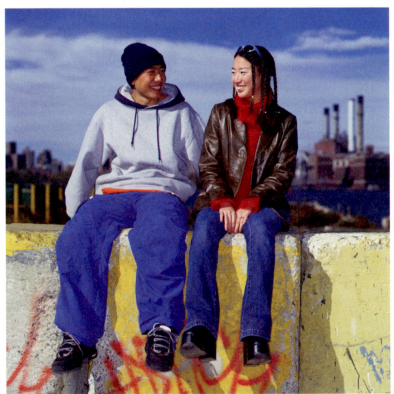

Courtesy of Photodisc

FIGURE 4-5 • People who are comfortable with themselves and are able to express their feelings while respecting the feelings of others are capable of creating intimate relationships.

Creative

You may not think that you're the creative type, but all of us are the artists of our own lives. Being creative means being open to new experiences. Instead of staying safe and secure in what they already know, creative people are curious and adventurous. Even if they don't demonstrate great talent in a particular area, they may participate in an activity just for the sheer enjoyment. In Figure 4-6, a young woman is demonstrating her creativity, but we have no sense of what beautiful creation she is working on; it doesn't really matter as long as she is enjoying what she is creating. Think about how you would feel if you were given a box containing the following items, all brand new: finger paints, Play-Doh, a box of 64 colorful crayons, 24 markers, assorted colors of pipe cleaners, scissors, assorted colors of construction paper, and a tablet full of blank white paper. What about if you were given a stack of wood and a toolbox with hammer, nails, and saw. Would you be motivated to create something with these materials?

Self-Esteem

Self-esteem is the personal opinion of your value and worth as a human being. If you have good self-esteem, you generally like yourself despite what others might say or do. Self-esteem continues to develop throughout life and is based on both our own experiences and feedback from others. Sometimes our self-esteem is threatened. Suppose you've always taken pride in your athletic ability. So far, you've mastered every sport you've

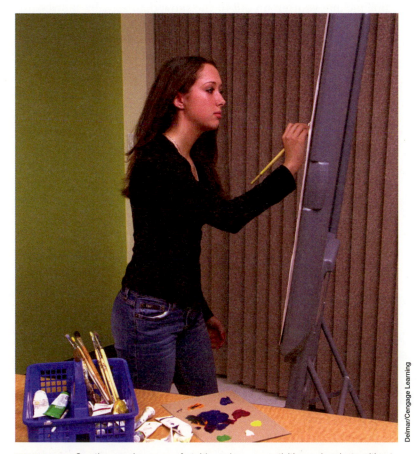

Delmar/Cengage Learning

FIGURE 4-6 • Creative people can comfortably explore new activities and projects without worry about the accuracy of the product.

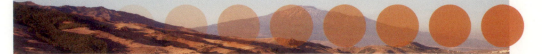

What's Your View?

Finding Your Purpose

Many people don't believe they have anything important to accomplish while they are young adults. They believe that significant accomplishments come later, after they've finished college or when they have a career. Yet, regardless of age, many people seem to enjoy helping others and describe it as a fulfilling, satisfying experience. Many colleges have thriving service-learning programs, campus committees, or clubs that add relevancy to one's learning. What about you? Have you thought about what your short-term purpose in life might be? What about your long-term purpose? How have these changed across your life span?

attempted. Other people always comment on what a great athlete you are. Your confidence in your athletic ability contributes to your self-esteem and how you see yourself. Last week a friend invited you to go snowboarding for the first time. You were confident that you wouldn't have any trouble learning. But after a whole day on the beginner slope, you still spent more time picking yourself up out of the snow than actually snowboarding. It was a real blow to your pride. People with good self-esteem are able to accept that they won't automatically succeed at everything they try.

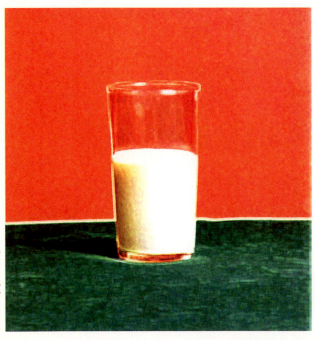

Delmar/Cengage Learning

FIGURE 4-7 • Do you perceive this glass of milk to be half empty or half full?

Have Value

People who are mentally and emotionally healthy are likely to value life and discover a purpose for living. In other words, they know why they are here on this earth. Sometimes it takes many years to develop a clear sense of your purpose in life. A good first step to finding your purpose is to consider all the things you have to be thankful for in your life. Take some time to consider how your actions affect others and how you can contribute to the good of others and to society as a whole. We all have opportunities to make a difference in the world.

Optimistic

Optimism is a way of looking at life. Look at Figure 4-7 and see why you have probably heard the question "Is the glass half empty or half full?" For people who are optimistic, most often the glass is half full. They see the possibilities and opportunities in life as opposed to the barriers and pitfalls. If something bad happens, they assume it's temporary

What's News

In 2005, Daniel Goleman, a psychologist and science writer, wrote a book titled *Emotional Intelligence*, which was on the *New York Times* best-seller list for more than a year and has now sold more than 5 million copies world-wide and been translated into 30 languages. He reported on new discoveries in brain research that indicated emotional intelligence to be more important than standard measures of intelligence, such as IQ tests, in determining an individual's success in life. It seems that when an event occurs, emotional memories are stored for future use. If the memories are mostly positive, such as self-awareness, self-restraint, hope, optimism, and empathy, we develop an "emotional intelligence" that serves us well in meeting future challenges. If the memories are mostly negative, such as fear, anxiety, frustration, anger, and depression, we may find ourselves reacting to future situations with similar negative responses. Goleman believes that emotional intelligence can be taught, both at home and in schools, to help both children and adults learn to identify and manage their emotions in positive ways.

and won't last forever. They also believe that one unfortunate event is simply one event, and they don't complain that "everything is always going wrong." According to Martin Seligman (1998) and other researchers, there may be a genetic predisposition toward optimism or pessimism. But we can all learn to approach life in a more optimistic way.

Comfortable Being Alone

People with good mental and emotional health are comfortable spending time alone as well as with others. They don't feel helpless. They can satisfy many of their own needs without depending on others. For example, imagine you've had a hectic week and have been looking forward to spending Friday night relaxing on your own listening to music or reading. You want to relax quietly. Then your friend or coworker calls on Friday afternoon and wants you to go to a party. You feel comfortable saying that you really just want to hang out on your own tonight. On the other hand, you may decide to accept the invitation because you really want to go but not because you're worried about being alone.

●●● Defense Mechanisms

Defense mechanisms are mental strategies and behaviors used to avoid painful feelings caused by difficult situations. They provide a distraction or escape from having to directly confront and deal with events or circumstances we find upsetting. They

defense mechanisms
mental strategies and behaviors used to protect ourselves from situations that cause conflict or anxiety

WEB LINK

Emotional Intelligence

http://www.6seconds.org

For more information on emotional intelligence, check out this Web site, which includes an explanation of emotional intelligence as well as related stories, articles, and cartoons.

SEARCH TERMS: emotional intelligence, emotional competency

also serve as protection when we are faced with unpleasant thoughts, emotions, or situations that threaten our self-esteem or contradict our perception of reality. The occasional use of defense mechanisms is common. But using them as a regular means of dealing with life is unhealthy. They may help us escape temporarily from our bad feelings, but they can also prevent us from doing something about solving the problems that caused those feelings. People usually have a few regular defense mechanisms that they resort to when they feel threatened. Reflect on whether there are any of these that you use often to try to protect yourself.

Repression

Repression involves pushing upsetting thoughts, feelings, or circumstances from conscious memory. This usually happens without the individual making a conscious decision to repress the memory. When an individual represses an event, he or she may not even remember it happened. This is particularly true if the situation was extremely traumatic.

Denial

Denial is one of the most commonly used defense mechanisms for many people. It means consciously rejecting an obvious truth or reality. For example, if someone close to you is seriously injured in a car accident and is not expected to live, you may refuse to believe the seriousness of the situation in order to protect yourself from feeling devastated. While denial can be a healthy defense mechanism that allows time to adjust to a difficult situation, it can also be unhealthy, such as when alcoholics deny that they have a drinking problem even when it has persisted for years and is obvious to others around them.

Rationalization

Rationalization involves creating a possible but false reason to explain a situation. For example, if you want to buy a big-screen television that you know you don't really need, you might rationalize your purchase by telling yourself or someone else that your current television is worn out and no longer working properly even though that's not completely true. In truth, perhaps you simply want a newer, bigger television to watch sports and movies.

Daydreaming and Fantasy

Daydreaming and fantasizing are ways to escape from your real life into a more pleasant, imaginary world. It is another of the most commonly used defense mechanisms. All of us engage in daydreaming and fantasizing from time to time. This can be a healthy and creative way to add pleasure to our lives. But daydreaming can be destructive if it interferes with daily functioning and becomes a habitual way of responding to any situation we find disturbing.

Humor

Using humor and laughing are two of the best things we can do for ourselves. But, like other defense mechanisms, they can also be misused. Sometimes we poke fun at others in a way that is hurtful. Then if they get upset, we protest, "But I was only joking!" Humor that takes advantage of another person in order to get a laugh is unkind. Sometimes we use humor to make fun of ourselves. This can be a cover-up for our true feelings when we're upset about something. For example, someone who failed an important exam might make fun of a classmate who did well by saying, "Well, it's a good thing you're smart and don't have to depend on your looks." Or they might make fun of themselves by saying, "I guess I must have been at the back of the line when brains were handed out."

Projection

Projection is attributing your own thoughts and feelings to someone else. For example, suppose you really want to see a particular movie and your friends don't, but you don't want to take responsibility for expressing your feelings directly. Instead, you might say, "Let's go see that new movie that started this week. It's supposed to have great special effects. Luis really wants to see it and I know he'll be mad if we don't see it this weekend."

Displacement

Displacement occurs when you transfer the root cause of an emotion to something or someone else. If you've had a bad day at work, you may come home and argue with someone at home. Those you may argue with are not the cause of your frustration, but you use them as the target for your frustration. Displacement is the defense mechanism that has given rise to the old adage about "coming home and kicking the dog."

Using Defense Mechanisms

Everyone uses defense mechanisms at one time or another. However, regularly relying on defense mechanisms to avoid dealing with negative feelings is not healthy, nor does it resolve the original problem. Table 4-1 illustrates some examples of common defense mechanisms and how they are often used.

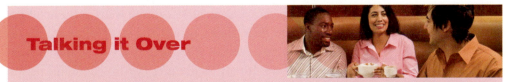

Talking it Over

How have you used defense mechanisms in the past? In some ways, using them may have been useful to you at the time. In some ways, using them may have caused problems for you. Which defense mechanisms are harmful to you, and which ones are mostly useful to you? When you are faced with a difficult situation, what are some healthier ways to resolve daily problems other than using a defense mechanism?

TABLE 4-1 • Common defense mechanisms.

Defense Mechanism	Definition	Example
DENIAL	Refusing to acknowledge a painful reality, pretending the event did not happen or does not exist	Someone is presented with a serious cancer diagnosis, but never admits to receiving the diagnosis from the doctor
ACTING OUT	Performing an inappropriate behavior rather than verbally expressing one's thoughts or feelings	One of the partners in a romantic relationship is told by the other person that the relationship is going to end, throws a lamp in anger rather than verbally expressing their pain of the news
PROJECTION	Redirecting one's uncomfortable thoughts or feelings onto someone else	Someone who is not selected for a job, and telling friends that he/she was told by some members of the selection committee that he/she was the top candidate
RATIONALIZATION	An effort to replace or justify acceptable reasons for the actual feelings, beliefs, or behaviors	An individual wants to stay home from work and tells himself that the work he had to do that day was unimportant and can wait until tomorrow
REPRESSION	Unconscious forgetting or blocking of painful or dangerous thoughts	A woman loses her mother in a tragic automobile accident states to friends one month later that she does not feel any sadness
DISPLACEMENT	Redirecting thoughts or feelings to someone who had nothing to do with the actual incident	Someone has an argument with a roommate, and mistreats a co-worker

Delmar/Cengage Learning

●●● Developing Communication Skills

Identifying and clearly expressing your thoughts, feelings, and emotions are important skills for maintaining good mental and emotional wellness. Everyone can talk, but not everyone is a good communicator. Your mental and emotional health is stronger if you have the motivation and skill to be an effective communicator.

Honesty

Emotionally healthy people are honest with themselves and with others. Sometimes it's easy to communicate honestly; sometimes it's much more difficult. It's often difficult to be honest when we don't want to hurt someone's feelings or we aren't sure how to deliver bad news. For example, suppose you've been dating someone exclusively for several months, but now you find yourself attracted to someone new. You want to break off the relationship, but you don't know how to do it. Being honest and straightforward means talking to the other person and explaining as kindly as possible that you no longer want to be involved in an exclusive relationship. It may seem easier just to ignore this person or to act badly and hope that he or she will end the relationship. But that's not an honest way of handling the situation. It is fairer to others to tell the truth, as painful as it might be for both of you at the time.

Self-Reflection

Sometimes it's difficult to even identify exactly what you're feeling, let alone express the feeling to someone else. Self-reflection means looking into yourself to discover your true feelings and look for the courage and characteristics that contribute to good communication. This is a necessary first step before meaningful communication can take place. Let's say you have just found out that you were unsuccessful in your attempt to make a sports team or get a job that you really wanted. It might take some time and self-reflection to determine what you're really feeling. Are you disappointed? Embarrassed? Angry? When you can identify your innermost feelings, you have a better chance of communicating them clearly to someone else. You may have to tell friends, "You know, right now I think I'm just really disappointed, and I don't feel like talking about it. Could we just talk about something else? I'll let you know later when I feel more like talking about it."

Assertiveness

Assertiveness means respecting yourself and letting others know what you need or what your position is on an issue. It also means respecting the rights of others, even when you disagree. When you communicate assertively, you try to find the balance between giving up your own rights (being too passive) and forcing your beliefs or desires on others (being too aggressive). Suppose you're in a restaurant with friends, and they start making fun of a person at the next table who appears to be very overweight. You believe their behavior is cruel. Telling your friends, politely and with conviction, that you think comments are unkind would be an example of assertive behavior.

Did You Know...?

We usually think about communication as something that takes place between two or more people. But have you ever thought about the way you communicate with yourself? It's called self-talk, and many of us say things to ourselves we would never say to someone we care about. When we're talking to ourselves (and this "talk" can be out loud or just our internal thoughts), we tend to be harsh and critical, focusing on our flaws and failures. You can learn to change your self-talk to be more encouraging and positive toward yourself. You'll be surprised at what a big difference it makes in the way you feel about yourself.

●●● Managing Feelings

It's normal and healthy to have a wide range of feelings. Managing our positive feelings is usually not a problem. People rarely complain because we are happy or excited, even if we're overdoing it a bit. But managing our negative feelings can be more difficult. Even though feeling sad, anxious, depressed, or angry is completely normal, most people aren't as comfortable with these feelings as they are with more positive feelings. Our negative feelings can also be upsetting to the people around us.

Many studies show that it's best to acknowledge your feelings rather than hide them or pretend they don't exist (Figure 4-8). An important wellness skill is learning to express your feelings without overreacting and behaving inappropriately. While it may be difficult to handle your feelings well all the time, you can work toward recognizing and managing them well most of the time.

Anger

Statistically speaking, one out of five Americans has an anger management problem, indicating that anger is one of the most difficult feelings to manage because it often catches us off guard. We may find ourselves angry before we're even aware of what's happening. In the heat of the moment, it's hard to step back and think clearly about the best way to respond to a situation.

WEB LINK
Anger Management

http://www.angermgmt.com

This Website is a wonderfully interactive site containing numerous resources for addressing anger. From the homepage you can link to an an "anger tool kit" with tips for managing anger in constructive ways: You can also go to **http://www.insyncsurveys.com.au/**. Enter the term "quizzes" in the search bar and take the anger management quiz with feedback.

SEARCH TERMS: anger management, anger management quiz, anger management assessment

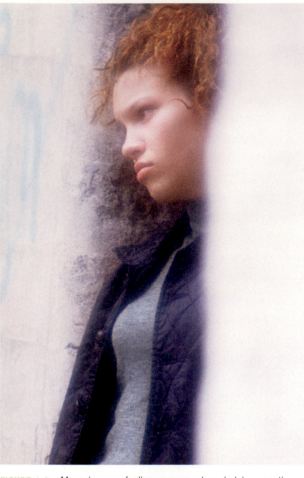

FIGURE 4-8 • Managing your feelings means acknowledging negative emotions like anger, sadness, or anxiety.

Anger usually occurs when we face an actual or imaginary situation that causes us to experience harm, loss, or blame. Catching yourself before your anger gets out of control is a skill you can learn.

Depression

Depression is another feeling that can be difficult to manage. Sometimes we can identify the factors that contribute to depression, but it's common for people to feel "blue" without any specific reason. Part of depression is feeling unable to cope with the problems of daily life. Another symptom is feeling paralyzed and unable to take action to resolve life's problems. Depression is one of the most common mood disorders in the United States. It is discussed more fully later in this chapter.

Anxiety and Fear

Anxiety and fear are useful when they help us avoid potentially dangerous or harmful situations. But sometimes we spend a lot of time worrying about things that aren't actually harmful or that never happen. Fear of an unpleasant outcome can keep us from taking a risk that might turn out well. Suppose you want to apply for a new job or ask someone new out on a date, but you are afraid of failing or, worse yet, of making a fool of yourself. Just thinking about the situation causes you anxiety. When faced with this kind of situation in which there is something to gain, as well as something to lose, it might be helpful to ask yourself these questions:

- What's the worst thing that can happen?
- How will I respond if that thing happens?
- How will I feel if the situation turns out well?
- Am I willing to take the risk?

Effectively managing anxiety and fear means developing personal wellness skills to help you assess what your feelings tell you and when to take action despite the negativity you may feel.

Loneliness

Everyone feels lonely at one time or another. No matter how close we are to our family or how many friends we have, part of our human experience is to occasionally feel alone and unsupported. Loneliness can be an indicator that we need to spend more time developing a good

Did You Know...?

Data from a large number of research studies indicate that regular exercise can help alleviate depression and anxiety. Researchers believe that exercise increases the levels of serotonin, a brain neurotransmitter. Serotonin is one of the brain chemicals responsible for positive mood. In some of the studies, exercise was just as effective as psychotherapy and antidepressant drugs in relieving depression.

relationship with ourselves. It can also be an indicator that we need to spend more time developing social connections with other people.

Although loneliness is not always negative, it can be quite painful. When you experience loneliness, ask yourself what would make you feel more connected to yourself or to others. For example, if you often find yourself spending your weekends alone and you feel lonely, develop a plan to make some new friends with whom you can share some activities. This may require stepping outside your comfort zone to initiate an invitation to someone else who might be interested in some of the same activities in which you are interested.

●●● Understanding Mental Illness

Your overall health status is related to the quality of your mental and emotional health and the extent to which you are practicing wellness in these areas. Unfortunately, mental health problems are quite common, and sometimes things go seriously wrong. In fact, in 20 percent of American households, there is at least one person who is affected by a mental health problem at some time in their life. It's important to understand that mental disorders can be treated. People should be able to recognize common disorders and be prepared to seek help, if necessary, for themselves or for the people they care about. Mental disorders should not be suffered in silence, nor should they prevent people from enjoying their lives. The following sections include information that will enhance your understanding of the causation of mental illness.

The Human Brain

To comprehend mental disorders, it may first be necessary to have a better understanding of the brain (Figure 4-9). The brain is the most complex organ in the body. It contains more than 100 billion nerve cells, or **neurons** (Figure 4-10). Whereas the other organs

neuron
a specialized body cell that is the basic unit of nerve tissue

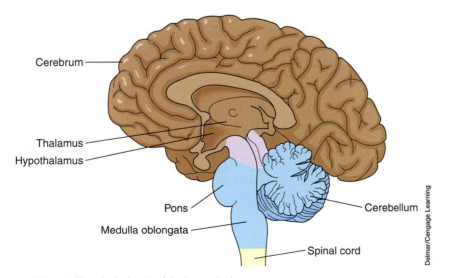

FIGURE 4-9 • The principal parts of the human brain.

Cerebrum

Thalamus

Hypothalamus

Pons

Medulla oblongata

Cerebellum

Spinal cord

Delmar/Cengage Learning

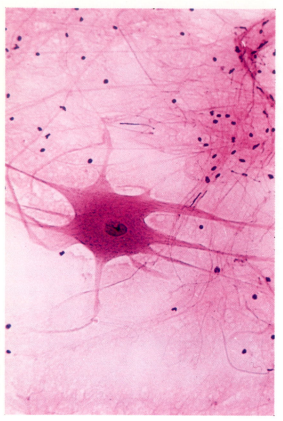

Delmar/Cengage Learning

FIGURE 4-10 • The brain contains more than 100 billion neurons.

are composed of only a few different cell types, the brain contains *thousands* of different cells. These neurons are organized in different parts of the brain to control the functions needed for life support, survival, and daily activities. These functions include thought, memory, speech, vision, hearing, decision making, and muscle movement. Adding to the complexity, each neuron has thousands of connections with other neurons that enable the cells to communicate with each other. This communication takes place because of chemicals called **neurotransmitters**, which provide complex electrical pathways for impulses to move within and among neurons. These connections allow communication to take place so rapidly that we aren't even aware of the process.

Let's look at an example. Suppose you enter a room and discover a fire. In an instant, you *see* and *smell* smoke coming from a trash can. You *remember* where the fire extinguisher is in the kitchen, so you turn to the hallway and *yell* to your roommate in the kitchen to bring the fire extinguisher to you quickly! The neurons in your brain work together to take in and process information, take advantage of what's stored in your memory, and suggest the appropriate action. And your brain can do all this in less time than it's taking you to read about it!

Mental illness is related to brain function. The complexity of the brain that allows us to do amazing things can also be the cause of problems when these complex functions are disrupted or not working in a coordinated fashion. Many of us take the brain for granted and believe that we can control both our thoughts and other brain functions. The truth is that our brain function depends on a complicated arrangement of structures, **receptors**, and chemicals that are constantly performing billions of functions. Malfunctions in this complicated system can result in mental illness.

neurotransmitters
chemical substances that enable transmission of information among neurons

receptors
nerve endings that receive stimuli, as from the sense organs

outpatient
refers to treatment given to a patient during periodic visits to a health care facility or physician's office

inpatient
refers to treatment given to a patient who has been admitted to a health care facility

●●● Treating Mental Illness

In 1952, the American Psychiatric Association began publishing the *Diagnostic and Statistical Manual of Mental Disorders* (*DSM*). The *DSM* is now in its fourth edition, text revision (*DSM-IV-TR*; American Psychiatric Association, 2000), and contains classifications of many varieties of mental illness. The *DSM-IV-TR* is written to serve as a manual to help professionals diagnose mental conditions. It does not include suggestions for treatments.

It is important to understand that mental disorders are *illnesses* and not conditions that happen to bad people. In that regard, just like physical illnesses, mental illness can be improved with professional treatment. To help someone recognize the mental health problem and encourage them to seek treatment is important. We express concern for somebody who has the flu and needs to stay in bed. We have compassion for the person with cancer who undergoes chemotherapy or surgery. The same level of concern and compassion should be given to someone with mental illness.

As with other forms of illness, mental illness is treatable with counseling or medication or both. Some mental health problems can be treated very well on an **outpatient** basis, whereby the individual goes to the mental health care facility, obtains treatment, and then goes home. Outpatient treatment may require a number of visits as determined by the health care provider. More serious mental illness may require **inpatient** treatments.

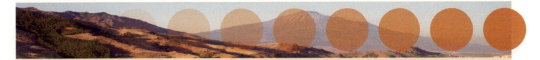

What's Your View?

Factors Affecting Mental Health

Mental health problems can range from being almost unnoticeable to quite severe. Some of these problems are related to chemical changes in the body; some may be influenced by things that a person experiences in his or her environment. In the same regard, there may be circumstances that encourage good mental health:

- Make a list of environmental factors that you think affect your mental health in both positive and negative ways.

- Do you think your friends or colleagues would have the same items on their list if they created one?

- Talk to other people who are close to you about the items they would include on their list.

Unfortunately, even when a person wants help, it can be difficult to access good mental health treatment, especially if the individual does not have insurance. Even with insurance, there is often a shortage of mental health treatment options, particularly in rural areas. It can take a great deal of perseverance to access mental health treatment, and often the person with a mental illness does not have the energy or the ability to face this challenge alone. Friends and family can support the person who needs help by working with the patient to gain access to appropriate mental health treatment.

Did You Know...?

It is estimated that 26 percent of adults (about one in four) in the United States have a diagnosable mental illness in any given year. A smaller number, about 6 percent, or 1 in 17 adults, have a serious mental illness.

⬤⬤⬤ Causes of Mental Illness

There are a number of factors that may influence mental health. Among them are physical conditions, genetic factors, or environmental causes. It is believed mental illness is somehow related to poor functioning among the brain's neurotransmitters.

- *Heredity.* A person may inherit the predisposition for mental illness. The role of genetic factors in mental illness is very complex. Characteristics such as gender, age, and race can play a part in genetic influence in mental illness. Current research on mental illness suggests that it is the interaction among many genes that contributes to the development of mental health problems.

- *Physical health problems.* Some physical conditions have been associated with mental illness. For example, many children who had a certain bacterial infection of the throat in the 1980s later developed a mental illness known as obsessive-compulsive disorder.

  There are other disease conditions, such as HIV infection, syphilis, and measles, that can cause brain changes, possibly leaving a person vulnerable to mental illness.

- *Injury.* Head injuries resulting from accidents and violence can damage the brain and create conditions for impaired mental functioning.

- *Environmental conditions.* Exposure to toxic materials can lead to mental impairment. House paint, for example, used to contain lead. Small children sometimes chew on painted surfaces, such as bed rails or windowsills, and then swallow the paint flakes. In older houses that contain leaded paint, this behavior can result in brain damage from lead.

- *Stress.* A vulnerable person, under stress, may exhibit some form of mental illness. Stress, however, is not itself the primary cause. Stress contributes to the magnification of underlying mental illness behaviors.

- *Drugs.* Use of both legal and illegal drugs can contribute to the onset of mental health problems. Drugs such as stimulants ("uppers") and barbiturates ("downers") that stimulate and then depress the nervous system are especially dangerous.

⬤⬤◐ Forms of Mental Disorders

People suffering from mental disorders often overlook the symptoms because the signs associated with mental illness may not be as obvious as the symptoms associated with physical illness. It's easier to know you are suffering from a throat infection than to recognize that you have clinical depression. The *DSM-IV-TR* lists diagnostic information for more than 450 mental conditions. Some of the conditions, such as "major depression," are well known. But there are also lesser-known disorders, such as "identity problem" and "sleep disorders." The following sections present some of the more common conditions.

Anxiety Disorders

There is nothing wrong with feeling anxious. It happens to everyone from time to time. It's natural to experience the "butterfly feeling" in your stomach when you'll be meeting someone new, getting ready for a big test, or starting a new job. Mental health problems arise when feelings of anxiety become more frequent or even permanent. Anxiety may be considered a problem when the feelings are not associated with specific stressful events or when the feelings are so intense that they interfere with daily activities.

Anxiety disorders are real medical illnesses affecting approximately 19 million adults in the United States. Anxiety disorders are the most common mental health problems. There is no clear, single cause of anxiety disorder. In fact, causes appear to be both biological and psychological in nature. Anxiety disorders tend to run in families, and it appears that excessive stress can trigger anxiety disorders.

Phobias

Phobias are overwhelming, irrational fears related to specific events or things. Phobias are currently the most common classification of psychiatric disorders in the United States. They are also the most common psychological disorder among females of all ages.

People with phobias experience both physical and emotional reactions to an object or a situation. These reactions may include feelings of panic, dread, or horror; a rapid

phobias
overwhelming, illogical fears of an event or object

heartbeat; and an intense desire to flee the situation or avoid the object. People with phobias realize that their feelings are stronger than what might normally be expected. The causes of phobias are not well understood, but there is some evidence that they may relate to a frightening experience that occurred in childhood related to the object of the phobia. Phobias come in many forms. How about "paralipophobia," or the fear of neglecting duty or responsibility? The Phobia List Web site (http://phobialist.com) verifies 530 different phobias. As described in *DSM-IV-TR*, two main types of phobias and a number of examples are presented in Table 4-2.

Phobias are usually treated in one of two ways: **cognitive-behavioral therapy** or medication. A mental health professional recommends the most appropriate method of treatment after interviewing and examining the patient. In cognitive-behavioral therapy, the patient meets with a trained therapist and learns to control the physical reactions caused by the fear. The patient gradually confronts the phobia in a carefully structured way in order to identify the trigger that causes the phobia; each confrontation with the phobia trigger is followed by relaxation techniques. The patient first imagines the feared object or situation. The next step is to look at pictures of the object or situation. Finally, the patient actually comes into contact with the feared object or experiences the situation. By facing rather than fleeing from the source of fear, the patient eventually becomes free of the anxiety and dread associated with it.

Medication may be prescribed to control the extreme anxiety or panic experienced during a phobic encounter by reducing the anxiety associated with just thinking about dealing with the object or situation. For patients suffering from agoraphobia or social phobia, medication tends to be the first choice, although they may also need cognitive-behavioral therapy. With treatment, the vast majority of phobia patients can be relieved of their fears and live a symptom-free life.

cognitive-behavioral therapy
used by a trained mental health professional to help a patient alter his or her response to a stimulus

TABLE 4-2 • Classification and types of phobias.

Phobia	Description
1. Social phobias	**Intense excessive fear of being observed in one or more social situations. The fear is that the individual will perform in a way that will cause extreme personal humiliation.**
Fear of going to social events alone	Distress about being looked at thinking everyone is being critical.
Fear of going to meetings at work	Anxiety about saying something embarrassing in front of coworkers.
Fear of standing in lines alone	Concern that people are watching and talking about you.
2. Specific phobias	**Extreme fear of a specific object or situation.**
Acrophobia	Fear of heights.
Agoraphobia	Fear of being in open or public places.
Arachnophobia	Fear of spiders.
Ergophobia	Fear of work.
Pedophobia	Fear of children.
Hydrophobia	Fear of water.
Gamophobia	Fear of marriage.

Delmar/Cengage Learning

Posttraumatic Stress Disorder

Posttraumatic stress disorder (PTSD) can happen after a person is involved in or witnesses an extremely frightening event such as an accidental death of a loved one, war, or physical or sexual abuse. These types of experiences leave a deep impression that results in mental reactions to the experiences that can take place weeks, months, or even years later.

The person does not have to be physically injured in the event to suffer PTSD. Even people who are not directly involved but who witness a traumatic event can be affected. In recent years, many people of all ages have experienced posttraumatic stress as a result of the terrorist attacks of September 11, 2001; the Iraq War; and Hurricanes Katrina and Rita.

PTSD is a serious condition that can interfere with a person's ability to engage in many daily activities. Signs of posttraumatic stress disorder include the following:

- Nightmares and sleep disorders

- Frightening memories of the event

- Difficulty concentrating

- Not wanting to be with friends

- Discomfort with situations related to the traumatic event

The effects of PTSD can last for years. For example, a person who was abused as a child may be fearful of engaging in a normal intimate relationship as an adult and will often need counseling to manage his or her disorder.

Generalized Anxiety Disorder

Generalized anxiety disorder is characterized by excessive worry about a variety of things over a period of at least six months. This mental health condition often develops during childhood or the teen years. People with generalized anxiety disorder may also exhibit physical symptoms such as headaches, tiredness, and muscle tension. They may complain of having difficulty sleeping or feeling a lump in their throat. Generalized anxiety disorder usually runs in families and can become worse when a person is stressed. The condition can be treated with medication and/or counseling.

Panic Disorder

Panic disorder is characterized by unexpected and repeated feelings of fear. The panic attacks become full blown in about 15 minutes and can include physical symptoms such as rapid heartbeat, sweating, dizziness, and a feeling of not being able to move or breathe. Panic disorder is relatively rare in children. It is most likely to develop during adolescence or young adulthood. Research indicates that both heredity and stressful experiences may play a role in causing panic disorder. Knowing that an attack can happen at any time adds to the fear and stress and may actually contribute to future episodes. Depending on the level of intensity experienced by the patient, the mental health professional can treat the disorder with counseling, drug therapy, or both.

Obsessive-Compulsive Disorder

Obsessive-compulsive disorder is characterized by repeated disturbing, seemingly sense-less thoughts (**obsessions**) or ritual behaviors (**compulsions**) that cannot be easily controlled or stopped. For example, someone who has an uncommon fear of germs (obsession) may constantly wash his or her hands (compulsion). Another example is someone who repeatedly checks the lock on the door (compulsion) from a fear that someone will try to enter the room or home (obsession).

Mood Disorders

In a psychological sense, *mood* refers to emotions over a period of time. Our mood influences our attitudes and how we view the world. Mood disorders are characterized by a disturbance of normal mood, which can result in symptoms such as depression, euphoria, and hyperactivity.

Mood disorders are the source of much human suffering and occur throughout the life span. They are the cause of lost productivity and many suicides. They rank among the top 10 causes of disability *worldwide*. When mood disorders are not recognized and treated, they can cause physical symptoms. The physical symptoms caused by untreated mood disorders result in unnecessary health care expense and, worse, may prevent the patient from being treated for the real cause of the symptoms.

Depression

One thing is very natural about the mental states of human beings: they are not consistent. We are capable of experiencing a wide variety of emotions. Sometimes we are happy, sometimes angry, and sometimes sad. These emotional states are usually temporary, and it's normal to feel sad or depressed from time to time. What is not normal is depression that is extreme and lasts for a long period of time.

Severe depression often begins in the teen years, with females twice as likely to be depressed as males. Studies also suggest that the number of cases of depression has risen sharply among children and teens. Symptoms of depression in children and youth are often different from those in adults. There is evidence that many young people who suffer from depression continue to suffer from depression as adults. There are also gender differences between males and females in the way that depression is expressed. While women often express depression as sadness and lethargy, men may also appear angry when the root cause of the anger is actually depression.

Depression can interfere with school and work performance and family and social activities. Identifying and treating depression as early as possible is important so a person can live a full life now and in the years to come.

Depression is a treatable disorder. It is important for people to seek help from a mental health professional as soon as they suspect they may be suffering from depression. If you or anyone you know exhibits some of the following symptoms for more than a couple of weeks, it's a good idea to arrange a visit with a health care professional who has expertise in mental disorders.

- Withdrawal from friends, family, and normal activities

- Violent actions or rebellious behavior

obsessions
unwanted and distressing thoughts or impulses that occur repeatedly

compulsions
repetitive behaviors that are performed in response to obsessive thoughts

- Feelings of hopelessness

- Drug and alcohol use

- Persistent boredom

- Difficulty concentrating

- A decline in the quality of schoolwork or professional work

- Frequent complaints about physical symptoms, often related to emotions, such as stomachaches, headaches, and fatigue

- Loss of interest in what were previously pleasurable activities

- Inability to accept praise or rewards

Psychologists don't have a clear picture of what causes depression. It appears that biological and social factors interact to play a role. Because the exact causes are unknown, there is not one specific treatment. People who exhibit major depression are usually treated with counseling interventions that are combined with medications to address the biological causes and behavioral interventions, thus increasing one's behavioral skills and coping resources.

Bipolar Disorder

Bipolar disorder is a serious mental illness that includes extreme shifts in mood ranging from depression to **manic** highs (excited, mostly happy episodes and increased alertness and hyperactivity) and mixed conditions. For this reason, some time ago the condition

manic
referring to mania, excessive mental and physical energy often associated with mood disorders

What's News

About a third of all patients diagnosed with severe depression do not respond to medication. These individuals may be helped by a new treatment on the horizon. A device already approved by the U.S. Food and Drug Administration to help control seizures is now being tested to see if it is effective in treating severe depression. The device is implanted under the skin much as a heart pacemaker and gives off electrical signals every 30 seconds. The impulses stimulate the brain and improve mood.

What's News

A 2001 movie, *A Beautiful Mind*, was based on an unauthorized biography of mathematician John Forbes Nash. In spite of his schizophrenia, Nash was awarded the Nobel Prize in Economics and made valuable contributions to the field of mathematics. This example provides concrete evidence that although schizophrenia can present serious difficulties in cognitive processing, significant contributions to others are still possible.

was commonly referred to as manic depression. Everybody has ups and downs in their lives. It is when these episodes become constant and interfere with everyday functions that bipolar disorder might be suspected.

Schizophrenia

Schizophrenia is a persistent, serious, and disabling **psychotic** brain disorder. It affects about 1 percent of the population. Schizophrenia usually appears in adolescence or young adulthood. Symptoms of the disorder are many and varied. In fact, many psychological experts believe that schizophrenia is not one condition but many.

Some of the symptoms of schizophrenia can be terrifying, such as hearing internal voices not heard by others. Schizophrenic patients may believe that people are reading their minds, controlling their thoughts, or plotting to harm them. The condition can cause patients' speech and behaviors to become so disorganized that they are incomprehensible and frightening to others. Many patients also experience hallucinations, that is, disturbances of sensory perception in which they believe they see things that don't really exist.

While the cause of schizophrenia is not clear, it appears there is a genetic link because someone from a family with a history of schizophrenia is 10 times more likely to exhibit the symptoms of schizophrenia than is someone from a family that has no such history. There is no single treatment for schizophrenia because the disorder may include more than one condition. It is often necessary to prescribe antipsychotic drugs, so schizophrenia is best treated by a psychiatrist.

schizophrenia
a brain disease that is perhaps the most severe of the mental illnesses

psychotic
referring to a mental disorder in which the patient loses touch with reality by way of hallucinations, paranoid behavior, and fantasy thoughts

●●● Treating Mental Illness

It is not easy for people to recognize that they have any form of mental illness. At some point, a trigger is necessary for someone to realize that they have a mental health problem serious enough to require professional treatment. It may be that significant people in their lives will try to convince them that there is a problem, or there may be a legal incident ordering them to treatment, or some other personal event, such as job loss, can serve as a trigger.

Barriers to Treatment

Even with triggers, there is no assurance they will be treated. There are a number of barriers that prevent people from seeking and continuing with mental health treatment.

Personal Perception

Many people who need treatment deny that they have a problem. Remember, their view of the world and their place in the world is defined by their own cognitive framework. One study reported that among people who had a diagnosable condition, 55 percent of those subjects did not believe that they had a problem serious enough to require treatment. Research indicates that the number one barrier to treatment reported by people who need it is that "it's nothing serious, I can handle it." People tend to believe that as long as they admit to others that they are aware of the problem, they can resolve the condition on their own.

Financial Conditions

Many people who need treatment cite their financial situation as a reason for not receiving treatment. The cost is beyond their ability to pay, and they may lack any support from an insurance program. There is also the issue of the personal cost of treatment. Some individuals may need to take time from their jobs, and the potential loss of income is a barrier to treatment. This condition may also prevent the continuation of treatment, especially if the patient has the impression that they are "cured enough."

Stigma

In addition to the effects of the mental illness itself, a problem for patients is the **stigma** that many people attach to mental illness. There are people who feel that persons with mental illnesses are abnormal. This attitude sometimes makes it difficult for people who feel that they may have a mental disorder to seek treatment. About two-thirds of all people with diagnosable mental disorders do not seek treatment. Stigma surrounding the receipt of mental health treatment is among the many barriers that discourage people from seeking treatment. Concern about stigma appears to be greater in rural areas compared than in larger towns or cities.

stigma
a belief that most people will devalue and discriminate against individuals who have a mental illness or seek treatment

psychotherapists
mental health professionals who are trained to treat mental disorders using psychological counseling techniques

psychiatrists
medical doctors who specialize in treating mental illnesses

●●● Treatment Professionals

Just as there are many types of mental health disorders, there are many types of treatment. Getting effective treatment for a mental disorder starts with realizing that help is needed. Recognizing that help is needed may sound very simple, but it is not. All too often, the signs of mental illness are not recognized, or the person with the disorder refuses to admit that there is a problem. It is common for people to believe that their symptoms will take care of themselves and go away. Some people are reluctant to seek treatment because of perceived stigma associated with mental illness. Still others are afraid of the discomfort they might experience as they go through the changes necessary to correct the disorder.

There are two main types of mental health treatment experts. **Psychotherapists** (counselors) are trained to diagnose and treat mental disorders using special counseling techniques (Figure 4-11). **Psychiatrists** are medical doctors with special training in treating mental disorders. They use counseling techniques and may also prescribe medications. Both psychotherapists and psychiatrists must be licensed by the state in which they practice.

Did You Know...?

Treating mental health problems is costly in both human and financial terms. Statistics show mental illness to be the second most burdensome health condition after heart disease. This burden is measured in years of life lost to premature death as well as years of living with a disabling condition. The financial costs of treating mental illness are high. In the United States, we spend about $70 billion annually to treat mental illness, and this figure does not include the costs of drug abuse treatment.

●●● Understanding and Preventing Suicide

Sometimes people come to feel that life is no longer worth living. People might reach this conclusion for a variety of reasons. They may feel so depressed that they don't believe they'll ever be happy again (Figure 4-12). Perhaps experienced a great loss and don't think they can live through it. Or maybe they've been so bitterly disappointed that they don't feel they'll be able

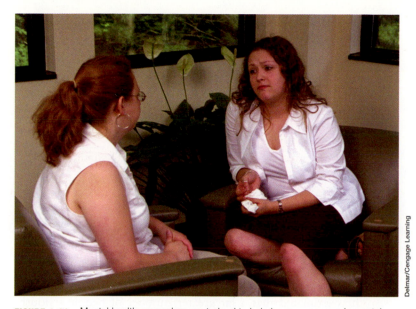

Delmar/Cengage Learning

FIGURE 4-11 • Mental health counselors are trained to help improve a person's mental health condition.

to bounce back. Fortunately, even in the most desperate situations, there is always hope for improvement with the help of trained professionals and the support of friends and family. Preventing suicide is possible if individuals learn the skills to deal with hopelessness and despair, identify helpful resources, and then take the time to develop solutions to problems.

You may have heard the saying, "Suicide is a permanent solution to a temporary problem." A person who is facing a serious problem may not believe it is temporary, even though it really is. Developing the ability to cope with serious problems and understanding that they *are* temporary can mean the difference between life and death. In this section, we explore the reasons people consider taking their own lives and what can be done to prevent this tragic loss of life.

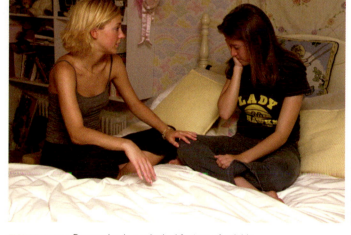

Delmar/Cengage Learning

FIGURE 4-12 • Depression is a principal feature of suicide.

Suicide is a deliberate, intentional, self-inflicted act that results in one's own death. It is probably not possible to fully understand why a person decides to end his or her own life. There are usually many factors that contribute to this decision. The underlying reason for most people deciding to commit suicide is that they don't believe they can continue living with the emotional pain they're feeling. It doesn't seem as if the pain will ever pass, and they don't believe they'll ever feel any better. Simply put, they have lost all hope that things can ever be better. Although this is the way the person feels at the time, there are really many ways to resolve emotional pain without ending one's life. Understanding this pain and identifying options for hope for the future are keys to preventing suicide.

Although suicide affects all age-groups, it is a major cause of death for teens and young adults as well as for adults 65 and over. According to the Centers for Disease Control and Prevention, in 2006, suicide was the third-leading cause of death for young

suicide
a deliberate, intentional, self-inflicted act that results in one's own death

WEB LINK
Suicide

For more detailed information about suicide, see the following Web sites:

- American Association of Suicidology: **http://www.suicidology.org**
- Centers for Disease Control and Prevention: **http://www.cdc.gov**. At the home page, enter "suicide" in the search bar
- National Institute of Mental Health: **http://www.nimh.nih.gov**. At the home page you can enter "suicide" in the search feature

SEARCH TERMS: suicide, self-harm

attempted suicide
a deliberate, intentional, self-inflicted act that is intended to cause death but does not

completed suicide
a term used to describe a suicide attempt that results in death

people aged 15 to 24. The highest rates of suicide occur among the elderly, particularly among older white males, and the rates of suicide are disproportionate among racial groups. The following 2006 suicide rates were reported by the National Institute for Mental Health (2009) for every 100,000 people in each of the following ethnic/racial groups:

- Highest rates:
  American Indian and Alaska Natives—15.1 suicides per 100,000 people
  Non-Hispanic whites—13.9 suicides per 100,000 people
- Lowest rates:
  Asian and Pacific Islanders—5.7 suicides per 100,000 people
  Non-Hispanic blacks—5.0 suicides per 100,000 people
  Hispanics—4.9 suicides per 100,000 people

It is estimated that a far greater number of people seriously consider suicide or make a suicide attempt. An **attempted suicide** is a deliberate, intentional, self-inflicted act that is intended to cause death but does not. **Completed suicide** is a term used to describe a suicide attempt that results in death.

It's not possible to know for certain whether someone who attempts suicide really wants to die. We *can* be certain that *all* attempted suicides are cries for help. The person is in such intense emotional pain that death seems the only way to remove it. The person may not really want to die but desperately wants the pain to stop.

Contributing Factors

There is no single factor that explains why people attempt suicide. Even in a single suicide attempt, there is likely to be more than one factor contributing to the person's decision. One single factor is probably not enough to cause a suicide attempt. But when many problems pile up, they may seem overwhelming. The person can't see any way of dealing with his or her problems. It is this sense of hopelessness and utter despair that can lead to a suicide attempt.

The factors discussed in the following sections have been identified as factors that increase the likelihood an individual will attempt suicide. It is true, however, that many people have one or more of these contributing factors and yet are not suicidal. Just because a person experiences one of the contributing factors does not mean that he or she is likely to attempt suicide, but these factors are present more often in those individuals who attempt suicide.

Mental Disorders and Substance Abuse

Many suicide victims have at least one mental disorder, most commonly depression, or a history of substance abuse. Although the person may have been in treatment for these conditions at some point, relatively few are actively in the care of a mental health professional at the time of death.

Substance abuse can occur as an attempt to medicate emotional pain. Alcohol and other depressant drugs depress the central nervous system. Depression of the central nervous system can lower inhibitions and impair judgment, making it more likely that an individual will act impulsively to end his or her life. Autopsy reports of suicide victims show that many of the victims were under the influence of alcohol or other drugs during the time shortly before they killed themselves.

Although females are about three times more likely to attempt suicide than males, males are four to five times more likely than females to actually complete suicide. In large part, this difference is because males choose more lethal methods for attempting suicide than do females. Males are more likely to choose shooting or hanging, whereas females are more likely to choose poisoning, overdose of pills, or other less lethal methods. A reason females may attempt suicide more frequently is that they use a suicide attempt as a way to communicate their feelings of desperation. Males, however, may be so ashamed of their feelings that they think they are better off dead than admitting to feeling so depressed or overwhelmed.

Situational Stressors

Situational stressors, such as family, school, employment stressors, and relationship problems, are often associated with suicide. These stressors are not the cause of the suicide but rather are triggers that make it likely the person will attempt suicide. Sometimes, people who have difficulties at home, at school, at work, or with law enforcement authorities see suicide as the only way out.

Many college students feel tremendous pressure to succeed academically, athletically, or socially. They may have experienced a major disappointment or loss, such as breaking up with a boyfriend or girlfriend, the death of a child or close family member, domestic problems, or large financial burdens. Most people are able to eventually resolve these difficulties, but those who have other risk factors, especially compounding stressors, depression, and/or substance abuse, may not have the coping skills to deal with their problems.

Access to Lethal Methods

A completed suicide is much more likely when a firearm is available in the home than when one is not. The reason is that gunshots are more likely to cause death than are other methods used to attempt suicide. In 2009, the CDC reported that 53 percent of all suicides were committed using a firearm (Karch, et al.). Combined with lethal weapons, distorted thoughts and impulsive behaviors can have deadly consequences. Guns are chosen as a suicide method more frequently by males than by females.

Previous Suicide Attempts

A suicide attempt increases the likelihood that a future attempt will result in a completed suicide, unless the person receives successful treatment to cope with the underlying emotional pain. Every attempt becomes a more significant risk factor in the chain of events leading to a completed suicide.

Exposure to Suicide of Others

The risk of completed suicide increases for an individual who has a family member or close friend who has attempted or completed suicide. Even a news report about a suicide or a movie that shows a fictional suicide can increase the probability of a suicide attempt

Did You Know...?

Suicide statistics may be significantly underreported. Families of suicide victims may try to avoid having the death classified as a suicide because they are ashamed or embarrassed or want to protect their family's privacy. Some medical examiners will classify a death as a suicide only if a suicide note is found, but notes are found in less than a third of all cases. Even law enforcement officers may classify a suicide by automobile as an accident. Medical personnel have created a word for these single-car "accidents," including those showing no skid marks on the pavement: *autocide.* When you combine all the opportunities for faulty reporting of suicides, it seems clear that confirmed suicides are only the tip of a large iceberg.

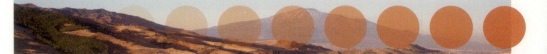

for individuals who already have other risk factors. Seeing or hearing about other people who choose suicide makes it seem like a reasonable solution for problems. What the victims don't comprehend at the time is that there are *always* options for solving problems other than suicide, even if they are not readily apparent.

Protective Factors

Just as there are factors that make it more likely a person will attempt or complete suicide, there are also factors that appear to act as protection against suicide attempts. Some of these protective factors may be genetic and unchangeable. But nongenetic factors, such as attitudes, behaviors, and environmental characteristics, can be changed. Developing a wellness lifestyle to include learning how to solve problems, control impulses, and resolve conflicts can help reduce family, school, work, and relationship problems before they reach the crisis point. Families and communities can provide support by ensuring access to mental health professionals when people become depressed or distressed. Friends can be part of the solution by knowing where to get help and keeping this information easily available in case they know someone who needs help. The restriction of easy access to lethal means, such as guns and pills that can be used for an overdose, can prevent impulsive deadly actions. Family, cultural, community, and religious beliefs that stress the value of life can influence attitudes about suicide. Recognizing and treating depression, substance abuse, and aggressive behavior can also help reduce the likelihood that a troubled person will consider suicide as a solution.

Warning Signs

There is no such thing as a typical suicide. Certain factors make people more vulnerable to suicide, and certain factors tend to protect against suicide. Even so, people of all ages, ethnic backgrounds, geographical locations, and socioeconomic conditions are represented in suicide statistics. There are some common warning signs exhibited by people who are going to attempt suicide. In fact, it is unusual for a person to attempt suicide without ever exhibiting any of the warning signs. Research indicates that the risk factors for non-fatal suicide attempts by adults include depression and other mental disorders, alcohol abuse, cocaine use, and separation or divorce. It is important to understand that a person who exhibits one of the warning signs is not necessarily suicidal. He or she may just be experiencing a high level of temporary stress. However, because the warning signs *can* be indications of a planned suicide attempt, you should learn to recognize them. These signs may be calls for help from someone who is suffering overwhelming emotional pain. Being aware of these signs can make the difference between life and death. These warning signs are described in Figure 4-13, and they are presented in more detail in the following sections.

Talking about Suicide

There is a common misconception that people who talk about suicide don't really do it. In fact, talking about suicide before actually attempting it is quite common. Talking about suicide may occur either directly or indirectly. An example of a direct comment is, "I wish I were dead." An example of an indirect comment is, "Things would be better if I just wasn't around anymore." Whether the comments are direct or indirect, anyone who talks about suicide should be taken seriously. Moreover, referencing the specific method to be used indicates a need for immediate help. Later in this chapter, we'll discuss what you should do if someone begins to talk about suicide.

Talking about suicide
- Direct comments
- Indirect comments

Behavioral changes
- Trouble eating and sleeping
- Withdrawing from friends or becoming unusually social
- Preoccupation with death and dying
- Losing interest in hobbies and activities
- Giving away cherished possessions

Emotional stressors
- Depression
- Rejection, loss, or humiliation
- Hopelessness

Delmar/Cengage Learning

FIGURE 4-13 • Warning signs of suicide.

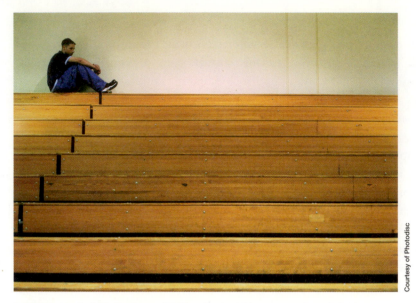

Courtesy of Photodisc

FIGURE 4-14 • Individuals who are thinking about suicide may experience behavior changes, such as withdrawing from friends and family.

Behavioral Changes

Individuals who are thinking of attempting suicide may have trouble eating or sleeping. Their normal behavior may change. If they are usually outgoing, they may withdraw from friends and social occasions (Figure 4-14). On the other hand, if they are normally a loner, they may become more social. They may lose interest in hobbies, work, school, or relationships. They may seem preoccupied with death and dying. Giving away possessions that are important to them can also be an indicator that they are thinking about suicide.

Emotional Stressors

Depression is one of the most common warning signs of suicide. When people are depressed, it's hard for them to believe that they'll ever feel any better. Severe loss, humiliation, or rejection can increase the risk for a suicide attempt, especially if the person is already emotionally distressed. If a loved one has recently died or the person has been rejected by a friend or romantic partner, feelings of hopelessness may trigger thoughts of suicide as a way to escape the emotional pain.

Did You Know…?

The highest rates of suicide actually occur among the elderly, particularly among older white males. Historically, men over the age of 75 have had significantly higher rates of suicide than the rates in the general population.

Preventing Suicide

Most people who attempt suicide are desperately crying out for help. It is common for them to give many clues and exhibit warning signs that they are considering suicide. They may not fully realize it, but they want help; they want someone to save them from themselves. Understanding the factors that can lead to suicide and being aware of the warning signs are the first steps to preventing it. Each of us can learn ways to help people we know who may be at risk. If you know or suspect someone who exhibits risk factors for suicide, there is something you can do. You can listen to them and help get them to a competent health professional as soon as possible.

What's News

There is no evidence that the tendency to commit suicide is inherited. However, according to the National Institute of Mental Health (2006), there is increasing evidence that major psychiatric illnesses, which can have an inherited component, increase the risk for suicide. Depression, bipolar disorder, schizophrenia, alcoholism, and substance abuse all tend to occur more frequently in some families than in others. Researchers have linked both depression and suicidal behavior to decreased levels of serotonin, a brain neurotransmitter. Understanding more about the biology of suicidal persons can help improve treatment and save lives.

If necessary, call 911, and be sure they have no access to weapons or drugs. You can make the difference between life and death for someone who is having thoughts of suicide. The following sections describe some actions to take to help a person who is threatening to attempt suicide.

What You Can Do

The person who wants to commit suicide is ultimately responsible for his or her own actions, but those of us who interact with him or her may have the opportunity to influence that person's actions. The following suggestions can help you be more aware of those around you who may be silently asking for help.

Communicate

Be willing to talk openly and nonjudgmentally. If a person begins to talk about suicide or wanting to die, there is no need for you to feel uncomfortable, embarrassed, or awkward. Sometimes we try to pretend that they are only joking, fearful that if we talk about suicide, the person will be more likely to actually do it. Experts recommend, however, that the best response is to talk openly about the situation.

Listen carefully and allow the person to express his or her feelings. Do not offer advice or try to convince the person that he or she is wrong and don't *ever* challenge a person to attempt suicide just to see if the person is serious. It's more effective to ask direct questions to learn about the person's thoughts and intentions:

- "Are you thinking of hurting or killing yourself?"

- "Have you thought about how you would do it?"

- "Do you have the means to do it?" (e.g., does the person have a gun or pills?)

- "Have you decided when you will do it?"

If the answer to all these questions is yes, the risk for a suicide attempt is extremely high, and you should take the following actions:

- Get professional help for the person immediately.

- Do not leave the person alone, even if he or she promises to get help.

- Don't say you won't tell anyone. Experts concur that many lives could be saved if only their friends would break the "code of silence" that exists.

Even if you have misjudged the seriousness of the situation, it is better to be safe than sorry. A life hangs in the balance.

Suggest Alternatives

People who are contemplating suicide are not able to think clearly and rationally. They may believe that they have no other option for ending the pain they are experiencing. Although it is true that time has a way of healing emotional pain, when the pain is intense, it can be very difficult to believe that things will get better.

Help the person identify other options for dealing with the situation. Ask the person to agree not to try to hurt or kill him- or herself without first talking with a professional. Delaying a decision can be very important because many suicide intentions are short lived. This tactic can buy valuable time to connect the person to skilled resources.

Connect the Person with Helping Resources

You can be supportive to someone who is hurting emotionally, but you probably don't have the skills needed to help a person who is suicidal. Encourage the individual to get professional help and offer to go with him or her. People in crisis are not always capable of taking action without support from someone else. If the situation is critical, call 911 immediately.

Most cities and towns have a suicide crisis hotline. The National Suicide Prevention lifeline number is 1-800-273-TALK (8255). Trained telephone counselors are available at this number 24 hours a day, seven days a week. This number can also be used to locate a suicide crisis center in your area. Offer to take your friend to the center where trained mental health professionals are available to work with people in crisis who may be thinking of suicide.

One of the ways you can help yourself and others avoid the pain and grief associated with a completed suicide is to take action ahead of time by developing resources to be used in a crisis situation. Just as having a first-aid kit can be a lifesaver in the event of an emergency, you can compile the information and resources you would want to have easily available in the event that you or someone close to you had thoughts or suicide attempts. Planning ahead can make a difference.

There are many ways you can try to help someone who is threatening suicide, but each person ultimately has responsibility for his or her own actions. If someone you know commits suicide, it is not your fault regardless of whether you did or did not try to help. It not uncommon to feel guilty or at fault if someone close to you commits suicide. In the grief at the person's death, it may be difficult to remember that you are not responsible for their actions. You may need to seek professional help if you are unable to accept the fact that it's not your fault.

> **WEB LINK**
> ## Suicide Prevention Resources
>
> For more information on suicide prevention, see the following Web sites:
>
> - American Foundation for Suicide Prevention: **http://www.afsp.org**
> - Suicide Awareness Voices of Education: **http://www.save.org**
> - Yellow Ribbon Suicide Prevention Program (preventing youth suicide): **http://www.yellowribbon.org**
>
> **SEARCH TERMS:** suicide prevention, suicide awareness

What Mental Health Professionals Can Do

Mental health professionals are trained to assess risk for suicide and to help potential victims manage the crisis until it passes. These professionals can arrange for medications, such as antidepressants, if appropriate. Because antidepressant drugs take a few weeks to become fully effective, it is sometimes necessary to refer the patient for inpatient hospital treatment until the immediate danger of a suicide attempt passes. Mental health professionals also use behavioral therapy techniques to help the person resolve the crisis. If you suspect that a person is thinking about taking his or her life, you should always ask that person to seek help from a mental health professional. If you knew someone had a broken leg, you would insist that he or she seek medical treatment. If you know someone with a broken spirit, that situation should not be treated any differently.

What Communities Can Do

Communities can establish support systems to assist people with depression and suicide. For example, they can set up programs to promote nonviolent conflict resolution and teach skills in problem solving. Community members can also work to ensure that adequate help from mental health professionals is available for all members of the community regardless of ability to pay and that community members know where to go to get this help.

Are You at Risk?

This section covered suicide in the United States, common warning signs for suicide, and ways to help a person who may be thinking about suicide. If you feel you may be at risk, take action to get help. Talk to someone you trust and tell that person you need help. Many people have thought about committing suicide at some time in their lives. Fortunately, most of them didn't act on their thoughts. They eventually came to realize that the crisis was temporary but that a choice of suicide would be permanent. Now more than ever, help *is* available for anyone considering taking his or her own life. You need not suffer alone. Get help *today*.

BUILDING YOUR LIFETIME WELLNESS PLAN

Many factors influence mental and emotional health. Some factors are genetic; others are the result of life experiences. Some people have developed a sound foundation for creating and maintaining good mental and emotional health. Others have already experienced some serious roadblocks or bumps in the road. The good news is that regardless of your past experiences, you can begin now to create a plan that contributes to mental and emotional wellness. As you begin to develop your wellness plan, you might want to begin with a realistic personal assessment of your emotional and mental assets at the present time. The following key points may help you reach that point:

- Monitor your feelings and reactions to stressful conditions.

- Identify the characteristics of mental and emotional health that you'd like to develop more fully.

- Explore ways you can make these improvements.

- Practice behaviors that maintain your general wellness level, such as eating well, exercising, and getting enough sleep.

- Know where mental health caregivers can be found and how to contact them.

●●● **End-of-Chapter Activities**

Opportunities for Application

1. Duplicate the table illustrated in Table 4-1 and add a fourth column labeled "healthy alternatives." Complete each of the cells in column 4, describing a more healthy way of dealing with the examples given for each defense mechanism.

2. If someone whom you knew exhibited signs and symptoms of a mental illness, what resources could you suggest for him or her? Describe how you would approach him or her to offer your help.

3. Identify the resources for suicide prevention that are available in your community. If you thought that someone you knew might be having thoughts of suicide, what would you do?

Key Concepts

1. Describe the characteristics that you possess that demonstrate good mental and emotional health. Describe the characteristics that you would like to develop to improve your mental and emotional health. How will you go about doing this?

2. Compare and contrast the characteristics of a mentally healthy person and an emotionally healthy person.

3. Explain what factors might help you identify a person who is considering suicide.

Answers to Personal Assessment: Mental and Emotional Health Quiz

1. Score one point if you agree with this statement. People who are mentally healthy see life events and behaviors without distortion.

2. Score one point if you agreed with this statement. Mentally healthy people do not hold prejudicial views.

3. Score one point if you disagreed with this statement. We all feel lonely at times. Of greater significance is if the loneliness develops into continued depression.

4. Score on point if you disagreed with this statement. As an adult, many circumstances will affect your personal identity; having children is an example.

5. Score one point if you disagreed with this statement. You need the help of a trained professional. Would you want to surgically remove your own cancerous tumor?

6. Score on point if you disagreed with this statement. They may in fact be just the opposite: quiet and withdrawn.

7. Score one point if you disagreed with this statement. Data indicate just the opposite: those who are depressed and considering suicide benefit from discussions with trusted people until they can get to a trained therapist.

8. Score one point if you agreed with this statement. A person who attempts to take his/her life is not acting in a healthy way.

9. Score one point if you disagreed with this statement. Having access to such devices can increase the likelihood of suicide.

10. Score one point if you disagreed with this statement. A potentially suicidal person can benefit from conversation with close family and friends.

If you scored more than 8 points on this assessment you already have a understanding of mental/emotional health issues. More importantly, if your correct answered were "strongly" in the right directions, your level of understanding is even better.

References

American Psychiatric Association. (2000). *Diagnostic and statistical manual of mental disorders* (4th ed., text revision). Arlington, VA: Author.

Centers for Disease Control and Prevention. (2006). *10 Leading causes of injury death by age group highlighting unintentional injury deaths, United States—2006.* National Vital Statistics System. Retrieved May 12, 2010, from http://www.cdc.gov/Injury/Images/LC-Charts/10lcUnintentional-Injury2006-bw-a.pdf

Goleman, D. (2005). *Emotional intelligence.* New York: Bantam Books.

Karch, D.L., et al.(2009). Surveillance for violent deaths—National violent death reporting system, 16 states, 2006. *MMWR Surveillance Summaries,* 58(ss01), 1-44.

National Institute of Mental Health. (2006). *Suicide in the U.S.: Statistics and prevention* (NIH Publication No. 06-4594). Bethesda, MD: Author. Retrieved October 2007, from http://www.nimh.nih.gov

National Institute of Mental Health. (2007). *Anxiety disorders.* Bethesda, MD: Author.

National Institute of Mental Health. (2009). *Suicide in the U.S.: Statistics and prevention.* Retrieved May 01, 2010, from http://www.nimh.nih.gov/health/publications/suicide-in-the-us-statistics-and-prevention/index.shtml

Seligman, M. (1998). *Learned Optimism: How to Change Your Mind and Your Life.* NY: New York: Simon and Schuster.

CHAPTER 5

Resolving Conflict

CHAPTER OBJECTIVES

When you finish this chapter, you should be able to:

- Describe why conflict can be considered either positive or negative.

- List and describe the difference between various levels of conflict.

- List and briefly describe several potential causes of conflict.

- Identify four broad sets of skills that support conflict resolution.

- Explain the difference between negotiation, compromise, and mediation.

- List and briefly describe the six general steps for resolving personal conflict.

- Create a personal wellness plan to assess and develop your conflict management skills.

KEY TERMS

boundaries	conflict	interpersonal conflict	negotiation
bullying	conflict resolution	intrapersonal conflict	tolerance
coercion	cyberbullying	mediation	
compromise	deterrence		

●●● Introduction

Experiencing conflict is a normal part of life. It is impossible to go through life without experiencing conflict on a regular basis. Conflict is not a bad thing, though that is the way many people perceive it. Many great things began as conflicts, only to pave the way for change that resulted in something truly exceptional. One example is the conflict that many English citizens, known as Puritans, had with religious doctrines of the Church of England. The Puritans felt that the Church had become too politicized. Unable to encourage the Church to change, the conflict led to the Puritans leaving England to settle in America. Whenever someone disagrees with us, a conflict is formed. The conflict is not bad, but how it is dealt with can be harmful.

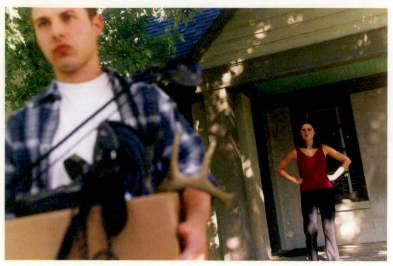

Courtesy of Photodisc

FIGURE 5-1 • Developing good conflict resolution skills will help you handle the conflicts that arise in your life.

Sometimes the conflict is with someone in your family or a partner in a romantic relationship. Sometimes it is with a coworker or someone else with whom you interact. More serious conflict can occur with legal authorities. You can even have conflict within yourself, such as when you feel confused when making an important decision or choosing to take on a new behavior. By developing an awareness of situations that are likely to cause conflict, you can prevent possible trouble and move toward a successful resolution of the conflict. If you learn and practice good conflict resolution skills, you will be prepared to handle minor and major conflicts in your life (Figure 5-1). In this chapter, you will learn what conflict is, how to recognize situations that might cause conflict, and what you can do to make sure you stay in control instead of letting your emotions or other people control you.

PERSONAL ASSESSMENT
Resolving Conflict

Before reading this chapter, take this personal assessment to discover more about the way you currently handle conflict. In the space provided, respond to the statements below on the basis of the way you respond **most** of the time. Rate your answers using the following scale: 1 = Definitely True, 2 = Mostly True, 3 = Mostly False, or 4 = Definitely False. An interpretation of your results is located at the end of the chapter.

1. I avoid conflict whenever possible.

2. I think I'm pretty good at handling conflict with my supervisors at work.

3. I don't think I'm very good at handling conflict with my peers.

4. If I have a conflict with someone, I can usually resolve it by talking with the person about it.

5. I often give in to someone else rather than face an argument or disagreement.

6. I stand up for what I believe in, even if doing so might cause an argument or disagreement.

7. There are very few things I believe are worth an argument or disagreement.

8. If I can't resolve a problem with someone by myself, I ask others for help.

9. I often respond to a confrontation with someone by getting angry.

10. If I get angry with someone, I give myself time to cool down before approaching the person.

● ● ● Understanding Conflict

Conflict is a struggle that results from incompatible or opposing interests, values, needs, or desires. Conflict can occur whenever two or more people or groups view a situation differently. Conflict is a normal part of adult life as well as a critical element of a person's growth and development. In the Mandarin Chinese language, similar characters are used to represent *crisis* and *opportunity* (Figure 5-2). Many people, especially those who are in tune with conflict management, believe that a crisis also presents an opportunity for growth. The same is true for conflict. Situations resulting in conflict present opportunities to expand your knowledge and improve your ability to see multiple sides of issues. A certain amount of conflict is necessary for us to learn and develop emotionally and socially. The problem is not that a conflict occurs. Rather, the problem results when the parties involved are not able to resolve the conflict in a mutually satisfying way. The way conflict is handled is often the key to whether it has a positive or a negative outcome.

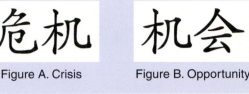

危机	机会
Figure A. Crisis	Figure B. Opportunity

Delmar/Cengage Learning

FIGURE 5-2 • Mandarin Chinese characters representing crisis and opportunity.

conflict
a struggle caused by incompatible or opposing interests, values, needs, or desires

Forms of Conflict

Conflict can occur at many levels. It is easy for us to recognize periods of conflict when we are personally involved. But with our personal perceptions and attitudes, we can become blinded to what is going on in the world around us. The following sections define the various levels of conflict and describe the dynamics that contribute to causing and alleviating conflict.

Intrapersonal Conflict

Have you ever felt as if you were in conflict with yourself? Most likely, your feelings were accurate. This is called **intrapersonal conflict**. It can happen when you have contradictory feelings about a situation, a decision, or other issue, and it can happen no matter what your age. For example, an intrapersonal conflict might occur if you really want to accept an invitation to a party but you have already agreed to go to a movie with a friend. You want to go to the party, but you don't want to hurt your friend's feelings. The other people involved might not even be aware of your conflict, but the conflict exists for you. If you decide to accept the party invitation and back out of your commitment to go to the movie, your friend might get angry with you. On the other hand, if you go to the movie, the person who invited you to the party might be upset with you for not coming.

It may sound strange, but being able to resolve intrapersonal conflict requires certain skills. To begin with, you need to be comfortable with your own "self-talk," meaning that your underlying thought process should contain an optimistic tone. A pessimistic thought process prevents you from being open to developing a healthy response to your conflict. In addition, you should possess good decision-making skills. Being able to see both sides of a dilemma is an asset to developing a value-creating resolution to the conflict.

intrapersonal conflict
confusion or struggle within yourself

Interpersonal Conflict

Continuing with the previously mentioned example, what happens when you tell those who invited you to the party about your decision to go to the movie? At this point, you might find yourself involved in an **interpersonal conflict**, a conflict with another

interpersonal conflict
disagreement or argument between persons or groups

Did You Know...?

Experts agree that conflict is a positive aspect of life. If you never experienced conflict, life would probably be pretty boring. Humans need to face challenges so that they can learn and develop physically, emotionally, and socially. Handling conflict effectively is a fundamental competency needed for healthy relationships.

person or individual members of a group. Interpersonal conflicts can occur with family members, peers, people you are acquainted with through school or work, and sometimes even strangers. How we respond to interpersonal conflict varies with a number of factors, such as our emotional state at the time, the intensity of the issue relating to the conflict, and the person with whom we have the conflict. We respond and are treated differently when our conflict is with someone close to us, such as a caring family member, a spouse, or a good friend. People such as coworkers, sales clerks, and people we meet in public care less about our needs than our close friends and family members. Perhaps the most important consideration when negotiating conflict, regardless of the opposition, is the underlying assumption that *both parties* must take the position that resolving the conflict is in their mutual best interest.

Family Conflict

Family conflict is inevitable. All human organizations, be they political bodies, corporations, athletic teams, governing boards, tribes, and so on, all encounter opportunities deriving from conflict, and families are no exception. Family conflict can occur for any number of reasons. Almost two decades of research on this topic has clarified one thing, namely, that familial behavior problems and social deviance are rooted in dysfunctional, problematic family conflict. The behaviors of children in the family are directly related to the quality of parenting. Many parents raise their children by the manner in which they were raised. If their family dynamic was dysfunctional, they will bring that model to their own family—unless they learn new strategies. Failure to develop value-creating strategies will only perpetuate ill-defined behaviors into future generations.

There are a number of qualities that characterize a family unit. Effective parenting creates children who feel good and comfortably protected. This in turn makes parenting easier because of the relational bond between parent and child. The family expresses cohesion, where family members are respected and nurtured and everyone is unified to advance the image of the family unit. Another quality of the family is the balance of power. During childhood, children need to be nurtured, protected, and have their physical needs cared for. At that time, it is easier for the parents to "parent" because they "have the power." The problem with this model is that children are not well prepared with the transition to their own independence. When the child becomes an adolescent and develops the need for independence, a power struggle develops between parent and child because the child has not been permitted to transition into independence with a sense of empowerment to be a member of a cohesive unit.

Assuming that the family unit includes children, the physical and psychological health of the family unit rests with the parents. Both parents must have the necessary qualities and skills to raise the children in an environment that empowers the kids with a sense of security, trust, and appropriate level of independence. The parents need to cultivate a family structure that inoculates the children from the social threats they may be exposed to as they pass through their school years. For whatever reason, if the parents don't feel prepared to raise their children in this manner, it is advisable for the parents to consult some parenting self-help texts or use their health literacy skills to obtain some

For this strategy to work, all family members need to feel they are respected and have something to contribute to the discussion. This technique should be introduced to the family unit as soon as the children can understand a problem-solving process.

Surface the problem. The parent/moderator introduces the general overview of the apparent problem. Then give each person in the family the opportunity to present their view of the problem.

Every family member should listen carefully to the views presented. Write down significant items. Don't allow anyone to interrupt the speaker during this phase. Continue until the group has clearly stated the problem.

Brainstorm solutions. This means anyone stating anything that comes to mind Don't analyze the solutions now. Just write them all down.

Go through the list of possible solutions to narrow them down to the best solution for all family members. To assure this, use the technique in step one to allow each person's view on what is the best solution for everyone.

Select the best solution. Get commitments from each person that they will help make the solution work.

Decide what each person will do to implement the solution. Children can help identify responsibilities, rewards, limits, consequences, and other agreed upon commitments.

Delmar/Cengage Learning

FIGURE 5-3 • Family conflict management strategy.

appropriate child-rearing advice. The skills children need to address life's problems and potential conflict in and out of the family must begin in childhood, not during adolescence. There are strategies parents can use to develop some of the qualities in their children; one is presented in Figure 5-3.

Group Conflict

Conflict doesn't just occur between two individuals who can't agree on a particular issue. Differences occur between and among organizations, communities, religious groups, political groups, and even entire nations. Sometimes we feel as if we are in conflict with people we don't even know. Racial animosity, religious violence, and misdirected feelings among political rivals are all examples of conflict between groups. Disagreements among coworkers and teammates would exemplify within-group conflicts.

Within-Group Conflict

Much of our professional experiences are likely to involve group work. You may even experience group activities as part of your educational experiences. With all the opportunities available for group work, there are bound to be occasions when differences of opinion will arise. Understanding the dynamics of group conflict may help you get through the tensions that come with the conflict and allow you to use the conflict as a constructive force. Research indicates that the main sources of conflict in work groups are the following:

- *Miscommunication and misinformation.* Communication is important to all business enterprises. Because business and clients are made of people, communication is essential. In our current business environments, employees and clients demand timely and well-presented information. Miscommunication occurs when messages are not constructed and delivered properly. Misinformation results when the messages that are delivered do not contain the correct information or when important elements are omitted.

- *Differences in individual needs and personal priorities.* The differences that exist among the individuals forming the work groups may be varied. People have different opinions and have their own motives for attempting to press for their own point of view.

- *Real or imaginary psychological differences.* There may be real differences among participants on any number of psychological characteristics, such as cultural factors, beliefs, attitudes, and so on.

- *Structural factors.* Structural factors are those conditions in the environment or the meeting logistics that can pave the way for conflict. An example would be a company having a vague or incomplete pathway for communications between employees and supervisors or among supervisors.

It is inevitable that conflict will arise within a group. Once the conflict is identified, it will begin to affect group performance. In that regard, researchers Thomas and Kilmann (1974) have identified five basic approaches for managing the conflict. These five approaches are based on two dimensions: assertiveness and cooperation. In Figure 5-4, you can see how these dimensions interact to form the five approaches according to the levels of assertiveness and cooperation. Given the five approaches and what you know about cooperation and competition, which of the five do you think is the most productive? It would be surprising if you were to choose "avoidance." While it may be a common approach that many people use, it can't lead to a successful resolution to the source of the conflict. If you answered "collaboration," you are correct. If your choice was "compromising," you chose an okay but not a good selection. What separates the two choices is not just the resolution of the conflict but also the type of process involved to get to the resolution. On the surface, compromising seems like a balanced approach to a solution. The problem is that when a compromise becomes the course of action, it means that one party did not get the solution that he or she was looking for. The result is that in a subsequent conflict, that party will be in a weak negotiating position because the compromise went to the other party. The better approach is for both parties to work cooperatively toward a solution that becomes the "third alternative" from the original two positions.

One of the challenges in group settings is being able to negotiate effectively. Negotiation is a process whereby two or more people with differing needs and goals work to develop an acceptable solution to the matter being discussed. Negotiation is a skill that can be learned, but it should be noted that there are personal barriers that may prevent successful negotiation. For example, some people view negotiation as confrontational and take the position that it should be avoided. Negotiation does not have to

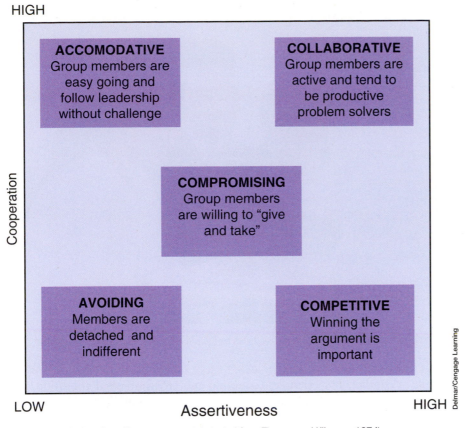

HIGH

Cooperation

ACCOMODATIVE
Group members are easy going and follow leadership without challenge

COLLABORATIVE
Group members are active and tend to be productive problem solvers

COMPROMISING
Group members are willing to "give and take"

AVOIDING
Members are detached and indifferent

COMPETITIVE
Winning the argument is important

LOW   Assertiveness   HIGH

Delmar/Cengage Learning

FIGURE 5-4 • Styles of conflict management (adapted from Thomas and Kilmann, 1974).

be confrontational, nor should it ever be avoided. In fact, the real purpose of negotiation is to find the solution that is best for all parties, *not* to ensure that one position is in a *winning* position. If someone approaches conflict in this manner, for every winner, there must be at least one loser.

Another barrier to negotiating is bringing your emotions to the table. It is okay to be passionate about your position, but it is very important to keep your emotions in check so as to present your point of view in a constructive way. Finally, it is helpful to understand your opponent in the conflict. Try to understand who your opponent is and get a sense of his or her needs and wants. If you find you don't care for that person, you will be more successful if you refrain from focusing on his or her personality. Keep your focus on the issue at hand. Don't argue with your opponent. Remember that negotiating is about finding solutions to a problem, not proving the other person wrong (Figure 5-5).

Community Conflict

The potential for community conflict exists whenever and wherever individuals are in contact with one another. The magnitude of the conflict will vary depending on the conflicting situations and the level of anger that arises. There are a number of circumstances

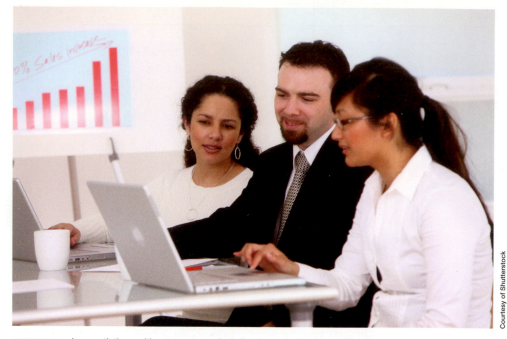

Courtesy of Shutterstock

FIGURE 5-5 • In negotiations with a person you don't like, focus on the issue at hand rather than the individual.

that contribute to conflict. For example, economic and environmental conditions can raise stress levels among those people most impoverished, especially if those people feel that their needs are not being met by the community or state. Community conflict also can occur when individuals or groups perceive or experience discriminatory behavior directed at them by an agency or its representative, by members of another group, or by members of their own group. Perceived police brutality directed to a member of a particular community group can raise anger that sometimes becomes misdirected and violent. Healthy communities are those that work together to prevent potential conflicts and/or address conflict quickly and fairly.

Community Conflict: Gangs

One of the current noteworthy aspects of community conflict is gangs. The word "gang" is likely to bring up many connotations and stereotypes for people depending on where they live. Names like "Mara Salvatrucha or M-13," "Bloods," and "Crips" have become familiar in some cities, especially when discussing community-based conflicts. Since most gang members are not born into gangs, it is a choice that has become an option for many young people in the United States. A gang can be described as a specific collection of individuals who organize themselves and exclude other people, have a group name, a specific territory, and regularly participate in criminal and/or antisocial behavior. Gangs bring community tensions between the gang members and rival gangs, confrontations with law enforcement, and threats to the personal property and physical well-being of community citizens. There is also the stress associated with possible recruitment of family members into gang activity.

The issue of gangs is not a new one. Gangs have been noted throughout recorded history. The phenomenon is relatively new to the United States. They were a part of American society as early as the late 1800s and very prevalent in the 1920s. Most American gangs emerged from social ethnic groups, such as Irish, Italian, and Jewish immigrants, and have evolved to include those that represent Hispanics and African Americans. The ethnic gangs banded together for protection, social events, and monetary gain. In fact, research shows that gangs are the number one venue for distributing drugs throughout the country. There are many reasons why a young person might be attracted to joining a gang. In his book, *Gangbusters: Strategies for Prevention and Intervention* (1998), Lonnie Jackson (1998) identified many factors that contribute to the increasing prevalence of gang youth. Factors include early exposure to crime and violence, lack of positive role models, lack of parental control, living in communities with lower socioeconomic conditions and few social or recreational activities, a sense of hopelessness or lack of self-esteem about the future, and a sense of feeling powerless. Another very compelling lure for young people is the need to feel physical security, a place to belong, and an opportunity to form emotional connections. Unfortunately for many young people, gang membership becomes a substitute for a family dynamic that they so desperately long for. Social scientists have also noted that gangs are a social indicator that communities are not well organized or are disenfranchised to a level that is out of control by local institutions.

There is a considerable amount of conflict surrounding gang activities. Research indicates that gangs often form initially as social groups, such as a break-dancing social club, and eventually get to where they band together or are recruited to gangs for protection against rival gangs. Thus, there is conflict between rival gangs for territory and respect. Gang activity tends to have a terroristic effect on the local community because gang members engage in antisocial activity in the local community in order to obtain money and stolen property that they can use to fund gang activities and drug purchases. In turn, conflict develops as community agencies (police, city councils, and so on) develop and implement gang prevention strategies.

While there are gangs in rural areas, the 2006 National Youth Gang Survey from the U.S. Department of Justice (Egley and O'Donnell, 2008) found that, for the most part, gangs, gang membership, and gang-related homicides are concentrated mainly in larger cities. It is estimated that there are at least 785,000 gang members affiliated with approximately 26,500 gangs in the United States. In 2007, 23% of students reported the presence of gangs in their schools (Department of Education, 2008). Gang attacks can be anything from machete attacks, gang raping or other forms of sexual assault, car theft, drug trafficking, or vandalism, depending on the region of the country and how well established the gang is the specific community.

While the majority of gang members are males, in the past decade there has been a significant increase of young women joining gangs. Research has been done to identify

What's News

A report by the National Alliance of Gang Investigators Associations (2005) described the status of gang activity and prevention across the country. One of the significant findings was that approximately 31 percent of survey respondents indicated that their communities refused to acknowledge the gang problem. Many of those communities only began to address gang issues when high-profile gang-related incidents occurred.

the specific pushes of young women into gangs. Most female gangs start out as auxiliary entities to male gangs. It has been suggested that young women, especially of ethnic minority groups, who are drawn to gangs are rejecting traditional social norms that have been placed on them because of their gender, such as passivity, femininity, and loyalty. Instead, they have embraced the individualistic mentality that is intrinsic in U.S. society and chosen to attach themselves to a gang to somehow advance their situation in life. For these girls, the gangs represent a place where they will experience true friendship, loyalty, protection, and understanding. Those assets are so attractive to some young women who might not have these aspects in any other part of their lives that they are willing to be beaten up as part of the initiation to the gang or risk their lives to defend other gang members. For some young women, it also means separating themselves from their families.

Sometimes, in the initial formation of a gang in a community, it might be difficult to detect gang activity or differentiate between a group of friends hanging out and gang activity. Some gangs place value on the adherence to certain rituals or rules, while other gangs are more concerned with clothing, colors, and symbols, all of which are associated with social identity. Often gangs will use mood-altering substances such as alcohol and illegal drugs or inhalants, but the most consistent indicator of a gang is the violence that they perpetuate.

For many years, youth advocates, law enforcement officials, school administrators, and religious leaders have formed coalitions and task forces to address the increase in gangs and to counteract the negative influences that gangs have in a community. Similar to other social ills, before a problem can truly be addressed, it must first be understood. To be entirely effective in addressing such a widespread phenomenon, experts on gangs seem to agree that there are certain tenets that must be in place to prevent future gang membership, help someone leave a gang, or address the key societal issues that make gang membership so attractive.

Similar to the D.A.R.E. (Drug Abuse Resistance Education) prevention program that became so popular in the 1980s, there are many gang prevention programs that target middle school learners. Since most gang members join a gang between the ages of 12 and 15, it is important to reach them before this time period. These prevention efforts attempt to reach learners before they are involved in gangs and address the risk factors that might lead to gang membership. The programs also attempt to change attitudes that youth might have about law enforcement. The Office of Juvenile Justice and Delinquency Prevention, through the U.S. Department of Justice, is implementing a Gang Reduction and Intervention Program in neighborhoods that have high rates of crime and gang activity. The program's success is based on activities relating to prevention, street outreach and interventions, suppression of gangs by law enforcement and community-based groups, and reentry activities that help gang members become self-sufficient outside their gang membership.

One specific example of the seriousness of gang activity is in Los Angeles, California, where the prevalence of gangs has increased in the past 20 years. The California Association of Human Relations Organizations (CAHRO) is working on conflict resolution between gangs and for individual members. The CAHRO believes an important asset to conflict resolution is to have mentors whom gang members can trust and identify with so that conflict resolution can be achieved. Gang members must feel that they can trust the mentors and know that they will listen. CAHRO has found that many of the gang members with whom they work want to be treated with respect from law enforcement officials, have a safe place to hang out, find employment, and not be pressured to drop out of the

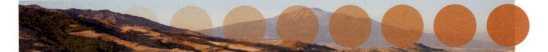

What's Your View?

In the country of El Salvador, home of one of the largest gangs in the world, the Mara Salvatrucha, or M-13 , a temporary law was passed stating that anyone displaying a gang tattoo will be arrested. Would a similar law in the United States help the increasing problem with gangs? What do you think?

gang. It is the hope of CAHRO that, through dialogue and meeting the needs previously mentioned, the need to stay in the gang will diminish over time as other opportunities open up for the youth.

International Conflict

The ultimate level of conflict is exhibited when countries engage in conflict. For some, the conflict emerges as individuals within a country are in conflict with individuals in another country, such as the ongoing conflict between the Israelis and the Palestinians; other circumstances have one country attempting to take over another country for political reasons, as was the case when Iraq invaded Kuwait.

These international conflicts are disagreements concerning nationalistic values, that is, issues or territory, regional dominance, or resources (natural and otherwise). Generally, these conflicts are limited in time and scope, but there are those that last for generations, as is the case of the Israeli/Palestinian conflict. In the initial phase, countries will use **deterrence** to threaten a country with sanctions or war in an effort to gain some form of compliance. This was the basis of the Cold War philosophy between the United States and Russia between 1947 and the early 1990s. The two powers engaged in political and social activities to become world superpowers. Deterrence was also employed by President John F. Kennedy during the Cuban missile crisis in the early 1960s. Cuba was threatened with war if it did not convince the Russians to remove their missiles from Cuba.

Although deterrence is one method of addressing conflict, nations often resort to armed conflict to achieve their objectives. On the surface, war seems like an appropriate alternative to many, but experiments in social psychology have long shown that armed conflict generally leads to escalation of hostility, regardless of the outcome.

deterrence
the use of threats by one party to intimidate another party from exercising a particular behavior

●●● Creation of Conflict

Conflict usually occurs because one or both parties in the conflict are not getting their needs met. There are numerous sources of conflict, just as there numerous situations where we may encounter conflict, be it with coworkers, colleagues, family members, neighbors, significant others, and so on. The following list of characteristics tends to exacerbate conflict:

1. *Poor communication.* Not having good information, written or verbal, is one source of conflict. Information may be lacking because other people withhold

information, give incorrect information, or communicate in a way that we do not understand their meaning.

2. *Relationship issues.* Distrust may evolve as the relationship progresses. One person may make false statements or not follow through on commitments. Stereotypes and misperceptions will interfere with good communication. It is also difficult to resolve conflict if the other person can't be counted on to avoid conditions that create conflict.

3. *Structural factors.* The competition for resources may be a source of conflict. This competition is born out of needs we and the people around us have. Under certain conditions, one party may have the majority of power in the relationship, such as a supervisor with whom you have a conflict, or in a marital relationship where one spouse produces the lion's share of the income.

4. *Conflicting values.* People may have different ideologies or life views. It is not uncommon for people to have different life experiences and/or psychological states that influence the criteria used to evaluate ideas.

When you were a child playing with other children, someone may have taken your favorite toy. Feeling frustrated, you may have cried and screamed until an adult came to your aid and corrected the situation by teaching you how to use words to express yourself and negotiate a solution. In some instances, you may have responded physically by shoving the other child away or hitting him or her. The outcome of either behavior was that you probably got your toy back. Crying, screaming, and hitting might work for infants and toddlers, but such behaviors do not work well for adults (Figure 5-6). As most people mature, they find out that there are healthier ways to solve conflicts. Individuals learn that there are better, more effective and socially acceptable methods of getting one's

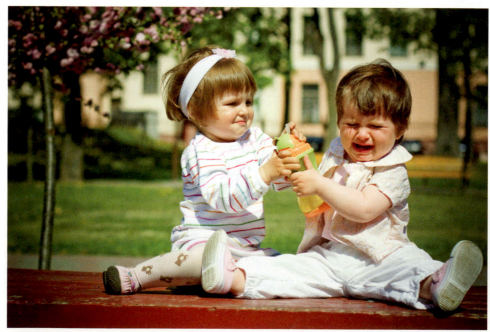

FIGURE 5-6 • Crying, screaming, and hitting may be a young child's only tools for getting what he or she wants, but they are not effective tools for conflict resolution.

needs met. Unfortunately, there are some people who never advance past the toddler stage in learning to resolve problems. They still use some form of **coercion** to get what they want. Coercive behaviors include psychological manipulation, such as withholding affection or presenting a threat, and sometimes it may be direct physical force such as shoving, hitting, or using other forms of violence. But "winning" in this manner is likely to feel like an empty victory because no one feels truly satisfied with the outcome except the individual who was successful in coercing the outcome.

Bullying

One particular type of coercion that happens more overtly among children and teens than among adults is bullying. **Bullying** is the use of threats or force by one person or group to intimidate another person or group. Bullying can be something as simple as making fun of someone or trying to intimidate another person in a restaurant or at a social event. Bullying often occurs when there is an imbalance of strength, power, or prestige.

An emerging form of bullying is that of **cyberbullying**. Research indicates that almost one-third of young people have experienced some form of cyberbullying. Moreover, teachers have reported being cyberbullied by students and/or parents. Cyberbullies are perhaps the most deceitful of bullies because the technology offers them a degree of anonymity. They do not have to look their victims in the eye; they think they are untraceable. With current technology, however, it is possible to trace the source of the bullying messages to a particular computer or cellular phone.

If ignored, bullying can lead to violent acts that result in physical injury or serious emotional damage. Many elementary schools now have programs designed to teach learners who bully other children how socially unacceptable it is to bully others in hopes of preventing bullying behavior. Although bullying is most common in childhood and adolescence, there is evidence that when bullying is allowed early in life, the learned behavior is then repeated throughout later life. Even whole countries have been accused of bullying behavior. The use of threat or force by a large, powerful nation to intimidate a smaller, less powerful nation is an example of bullying on a large scale.

coercion
the use of physical or psychological threat or force to obtain a desired outcome

bullying
the use of threats or force by one person or group to intimidate another person or group

cyberbullying
the use of electronic information and communication technologies, such as the Internet or text messaging, to harass and intimidate

WEB LINK
Bullying
http://www.bullying.org
http://www.dontlaugh.org
These Web sites focus on avoiding bullying from the earliest ages and provide general information in a user-friendly format that can be helpful to parents and educators as well as children.
SEARCH TERMS: bullying, coercion, intimidation

What's News

In a landmark study, the Workplace Bullying Institute and Zogby International completed the first national study of workplace bullying (2007). Among the key findings reported in the study, 37% of the respondents said they had experienced bullying in the workplace, and that the vast majority of bullies (72 %) were bosses. Moreover 62% of the employers tended to ignore the problem. Approximately 45% of the targeted individuals reported stress related health problems.

TABLE 5-1 • Facts and myths about bullying.

Myth	Fact
"Bullying is just stage; a normal part of life."	Bullying is not "normal" or socially acceptable behavior. We give bullies power by our acceptance of this behavior.
"People are born bullies."	Bullying is a learned behavior, and behaviors can be changed.
"If I tell someone, it will just make it worse."	Research shows that bullying will stop when adults in authority and peers get involved.
"Just stand up for yourself and hit them back."	While there are some times when people can be forced to defend themselves, hitting back usually makes the bullying worse and increases the risk for serious physical harm.
"Bullying is a school problem; the teachers should handle it."	Bullying is a broader social problem that often happens outside of schools, on the street, at shopping centers, at the local pool, at summer camp, and in the adult workplace.

Source: Adapted from http://www.bullying.org.

Recognizing Potential Conflicts

Many types of life events have the potential for conflict. In general, the likelihood of conflict is highest when people feel strongly about their issues When an issue isn't very important to someone, they are likely to give in or work toward a solution, even if it means not getting everything they wanted. But if the issue involves something very important to people, they are likely to have strong emotions about the issue. These emotions can interfere with one's ability to see different points of view. People may be blind to certain solutions because they can see the solution from only their own point of view. This narrow perspective makes it very hard to find pathways to conflict resolution.

At the most personal level, conflicts often arise when your feelings have been hurt or when you feel there is no way you can accept the way another person feels or thinks. In these situations, you may feel overwhelmed by anger, sadness, loneliness, or rejection. Using creative ways to express your emotions—such as writing in a journal, drawing sketches, painting pictures, dancing, or listening to music—can help you release your emotions and see and think more clearly. Then you can reframe the situation and see it in more neutral, less emotional terms. You may also find comfort and support if you have a good friend you can speak with about the conflict.

Strong feelings you are unwilling to change are one cause of conflict. Some other common causes are unequal levels of power and status, different points of view, and miscommunication.

Power and Status

Often, the desire to establish power or gain status is a source of conflict. Feeling in control of your life and circumstances you encounter is a very important component of mental and emotional health. Sometimes your need to be in control is so strong that you resort to negative behaviors to establish a position of power and dominance. Have you ever wanted to do something just so other people would pay attention to you or look up to you? Status gives you a positive reputation among your peers and results in feelings of importance. Any threat to the satisfaction of those needs can be a cause for conflict.

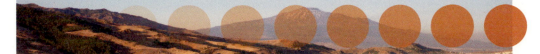

What's Your View?

When conflict occurs, those involved in the conflict have to decide on an appropriate course of action. This is especially true if the conflict is a serious one, such as a bullying relationship. There are some who believe that it's important to stand up against the bully and fight. Other people think that the parties involved should attempt to resolve differences peacefully. What are your feelings about a situation like this? What approach would you advise?

The first step to resolving conflicts is to be aware of the underlying, unmet needs of the people involved, including you. In fact, after thinking it over, you may decide that your needs for power and control in a particular situation are hurting you rather than helping you.

Perception and Point of View

Even people who are very much like you don't always share your perceptions of certain issues. Or they may disagree with you about what action to take in a particular situation. When you consider the vast diversity of our world today, it isn't surprising that people and groups have different perceptions and points of view.

Tolerance means promoting respect for differences and appreciating diversity. Tolerance doesn't mean that you give up your own views. It simply means that you understand and respect the fact that other people have opinions that are different from your own. Tolerance means being open minded enough to try to find common ground between yourself and persons with whom you disagree instead of insisting that everyone agree with you.

tolerance
respect for people whose beliefs and practices differ from yours

Miscommunication

Despite your best efforts to clearly communicate your thoughts and feelings, misunderstandings do occur. You can decrease the likelihood of communication misunderstandings by learning and practicing effective speaking and listening skills. Some of these communication skills are discussed in chapter 4. You can also become aware of your own personal emotional triggers. These triggers are words, behaviors, and attitudes that "push your buttons" and cause responses out of proportion to the incident. If you can recognize these "buttons," you can take deliberate steps to be especially calm and careful with your communication when the buttons are pushed.

WEB LINK
Southern Poverty Law Center
http://www.tolerance.org

This organization seeks to fight hate and promote tolerance. Although there is a strong focus on the educational setting, there are resources here that are useful to all ages. You can even take some self-assessments to help identify hidden biases that may prevent tolerance.

SEARCH TERMS: tolerance, social justice

●●● Experiencing Conflict

As we have stated before, conflict is a normal part of life, and this is particularly true during your college years. Perhaps you are in the process of becoming more independent of your family and making more independent choices or are struggling with some of the choices you have yet to make, or perhaps you are required to make some choices on behalf of your family. Independence and decision making can be sources of both interpersonal and intrapersonal conflict. You may find yourself getting into arguments with parents, friends, or family members about your choices even when you aren't sure yourself what choices you want to make. Your social relationships may cause you both interpersonal and intrapersonal conflict. And your own changing viewpoints and values may result in conflict both with other people and within yourself.

You may experience more conflict when you're not feeling well, physically, emotionally, or socially. When you're feeling bad, it's tempting to take it out on those around you. Of course, lashing out doesn't solve the problem. It usually ends up making you feel worse instead of better. When you're not feeling well, you may also have less patience and tolerance than normal. Things that usually wouldn't bother you become annoying. During these times, other people may accuse you of "blowing things out of proportion" or "making mountains out of molehills." Later, when you're feeling better, you may even come to the conclusion that they were right!

Here's a brief acronym to help you remember to check in with yourself before you get involved in an unnecessary conflict with someone else when the core problem may really be within yourself. HALT:

- *Hungry.* Have you eaten healthy foods recently, or are you hungry or subsisting on a diet of sugar and caffeine? Fluctuations in blood sugar can make you feel out of sorts and easily irritated in situations that you would normally be able to handle just fine.

- *Angry.* Is the situation triggering some type of underlying anger in you that exists under the surface, out of your conscious awareness? Is your anger clearly related to the current situation, or is it possible that it has roots in experiences of the past or fear of the future? Regardless, it is almost never a good idea to try to resolve conflict when you are really angry. Give yourself time to cool off and think more clearly before trying to resolve the problem.

- *Lonely.* How are you feeling emotionally? Are you getting along well with others in your life, or are you feeling disconnected? Is your emotional state affecting the way you feel about the current situation?

- *Tired.* How much restful sleep have you had recently? Are you well rested, or have you been pushing yourself too hard to do too much? Even when we aren't consciously aware of being sleep deprived, it can affect the way we feel—and the way we respond to stressful situations.

●●● Approaches to Conflict

When you find yourself in a situation in which conflict is likely to occur, there are three possible approaches you can take to resolve it. These are often called "win-win," "win-lose," and "lose-lose." Let's consider a typical conflict using each of these three approaches. Suppose that Robert and Juan have been assigned to work together on a project in history. They really didn't know each other very well before beginning the project. They have gotten along okay so far, but Juan feels as if he has been doing most of the work. He decides to tell Robert how he feels (Figure 5-7).

Win-Win

In a win-win (both parties win) approach, Juan wants to accomplish his purpose—to get Robert to do more of the work—but he doesn't want to make Robert angry or hurt him. Juan wants Robert to contribute more to the project, and he wants to get a good grade on the project. He might say, "Hey, Robert. I've been working really hard on this project because I want to get a good grade. But I need your help. We have to work on this together so that when we present our project, our presentation will go well. That way we'll both get a good grade. When can you and I get together to plan our presentation?" If this request is presented in a positive way, Robert is more likely to cooperate. The attempt is made to create a situation where both participants gain from doing the work.

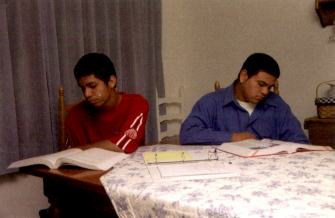

FIGURE 5-7 • When approaching conflict resolution, look for a win-win approach.

Win-Lose

In a win-lose approach, one person wins, and the other loses. This method is often used when one of the parties takes an extremely competitive approach. If Juan were to use this approach, he wouldn't care if Robert gets angry or hurt in the process. In a win-lose approach, Juan might tell the teacher that Robert hasn't done any work on the project and doesn't deserve credit for the project. Maybe the teacher will agree, and Juan will get a good grade without Robert's input. But if Juan denies Robert a chance to contribute more before Juan approaches the teacher, this could lead to an ugly confrontation between Juan and Robert and almost certainly would hurt Robert.

Lose-Lose

People don't approach a conflict situation intending to lose. A lose-lose outcome (both parties lose) is evidence that neither person had the skills to find a good solution to the problem. This condition would occur if both parties were intensely competitive and unwilling to collaborate on a solution. Suppose that Juan tells Robert that he had better do his part of the project, "or else." Robert gets mad and tells Juan that he can't make him do anything. This remark makes Juan angry, and he decides to walk out on the project. Not only has more trouble been created, but the original problem still hasn't been solved.

●●● Conflict Resolution

Some problems can be resolved rather easily; others are extremely difficult to resolve. But all problems have the potential for resolution if the parties involved are seriously committed to seeking a solution instead of simply trying to win. When people are genuinely interested in solving a problem, they have the opportunity to employ **conflict resolution** skills to create win-win outcomes. Conflict resolution is a structured problem-solving process that uses reflective awareness, communication skills, problem-solving skills, and decision-making skills to prevent, manage, and peacefully resolve conflicts.

conflict resolution
a structured problem-solving process that uses reflective awareness, communication skills, problem-solving skills, and decision-making skills to prevent, manage, and peacefully resolve conflicts

The basic skills needed to resolve conflict at the group level are the same skills needed to resolve problems between individuals. However, the more complex the conflict and the greater the number of people involved in the conflict, the more challenging it is to use these skills effectively. Practicing the use of conflict resolution skills at the individual level with daily conflicts can help you improve your skills. If you ever need to use these skills in a complex conflict that involves a lot of people, you will be better prepared.

In a conflict, one person weakly committed to win-win problem solving may label the other party as the enemy. But identifying the other party as an enemy eliminates many possible options for resolving the conflict. It is likely to end in either a win-lose or a lose-lose outcome because the "enemy" becomes someone to be beaten at all costs. This attitude can cause even minor problems to escalate into major ones. Sometimes, people or groups resort to violence to get rid of the enemy. Although it's tempting to think that this will solve the problem, violence is never the best solution to a problem. Learning to resolve conflict peacefully and effectively is one of the most important skills you can acquire on your journey.

Conflict Resolution Skills

Good conflict resolution skills build on the other important life and wellness skills presented in this book. Some of the skills we have already looked at include the following:

- *Reflective awareness to help you to identify what you are feeling before you react.* It may be helpful to maintain a personal journal and record personal reflections as you encounter tense situations.

- *Communication skills to help you present your thoughts and feelings clearly and effectively.* Choosing to not talk about a conflict is not a healthy option.

- *Problem-solving skills to help you identify possible solutions to problems that cause conflict for you.* You can use the personal journal strategy to help you think through the problems.

What's News

Seeds of Peace is a not-for-profit, nonpolitical organization that helps teenagers from regions that have a lot of conflict learn the skills for making peace. The organization was founded by author and journalist John Wallach in 1993. The organization's first project was bringing together Arab and Israeli teenagers to train them in conflict resolution and help them discover the human face behind "the enemy." In 1998, the project expanded to include other regions experiencing conflict. Since 1993, more than 2,000 teens from 22 nations have graduated from the Seeds of Peace program and returned to their home countries. They leave the program having made friends among "the enemy." It is hoped that these bright young teens will become the leaders of tomorrow and eventually bring about peace in their own countries.

- *Decision-making skills to enable you to work through possible options and select a course of action that is right for you in a given situation.* Sharing your thoughts and decisions with a close personal friend or family member can help validate the choices you are considering

- *Stress management skills, such as those you developed in chapter 3.* These skills allow you to access inner calmness when the external situation is stressful and uncertain.

WEB LINK
Seeds of Peace
http://www.seedsofpeace.org
This organization teaches the skills of peace for the next generation of world leaders using an experiential model.

SEARCH TERMS: world peace; world conflict; peace

Practical Steps for Resolving Conflict

There are many strategies for resolving personal conflict. The following six steps provide some general guidelines for resolving conflict. The first three steps involve preparing the ingredients for a successful outcome, just as you would do if you were following a recipe. Successful completion of the first three steps provides a good basis for resolving the conflict. The last three steps focus on actively resolving the conflict and reaching an agreement acceptable to all parties:

1. *Set the stage to meet and establish ground rules.* It will be impossible to solve a problem unless the parties involved are willing to talk about it and agree to work together to find a solution. The first step, then, to resolving a conflict is to agree to meet peacefully to establish the ground rules for your discussions. Sometimes this is a simple process, but other times it is very difficult. In situations of serious conflict, this first step can be a very large step indeed.

2. *Gather perspectives of the parties involved.* In this step, the focus is *not* on solving the problem. It is on each party's making an effort to *hear and understand* what the other one thinks and feels about the problem. It is very important to try to be non-judgmental. At the end of this step, there should be a clear understanding of the perspectives of the people involved and exactly why this issue is important to them.

3. *Identify interests, needs, wants, and desires.* During this step, the parties are given the opportunity to clearly state what their interests are and what they feel they need to resolve the conflict. They also have a chance to state what they want to see happen and describe how the situation would look if their desires were met. It is important to separate the demands that people make—what they say they want—from their underlying needs, which are often left unexpressed. For example, your roommate may demand that she be included whenever you go out with your friends. That is her demand. Her *need*, however, is to feel a part of the group. There may be a solution that meets the underlying need and resolves the problem without meeting the demand.

4. *Generate creative options.* With the first three steps completed, the stage is set to begin actively working to resolve the conflict. At this stage in the process, it's important to think "outside the box." This means that the parties don't just rely on what may seem to be the obvious solutions. One way to think of a problem is as a jigsaw puzzle to be solved. It's important to have all the pieces of the puzzle on the table for it to be put together properly. If potential pieces are left out of the problem-solving process, the parties may miss opportunities to find win-win solutions. It's important to stay focused on this step until several options have been identified that seem to have a potential for success.

5. *Evaluate options.* Once the parties have brainstormed as many potential options as possible, it's time to evaluate them to see which have the most likelihood for success. The parties should be willing to try a lot of different puzzle pieces to find the solution that fits best. If none of the options seems to be workable, it may be necessary to start over and go through the steps again. The goal is to create a win-win agreement for everyone involved.

6. *Create a formal agreement.* Once an agreement has been reached, it's a good idea to formalize the agreement by a specific action. This may be an action as simple as shaking hands. Or it may be a written document that contains the agreement and lists the consequences if the agreement is violated. Formalizing the agreement acts as a reminder to the parties, in case of future conflict, that there was agreement on this issue's resolution.

In efforts to resolve a conflict, the previously described steps may be used in a **negotiation**. In negotiation, people work out their problems by talking them through. The parties reach a resolution without help from anyone else. Many problems can be resolved through negotiation.

If, after trying negotiation, the parties are still unable to resolve their conflict, they may invite **mediation**. In mediation, a third party steps in to help facilitate the discussion so that the two disputing parties can reach an agreement. The third party could be a trained mediator, or it could be an uninvolved third party agreed on by the two disputing parties. Mediation is used in conflict resolution with individuals, groups, and nations.

It is usually impossible for both parties to get everything they want and need. If both could get everything they wanted, there probably wouldn't have been a conflict in the first place. Consequently, a common outcome of negotiation and mediation is **compromise**. Compromise involves giving up some of the things that each party wants in order to reach a solution that satisfies both parties. Compromise does *not* mean giving in and accepting a solution that doesn't satisfy you. Rather, it means recognizing that there are things you are willing to give up in order to get something else you want more. Through compromise, you can create a win-win situation for both parties and a peaceful resolution to the problem.

The only way to become really effective at resolving conflict is to practice conflict resolution skills at every opportunity. Each time you practice your conflict resolution skills, you will gain insights about what works and what doesn't work for certain conflicts in particular situations. Over time, you will increase your confidence in your ability to reach positive solutions to conflict.

Practicing your conflict resolution skills will help you develop a number of potential conflict resolution "tools" at your disposal. If you are building a house, you need more tools than just a hammer and a saw. In the same way, if you want to become gifted at managing conflict, you will need to have multiple tools available to you. Think about all the possible choices that you have available and choose the ones that are likely to work best.

Did You Know…?

History contains many examples of people who have used peaceful, nonviolent means to address social issues about which they felt strongly. Two of the most famous of these are Mahatma Ghandi and Martin Luther King Jr. In South Africa and then in India, Ghandi sought to help end prejudice and achieve equality for people of all races. King focused on using nonviolent means to help increase civil rights for African Americans and decrease racial discrimination against them. His efforts laid the groundwork for progress toward equality for African Americans.

negotiation
a process in which two disputing parties work out their problems by talking through them without the assistance of an outside party

mediation
a process in which two disputing parties work out their problems by talking through them with an outside person who facilitates the discussion

compromise
a conflict resolution in which both parties give up something

When you find yourself having difficulty resolving a particular conflict, it may be an indication that you need to develop some new "tools." Just as we often don't recognize all the tools that we need until we find ourselves in the middle of the situation when we are building something, the same is true for conflict resolution. Conflicts are opportunities to acquire and learn to use new tools for a successful outcome.

Creating Peace without Giving In

One of the most difficult aspects of conflict resolution is learning how to reach a peaceful solution without giving in and surrendering your values and principles. When a conflict is resolved successfully, all the people involved feel that their interests, needs, and desires have been respected (Figure 5-8). It may not be possible to get everything you want in a solution, but you should not feel as if you had to give up everything that's important to you just to end the conflict. Giving up everything is not really a resolution. It is a passive acceptance of defeat and ignoring what you believe, need, and want. Giving in can have a negative impact in the long term because people who give in easily eventually find themselves feeling resentful and angry. The immediate conflict may *appear* to have been resolved, but it simply resurfaces later in another form.

At the same time, it is also important to recognize that sometimes it can be useful to surrender short-term desires to reach a long-term solution. Even though a certain situation may be really undesirable, it may not be worth fighting about, verbally or physically. There are certainly times when it makes more sense to give in than to escalate a conflict. Of course, you also need to be sure that you are not violating your most basic values in the process. There is a difference between being a "doormat" and occasionally giving in to contribute to the greater good. Peaceful resolutions are more likely to occur if you make it a priority to separate the emotional issues of the conflict from the intellectual issues.

Personal Boundaries

Healthy people have appropriate physical, emotional, and social **boundaries**. Boundaries are imaginary lines that indicate a limit beyond which you will not go. Boundaries help keep you safe. They help keep you connected to your basic values and priorities. When you are faced with a conflict, take some time to identify what your current boundaries are for that particular situation. You can then determine what you can compromise on and what you cannot. When you decide that your boundary cannot or should not be compromised, you can clearly explain your position to the other person.

There are times in your life where you will be pressured to change your boundaries. Colleagues, friends, or influential others might encourage you to perform unethically,

WEB LINK

The M. K. Ghandi Institute for Nonviolence

http://www.gandhiinstitute.org

The M. K. Ghandi Institute for Nonviolence was founded in 1991 by the grandson of Mahatma Gandhi, Arun Gandhi, and his wife, Sunanda. Many of the institute's educational programs are aimed at conflict prevention, anger management, diversity training, and relationship and community building.

SEARCH TERMS: peace strategies, nonviolent peace strategies

Did You Know…?

Throughout history, many countries have developed proverbs related to conflict resolution. A proverb is a saying that paints a vivid picture to help people understand a complex idea. Give some thought to how the following proverbs apply to conflict resolution:

- "Without retaliation, evils would one day become extinct from the world." (proverb of Nigeria, West Africa)
- "To engage in conflict, one does not bring a knife that cuts but a needle that sews." (adapted from a Bahumbu proverb of Zambia, East Africa)
- "A frog in the well does not know the ocean." (proverb of Japan)
- "Lions believe that everyone shares their state of mind." (proverb of Mexico)

boundaries
imaginary lines that indicate a limit beyond which you will not go

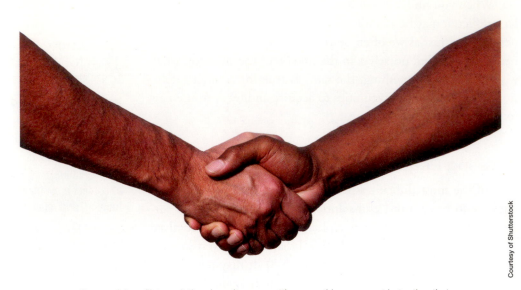

Courtesy of Shutterstock

FIGURE 5-8 • Successful conflict resolution doesn't mean getting everything you want but rather that everyone involved feels their interests, needs, and desires have been respected.

cheat, or give up a preferred political stance. There are many good reasons why you might choose to be flexible in your personal boundaries, but pressure from someone else is *not* one of them. By identifying your boundaries *before* you are faced with a difficult decision, you ensure that you are making your own choices about your life rather than being controlled by others.

When All Else Fails

Most conflicts can be resolved using the skills and techniques we have discussed. But sometimes, despite your best efforts, you just can't seem to reach an agreement with another person or group. These instances require you to reach deep within yourself for the patience and commitment to step back and give yourself some time to consider new approaches or to develop new skills to help you resolve the conflict.

When you don't seem to be making any positive progress toward a solution, a good initial step is to ask your adversary for a cooling-off period before you address the situation. This is one way to allow all parties more time to look for solutions they may have missed. When you're in the heat of the moment, it's hard to see solutions, even when they do exist. Even if a formal agreement to a cooling-off period isn't made, it can help to say something like "I am too upset (or hurt) to really engage in this issue right now. I need to have some time to myself to gather my thoughts." Many people find that it is helpful to go for a walk and allow some of their emotional energy to be dissipated in physical activity. The goal of this cooling-off period is not to avoid the situation or simply to distract you but rather to give yourself time to review the situation more calmly and see different perspectives. Once you have calmed yourself and gained some perspective, you can go back to the discussion and work toward a thoughtful resolution.

Not all conflicts can be resolved in ways that please everyone. However, with patience and commitment to peaceful solutions, conflicts can be resolved without resorting to violence. Acting violently, whether the violence is physical or verbal, is not a real solution but only creates new problems and conflicts. Violence should be avoided at all costs.

BUILDING YOUR LIFETIME WELLNESS PLAN

You have the opportunity to learn skills and make choices for the peaceful resolution of conflict now that can make important changes in your personal life, the community, and possibly the world. These skills are important parts of your wellness plan because they can influence so many aspects of your life and the lives of those around you. As you embark on developing your wellness skills, keep in mind a few basic premises. You must be able to recognize conflict when it occurs. It is unhealthy to take the avoidance approach to conflicts and disagreements. Do all you can to create collaborative win-win outcomes.

● ● ● End-of-Chapter Activities

Opportunities for Application

1. Visit http://www.bullying.org and click on "I Want to Learn." Search the site for "Bullying Myths and Facts." There you will find research summaries related to forms, causes, and characteristics of bullying. Choose four of the research facts and describe some possible strategies for preventing the situation from occurring.

2. Using your local daily newspaper, research and report on a recent conflict that affected your community. In your report, explain the possible source of conflict and suggest how the conflict might have been resolved or prevented.

3. Imagine that you are experiencing a conflict with a colleague and that you will soon have to surface the disagreement. Describe the HALT strategy and, for each of the components, describe what you would do to prepare yourself for the confrontation.

Key Concepts

1. Describe examples of cyberbullying and discuss possible solutions for preventing those that you describe.

2. List and describe the practical steps for resolving conflict.

3. List personal skills and qualities that can help with conflict resolution.

4. List and describe four characteristics that can contribute to the escalation of conflict.

Answers to Personal Assessment Quiz: Resolving Conflict

Answers will vary. A higher proportion of "Definitely True" or "Mostly True" responses to questions 2, 4, 6, 8, and 10 and "Definitely False" or "Mostly False" answers to questions 1, 3, 5, 7, and 9 indicates that you have skills and qualities that increase the likelihood you will be able to cope with conflict effectively. It is important to note that responses to these questions will vary over time, depending on circumstances and moods. A pattern of "Definitely True" or "Mostly True" responses to questions 1, 3, 5, 7, and 9 and "Definitely False" or "Mostly False" responses to questions 2, 4, 6, 8, and 10 reveals difficulties in resolving conflict effectively.

●●● References

Department of Education. (2008). *Indicators of school crime and safety*. NCES 2009-22. Retrieved May 17, 2010 from http://www.cdc.gov/violenceprevention/pdf/School Violence_FactSheet-a.pdf

Egley, A. and O'Donnell, C. E.(July 2008). *Highlights of the 2006 National Youth Gang Survey*. U.S. Department of Justice: OJJDP Fact Sheet.

Jackson, L. (1998). *Gangbusters: Strategies for prevention and intervention*. Lanham, MD: American Correctional Institute.

NAGIA. (2005). *2005 National Gang Threat Assessment*. National Alliance of Gang Investigators Associations.

Retrieved April 28, 2010 from http://www.ojp.usdoj.gov/BJA/what/2005_threat_assesment.pdf.

Thomas, K.W., and Kilmann, R.H. (1974). *Thomas-Kilmann Conflict MODE Instrument*. Tuxedo, NY: Xicom.

U.S. Department of Education. (2009) Indicators of school crime and safety: 2008. NCES 2009-022. Washington, DC: U.S. Government Printing Office.

Workplace Bullying Institute. (2007). *U.S. Workplace Bullying Survey*. Retrieved May 18, 2010 from http://www.workplacebullying.org/research/WBI-Zogby2007Survey.html

CHAPTER 6

Developing Healthy Relationships

CHAPTER OBJECTIVES

When you finish this chapter, you should be able to:

- Describe the importance of social support for overall health and wellness.

- List and describe several qualities of healthy family relationships.

- Explain the difference between family support, social support, and social network.

- Identify some of the factors that influence the development of friendships.

- Identify five skills for building healthy relationships.

- Briefly explain Sternberg's three components of love.

- Describe the similarities and differences between friendships and romantic relationships.

- Identify several characteristics of addictive and abusive romantic relationships.

- Create a personal action plan to assess and develop your relationship skills.

KEY TERMS

abusive relationship	extended family	reciprocity	social support
addictive relationship	infatuation	reflective awareness	stepsiblings
blended family	intimate partner violence (IPV)	self-disclosure	toxic relationship
dysfunctional family	personal identity	social network	traditional family

●●● Introduction

When you were younger, it is likely that most of your thoughts, feelings, and activities revolved around your family. The relationships you developed with members of your family are among the most important connections you will ever establish. These relationships provide you with many of your earliest models for establishing relationships with people outside the family. The qualities and skills necessary to build successful relationships are directly related to the kinds of experiences you formed within your own family (Figure 6-1). Now you are probably much more involved in social interactions

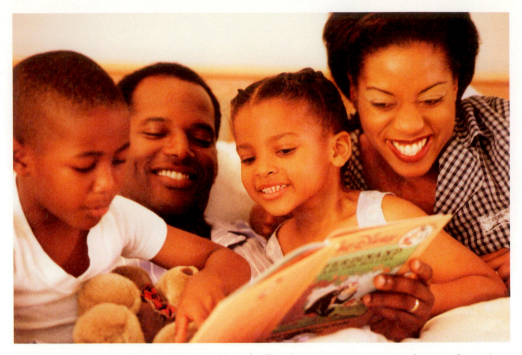

FIGURE 6-1 • The relationships we all develop with our families when we are young are not only among the most important relationships we will have but also the models for future relationships with people outside the family. Courtesy of Adobe Image Library

with friends, coworkers, and organizations you are involved in. Just like family relationships, sometimes your peer relationships run smoothly and make life fun, interesting, and exciting. Other times, they can cause you a great deal of anxiety and make your life very stressful.

Over the course of an adult life, most people are involved in a romantic relationship at one time or another. Countless books, poems, and songs have been written about romantic love. Countless more plays, movies, and television episodes have used love as their central theme. Almost everyone searches for it. Some people claim to have found it, only to have it disappear later. Despite searching, some people never find it. Others find it when they're least expecting it and remain in love with the same person throughout their lives. As a young adult, you may find that a lot of your thoughts and actions revolve around romantic relationships. Or you may not be at all interested in having a romantic relationship. Both of these circumstances are normal. Dating is one of the ways in which we gain experience in romantic relationships. In this chapter, you will learn about the importance of family, social, and romantic relationships and how they affect your health. You will also learn more about the qualities and skills you can acquire to help you develop strong, healthy relationships that are satisfying and mutually beneficial.

●●● What Is a Family?

What are the first images that come to your mind when you hear the word *family*? Before reading any further, take a minute to construct a mental picture of your impressions when you hear the word *family*. As you read further, compare your mental picture with the following description of what it means to be a family.

Throughout history, families have formed the basic unit of society. Families provide resources and support for children as they make their journey toward adulthood. These

PERSONAL ASSESSMENT

Healthy Relationships Quiz

Before reading this chapter, take this personal assessment to discover more about how you relate to others. Read the statements below and, in the space provided below, rate your answers on the basis of the way you respond *most* of the time. Use the following scale: 1= Definitely True, 2 = Mostly True, 3 = Mostly False, or 4 = Definitely False. An interpretation of your results is located at the end of this chapter.

1. I treat other people with respect.

2. I can be trusted to keep my word and not betray a confidence.

3. I do not have to pretend to be someone I'm not.

4. I am able to express my love for those who are important to me, both physically and verbally.

5. If I have a problem with someone, we are usually able to work it out.

6. I have both male and female friends with whom I get along well.

7. I am comfortable with myself and who I am.

8. I am able to stand up for myself and not "lose" myself in a relationship with another person.

9. I am able to accept other people as they are and not want them to change to meet my expectations.

10. I can communicate my needs, desires, and feelings accurately and appropriately.

resources include both material resources, such as food, clothing, and shelter, and emotional resources, such as love, attention, and belonging. Families try to ensure the safety and security of their members. They communicate values for decision making, model skills for social relationships, and generally help children develop the skills they need to someday live successfully on their own. Although many families today may look different from families of the past (Figure 6-2), children still depend on families to provide these necessary resources and support.

Each person in a family is both an individual and a member of the family unit. Each family member affects and is affected by the other members. Family members share joys, sorrows, challenges, and chores. Just as in any other relationship, sometimes getting along well is easy and enjoyable, and sometimes it requires a good deal of effort. Developing and practicing skills for building healthy relationships within your family can make a big difference in the quality of your relationships with all the other people in your life.

At its best, a family provides a web of support that encourages the growth and development of each member while also maintaining the importance of the bonds between them. A healthy family celebrates individual and family successes and accepts mistakes and failures as inevitable parts of growth. Healthy families are not families that never have problems. Rather, they are families that develop the qualities and skills necessary for successfully resolving problems when they occur. Despite the difficulties they experience, healthy families continue to seek positive ways to remain connected to each other.

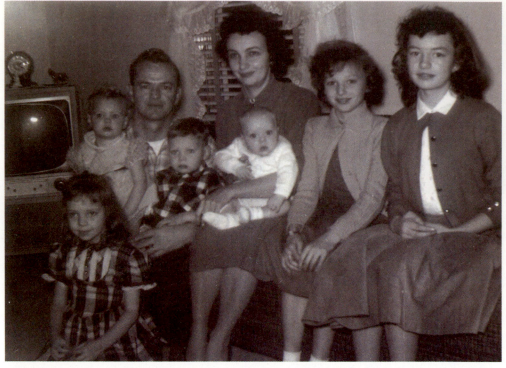

FIGURE 6-2 • Families may look different today than they have in the past, but they form the basic unit of human society, with family members depending on each other for safety and security.

Qualities of Healthy Family Relationships

For children, families provide the earliest model for the future relationships with other people. Healthy families will exhibit the same qualities that are present in healthy relationships with friends, romantic partners, and members of the extended community (Figure 6-3). Have you ever thought about what makes a healthy relationship? The characteristics common to healthy families include mutual respect, trust, honesty, and authenticity. Strong, healthy family relationships also demonstrate love, acceptance, commitment, and loyalty. Communication and problem solving are other important relationship skills that can be learned and practiced within the family.

Although there will always be occasional lapses, the members of successful families exhibit the following 10 qualities *most* of the time:

1. *Respect*. Family members do not belittle or demean each other. Both adults and children demonstrate courtesy and consideration for the other members of the family.

2. *Trust*. Family members do not intentionally hurt each other. They can be relied on to keep promises and not to share confidential information.

3. *Honesty*. Family members tell you the truth. They do not say anything behind your back that they would not say to you personally.

4. *Authenticity*. Family members are real and genuine. They do not put on an act, pretending to be someone they really aren't.

5. *Love*. Family members are able to express their positive feelings for each other, physically and verbally. They sincerely want the best possible outcomes for other members of the family.

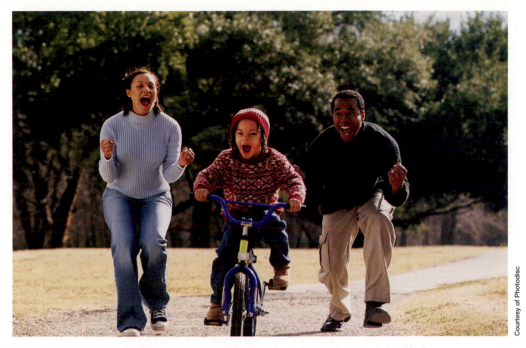

Courtesy of Photodisc

FIGURE 6-3 • Healthy family relationships have the same attributes that any healthy relationship does.

6. *Acceptance.* Family members allow the other family members to be themselves. They allow each other to be spontaneous and genuine, without ridicule or criticism.

7. *Commitment.* Family members are committed to the well-being of all the family members and work to ensure the best possible outcomes for each other. Families who demonstrate commitment don't give up just because there are problems or something is difficult.

8. *Communication.* Family members learn and use good communication skills, not just by talking but also by listening and reading body language.

9. *Problem solving.* Family members make the effort to acquire or develop good skills in problem solving. When they are confronted with a difficult problem, family members work together to discover new ways to solve the problem so that everyone comes out a winner.

10. *Conflict resolution.* When conflicts occur between or among family members, they have the necessary skills to work through the conflict and reach a solution that is mutually acceptable to everyone involved. Conflicts can be addressed without producing lasting bitterness and resentment, characteristics that can permanently destroy family harmony.

●●● Current Family Structures

If you ask your grandparents about their families, you will find a description of the family structure much unlike the one you are currently living in. The roles in their families may be very different than those you are accustomed to. The changing family dynamic has changed over the years, mostly because of economic challenges to families. For example, your grandparents may have been able to afford a home on only one person's salary, but today that is almost impossible given the cost of housing.

Changing Family Structures

Today's families are more diverse than ever before. You may be a part of a **traditional family**, in which you shared a home with your parents and possibly brothers and/or sisters. It is possible you may be part of an **extended family**, where you may share a house with aunts, uncles, or cousins. Or you may be part of a **blended family** that includes a stepparent and possibly **stepsiblings**. You may be an only child, or you may have several siblings. Perhaps you live with only one of your parents, with a grandparent, or in some other type of family situation. Regardless of the family situation in which you currently live, your "family" is the group of people you count on to provide the basic love, understanding, and material resources you need to make a successful transition from the dependency of childhood to the independence and self-sufficiency of adulthood.

The U.S. Census Bureau keeps statistics on the number of households in the United States and the individuals living in those households. The bureau conducts a census once every 10 years. The most recent census was in 2000. The U.S. Census Bureau has two broad categories of households: family households and nonfamily households. A **family household** is defined as a householder and persons who live in the same household who are related to the householder by birth, marriage, or adoption.

According to the U.S. Census Bureau's 2009 *estimates*, 50 percent of all households were headed by a married couple, about 12.4 percent were headed by a single-parent female, and about 5 percent were headed by a single-parent male. The remaining 32 percent of households were considered nonfamily households, in which persons lived alone or with others who were not relatives. The U.S. Census Bureau (2009) confirmed that the size of households remains stable since 2000, with an average of just over three people per family. At the same time, the percentage of single-parent households and nonfamily households continues to increase.

More children today live in single-parent households for at least part of their childhood and teenage years than they did in the past. More than half of all American children do not live in traditional two-parent families with both biological parents. Data consistently reveal that in the U.S. about 43 percent of first marriages end in separation or divorce within 15 years. Almost 70 percent of people who divorce will eventually remarry, often bringing children from the first marriage into the second marriage to form a blended family. In fact, it is likely that about a third of all U.S. children today can expect to live in a blended family before the age of 18. In addition to all the challenges facing a traditional family, blended families are confronted with special challenges that occur as a result of taking two separate family units and combining them into one larger unit.

Changing Roles and Responsibilities

One of the key functions of families is to provide physical, emotional, and social support for its members. Each person in the family has roles and responsibilities that contribute to providing this support. These roles and responsibilities are not usually created consciously. They are naturally assumed by the members without much thought or notice.

---

traditional family
a family that consists of two parents and their biological or adopted children

extended family
sharing a home with numerous relatives

blended family
a family created when one or both of the partners who remarry bring children from a previous marriage into the new family unit

stepsiblings
brothers and/or sisters who joined your family when one or both of your parents remarry

family household
a householder and persons who live in the same household who are related to the householder by birth, marriage, or adoption

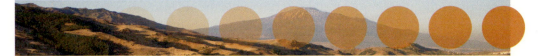

What's Your View?

Who's Watching the Kids?

In the past, two-parent households were much more common than they are today. In many of these families, there was a parent who did not work outside the home. It was also likely that there was a much larger extended family, such as grandparents and aunts and uncles, who lived in the same geographical area than is true for most families today. In a small town, other community members may have taken significant amounts of responsibility for children who were not their own. So there was always someone watching the kids. Today, however, circumstances have changed dramatically. There are more mothers working full-time away from the home. There are more single-parent households and fewer grandparents and other family members living close by. What are your thoughts on the following questions?

- Who watched you when you were younger and your parents weren't available?

- Do you think that changes in family structure have resulted in positive or negative consequences for children growing up today?

- What value is there in having extended family members living close by?

Think back to the earliest time you can remember in your childhood. What were your roles and responsibilities in the family? You were probably primarily a "taker" because you were too young to assume many responsibilities. Maybe some of your earliest responsibilities were to make your bed, take out the trash, or set the table for supper. As you grew older, your role changed within the family, and you assumed more responsibilities. As a teenager, your role and responsibilities changed once again and became more like those of the adults in the family.

Perhaps you noticed that sometimes the adult family members make personal sacrifices for the good of the entire family. In the process of becoming an adult member of the family, you may sometimes have to choose between doing what you personally want to do and what is best for your family. Making these choices will help define your maturing role within your family. If you don't already have one, once you have a family of your own, your choices and responsibilities will change yet again.

Establishing a Personal Identity

Establishing **personal identity** is a key challenge of young adulthood. As a child, your early identity was strongly influenced by your family. As you accumulated life experiences outside the family unit, you begin constructing your own personal identity. Adolescence was a time of "trying on" different identities to see what "fit" best for you—much like trying on a new hat or pair of shoes. Perhaps you discarded some of these trial identities as you would a pair of shoes you have outgrown after a growth period. You kept

personal identity
a unified sense of self, expressing attitudes, beliefs, and actions that are uniquely characteristic of you

developing other parts of your identity as you would the old hat that feels so comfortable. It is likely that the adult identity you eventually established will retain some characteristics of your childhood and adolescent identities and that you'll add new elements as the years go by. Even as an adult, you will continue to shape and add to your identity in ways that provide a unique fit for the person you are.

●●● When Trouble Strikes

All families go through times of chaos and upheaval. Your family life, like other aspects of your life, has ups and downs and good days and bad days. Some families, however, have many more relationship difficulties among their members than average. Sometimes you hear such a family referred to as a **dysfunctional family**. What does it mean to be a dysfunctional family? Experiencing occasional problems in family relationships, even if those problems are serious, doesn't make a family dysfunctional. A dysfunctional family is one in which family interactions continually negatively affect the physical, emotional, and social development of the individuals in the family. In a dysfunctional family, the sum total of all the relationship experiences in the family over time creates pain rather than pleasure.

There can be many causes of dysfunction within a family. Sometimes alcohol or drug abuse by a family member is the problem. Physical abuse and emotional neglect are other causes of dysfunction. Sometimes family members just don't have good communication, conflict resolution, and problem-solving skills. There are people who never learned good parenting skills. They parent using the same skills they witnessed in their families; thus, poor parenting can be passed down from generation to generation unless the cycle is broken. Poor parenting skills produce a family unit that does not get along well and that doesn't want to spend much time together.

At its most basic level, a functional family is one that works well; it functions effectively. A dysfunctional family, on the other hand, has one or more elements of family life that are not working well. It's important to remember that even in the healthiest families, a certain amount of dysfunction may exist.

When family relationships don't seem to be working, members of a healthy family have a problem-solving process they use to try to seek a solution. If they can't resolve the problem alone, they may seek assistance from resources outside the family. They may read some books on improving family relationships, seek advice from someone they trust, or make an appointment with a professional therapist. A family is not a dysfunctional family just because it is having problems. Dysfunctional families are those in which no one acknowledges that problems exist and in which no one is willing to seek solutions to help the family function more smoothly.

dysfunctional family
a family in which family interactions negatively affect the physical, emotional, and social development and well-being of the individuals in the family

WEB LINK
Healthy Parenting

http://www.lifescript.com

You can learn more about family dynamics, characteristics of dysfunctional families, and suggestions for good parenting at this Web site. At the home page, you can enter any of the search terms below to obtain helpful parenting information.

SEARCH TERMS: dysfunctional families, parenting, healthy families

●●● Succeeding in Family Relationships

Your most personal and intimate relationship is the relationship you have with yourself. Sometimes it's easy to forget that the relationship you have with yourself affects all the relationships you have with other people. So one of the most positive actions you can take to develop successful associations with others is to learn to value and nurture your relationship with yourself.

Families provide the "testing ground" for all the skills you are using now or developing to serve you in your lifelong relationships. It is within the family that you learn what works and what doesn't with respect to relationships. You have opportunities to observe the qualities that make family relationships satisfying and enjoyable—and those that don't. Family life also provides your earliest opportunities for learning and practicing skills in communication, problem solving, and conflict resolution. People who are fortunate enough to have good role models for these skills as they grow up have a head start in developing healthy relationships later in life.

●●● Social Relationships

From our earliest days as infants, we need social contact with other humans. Documented cases of children raised in social isolation (orphanages, poor home environments) where they are deprived of nurturing human contact attest to their poor physical and psychological development. In some cases the children died. Those who did survive often suffered serious psychological damage.

Importance of Social Relationships

Social relationships help to meet some of our most basic human needs: the needs for affection, love, and belonging. In Maslow's hierarchy of needs, having these needs met provides the basis for becoming a self-actualized individual, which means functioning at or near your optimal level of mental and emotional health.

Developing relationships with other people also provides opportunities for you to learn more about yourself. In fact, some experts have suggested that most of what we know about ourselves comes from what we learn about ourselves from others. Our social interactions act as "mirrors" to provide feedback about how other people see us. We then use this feedback to guide our future behavior. So, in addition to making life more enjoyable, social relationships make life more meaningful. Research indicates that social relationships also help protect your physical health. Strong social relationships help protect you against stressors that can predispose you to certain diseases. These relationships also increase your sense of well-being, stability, and control, contributing to good mental health. Interestingly, numerous research studies revealed that people who have good relationships with other people live longer and healthier lives than do people who have negative or no social relationships.

> **Did You Know...?**
>
> A famous 10-year study of almost 3,000 residents of Tecumseh, Michigan, revealed that people who were the most socially isolated had four times the death rate of those who were more socially involved (House, et al. 1982). When social ties were broken or disrupted, the incidence of disease increased. Researchers concluded that the interruption of social ties suppresses optimal functioning of the body's immune system.

Social Support

As you develop your own identity as an adult, you select your own friends and develop your own social relationships with others. **Social support** is a term used to describe the degree to which a person's basic social needs are met through relationships with other people. Relationships with other people provide both tangible and intangible resources

social support
aid and assistance exchanged through social relationships

that can be used to meet our needs. Tangible resources include things such as money, transportation, or physical help of some kind. Intangible resources help to meet our emotional needs for affection, acceptance, and understanding. For example, suppose that Kim's child was in a serious accident and required emergency blood transfusions and close friends came forward offering to donate their blood; this would be an example of providing a tangible resource— blood donation. Kim might also need some emotional support. Extended family members and/or close friends could come forward to offer personal comfort. Doing so would be an example of an intangible resource—caring and comfort.

Social Networks

A **social network** includes all the people with whom you have relationships. There are many kinds of relationships in your social network. Picture yourself at the center of a wheel, with the spokes of the wheel representing the various types of relationships you have. For example, your social network might include spokes of family, friends, classmates, and coworkers. Figure 6-4 shows an example of a social network wheel. Your network is constantly changing as you gain more life experiences.

The size of your social network is the number of people in the network and may range from small (fewer than 10 people) to large (possibly hundreds). Frequency is the amount of time you spend with the members of your social network. You may spend a

social network
a person-centered web of social relationships

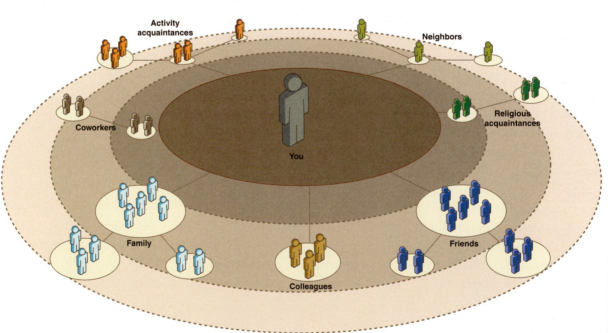

FIGURE 6-4 • A social network is similar to a wheel with you at the center and your relationships as the spokes.

Delmar/Cengage Learning

great deal of time with some members and relatively little time with others. Intensity is the depth of interaction and closeness you have with the people in your social network. You may have strong, intimate relationships with some members, such as your closest and best friends. And you may have very casual relationships with others, such as people who live in your neighborhood.

Reciprocity is another important aspect of a social network. Reciprocity is the "give-and-take" of a relationship, with this give-and-take being approximately equal among the people in the relationship. The members of your social network often provide social support but not always. Some people in your social network may not offer any particular resources to you—tangible or intangible. That is, there is no reciprocity.

> **reciprocity**
> the "give-and-take" of a relationship; the evenness of exchange between the people involved

Loneliness

Loneliness is often a problem in young adulthood. Many college learners have a large social network, but they often have unrealistic expectations about what friendships should provide. For example, they may think that friends should always be available to each other or that true friends should always be able to meet their needs and make them feel good. It is not realistic to expect friends to meet all your social and emotional needs. Have you ever had the experience of feeling lonely in a crowd? This is how it feels to have social relationships with a large number of people without getting your needs met.

Loneliness is not the same as being alone, which means choosing to be by yourself. And loneliness is not determined by the size of your social network. Loneliness occurs when your current relationships don't match the quantity and quality of your expectations for ideal social relationships. Some people have a hard time forming relationships because they are too shy to reach out to other people or because they lack some of the qualities and skills needed to form good relationships. It is normal to feel lonely sometimes. But if you feel lonely a lot of the time, you may want to rethink your expectations of relationships or take steps to enhance your relationship skills.

Factors Influencing the Development of Relationships

Considering all the billions of people in the world, throughout the years of your life, you will develop social relationships with relatively very few people. In addition to your own choices about who you want to develop relationships with, there are other factors that may determine the influential people in your life. Three important factors are geographical closeness, shared interests, and reciprocal self-disclosure.

1. *Geographical closeness.* Modern advances in transportation and communication have reduced our perceptions and the effects of distance. Today, it is easier than ever to develop and maintain long-distance relationships. It is more likely, however, that you will develop relationships with people who live, go to school, and work with you. Sharing a common physical space makes it easier for people to get to know each other and participate in the common activities that help a friendship thrive.

2. *Shared interests.* Social relationships often develop around a shared interest. For example, you may share with some of your friends an interest in a particular

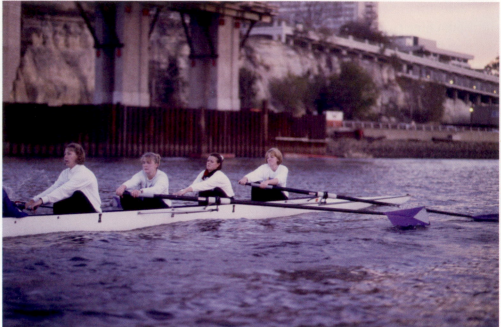

Courtesy of Photodisc

FIGURE 6-5 • Any number of interests can be a source of relationship building.

musical group or sport (Figure 6-5). These shared interests provide the "glue" that helps sustain the relationship through those early, awkward moments of trying to get to know someone.

3. *Reciprocal self-disclosure*. Social relationships may develop because of geographical closeness or shared interests, but they are maintained and deepened by reciprocal **self-disclosure**. Self-disclosure is a process of being increasingly open about who you really are as a person. Through self-disclosure, you gradually allow the other person to see you as you really are. If you disclose something about yourself to someone else, a sense of closeness between you and the other person develops. If that person does not reciprocate by sharing with you, however, you may begin to feel that the relationship is one sided, perhaps leading you to reduce the level of your disclosure.

self-disclosure
revealing personal information to others

●●● Types of Friends

Does it seem to you that current friends and friends from the past share similar characteristics? There are probably some differences among them, too. One way of describing types of friends is by the types of relationships you share with them. You may be amazed to see how many kinds of friends you have. The following are some of the most common friendship categories:

• *Convenience friends*. Convenience friends are people with whom you are friendly and with whom you exchange small favors. You usually present a great deal of self-disclosure with this type of friend. You may have a convenience friend with whom you may choose to work together on class assignments because both of you have complementary academic skills.

- *Special-interest friends*. Special-interest friends are people with whom you share common interests and activities. You probably see them on a regular basis, but you may not be especially close to them. Examples of these friendships include team-mates on a sports team, people with whom you work, or people who belong to the same organizations you do.

- *Historical friends*. Historical friends are those with whom you used to spend more time with but now do not see very often. If you lived in one town when you were growing up but moved away after high school, one of your high school friends might be a historical friend.

- *Crossroads friends*. Crossroads friends are friends who were significant to you at one time in your life. You might have little contact with them now. But if you have an opportunity to spend time together, your closeness can be rekindled. An example would be a high school friend who stayed in your home town while you went away to college. When you return home for holidays or class reunions, you pick up where you left off.

- *Cross-generational friends*. Cross-generational friends are friends who are younger or older than you are. You might have a friendship with an older neighbor or with a younger couple living next door in your townhouse complex.

- *Close friends*. Close friends are people you trust enough to share your deepest thoughts and feelings with. These are people who make you feel accepted and valued just the way you are. Close friends can remain your friends throughout your lifetime, but it is also possible that your close friends will change over time.

●●● Qualities of a True Friend

There is a wise saying: "If you have three true friends in your life, you are a rich person indeed." We usually think of true friends as those friends who are close to us and who have been our friends over a long period of time. But we might find the qualities of a true friend in any of the types of previously listed friends. True friends play many important roles in our lives. They laugh with us, cry with us, play with us, and try to understand us when we don't even understand ourselves. Many qualities have been identified to describe true friends and true friendships. Here are some of the most frequently mentioned:

- *Companionship*. True friends feel comfortable around each other. They usually spend a lot of time together and enjoy just hanging out together. They also have common activities they enjoy sharing.

- *Trust*. Trust is one of the qualities always mentioned when people are asked about the qualities of a true friend. It is impossible to maintain a friendship without trust. Many relationships are damaged because one person betrays the trust of the other. Being a trustworthy person is one of the most important qualities you can develop if you want to have true friends in your life.

- *Mutual respect*. As with trust, friendships rarely survive if people do not have mutual respect for each other. Mutual respect involves more than just common courtesy. It is a sincere belief that the thoughts and feelings of the other person are as important and as valuable as yours.

- *Acceptance.* When we allow someone to begin to know us better, we need that person to be accepting of us—"warts and all." Regardless of how it appears from the outside, no one is perfect. The better we know someone, the more likely we are to discover his or her imperfections—and the more likely he or she is to discover our imperfections. True friends realize that human perfection doesn't exist. They accept others as they are instead of always trying to change them.

- *Loyalty.* True friends are loyal. They are able to count on each other for emotional and physical help. If you have a loyal friend, you know the person won't "trade you in" when something or someone who seems better comes along. True friends value you enough to stick with you, even in difficult times.

- *Reciprocity.* True friendships have a give-and-take that is relatively equal. At certain times, one person may give more to the relationship than another, but over time the contributions the two people make to the relationship tend to even out.

Thus far, the discussion has centered on the duality of a relationship, but, as you know, our relationships include numerous others. You may have one relationship with someone who is especially strong, but you may also have three or four people in your close friendship group. Everyone in the group has a relationship with each other person and with two or three others and so on. Relationships are complex.

●●● Common Stressors in Relationships

Although relationships can bring exceptional joy and pleasure, they can also bring a substantial amount of pain and heartache. The relationships you have can be stable, but there is a good chance that they will be dynamic and changing. Each of us has our own pace of growth and development. When your pace of growth and development differs from that of your friends, relationship difficulties can occur. You may discover that your

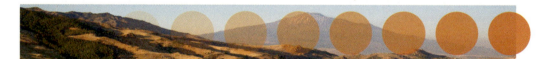

What's Your View?

Arielle Silverman is a normal American young adult who just happens to be blind. She also happens to be a very articulate and gifted writer who is attending college to earn her Ph.D. Arielle feels that, because she gets a sense of what people are really like. She gets to know them on the "inside". Arielle imagines a better world if no one could see at all; then the barrier between races would disappear. In such a world we would spend less time focusing on our own appearance, and dedicate ourselves to developing our character. There are many reasons why some friendships are permanent while others are fleeting, but all our connections leave an imprint in our hearts. How do you feel about these comments? Write a short summary of your thoughts and feelings.

values, attitudes, beliefs, and goals change. You may find that, over time, your friends no longer see things the same way you do. This is normal, but it can leave you feeling lonely and isolated. However, it can also give you the opportunity for growth.

Another change may be in the activities that were once really important to you. Perhaps you have developed new interests. For example, suppose you've played on a soccer team for several years. But this year, you don't want to play. You'd rather devote your energy to the student government association. As a result, you may not see your old soccer friends as much anymore, leaving all of you to adjust to the change in the relationships. There are numerous factors that can place a strain on even the best of relationships.

Unrealistic Expectations

To avoid being disappointed, you have to have realistic expectations about what a particular relationship can and cannot provide. It is unrealistic to think that any one relationship will meet all your needs. People who find themselves upset and disappointed when their expectations in a relationship are not met may have had unrealistic expectations to begin with. It is important to accept people for who they are, and not try to change them into who you want them to be.

Insecurity

Many people, young adults in particular, feel awkward and insecure about some aspects of their identity. To cope with this feeling, they try to find a group of friends who provide a ready-made identity and where they know they will fit in and be accepted. John Powell (1990), a gifted author, notes that many people play games with other people and are not true to who they really are. He believes that people play games because they think, "I am afraid to tell you who I am, because if I tell you who I am, you may not like who I am, and it's all that I have." (p. 12) Some level of insecurity is normal, but with maturity comes comfort in who you are and being able develop the personal strength to compensate for any previous insecurities.

Different Levels of Commitment

The level of commitment you want to give to relationships varies a lot. The young adult years are an ideal time to explore various relationship options. People may be able to sustain a strong level of commitment to a particular relationship, but others are not ready to make such commitments, or they may make a commitment and later break it. When two people in a relationship have different levels of commitment, the disparity can result in pain and confusion.

Sometimes when we begin a new romantic relationship, we begin spending time with that person exclusively, abandoning other friends. If the romantic relationship breaks up, we may have lost touch with our old friends. Another potential source of pain is when a relationship ends. Not every relationship will last forever, whether it's a friendship or a romantic relationship. Many relationships are temporary and exist only to fulfill a certain need or desire. Once that need or desire no longer exists, the commitment to maintain the relationship is no longer there. Even though it may be painful at first, telling the truth and being honest about your feelings about wanting to end a relationship or wanting to spend less time together is usually the least painful course of action in the long run.

●●● Skills for Relationship Success

Developing and maintaining good relationships can be challenging, but the rewards are worth it. Relationship skills are acquired over a lifetime, but they can be improved each day with practice. If you continually work on improving your relationship skills, you will increase your chances of having enjoyable and satisfying relationships. Let's take a look at some of the basic skills that contribute to relationship success.

Communication Skills

One of the most important skills you need to develop in order to build successful relationships is good communication. You may recall from Chapter 1 that communication means much more than just talking. In fact, there are a number of elements that create communication: the sender, the message, the channel, the receiver, and nonverbal body language.

The Sender

The sender is the speaker or composer of the message. You want others to understand you, so when you intend to compose a message, think it through, state it clearly, and take responsibility for your own feelings and thoughts. You want to communicate the message in a manner that is easily understood and accepted by the receiver. If you are communicating on personal issues or conflict, it's a good strategy to use "I" statements. For example, if you are upset about someone's behavior, don't say that "you are always late." A better strategy would be to say, "I worry about you when you are not here on time" or "I am embarrassed when we arrive late for dinner."

The Message

The chosen words in a message, written or spoken, are very important because they create an image in the receiver's mind of what you intend to say. The words must be chosen carefully, especially in times of stress or tension. It is a great skill to be able to express a position on an issue in a manner that creates value between you and the receiver.

The Channel

The communication channel is the manner by which a message is transmitted. An oral channel would take place in a face-to-face conversation. The same conversation delivered over the phone would use the phone as the channel. Other channels include e-mail, online chat rooms, social networking Web sites, letters, and newspapers. You can imagine what happens to the quality of a personal communication when it is delivered by way of channels that lack important elements of communication. For example, a message delivered via e-mail lacks a visual context of the sender and lacks the voice inflection of the speaker. Thus, it is essential to take important, emotionally laden messages directly to the receiver to ensure clarity.

The Receiver

The receiver is the listener who receives the message. Did you know that the human brain can process thoughts much faster than a person can speak? Maybe you've noticed how your mind wanders when you are listening to someone, such as when the teacher

---

WEB LINK

Relationship Communication

http://www.expertvillage.com

You can learn a lot about the positive and negative aspects of communication at this Web site. Search for "relationship communication," and you will have access to numerous short streaming videos that can help with understanding and communicating with a partner.

SEARCH TERMS: relationship communication, loving communications

lectures in class. As the listener, you have a lot of "free" brainpower. It's tempting to use this extra time and brainpower to evaluate the message and think about what you might say next, but this is a poor habit that can interfere with truly effective communication. Instead, a good listener will use this opportunity to pay close attention to the speaker and understand what he or she is trying to say. It is also helpful to make a mental checklist of the messages you are receiving so that you can respond accurately.

Other characteristics of a good listener include not interrupting, not giving advice while someone is speaking, providing nonverbal feedback, and asking for clarification of anything you don't understand. An easy way to remember your responsibility as a listener is to think of the word *understand* as being "under-where-you-stand." If you can imagine what it would be like to be in the same place as the speaker, you have a good chance of being able to communicate effectively.

Nonverbal Body Language

Much of our communication comes from our nonverbal body language. You may have had an experience when you wrote a letter or sent an e-mail to someone and your message was misunderstood. Misunderstanding can happen in these circumstances because these forms of communication don't provide us with nonverbal cues from body language. When you can't see the receiver, you need to pay special attention to making sure that you really understand the intended message before responding. And when you are face-to-face, keep in mind how much your body language is saying for you!

> **Did You Know...?**
>
> Communication research indicates that 55 percent of the impression we get about someone is communicated via body language. Another 38 percent comes from the tone, speed, and inflection of the voice. Only 7 percent actually comes from what is said!

Reflective Awareness

Reflective awareness is your ability to recognize what you are thinking and feeling at any given moment in time. To communicate well with another person and participate in a relationship, you have to know what you are bringing to the relationship. Reflective awareness means being able to identify your true thoughts and feelings about a particular situation. Knowing yourself allows you to communicate accurately, respectfully, and caringly with others.

> **reflective awareness**
> the ability to identify to yourself what you are thinking or feeling at any given moment in time

Self-Disclosure

Self-disclosure means revealing information about yourself to friends you wish to be close to. Revealing this information involves taking a risk, but it is part of establishing intimacy, a necessary part of a close friendship. Intimacy can be remembered as "into-me-see." This means letting another person see you as you really are. As trust and respect develop in a friendship, you begin to feel more comfortable letting the other person know more about you. In each relationship you have, you will face a choice of whether to reveal or conceal yourself. Which you choose will have a great influence on the final outcome of the relationship.

> **Did You Know...?**
>
> Positive mental health is characterized by high disclosure to a few significant others. Poorly adjusted persons tend to overdisclose or underdisclose to almost everyone.

Decision-Making Skills

Decision-making skills help us to stay on course so that our outer lives or actions are consistent with the information you have as well as your inner thoughts, feelings, and desires. As you make friends with a variety of people, you will have to make decisions such as how much time you want to spend with each person and how much you want to share with each one. Each decision represents a choice *and* has a consequence. Learning to make decisions that have positive consequences for your life is an important part of your progress toward responsible and satisfying adulthood.

Romantic Relationships

Our society uses the word **love** to describe our feelings for everything from candy and sports to marriages that last more than half a century:

- "I *love* chocolate."

- "I *love* playing soccer."

- "My grandparents have been married for more than 50 years, and you can tell that they still *love* each other."

We often use the word *love* when we're trying to describe a strong positive feeling for something or someone. There are many types of love. There is the love between members of a family, love between close friends, and love for humanity. In this section, we explore **romantic love** that develops between two people.

love
a feeling of strong affection and devotion, characterized by unselfish and loyal concern for the well-being of another

romantic love
a type of love that includes an attraction to another person based on affection and sexual interest

Characteristics of Romantic Relationships

Many of the characteristics that describe healthy romantic relationships are the same characteristics that describe good friendships. In fact, probably the most often cited recommendation for having a good romantic relationship is to "be friends first." Although this recommendation is often ignored, it is still excellent advice. Dating partners who take the time to be friends first give themselves time to get to know each other without being swept up in a rush of emotion. The same traits and qualities that are important to you in a friendship are the traits and qualities you should look for in a romantic relationship. For instance, if you expect your friends to be loyal and trustworthy, you will want those same qualities to be present in your romantic partner. It's a good idea to make a list of the qualities you want your romantic partner to have. You might also include a list of qualities you want to be sure to avoid.

Did You Know...?

Humans are fascinated with the topic of love. For example, the word *love* has more entries in *Bartlett's Familiar Quotations* than any other word except *man*. *Bartlett's Familiar Quotations* contains more than 8,000 quotations and is one of the best-known references for quotations from ancient to modern literature.

Attraction

The first step in developing a romantic relationship is to meet someone with whom you have an attraction. There is an entire scientific community that is now studying attraction, love, and arousal. While it seems to many of us that attraction is simply something that "just happens," there is a lot going on within us that leads to romantic interest in someone else. The notion of "love at first sight" is not so far-fetched. Research data point to the fact that from the time we are toddlers, significant people in our lives leave us with an imprint, a template, of the qualities we look for in those whom we would willingly take as a partner. For a man, the template may derive from the qualities he saw in any number of women in his life—mother, aunts, neighbors, friends, media types, and so on. A woman may develop her template from her father, male relatives, male movie stars, schoolmates, teachers, and so on.

Stages of Love

There is a sufficient amount of data to explain how a love relationship develops. It appears that there are five distinct stages through which the relationship passes before there becomes a permanent bond between the two partners. Obviously, not all relationships pass through all the stages, and not all relationships need to pass through the stages in the same sequence:

1. *Attraction.* As mentioned previously, there may be any number of characteristics a man or woman may be looking for. Foremost is the aspect of physical attraction. When we see someone who fits our template, body temperature increases, the heart beats faster, the stomach flutters, and so on. These are sure signs that the person we are looking at "turns us on." If we are drawn to the person in a physical sense, then we get close enough to see if there is an emotional/psychological attraction, meaning that we are looking for the mind–body connection that closely matches our template.

2. *Romance.* If the attraction is a solid one, the couple moves into a romantic period. Romance is the expression of fondness you share in the relationship. This is when people do what lovers do—they express themselves in caring ways, demonstrate their sexuality by kissing and touching, and court each other. Part of this period may include the feeling of limerence. Limerence is a feeling one person has for his or her partner who is psychologically his or her "love object." It is a sensation of seemingly swift and deep desire for the "love object," needing to be with him or her, always being in touch, always touching, and doing everything to express affection.

3. *Passion.* **Passion** is a deep physical desire for someone. It is an extension of limerence where the sexual, physical aspects of the relationship emerge. Of course, depending on values and attitudes, the couple may express the physical side of their passion in any number of ways, such as kissing, fondling, stroking, or intercourse. The couple can agree on how they will express their passionate side, and it should be mutually consensual.

4. *Intimacy.* Intimacy develops as partners feel comfortable enough with each other that they share their deepest thoughts with each other. They may discuss future life goals, family matters, fears, joys, and so on. The foundation of intimacy is communication.

5. *Commitment.* The relationship reaches a deep and trusting level with both partners become committed to one another. People who reach a deep level of commitment are ready to remain faithful and committed to that other person on a continual basis. If the commitment is deep enough, it will lead to marriage.

passion
a strong liking for, desire for, or romantic attraction to another person

●●● Sternberg's Three Components of Love

Robert Sternberg (1998), a psychologist at Yale University, developed a model describing the elements of a loving relationship. Using three dimensions of love (passion, intimacy, and commitment), Sternberg was able to provide a model explaining the many aspects of human love from "nonlove" through "consummate love" depending on the dimensions of love that are present/absent (Table 6-1). *Passion* is the dimension of a relationship that includes a level of arousal for the other person. It also includes the sexual interest and psychological level of lust that brings two people together. Generally, it is passion that brings two people together in the first place. *Intimacy* comes from the closeness and bonding effects between partners. It involves clear communication, reception and delivery of emotional support, and promoting the welfare of the loved one. Intimacy develops as the relationship grows past just passion. In addition, intimacy and passion can feed one another. *Commitment* plays a role in the length of

TABLE 6-1 • Sternberg's theory of love.

Type of Love	Passion	Intimacy	Commitment
Nonlove	0	0	0
Liking/friendship	0	X	0
Infatuated love	X	0	0
Empty love	0	0	X
Companionate love	0	X	x
Fatuous love	X	0	X
Consummate love	X	X	X

Source: Adapted from Sternberg (1998).

What's News

Research studies show that feelings of passion and infatuation are fueled by a natural brain chemical called phenylethylamine, which produces an amphetamine-like reaction within the body. Phenylethylamine is commonly called the "love drug" because it is thought to be responsible for many of the physiological reactions of the body at the beginning of a romance. Studies of the effects of this brain chemical reveal that it is impossible to maintain the passionate "high" that is experienced initially in a relationship. Over time (about 18 to 30 months), the body develops a tolerance to the effects of the chemical, and the intensity of the physiological effects diminishes and rarely returns during a relationship. This exciting period of time, however, gives a couple an opportunity to find out if there is more than passion to hold the relationship together.

the relationship. This element is important to the marriage decision, but it may satisfy aspects of short-term relationships and preserve monogamy.

Passion

Passion is a romantic attraction to another person. Passion derives from physiological and psychological sources. Research shows that we are physically attracted to specific people because of hormones and certain brain chemicals. Passion also involves emotional feelings and sexual urges. The physical and emotional feelings combine to create nervousness, excitement, and anticipation about the "newness" of a relationship. Passion does not have to disappear from long-term relationships, but it often feels less intense as time goes on than it did in the beginning.

Intimacy

Intimacy is a close, personal knowledge of another person. Intimacy can be physical, emotional, or both. Many people think that intimacy is purely physical. They think of intimacy as hugging, kissing, and other sexual activities. Those are certainly intimate behaviors, but intimacy is much more than physical acts. People in an intimate relationship feel very comfortable with one another. They know each other well and reveal to each other many things about themselves that they would never reveal to people outside the relationship. Intimacy is a characteristic of both friendships and romantic relationships. As passion decreases in a romantic relationship, the amount of intimacy that has been established often determines whether the relationship will survive.

Commitment

Commitment is necessary for a relationship to endure both the good and the bad times that are a part of every relationship. Commitment in a romantic relationship is just as important as commitment in families and in friendships. Commitment ensures that the partners will not walk out at the first sign of trouble. It means being willing and able to work through problems and to stand strong in the face of difficulties. Commitment is the "glue" that holds a relationship together. It is what enables people to remain faithful to a single romantic partner.

●●● The Process of Dating

Dating as we now know it evolved out of our American culture at the turn of the twentieth century. In the 1800s, young people "courted," meaning that a man and a woman would visit each other, generally at the woman's parents' house or in a public location. This was all done with the permission of the young woman's father. This changed with two historical events that occurred at the beginning of the century. The first was the

intimacy
a close personal knowledge of another person, characterized by feelings of warmth and closeness

Did You Know…?

Many studies report that males and females have differing viewpoints regarding the relationship among passion, intimacy, and commitment. Females are most comfortable with passion and intimacy in the context of a committed relationship. Males, on the other hand, seem to be more able to keep feelings of passion separate from intimacy and commitment. These findings can have important consequences for male–female romantic relationships.

Did You Know…?

An interesting fact is that the "love chemical" phenylethylamine is one of the key ingredients in chocolate. It has been theorized that this substance is responsible for our "love affair" with chocolate!

dating
going out with another person in whom you have a romantic interest

introduction of the automobile, a machine that gave young people more relationship freedom and led to the "dating" concept. The second event was a critical time for "women's liberation." Young women, known as "flappers," began dating, drinking alcohol, and rebelling against social stereotypes of women and courtship. Dating and attitudes favoring more independent partner relationships have been with us ever since.

Although the number of people who choose to remain single is growing, about 95 percent of adults will marry at some point in their life. Almost all married people went through a process of dating before getting married. Even people who have decided to remain single probably dated at some time. Have you ever thought about dating as having a purpose other than going out and having a good time? Some of the purposes are listed here:

- *Establishing a connection.* One of our most basic human needs is to establish meaningful connections with other humans. Dating provides a way for people to get to know each other better. Learning more about someone helps you decide whether you want to be more intimately connected and perhaps marry that person or to have a more casual relationship.

- *Self-discovery.* The process of dating allows you to discover more about yourself as you relate to others. Through dating, you can experiment with different roles and different types of relationships to discover the ones that are most satisfying to you. No relationship is perfect. Self-discovery can give you insights that help you develop empathy, tolerance, acceptance, and readiness for change.

- *Finding someone special.* Dating can be simply an opportunity to spend enjoyable time with someone else. But many people date with the hopes of finding someone special—someone with whom they can have a lasting and intimate relationship. This "someone special" may just be someone you want to date more than once or twice. You may seek a relationship that lasts much longer and might even lead to marriage.

Dating Ethics

Regardless of the type of dating you choose to do, it is important to show respect, caring, and consideration for the person you are dating. Partners have a responsibility to create a relationship that builds value and validates the worth of the other person. Dating partners can demonstrate their care for each other by being honest and by never trying to take advantage of the other person. Neither person should try to dominate the other

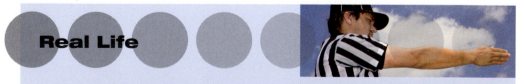

Real Life

Talk to your family, friends, and colleagues about the lessons they learned from their dating experiences. What things would they do differently? Is there a particular type of dating they would recommend or avoid? What can you learn from their experiences?

1. Always be honest with your partner. Sometimes the truth can be hurtful, but in the long run, it is best for both of you.
2. Share relationship details that your partner has a right to know, that is, what you expect out of the relationship. Are you looking for a life partner or just a short-term affair? Is your relationship going to be monogamous or open?
3. Be direct and forthcoming. If something in the relationship is bothering you, bring it up for conversation; don't stuff it away and get angry later.
4. Don't keep private issues that are important to the physical and psychological health of your partner. If you have or suspect that you have a sexually transmitted infection, discuss the matter with your partner.
5. Discuss sexual likes and dislikes with your partner. No one can give sexual pleasure to someone he or she cares about without knowing what works and what doesn't.
6. If the relationship needs to end for you, end it in an ethical manner. Your partner deserves to hear the truth in a timely fashion. It is unethical to go out with someone else with the intention that your partner finds out about it, and then expecting your partner to end the relationship.
7. If your relationship is a sexual one, be sure to have a conversation with your partner regarding a "what-if" scenario in the event of a pregnancy.

Delmar/Cengage Learning

FIGURE 6-6 • Ethical code of dating.

or always insist on having his or her way. Learning to treat romantic partners well is an important sign of maturity. For some important dating considerations, see Figure 6-6. Some of these things are evident for many people; others may need a reminder. Both you and your partner should subscribe to points that protect you and your partner both physically and emotionally.

Common Dating Issues

Dating can be awkward for people of all ages. Every new dating encounter brings with it a new level of excitement, anticipation, and anxiety. This holds true even for people with a lot of dating experience. At a time when divorce is not uncommon, those who are "newly singled" may need some time to adjust to going out with someone.

Fear of Rejection

Fear of rejection may be the worry that is most often mentioned by people when they are asked about dating-related problems. Fear of rejection can be a paralyzing force that stops you from moving forward toward something you really want. It takes a lot of courage to invite someone into your life while wondering if the commitment will be permanent or transitional. Perhaps you heard the saying that people come into your life for a purpose. Their time and purpose could be "for a reason, a season, or a lifetime." What this means is that you need to commit when the time is right, enjoy the immediate presence of that person, and let things work out for the best. Make a conscious decision to take a chance and not to let your fear of rejection keep you from enjoying potential new relationships.

Sexual Issues

A healthy, romantic relationship includes respect for yourself *and* your partner. It also includes being willing and able to take responsibility for your actions. Think through the sexual issues you might have and discuss them with the person you are dating. If sex is part of the relationship, talk it over. Define the boundaries, discuss sexual behaviors, and have predetermined strategies for birth control if sexual intercourse is within your relationship's boundaries. Be sure that both partners are clear on the issue, and if contraception is required, clarify who will be the responsible party for using it.

Jealousy

When some people feel insecure about themselves and their ability to be accepted and valued, they often try to control others. Jealousy is motivated by insecurity and demonstrated by possessiveness. You may think that your romantic partner's jealousy shows that he or she cares about you. In reality, however, jealousy is usually a sign of insecurity and the need to control the partner's contact with other people.

Did You Know...?

Many young adults believe that jealousy shows that their romantic partner likes them a lot. Sometimes people even try to make their partner jealous to prove that he or she cares. In reality, jealousy can be a danger sign in a romantic relationship. Jealousy can even be a predictor of dating violence, especially if the jealousy continues and the person becomes even more controlling. Jealousy in a partner should always be a warning sign that you may be in a potentially abusive situation.

Unrealistic Expectations

Sometimes people have unrealistic expectations of a romantic relationship. They "put all their eggs in one basket," expecting one person to meet all their social and emotional needs. This is an impossible task and can put a lot of strain on a romantic relationship. You may find, after you have been in a relationship for a while, that you want the other person to change and be more like you. But a necessary part of a healthy romantic relationship is respecting and honoring the differences between you and your partner. Another unrealistic expectation is that the relationship will be permanent. Although some relationships do last, most of them end within a few weeks or months. Recognizing this fact allows partners in a relationship to make decisions based on reality rather than on fantasy.

●●● Breaking Up Is Hard to Do

There are many reasons why relationships that seem so right in the beginning fall apart. A high percentage of breakups happen because the two people have different expectations about the three components that support relationships: passion, intimacy, and commitment. If a couple is unable to resolve these differences successfully, the relationship is likely to end.

Problems with Passion

At the beginning of a romantic relationship, passion is high. Indeed, it is often the driving force for the relationship. When passion is "in the driver's seat" of the relationship, one of the persons may be more interested in romantic or sexual activities than the other person is. No matter what the circumstance, to have both people in sync with the sexual desires 100 percent of the time is the exception rather than the rule. Negotiating when and how passion is expressed is part of the development of a relationship. Moving too fast or pushing another person into action before he or she is ready can cause stress in the relationship. Couples are encouraged to use their communication skills to resolve problems that occur, but there remains the possibility that issues cannot be resolved to both people's satisfaction.

Problems with Intimacy

Dating partners often have different ideas about intimacy—both physical and emotional intimacy. One partner may want a lot of physical intimacy but not be willing to be emotionally intimate. Some individuals, especially males, often find it much easier to establish physical intimacy than emotional intimacy. Because emotional intimacy requires the core of a person's identity to be exposed and vulnerable, it can seem very scary and risky. There are risks in both emotional and physical intimacy, especially if you don't feel you can fully trust your partner. To safeguard against taking risks you may later regret, moving slowly toward intimacy is the wisest course of action.

Problems with Commitment

One of the most difficult things for any adult to deal with when they are dating is the area of commitment. Recall that commitment is something that evolves later in a relationship. Some people may not be ready to make a long-term commitment to another person. When someone is just beginning to explore the world of potential partners, it's unfair to both you and the other person to make promises of long-term commitment that you aren't likely to keep.

Even so, a certain level of commitment is necessary to sustain a dating relationship. If the time comes that you or the other person wants to leave the relationship, the breakup can be very difficult for both of you. It's not a healthy choice to stay in a relationship that you no longer want to be in or to try to force another person to stay when he or she is ready to leave the relationship. It takes a great deal of maturity and honesty to leave a relationship or to allow the other person to leave with grace and dignity. Even in the best of circumstances, there are likely to be some hurt feelings for a while.

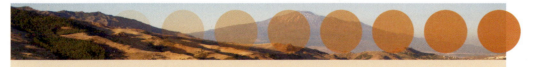

What's Your View?

Sexually Abstinent versus Sexually Active

As an adult, you will be faced with many opportunities for sexual relationships. Each of these opportunities is likely to challenge you to consider choices between sexual activity and sexual abstinence. Describe some of the factors that influence your decision. Clarify which of the two positions you favor and explain why you take that position.

● ● ● Unhealthy Relationships

A **toxic relationship** is a romantic affair that contains negative hurtful attitudes that result in negative consequences for one or both partners. In toxic relationships, there is an imbalance of need between two partners. As with alcohol and other drugs, relationships can be addictive. In an **addictive relationship**, one partner becomes the center of the world for the other person. In effect, the partner becomes the "drug of choice," someone the person depends on in an unhealthy way. Sometimes addictive relationships can also become abusive relationships. In an **abusive relationship**, one of the partners uses power and control over the other in order to get what he or she wants.

Addictive Relationships

Patterns of addictive relationships are quite common in young adult dating relationships. The initial fascination and attraction of a new relationship can cause people to give up other interests and friendships in order to spend more time with a particular person. In their desire to achieve closeness and belonging, people are often willing to give up important elements of their identity to be accepted by another person. A person who is addicted to a relationship, even when the relationship is healthy, allows the other person to control his or her life, just as addicts allow alcohol or drugs to control their lives. An example might be when one person in a relationship turns away from friends and things he or she enjoyed doing before the relationship began. The risk is that the relationship addiction becomes more important than reality. If the relationship doesn't last, it may be difficult to renew the relationship with old friends.

Avoiding the trap of an addictive relationship requires that you keep the relationship in perspective. Don't let the relationship become more important than other aspects of your life. Balance must be sought between things outside and inside the relationship. Each person in the relationship has his or her own life separate from the relationship. In a romantic relationship, there are actually three relationships: each partner's relationship with him- or herself and the partnership relationship.

Abusive Relationships

In an abusive relationship, one person controls the behavior of the other person. A person can be abused physically, emotionally, or sexually. This abuse is defined by the CDC as **intimate partner violence (IPV)**, which occurs between two people in a close relationship. An intimate partner is someone who is a current or former spouse or dating partners. IPV includes physical abuse, sexual abuse, threats of abuse, and emotional abuse that includes demeaning someone's self-worth or prohibiting the partner from going out or spending time with friends or family.

Each year there are more than 4.8 million women who experience IPV physical assaults and rapes. Approximately 2.9 million men experience assaults by their intimate partners. In 2005, there were 1,544 IPV deaths: 75 percent female and 25 percent male (Department of Justice, 2009). Not all effects of IPV are physical. Victims often develop poor self-esteem, and they have difficulty trusting others and maintaining relationships. Strangely enough, many women stay in abusive relationships in spite of the damage inflicted on them. Why would a person stay in an abusive relationship? There are many reasons, but it is usually the addictive personality of the victim. When asked why they don't leave such relationships, abused women are known to say "but he loves me." People who love you do not hit or abuse you.

---

toxic relationship
romantic involvement that results in negative consequences for one or both partners

addictive relationship
relationship in which the object of your affection is the center around which your world revolves or your "drug of choice"

abusive relationship
relationship in which one of the partners uses power and control over the other in order to get what he or she wants

intimate partner violence (IPV)
abuse that occurs between two people in a close relationship

The Cycle of Abuse

The use of alcohol and other types of drug use are frequently present in abusive relationships. The abuse may worsen when the abuser is under the influence of alcohol or a drug. Abuse often involves a predictable cycle of violence. Tension in a relationship increases, and the abuse gradually intensifies until an explosion of some type occurs. After the explosive incident, the abuser promises never to do it again and is especially nice to the partner. The abused partner tries to prevent another abusive incident by trying to control situations so that the partner doesn't get angry again. The abused partner is always "walking on eggshells" to prevent another conflict. Despite his or her best efforts, however, another episode of violence is sure to break out.

Dealing with Abuse

An abusive relationship can be changed or stopped through the efforts of either the abuser or the abused or both. People who are abusive need outside help involving psychotherapy to change their behavior. They are rarely able to change on their own and often don't admit the need for help or simply refuse to get it. Therefore, it is often up to the abused person to stop the abuse. Often, however, it is very hard for someone who is being abused to get out of the relationship and get help. An abused individual may love his or her partner, may believe that he or she will change, or may be afraid of what the partner will do if abandoned. At the first signs of abuse, including emotional abuse, it is extremely important for the abused person to demand that the abuse stop immediately and permanently. If the abuse continues or is repeated, the abused person must leave the relationship. Failure to leave may result in long-term emotional or physical injury or even death. The best time for both the abuser and the abused person to get help is while they aren't involved in the relationship. This may be after the relationship ends or just during a "time-out" period. This allows both parties to work on the issues that contributed to the abusive relationship. They can then consider beginning another relationship either with someone new or with the same partner. In most cases, professional assistance is necessary, but it is not uncommon to protect one's physical safety by way of legal intervention.

BUILDING YOUR LIFETIME WELLNESS PLAN

In this chapter, you learned about the importance of building successful relationships within your family and with friends and romantic partners. All these relationships are part of being a healthy adult. Your wellness plan should include information and strategies to help you gain additional insights and strategies to support your contributions to your family, your friends, and your romantic partner. Because we exist in a social network, we cannot avoid relationships and conflicts. We can go through life ill prepared to interact in a value-creating manner, or we can do all we can to hone our wellness skills, such as the following:

- Recognizing that you may have a variety of types of friends and that each of those relationships can be rewarding and fulfilling

- Understanding the different stressors that can affect your relationships with others and developing ways that you can cope with these stressors while maintaining good relations

- Developing certain qualities and skills that will help you establish and maintain successful relationships

- Work on developing good communication skills, including becoming a good listener

- Understanding the three components of romantic relationships: passion, intimacy, and commitment

- Recognizing the warning signs of unhealthy relationships and knowing strategies to avoid or leave them

●●● End-of-Chapter Activities

Opportunities for Application

1. List and describe at least six characteristics of a healthy family.

2. Much literature has been written about friendship and romantic relationships. Friendships and romantic relationships have also been the topics of countless songs, television shows, and movies. Locate some quotes, stories, poems, songs, or movies that express your feelings about friendships and romantic relationships.

3. Describe strategies for avoiding or ending toxic or addictive relationships.

4. Explain the value of developing a sexual code of ethics and list at least five ethical principles you intend to follow.

Key Concepts

1. Describe the various forms of family units in the United States at the present time.

2. Describe the role of limerence in a romantic relationship.

3. List and describe the three components of love relationships as presented by Sternberg.

4. Describe the differences among toxic, addictive, and abusive relationships.

Answers to Personal Assessment: Healthy Relationships Quiz

Answers will vary. A higher proportion of Definitely True or Mostly True responses to questions indicates that you have the skills and qualities necessary for healthy relationships. A higher proportion of Definitely False or Mostly False responses indicates that you may need to work on improving your skills in this area. It is important to note that responses to these questions may vary over time, depending on your circumstances.

References

Department of Justice. (2009). *Homicide trends in the United States*. Retrieved May 24, 2010 from http://bjs.ojp.usdoj.gov/content/pub/pdf/ipv.pdf

Divorce Rate (n.d.). *Divorce Rate for First, Second and Third Marriages*. Retreived May 19, 2010 from http://www.divorcerate.org/

Ferrante, J. (2008). *Sociology: A Global Perspective*. Belmont, CA: Thomson Wadsworth.

House, J.S., Robbins, C., Metzner, H. (1982) The association of social relationships and activities with mortality: Prospective evidence from the Tecumseh community health study. *The American Journal of Epidemiology*, 116, 123–140.

Powell, J. (1990). *Why am i afraid to tell you who i am?: Insights into personal growth*. Allen, TX: Thomas More Association.

Sternberg, R. J. (1998). *The triangle of love: Intimacy, passion, commitment*. New York: Basic Books.

U.S. Census Bureau. (2009). Households and Families. [From 2006–2008 American Community Survey] Retrieved May 18, 2010 from http://factfinder.census.gov/servlet/STTable?_bm=y&-geo_id=01000US&-qr_name=ACS_2008_3YR_G00_S1101&-ds_name=ACS_2008_3YR_G00_

CHAPTER 7

Sexual Wellness and Reproduction

CHAPTER OBJECTIVES

When you finish this chapter, you should be able to:

- Identify the major endocrine glands and explain the functions of each.
- Describe the endocrine glands that have important roles in human development and reproduction.
- Discuss the onset of secondary sex characteristics of males and females.
- Explain the major changes in the reproductive structures of males and females that are needed for reproduction.
- Explain the relationship between the menstrual cycle and fertilization.
- Discuss the importance of prenatal care during pregnancy.
- List and describe examples of the various birth control techniques.
- Discuss issues related to sexual preference.

KEY TERMS

adrenal glands
adrenaline and noradrenaline
androgens
basal body temperature (BBT)
blastocyst
bulbourethral gland
cervix
corpus luteum
ductus deferens
endometrium

epididymis
glans
hypothalamus
insulin and glucagon
labia
laparoscope
meiosis
melatonin
mitosis
myotonia

ovulation
ovum
parathyroid glands
pheromones
placenta
progesterone
prostate gland
semen
seminal vesicles
serotonin

spermicide
testes
testosterone
thymus
thyroid gland
urethra
uterine tubes
uterus

●●● Introduction

There is perhaps no other personal health issue as important to many Americans as their sexuality. In the popular press, articles abound about sexual desire, sexual behaviors, love, romance, partnership, and so on. In the previous chapter, you learned information to help you formulate healthy social and romantic relationships. In this chapter, we explore the biological side of human sexuality. It would be nice if everyone reading this text started this chapter with the same level of background information, but the reality is that among college learners, the depth and breadth of sexuality information vary tremendously. What sexual knowledge you or anyone else has at this point in time will depend on your family values, the amount of sexual information your parents transmitted to you, the quantity and quality of sexuality education you received in school, the amount of information you received from peers, and the reading, if any, you did on this topic. We say all this to let you know that this chapter may contain information that you already know (but some information that others in school with you may not know) and information that provides greater depth on the topic.

●●● Sexual Development

From the moment you were born, the growth and development of your body was controlled by the genetic blueprint you received from your parents. The genetic blueprint not only determines what your development would be like but also determines the time schedule. The steady controls of childhood are replaced by specific changes during the teen years, a time when chemical and physical changes transformed you from an adolescent to an adult. The sexual developments during adolescence are the physical and

---

PERSONAL ASSESSMENT

What Do You Know about Sex and Reproduction?

Read each of the statements below and indicate whether you think each statement is true or false. The answers are located at the end of the chapter.

1. There are male and female hormones present in every adult.

2. The pituitary gland controls all other glands in the human body.

3. Hormones are very important to the regulation and function of the reproductive process.

4. Males develop their secondary sex characteristics earlier than females do.

5. Identical twins are caused by one ovum being fertilized by two sperm cells.

6. A bone in a man's penis is responsible for his erection.

7. When a woman becomes pregnant, the fetus grows in her uterus.

8. It is possible for a woman to become pregnant without having sexual intercourse.

9. Ovulation takes place on the fourteenth day of a woman's menstrual cycle.

10. The only 100 percent effective birth control method is the contraceptive pill.

chemical changes that prepare the body for reproductive processes. The social side of sexual development comes from "learning" the sexual practices and customs of the culture in which one lives. In the United States, for example, young people go through a period of time where a male and female spend time together as part of a "dating pattern" (Figure 7-1). Dating is actually an American innovation. It evolved out of the "courtship" custom of the 1800s when the automobile appeared in the early part of the twentieth century. As the automobile became an accessible form of transportation, it gave young people more mobility and freedom to carry their relationships farther from home.

If you are a college learner reading this book, you have already gone through puberty. What do you remember about that period of time? Do you have a clear understanding of the physical processes that contributed to your sexual development? Imagine that you have children (if you don't already). Could you explain to them what happens during puberty? The following material may be helpful if you need to review the causes of the physical and psychological changes associated with puberty.

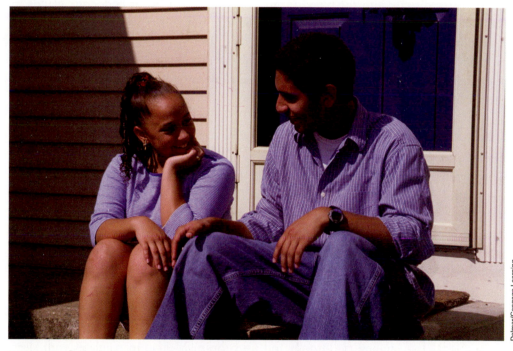

Delmar/Cengage Learning

FIGURE 7-1 • Dating in America is a period when young people explore the social side of sexual development when spending time together.

What's News

A research study of over 3,000 elderly adults, 57 to 85 years of age, revealed that elder adults are sexually active, though their frequency of sexual activity appears to diminish with age (Lindau, et al., 2007). Among subjects aged 57–64, 73 percent reported being sexually active while respondents 57–85 years of age, had a prevalence of 26%.

The Endocrine System

The chemical changes in your body that foster sexual development are controlled by the endocrine system, a collection of small glands exerting chemical control over many body processes. This control involves a very delicate balance of minuscule amounts of chemicals affecting the body as a result of a delicate partnership between the endocrine glands and the nervous system. These interactions are necessary to keep the body in homeostasis, which is the sum of the processes that keep the body's internal environment in balance.

The **hypothalamus**, an area of tissue at the very center of the brain, is the information-processing center that coordinates the activities of the endocrine system by way of its effect on the pituitary gland. The various body organs send information to the hypothalamus through the nervous system and bloodstream. The hypothalamus then processes this information and sends out messages resulting in chemical responses by the appropriate endocrine structures to regulate homeostasis.

The Endocrine Glands

The endocrine glands are ductless glands, meaning that the hormones produced by these glands enter directly into the bloodstream. There are eight major endocrine glands in the body. Each gland performs a specific function, but collectively they also work in a coordinated manner to regulate body functions. The major endocrine glands are the pituitary gland, the pineal gland, the thyroid gland, the parathyroid glands, the thymus, the adrenal glands, the pancreas, and the gonads, or reproductive glands, which include the testes and ovaries (Figure 7-2).

The Pituitary Gland

The **pituitary gland** is located in the very depths of the brain. Approximately the size of a pea, the pituitary is known as the "master gland" because hormones from the pituitary exercise control over many other endocrine glands. The front portion of the pituitary produces hormones that, in addition to other functions, regulate growth, the development of male and female reproductive structures during puberty, and the function of the reproductive organs throughout the life span. The back part of the pituitary helps maintain appropriate water balance in the body and produces the hormone that regulates the birthing process.

The Pineal Gland

The pineal gland is located in the base of the brain. It produces two hormones: **melatonin** and **serotonin**. Melatonin regulates your sleep cycles. The pineal body produces higher levels of melatonin in the mid- to late evening hours and maintains the level until morning. The triggering factor for melatonin production seems to be daylight. Serotonin assists with the transmission of nerve impulses and has some effect on sexual stimulation and appetite; low levels of serotonin are associated with depression.

The Thyroid Gland

The **thyroid gland** is located on the windpipe, just below the larynx (voice box). The thyroid produces hormones that regulate metabolism in the body. One of the principal functions is to convert iodine into thyroxine, a hormone needed for tissue growth. The principal source of

hypothalamus
an area in the center of the brain that exerts nervous system control over the pituitary gland and the rest of the endocrine system

pituitary gland
pea-sized gland in the center of the brain that regulates most of the endocrine glands in the body

melatonin
a hormone produced by the pineal gland to help regulate sleep cycles

serotonin
a hormone produced by the pineal gland to help regulate nerve impulses

thyroid gland
gland that produces hormones that influence growth and development by regulating metabolism

Did You Know…?

A lack of sufficient growth hormone from the pituitary can result in a form of impaired growth called dwarfism. Perhaps the most famous pituitary dwarf was known as Tom Thumb, who worked for the P. T. Barnum Circus. When Tom died in 1888 at the age of 45, he was only about 38 inches tall.

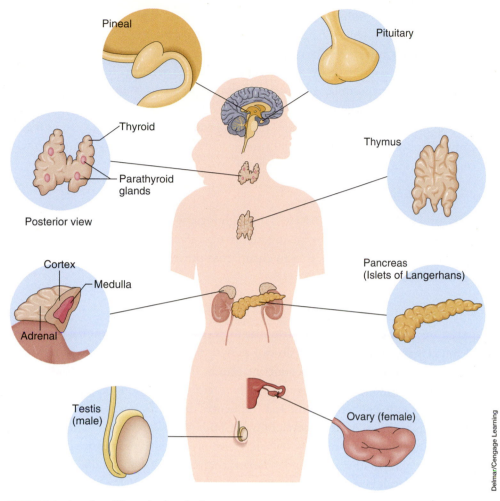

FIGURE 7-2 • Location of the endocrine glands.

iodine in the diet is seafood. If you are like most people in the United States, you do not consume a lot of seafood. For this reason, common table salt is "iodized" to provide a convenient source of iodine.

The Parathyroid Glands

The **parathyroid glands** are four pea-sized glands located on the back of the thyroid. The hormone from the parathyroid glands is necessary for regulating the distribution of calcium throughout the body. Calcium is essential for muscle contraction, development of female reproductive cells, formation of bones and tooth structure, blood clotting, nerve impulse transmission, heartbeat regulation, and fluid balance within cells.

The Thymus

The **thymus** is located behind the sternum (breastbone). The purpose of this gland is to assist in the development of a child's immune system. As an adult, your thymus has converted to a mass of fatty tissue.

The Adrenal Glands

The **adrenal glands** are attached to the top of each kidney. Each gland has two parts: the adrenal medulla (inner part) and the adrenal cortex (outermost part). The adrenal medulla

parathyroid glands
four very small glands located on the thyroid gland that help regulate calcium

thymus
endocrine gland that helps with the development of a child's immune system

adrenal glands
a set of glands on top of each kidney that produce two types of hormones that regulate the stress response and sexual development

**adrenaline and
noradrenalin**
hormones produced in
the adrenal medulla that
regulate blood pressure
and blood flow under
conditions of stress

androgens
male sex hormones
produced in the adrenal
cortex

insulin and glucagon
two hormones produced
in the pancreas that
regulate the level of blood
sugar

testes
male sex glands that are
located in the scrotum
and are responsible for
male sexual development
and sperm production

testosterone
the male hormone that is
produced in the testes

estrogen
the female hormone
produced by the ovaries
to repair the uterine lining
after menstruation and
to enhance feminine
characteristics

progesterone
the female hormone
responsible for
developing the uterine
lining during pregnancy

produces two hormones: **adrenaline and noradrenaline**. These two hormones work together to produce the physical changes that take place in the body when someone is under stress—changes such as increased heart rate and blood pressure, the distribution of blood throughout the body, and the production of sugar as a source of energy for the muscles.

The adrenal cortex produces male sex hormones known as **androgens**. Although androgens are male sex hormones, they are produced by both men and women. Androgens are responsible for the development of male sexual characteristics as young males pass through puberty. Adult women will produce androgens at lower levels than their male counterparts in order to stimulate their sex drive.

The Pancreas (Islets of Langerhans)

The islets of Langerhans are scattered throughout the pancreas, an organ found behind the stomach. The islets of Langerhans manufacture the hormones **insulin and glucagon**, which work together to ensure that the level of glucose (sugar) in the blood is in balance.

Testes (Males)

The **testes** are a pair of male reproductive structures covered by the scrotum, a protective layer of muscles and tissue. The testes do two things: they serve as endocrine glands, and they produce sperm. In their role as endocrine glands, the testes produce **testosterone**, the primary male hormone. The male produces testosterone throughout his lifetime, beginning at puberty. During puberty, testosterone influences the development of the male's secondary sex characteristics. After he develops his secondary sex characteristics, testosterone perpetuates things like muscle mass, body hair, sperm production, and sex drive. The time line for the development of male secondary sexual characteristics is shown in Table 7-1.

Testosterone levels begin decreasing after a man reaches age 30. The rate of decline is approximately 10 percent per decade throughout his lifetime. This decline in testosterone means that muscle strength and sex drive also diminish as he gets older. Note that the testes also produce very small amounts of estrogen and progesterone.

Ovaries (Females)

The reproductive endocrine glands of the female are the ovaries. The primary hormones produced in the ovaries are **estrogen** and **progesterone**. These two hormones influence

TABLE 7-1 • Male secondary sex characteristics.

Characteristic	Average Age of Onset
Hormone levels increase	10 years
Penis grows; pubic hair appears	12 years
Sperm are produced	13 years
Weight spurt begins; muscles develop	13 years
Height spurt begins	14 years
Voice lowers	15 years
Facial hair appears	16 years
Full adult height reached	21 Years

Delmar/Cengage Learning

What's News

Research is now showing that lower testosterone levels in older men are related to lower performance on memory tests. Scientists are not encouraging testosterone supplements to improve memory because of possible health concerns, but research is continuing.

TABLE 7-2 • Female secondary sex characteristics.

Characteristic	Average Age of Onset
Reproductive hormone levels increase	9 years
Internal sex organs enlarge	9 years
Breasts develop	10 years
Pubic hair appears	11 years
Weight spurt begins	11 years
Height spurt begins	12 years
First ovulation; menstruation begins	12 years
Pubic hair and breasts fully grown	16 years
Full adult height reached	18 years

Delmar/Cengage Learning

the development of the female's secondary sex characteristics (Table 7-2). As a young woman passes through puberty, these hormones influence the development of her reproductive structures and the development of her body. These developments include fat deposits on her hips, broadening of the pelvis, and retaining her high-pitched voice. The ovaries also make very small amounts of testosterone. Later in this chapter, you will learn how these hormones contribute to pregnancy.

Male Reproductive System

The male reproductive system consists of both external and internal structures. The external structures known as **genitalia** are the penis and the scrotum. The internal structures include the testes, epididymis, vas deferens, seminal vesicles, prostate gland, and bulbourethral gland (Cowper's gland) (Figure 7-3).

genitalia
the external reproductive sex organs

Penis

No other part of the human anatomy identifies a man's "maleness" as the penis. When a male child is born, everyone present at the delivery can look at the baby and quickly determine if it is a male. The penis is an external structure serving two functions. It is a passageway for urine to leave the body, and during periods of sexual excitement, it is the structure that can deliver sperm.

The penis has two main sections: the shaft and the glans. The **glans** is also referred to as the head of the penis. At birth, the glans is covered with a section of

glans
the rounded head of the penis

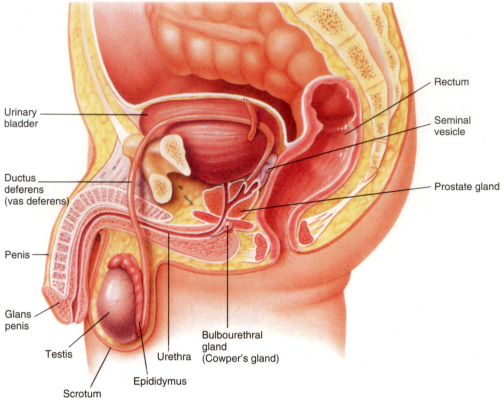

FIGURE 7-3 • The male reproductive system.

Delmar/Cengage Learning

circumcision
surgical removal of the foreskin

urethra
passageway from the bladder to the outside of the body

tissue known as the foreskin. In some cases, the foreskin is surgically removed during a process called **circumcision**. In the United States, the choice to have a child circumcised is a personal decision for the parents; it is not a required procedure. Data from the CDC (2008) indicate that circumcision rate have remained steady over a 20-year period, ranging from a low of 60.7 percent in 1988 to high of 67.8 percent in 1995.

The shaft of the penis contains three spongy tissue layers that are rich with blood vessels. Two of these layers are on the top side of the penis. The third is on the underside and has the **urethra** passing through it. The spongy layers are the "erectile tissue" in the shaft of the penis. Under a variety of conditions, such as sexual excitement, these tissue cause the shaft to become erect.

Scrotum

The scrotum is a pouch containing the testes, the endocrine structures where sperm cells are manufactured. Although the scrotum may appear to be only a pouch of skin, the scrotum is much more than that. In fact, the scrotum contains layers of tissue and muscle enabling it to perform a very important function. For the male to manufacture sperm, the testes must be at a temperature that is a couple of degrees cooler than the normal body temperature of 98.6 degrees Fahrenheit. The nerves and muscles inside and near the scrotum work together to draw the testes closer to the body when the external environment is cold or to allow the testes to drop lower from

Did You Know…?

Males are capable of obtaining an erection at any time after they are born. An erection is a physiological process that can occur in infants as well as children, teens, and mature men. In adulthood, males are socialized to have erections only during sexual arousal, but erection may still occur during sleep.

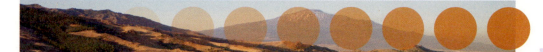

What's Your View?

Circumcision

The decision to perform circumcision on the penis is not without controversy. There are a variety of opinions surrounding this procedure. Over the years, research has disclosed reasons *for* circumcision, only to have later research report reasons *against* it. The debate continues today. Conduct some research of your own on the Web using the search term "circumcision." Read about the pros and cons of circumcision and give critical thought to the appropriateness of infant circumcision. If you or a family member had a male child, would you want him to be circumcised? Explain the rationale for your decision.

epididymis
structure adjacent to the testes where sperm are stored

ductus deferens
duct that transports sperm from the epididymis to the penis

seminal vesicles
structures that produce a component of semen that nourishes and protects sperm

prostate gland
accessory structure of the male reproductive system that supports movement of sperm

bulbourethral gland
small gland near the base of the urethra that produces a fluid that conditions the urethra for the movement of sperm

the body when the body is overheated or in a hot environment, such as a hot tub. The scrotum and testes are a very sensitive part of a male's body. To protect these structures from injury, males are advised to wear protective equipment during contact sports and other activities in which a blow to that area might occur.

Internal Sex Structures

There are a number of important internal structures that make up the male sexual anatomy. The testes, mentioned previously, serve two important functions. As endocrine glands, they are responsible for producing testosterone and delivering it into the bloodstream. They also serve a reproductive function by manufacturing sperm cells. This function begins as the male goes through puberty.

The sperm cells manufactured in the testes are stored in the **epididymis**, just outside the testes. They are stored there until such time that they are ejaculated. Ejaculation occurs as a result of sexual arousal, or they may be ejaculated during sleep. The **ductus deferens** is the duct system that transports the sperm from the epididymis to the **seminal vesicles** and **prostate gland**. The **bulbourethral gland** sits at the entrance of the urethra. Bulbourethral fluid enters the urethra during conditions of sexual arousal and serves to prepare the urethra for the presence of sperm. The fluid reduces any acidic environment in the urethra to ensure that sperm survive as they pass through the urethra.

Reproductive Functions

Sometime in his very early teen years, a male enters puberty. The pituitary sends chemical messages by way of various hormones signaling the structures in the reproductive system to mature and become functional for reproduction. A male is born with millions of specialized cells (primary sperm cells) in his testes. But not until puberty is the male's body capable of changing these cells into sperm. This conversion is controlled by pituitary hormones that continue sperm production throughout the life span. Sperm are microscopic in size and consist of three distinct sections (Figure 7-4). The male's genetic material is contained in the head of the sperm.

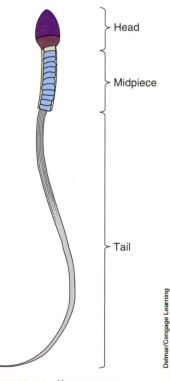

FIGURE 7-4 • Human sperm.

The primary sperm cells undergo some interesting changes as they become fully developed sperm capable of contributing to the reproductive process. All the cells in the human body contain 46 chromosomes—except for the male and female reproductive cells, which contain 23 chromosomes. The male and female each contribute 23 chromosomes necessary for human life. Therefore, the primary sperm cells, which themselves have 46 chromosomes, must reproduce themselves while reducing the chromosome number in each cell to 23. This is accomplished through a process called **meiosis**, or reduction division. (Meiosis should not be confused with **mitosis**, the process by which cells reproduce themselves. *Primary* sperm cells also go through mitosis in order to maintain their numbers.) Once the sperm cells have been reduced to 23 chromosomes, they grow tails and are moved to the epididymis, where they are stored as sperm. This entire process continues almost continually throughout the male's lifetime.

Sperm play half the role in reproduction. To carry out their function, they must get from the epididymis to the female. During sexual arousal, the sperm are moved from the epididymis through the ductus deferens to the penis. Along the way, fluids from the seminal vesicles and prostate are added to the sperm to produce **semen** (also known as seminal fluid). These fluids help nourish the sperm and ensure that they are mobile once they enter the female. The semen is pooled at the base of the penis until ejaculation.

Erectile Function

A male usually has an erection prior to ejaculation (although it is possible for ejaculation to take place without an erection). The penis becomes rigid when specialized muscles at its base push accumulated blood into its three spongy layers. An erection can result from either sexual arousal or urine retention while sleeping. Either way, the same mechanism causes the penis to become erect. This also helps explain why males occasionally ejaculate while sleeping. The penis becomes erect because of urine retention, and stimulation from bedcovers or clothing can

---

Did You Know…?

Sperm come in two sizes. The sperm carrying the genetic material to produce a male have a smaller head and longer tail than the sperm containing the genetic material to produce a female. Hence, only the father's reproductive cells can determine the gender of the child.

Did You Know…?

Whenever a male ejaculates, he ejects between 300 million and 500 million sperm. These millions of sperm occupy a space about the size of an aspirin tablet! The rest of the semen is composed of fluids to nourish and protect the sperm as they enter the female reproductive tract.

---

meiosis
the process of reducing chromosome numbers in reproductive cells to one-half the original number

mitosis
the process of duplicating living cells

semen
a translucent solution containing sperm and nourishing fluids from the seminal vesicles and the prostate

---

What's News

Recent research indicates that as men age, they are likely to produce damaged sperm. Evidence for causing this damage is leaning toward environmental effects such as tobacco, pesticides, and alcohol abuse. These factors appear to be damaging more sperm than the body can typically eliminate through natural processes, and though males produce millions of sperm, the increase in damaged sperm may have a negative effect on reproduction. For example, one study determined that the mutated gene contributing to dwarfism increases as men age; men in their forties were twice as likely to exhibit the mutation than men in their twenties.

trigger an orgasm, what people often refer to as "wet dreams." In the absence of sexual activity and wet dreams, older, unused sperm are absorbed by the body.

Male Reproductive Health

Erectile dysfunction (ED) is another issue in male reproductive health. ED is a condition where a man loses his ability to produce an erection suitable to perform sexual intercourse. This condition can occur in aged males simply because aging physiology just doesn't function well enough. Another cause could be a side effect from prostate cancer treatment. There are prescription medications available to help treat ED (e.g., Cialis, Levitra, and Viagra).

Male infertility is an issue for some couples attempting to conceive. In approximately 50 percent of the cases, male infertility is a major factor. The causes of male infertility are varied and include hormone deficiencies, physical obstructions, sperm deformities, and medications. Perhaps the most common cause is varicocele, a condition in which the veins in the scrotum are deformed, resulting in a poor blood supply and temperature control. It is one of the easiest causes of male infertility to diagnose and treat.

Although testicular cancer is not a common form of cancer in general, it is one of the most common cancers among males between ages 18 and 36. If detected early, this cancer is almost 100 percent curable. Males should know how to do a testicular self-examination so that early detection of testicular cancer is possible. You can learn more about testicular self-examination from the American Cancer Society.

Sexually transmitted infections (STIs) remain a significant health threats to sexually active males and females. More detailed information on STIs is presented in chapter 13.

Female Reproductive System

A woman's reproductive structures serve a number of purposes. Unlike the male's reproductive organs, the female's structures are almost entirely internal. Because everything is on the inside of the body, it can be difficult for a woman to detect any changes or diseases in her reproductive organs. Therefore, it is recommended that women learn as much as possible about their reproductive system so they can properly take care of themselves. Additionally, they should get an annual physical examination from a trained health professional such as a primary care physician, gynecologist, or nurse midwife. The same is true following a vasectomy.

Female Reproductive Structures

The most external parts of the female sex structures are the **labia**. The labia are folds of skin and tissue that appear at the entrance of the vagina. Where the labia meet at the front of the vagina, there is a small shaft of tissue known as the **clitoris**. The clitoris is structurally very similar to the male's penis in that it becomes erect during sexual stimulation and contains nerve endings that are a source of sexual pleasure for the woman. The **vagina** is a muscular yet flexible passageway, about four inches long, that extends from the labia to the **cervix**. The cervix is the opening between the uterus and the vagina (Figures 7-5 and 7-6).

The **uterus**, or "womb," is a major, pear-sized organ of the female reproductive system. The inner lining of the uterus, the **endometrium**, is where the fertilized **ovum** is implanted to start a pregnancy. This lining develops tissue and blood vessels to nourish

WEB LINK
Web MD

http://www.webmd.com

At this Web site, you can search for information on almost any health topic. If you want information on testicular examination, go to the home page and enter "testicular self-examination" in the search bar.

SEARCH TERMS: testicular self-examination, testicular cancer

labia
folds of skin at the entrance to the vagina

clitoris
A small mass of erectile tissue above the vagina which, when stimulated, is the source of sexual pleasure for a woman

vagina
a muscular, flexible passageway between the labia and the uterus

cervix
opening to the uterus

uterus
a pear-shaped, muscular organ that provides the proper environment where the fertilized ovum develops into a fetus and assists with childbirth

endometrium
the innermost lining of the uterus where a fertilized ovum becomes implanted and nourished during pregnancy

ovum
the female reproductive cell (the plural is *ova*)

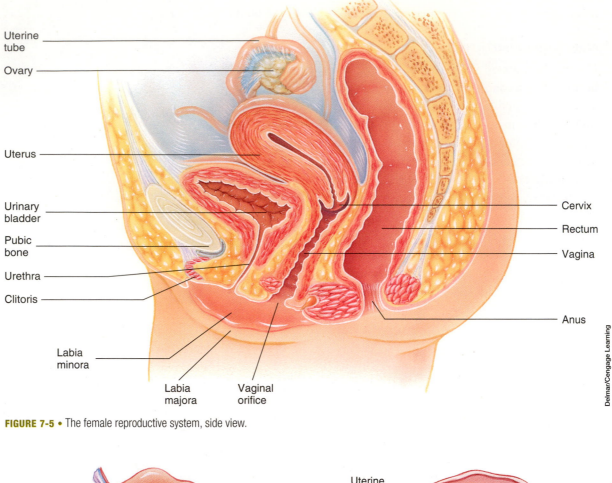

FIGURE 7-5 • The female reproductive system, side view.

Delmar/Cengage Learning

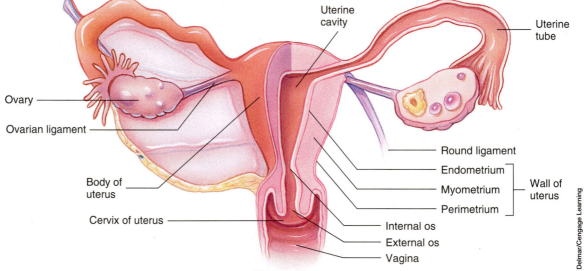

FIGURE 7-6 • The female reproductive system, front view.

Delmar/Cengage Learning

and grow the fetus. Other layers of the uterus are muscular and perform rhythmical contractions to squeeze the fetus into the vagina during childbirth.

Each month, through a process known as **ovulation**, a female releases an ovum from one of her ovaries; generally only one ovum is released, but there could be two or three. An illustration of an ovum is presented in Figure 7-7. Keep in mind that the ovum is

ovulation
the release of an ovum from one of the ovaries

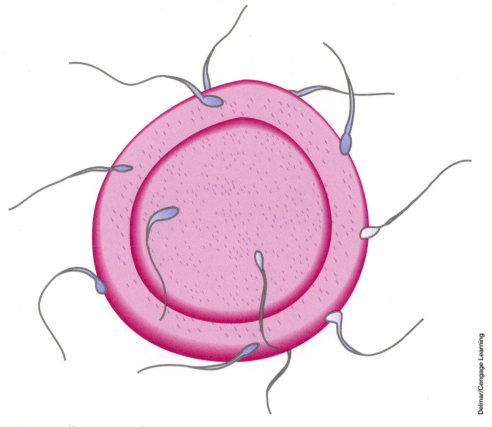

FIGURE 7-7 • Human ovum and sperm.

Delmar/Cengage Learning

actually smaller than the period at the end of this sentence. (The sperm cell in the figure illustrates its size in comparison to the ovum.) Ovulation begins when a young woman enters puberty and lasts until later in middle age, around age 50. The **uterine tubes** (also called fallopian tubes), which extend from each side of the uterus to the ovaries, are passages for transporting the ovum to the uterus. The ovum's journey from the **ovary** to the uterus takes three to five days. Because an ovum is capable of being fertilized by a sperm for about 24 hours, fertilization almost always occurs in the uterine tube.

The Menstrual Cycle

A woman's menstrual cycle is a uniquely significant event. When a female approaches puberty, her genetic makeup will direct her pituitary to produce hormones that influence the development of her secondary sex characteristics. One of the most significant of these characteristics is her ability to produce reproductive cells, or ova.

The ova are produced in the ovaries at the rate of about one each month. When a female is born, each of her ovaries contains almost 200,000 immature ovum cells. On entering puberty, the young woman's pituitary gland begins producing follicle-stimulating hormone (FSH), which directs her ovaries to cause an ovum to mature. At the same time, her pituitary will produce luteinizing hormone (LH), which stimulates the endometrium of the uterus to prepare to receive a fertilized ovum (Figure 7-8).

Once an ovum is mature, critical levels of FSH and LH trigger its release from the ovary, a process known as ovulation. Following ovulation, the ovum enters the uterine tube to begin its three- to five-day journey to the uterus. Following ovulation, at the location where the ovum left the ovary, another important hormone called progesterone is produced. Progesterone is responsible for developing the endometrium to receive a

uterine tubes
passageways that transport the ova from the ovaries to the uterus

ovary
structure responsible for producing reproductive cells and female sex hormones

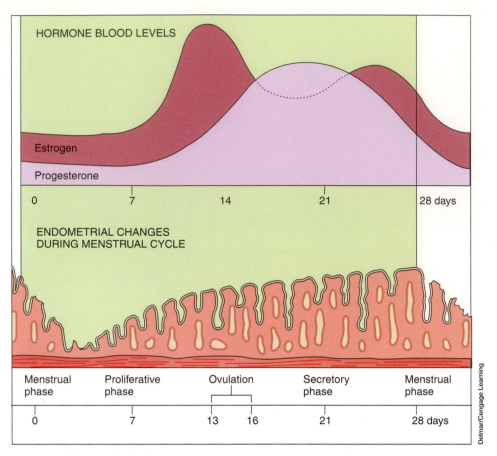

Delmar/Cengage Learning

FIGURE 7-8 • The menstrual cycle.

fertilized ovum. Once it implants in the endometrium, the fertilized ovum will need blood and nutrients so that it can grow.

If an ovum is not fertilized by a sperm cell on its way down the uterine tube, it will not implant properly on the endometrium. The failure to implant causes a hormone message to be sent back to the ovary to halt the production of progesterone. Without progesterone, the lining of the endometrium sloughs off during a three- to five-day period of bleeding, known as **menstruation**. If a fertilized ovum is implanted on the endometrium, a hormone is produced from the implantation site to signal the ovary to continue producing progesterone throughout pregnancy.

In order to use a physical marker to identify the beginning of the menstrual cycle, day 1 of the menstrual cycle is marked by the first day of blood loss. This time is used by medical personnel because menstruation is the only outward physical sign that occurs during the menstrual cycle. Many sexual reproduction textbooks and educational materials portray the menstrual cycle as being 28 days long. This is done as a matter of convenience, but doing so can contribute to confusion. The truth is that 28 days is the *average* length of the cycle for *mature* women. Teens and even young adult women may have considerable variability. Given the level of variability among women, especially younger and menopausal women, there is an element of unpredictability when trying to determine ovulation. The following information provides a more complete understanding of the relationship between ovulation and reproduction:

1. Not all women have menstrual cycles that are 28 days long. It is important to recognize that 28 days represents an *average* number among all women. Not everyone is average.

menstruation
a cyclical shedding of the uterine lining in response to changes in hormone levels

2. Menstrual cycles, especially among teens, young women, and menopausal women, are not regular. It is not uncommon for a teenager's cycles to vary from three to five days from cycle to cycle. A menopausal woman may even skip one to two months at a time.

3. Ovulation generally takes place about 14 days *before* the next menstrual cycle begins. We have no way of accurately predicting when the next cycle will begin, so we can't predict ovulation either. There are physical signs a woman might measure to determine if she *is* ovulating. These signs are discussed later in this chapter in the section on birth control.

Menopause

Normally, a woman will continue to menstruate during her lifetime until she enters **menopause**. Just as she began menstruating according to her genetic makeup, so will genetics play a role in menopause. During menopause, her ovaries will produce less estrogen and progesterone, the hormones that regulate the menstrual cycle. Although menopause may begin subtly in her late thirties, a woman will notice more obvious changes in her forties. Just as a woman had irregular and infrequent menstrual periods going through puberty, she will have the irregular and infrequent periods during menstruation. Additionally, she will not know when her last menstrual cycle will be. Medical personnel tell women that they are no longer fertile once they have gone 12 months without a menstrual period.

During menopause, a woman will notice a number of physical changes as her hormones adjust. Some of the symptoms include sleep disturbances, hot flashes, mood swings, and/or vaginal dryness. Each woman's symptoms and emotional state will vary, so it is best for her to contact her health care provider for recommended strategies for managing her condition during this time.

menopause
a time period in a woman's life when she no longer experiences a menstrual cycle

Conception

The timing of fertilization is very precise and is controlled by the woman's hormones. An ovum is released from the ovary and travels down the uterine tube toward the uterus. This journey may take up to five days, but the ovum is viable for only 24 to 48 hours. If it does not encounter a sperm cell and get fertilized within that 24- to 48-hour window, the ovum will deteriorate. On ejaculation into the vagina, sperm travel through the cervical os, the opening to the uterus that undergoes a molecular change at the time of ovulation encouraging sperm to pass through into the uterine tube. The sperm may survive up to five days in the uterine tube. If sperm are present in the uterine tube when the viable ovum arrives, the sperm will gather around the ovum and attempt to enter it. Each sperm cell is equipped with an enzyme that weakens the wall of the ovum, making it easier to enter. As soon as one sperm enters the ovum, another enzyme is released from the ovum and deters the remaining sperm cells from trying to enter.

Once the sperm enters the ovum, the head dissolves, and the 23 chromosomes from the sperm blend with the 23 chromosomes from the ovum to form a nucleus containing 46 chromosomes. The ovum will undergo a process of chromosome reproduction, and the ovum will split in two. The cells in this mass then begin to reproduce as it (now called the morula) tumbles down the uterine

WEB LINK
Pregnancy

http://www.pregnancy.org

This Web site contains current information on conception and pregnancy. You can search the site for everything from home pregnancy tests to baby's names. Another good site is **http://www.pregnancy.parenthood.com**.

SEARCH TERMS: conception, pregnancy, embryonic development

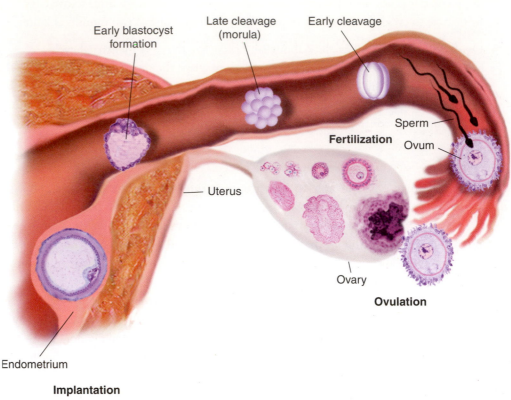

FIGURE 7-9 • Ovulation, fertilization, and implantation.

Delmar/Cengage Learning

blastocyst
a mass of cells that implants in the uterus after fertilization of the ovum

corpus luteum
structure formed in the ovary where the ovum was released (produces progesterone)

placenta
an organ that forms in the uterus to control the movement and exchange of nutrients and wastes between the fetus and the mother

prenatal care
all the things done to safeguard the health of the mother and fetus throughout pregnancy

tube to the uterus. Figure 7-9 illustrates ovulation, fertilization, and implantation. In the early stages of pregnancy, the cells reproduce approximately every 20 minutes. When the mass of cells arrives in the uterus, the mass (now known as a **blastocyst**) implants itself on the endometrium in the upper third of the uterus. The site where the blastocyst implants eventually evolves into the placenta, serving as the exchange point for oxygen and nutrients with carbon dioxide and waste materials between the mother and the fetus.

Once implantation occurs in the uterus, the messenger hormone (human chorionic gonadotropin [HCG]) is released into the bloodstream and transported to the ovary. The presence of HCG signals the **corpus luteum** to continue producing progesterone. This feedback loop of HCG and progesterone continues until the pregnancy is well established, and then the **placenta** takes over the maintenance of the pregnancy. For the first two months of pregnancy, the mass of cells is known as an embryo; from the third month until delivery, it is known as a fetus.

Detection of a pregnancy is linked to the production of HCG. Pregnancy tests measure the level of HGC in the woman's urine. Depending on the woman's genetic and chemical makeup, it is possible to detect HCG in the bloodstream roughly one week after conception.

Prenatal Care

Prenatal care (*prenatal* means "before birth") refers to all the medical attention a woman receives and the personal actions she takes to protect her health and the health of her fetus throughout her pregnancy. Prenatal care during the first three months of pregnancy is especially important because this is the time when many organs and structures are formed in the fetus, especially the brain and nervous system.

Good prenatal care includes having regular medical checkups, getting physical exercise, and eating well. It is also important for the mother to remember that anything she consumes will make its way into her bloodstream and therefore will also enter the fetus' bloodstream. That's why it is important for her to avoid tobacco, drugs, and alcohol, all of which can negatively affect the development of the fetus. The woman's nutritional requirements during pregnancy are the same as they normally would be for her except certain nutrients needed to support the pregnancy (Table 7-3). Use your health literacy skills to learn more about this important aspect of pregnancy.

A pregnant woman's exposure to environmental hazards such as environmental tobacco smoke, certain metals (such as lead, mercury, cadmium, and arsenic), pesticides, and organic solvents can also cause problems for the developing fetus. For example, a mother's exposure to lead may result in birth defects such as slow mental and physical development, depending on the level and time of exposure to the fetus. During pregnancy, a woman should be very careful to avoid environmental hazards that can affect the fetus.

Did You Know...?

When a man and woman conceive a child, each partner contributes 23 chromosomes from their pool of 48 chromosomes. But each chromosome contains many genes. Given the numbers of chromosomes and genes involved, scientists have calculated that there are over 69,949,000,000,000 different combinations of chromosomes that can result from fertilization!

TABLE 7-3 • Recommended dietary allowances (RDAs) for pregnant and nonpregnant women by age.

Female RDA	15–18	19–24	25–50	51+	Pregnant
Calories	2,200	2,200	2,200	1,900	+300
Protein (g)	44	46	50	50	60
Vitamin E (IU)	8	8	8	8	10
Vitamin K (µg)	55	60	65	65	65
Vitamin C (mg)	60	60	60	60	70
Thiamin (mg)	1.1	1.1	1.1	1.0	1.5
Riboflavin (mg)	1.3	1.3	1.3	1.2	1.6
Niacin (mg)	15	15	15	13	17
Vitamin B6 (mg)	1.5	1.6	1.6	1.6	2.2
Folate (µg)	180	180	180	180	400
Vitamin B12 (µg)	2.0	2.0	2.0	2.0	2.2
Iron (mg)	15	15	15	10	30
Zinc (mg)	12	12	12	12	15
Selenium (µg)	50	55	55	55	65
Calcium (mg)	800	800	800	800	1,100

Delmar/Cengage Learning

TABLE 7-4 • Selected birthrates per 1,000 people worldwide, 2009 estimates.

Country	Birth Rate	World Ranking
Worldwide	19.8	—
Niger	51.6	1
Gaza Strip	36.93	26
Honduras	26.28	62
Brazil	18.43	110
United States	13.83	154
Germany	8.18	220

Source: United States Central Intelligence Agency (2009).

Birth Control

Sexual behavior among human beings has long since evolved to where sexual intercourse is now part of romantic relationships and sexual pleasure; no longer is it intended solely for the purpose of reproduction. Our culture is more sexual than it is reproductive. It is a sociological reality that the more economically developed a society is, the more likely it is for that society to control the number of offspring in the family unit (Table 7-4). Not all cultures have the same view of human reproduction. In less economically developed countries, larger family units are desired in order to contribute to the labor pool in the family unit or community. In some cultures, large families are a sign of manhood. Every act of sexual intercourse between two fertile individuals carries with it a possibility for causing a pregnancy. This is why married couples choose to practice family planning. Family planning means having children when they are expected rather than having pregnancies occur according to chance. Some couples practice family planning for a number of reasons, most of which are economic in nature, such as having only the number of children they can afford to support comfortably or postponing having children until they can afford a house. Couples have a number of options available to help them practice **birth control** should they choose to do so. Birth control procedures include abstinence, fertility awareness, **contraception**, sterilization, and abortion.

Birth control methods carry various health risks. To help put the risks in perspective, Table 7-5 illustrates many of the more common forms of birth control in comparison to each other and the risk associated with pregnancy and childbirth.

As mentioned earlier, sexual values and behaviors among couples develop for a variety of reasons. As an adult, you make the decisions that guide your sexual health. You use information from your family, education, house of worship, and other reliable sources to help you develop your sexual values and behaviors. It means that you have already clarified the role sexual behaviors play in your life and recognize that any act of sexual intercourse carries with it a potential for pregnancy and in some instances the possibility of a sexually transmitted infection. It implies taking responsibility for your behaviors and protecting yourself and others from any physical or psychological harm. Ideally, decisions governing your sexual behaviors will include conversations with your partner to clarify values and behaviors that govern your partnership.

birth control
any behavior or method designed to prevent conception or childbirth

contraception
a method of preventing the union of sperm and ovum following an act of sexual intercourse

TABLE 7-5 • Mortality risks for selected birth control methods and childbirth.

Method	Risk of Death in Given Year
Fertility awareness, withdrawal	None
Barrier methods, spermicides	None
Intrauterine devices	1 in 10,000,000
Oral contraceptives	
Nonsmoker	1 in 66,700
Age less than 35	1 in 200,000
Age 35–44	1 in 28,600
Heavy smoker—more than 25 cigarettes per day	
Age less than 35	1 in 5,300
Age 35–44	1 in 700
Sterilization	
Laparoscopic tubal ligation	1 in 38,000
Hysterectomy	1 in 1,600
Vasectomy	1 in 1,000,000
Legal abortion	
Before nine weeks	1 in 262,800
9–12 weeks	1 in 100,100
13–25 weeks	1 in 34,400
After 15 weeks	1 in 10,200
Illegal abortion	1 in 3,000
Pregnancy/childbirth	1 in 10,000

Source: Adapted from Hatcher et al. (2007).

Abstinence

Sexual abstinence is practiced by some members of virtually every culture worldwide. In some instances, abstinence is practiced with the intention of preventing pregnancy; in some cultures, abstinence is practiced for religious reasons or avoiding sexual intercourse during menstruation or during certain religious events. American culture and many religions worldwide expect young people to remain abstinent until marriage. Moreover, parents don't want their children to get sexually transmitted infections or incur unwanted pregnancies. Underlying these expectations is the notion that young people should avoid sex until they are mature enough to take responsibility for a pregnancy that might arise from the sexual relationship. Among the methods of birth control, sexual abstinence is the only method that is 100 percent effective in preventing pregnancy and sexually transmitted infections.

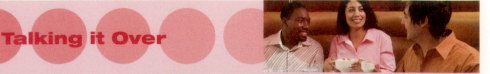

Talking it Over

Responsibility for Contraception

Among sexually active couples, the issue of birth control is a topic that must be discussed between the two partners. Two people in a sexual relationship share in the prospect of childbearing. There are methods of birth control that are used by the woman and some that are used by the man. Just who should take responsibility for preventing a pregnancy is a matter of debate. Some people think it should be the female's responsibility, while others believe the male should be held accountable. What do you think about this issue? Take the time to talk with your significant other, friends, or family members. After your discussions, write a statement of your position and the reasons you have for supporting it and place it in your wellness folio.

Fertility Awareness

Fertility awareness is a set of personal assessments a woman can make to determine when she is or is not ovulating. This information allows her to avoid or promote pregnancy. There are a number of procedures the woman can follow to help pinpoint when ovulation has occurred or might be near. These assessments relate to her reproductive physiology. Remember, ovulation occurs 14 days before the next menstrual period, so she can use the calendar to track her cycles for several months. Using those data, she calculates what might be the earliest and latest times of her menstrual cycle when ovulation may be likely to occur. She can also monitor her **basal body temperature (BBT)**, the temperature of the body at complete rest. A special thermometer is needed to obtain precise measures of her BBT. The woman needs to take and record her BBT every morning before she gets out of bed. She will notice that her BBT will drop about one degree over a few days and then spike almost *two* degrees *after* ovulation takes place. A third measure is cervical mucus monitoring. The surface of the cervix changes in response to hormone levels during the menstrual cycle. For about five days after her period ends and for about 10 days before her next period, her cervix will be "dry." However, as she approaches ovulation, her cervical mucus will become more abundant, and on the day of ovulation the mucus will be about the consistency of egg whites and somewhat sticky. If the woman collects information on all three of these methods, she can get a fairly accurate assessment of when ovulation *has occurred.* This method of birth control is inexpensive, reversible, drug free, and sanctioned by religious doctrine.

Contraception

Anyone who is considering having sexual intercourse must carefully consider the meaning and possible consequences of this action. The two people involved should have a common understanding

basal body temperature (BBT)
the temperature of the body at complete rest

WEB LINK
Fertility Awareness

http://www.fwhc.org

When you get to this Web site, click the link for "birth control." In addition to fertility awareness, other contraceptive methods are described. All the birth control methods on the site are also available in Spanish.

SEARCH TERMS: fertility awareness, birth control

about whether they want to make a baby. Having sexual relations requires mutual acceptance of the responsibility that goes with sex, thus taking the appropriate measures to maximize the potential for pregnancy if a pregnancy is desired or ensuring that a suitable and agreed-on contraceptive is used if a pregnancy is not desired.

Contraception is not practiced by all sexually active couples. Some people have personal or religious values that influence their decision to use or not use birth control, especially contraception. For those who do decide to use contraception, choosing a method is a highly personal decision that is based on individual preferences, medical history, lifestyles, motives, religious values, and economics. The fact is that there is no perfect contraceptive. Each method carries with it both risks and benefits. There are some contraceptive practices that are more effective than others. And certainly for any method to be effective, it must be used correctly and consistently. Correct use requires motivation and knowledge.

The methods discussed in the following sections and listed in Table 7-6 are the most common contraceptive methods. They are listed in reverse order from the least to the most effective. The effectiveness of each method is reported according to its **failure rate**, or the percentage of unintended pregnancies expected among couples who use the method for one year. Notice the differences between typical use and perfect or theoretical use. These rates are based on research conducted on human subjects over a particular length of time. For comparison, in one year, 85 out of 100 women who use no birth control during regular intercourse and intend to get pregnant will become pregnant.

failure rate
the number of pregnancies per 100 women using a particular birth control method during a one-year period

TABLE 7-6 • Types of contraceptive methods.

Method	Description	Effectiveness	Protection against STIs
Coitus interruptus	Withdrawal of the penis from the vagina just before male orgasm	About 25 percent	None
Spermicide alone	Can be a foam, jelly, or foam containing nonoxynol-9	About 50 to 80 percent	None
Female condom	A polyurethane sheath placed inside the vagina	About 80 to 85 percent	Yes
Diaphragm with spermicide	Dome-shaped rubber disk that covers the cervix	About 83 percent	None
Cervical cap with spermicide	Rubber cup that fits snuggly over the cervix	About 85 percent	None
Male condom	Latex or membrane sheath that fits over the erect penis	About 89 percent	Yes but not all
Oral contraceptives (combination)	Pill that prevents ovulation	99 percent	None (the pill makes it more likely for the female to get some infections)
Injection: Depo-Provera or (Lunelle)	Injectable progestin (and estrogen) inhibits ovulation and prevents fertilized ovum from implanting in the uterus	99.5 percent	None
Patch (Ortho Evra)	Skin patch of estrogen and progesterone replaced once a week for three weeks; acts the same as the pill	99 percent	None
Male contraceptive	Being tested but nothing approved as yet	99.9 percent and is reversible	None

Parental Sex Education Is Important

Research has clearly demonstrated that two things happen if parents talk to their children about sex and reproduction. First, children who have these conversations with their parents are more likely to delay their first sexual experience than children who don't have such conversations. Second, those children who have the talks are more likely to use contraception when they do become sexually active.

Using Contraception Effectively

Contraception is not a simple task because it requires planning and forethought. It also requires the individual to admit that he or she is sexually active. If a condom is used, for example, it must be available for use when the couple wants to have sex, and there must be an agreed intention to use it. Some types of birth control require a visit to the doctor and/or pharmacy. Two things must be considered to use contraception effectively: (1) a contraceptive method that matches each individual's or couple's needs as determined by personal motives, life goals, and interest in having a family and (2) a contraceptive method that can be used consistently and correctly.

Contraception Not Requiring a Doctor Visit

There are some contraceptive methods that do not require a visit to the doctor. As you will see in the sections that follow, some of these methods are more effective than others. Even when examinations are not required in order to obtain contraception, adults are encouraged to obtain regular physical examinations and to see their physician if they notice any changes in their reproductive system.

Coitus Interruptus

Also known as withdrawal or the "pullout" method, this is not a very good birth control choice for several reasons. The assumption behind the method is that the male withdraws his penis from the vagina at the time he is about to ejaculate. In that regard, the woman has to trust that her partner will withdraw. A problem occurs when the male holds off and withdraws at the very last moment or decides not to withdraw at all. Even if he does withdraw, he may begin to ejaculate as soon as he withdraws, and sperm can come into contact with the vaginal opening. When this happens, it is possible for sperm to move through the vagina and up into the uterus to fertilize the ovum. Another problem with this method is that before a man ejaculates, his bulbourethral gland is active, and preejaculatory fluid flows from the penis. Research evidence shows that 25 percent of bulbourethral fluid samples contained sperm. Can you see why this method is not very effective? In fact, the failure rate is high, with about 20 out of 100 women becoming pregnant. And this method offers no protection from STIs. All things considered, this is a high-risk form of contraception.

Spermicide Only

spermicide
a chemical that is harmful to sperm

A **spermicide** is a contraceptive foam, cream, jelly, film, or suppository that contains nonoxynol-9, a spermicidal chemical. The spermicide must be placed in the vagina prior to *each act* of sexual intercourse between five minutes and one hour before intercourse, depending on the form used. Following intercourse, the spermicide should not be disturbed for at least six hours. Studies report varying failure rates of 20 to 50 per 100. Failure can occur if a fresh application is not inserted prior to each act of intercourse. Because of the relatively high failure rate, it is recommended that spermicides be used in conjunction with other forms of contraception, such as the condom (male or female), diaphragm, or cervical cap. Spermicides should not be used during pregnancy.

Female Condom

Introduced in 1993, the female condom was marketed as a product designed to put barrier contraception under the control of the female. Barrier methods are helpful in reducing the risk of STIs because they prevent contact between the male and female structures and fluids. The female condom, which does not require a prescription, is made of polyurethane and fits as a sheath inside the woman's vagina. It helps prevent some but not all STIs. An advantage of this method it that it gives the female the opportunity to have control and protect herself since she is the one who runs the risk of getting pregnant. The failure rate, however, is 21 out of 100.

Male Condom

The male condom is a barrier contraceptive that separates the penis from the vagina. It is a sheath made from latex or animal membrane that fits over the erect penis to prevent sperm from getting to the vagina. A condom is placed on the penis after it becomes erect. It is essential to be very careful and not tear or puncture the condom when opening the package or rolling the condom on the penis. Following intercourse, the penis and the condom should be removed from the vagina while the penis is still erect to avoid spilling any sperm in or near the vaginal opening.

Condoms are second only to abstinence in preventing STIs. Some condoms also contain nonoxynol-9, which not only kills sperm but also is harmful to many disease-producing organisms. Condoms do not offer 100 percent protection, however, because there are some STIs, such as herpes simplex or human papilloma virus, that can be transmitted from infected tissue to tissue not covered by the condom.

Be aware that condoms come with an expiration date. Users should check the packaging for this date because latex deteriorates over time and will not offer protection. Deterioration is accelerated if condoms are stored in warm places, such as the glove compartment of a car or a man's wallet. Latex condoms should never be used with a petroleum jelly or any other form of petroleum product because these products cause latex to disintegrate quite quickly. If a lubricant is desired, it should be water based. Some condoms are sold as novelties, such as "glow-in-the-dark" condoms. These products are as not as resilient as standard condoms, nor do they offer protection from STIs.

Contraception Requiring a Doctor Visit

The contraceptives discussed in the following sections are used by the woman, and all require a visit to a doctor. There are a number of reasons for the visit. First, a doctor can conduct an examination to ensure that the woman is an appropriate candidate for particular contraceptive method. Second, the doctor can talk with the woman about the contraceptive method that is most appropriate for her. Finally, a doctor can write a prescription for the device if necessary. Some contraceptive devices need to be fitted to the woman, and oral contraceptives come in more than 30 different forms. While the methods in this section provide varying degrees of contraception, none provide protection from STIs.

Diaphragm with Spermicide

A diaphragm is a rubber dome-shaped device that the woman places in her vagina so that it covers her cervix. The diaphragm acts as a barrier to block the semen from entering the cervix. Before it is inserted, a spermicidal jelly is placed on the diaphragm to kill sperm and physically block the cervix. The device should remain in place for at least six hours but no more than 36 hours after intercourse.

A diaphragm requires a doctor's examination and prescription because it must be fitted to the size of the woman's cervix. For example, a young woman who has never been pregnant will have a smaller cervix than a 35-year-old woman who has had two children. If used correctly, the failure rate for the diaphragm is less than 10 out of 100, but research indicates that about 17 women out of 20 experience an accidental pregnancy during the first year of utilization because of improper use of the diaphragm. The cost, including the doctor's visit, the diaphragm, and spermicide, is about $150 for the first year.

Cervical Cap with Spermicide

The cervical cap is a soft rubber cup with a round rim that is put into the vagina to fit over the cervix. The cap is smaller than the diaphragm and sometimes more difficult to insert. A woman must visit a doctor or clinic to be fitted for the cervical cap and obtain a prescription to purchase it. As with the diaphragm, this device must be used with spermicidal jelly and inserted before intercourse. It can be left in place for up to 48 hours. After removal, it is cleaned and stored for use later. The failure rate for women who have never had a baby is 9 out of 100. For women who have given birth, the failure rate is 26 out of 100. The doctor's examination, cap, and spermicide cost about $125 for the first year of use.

Contraceptive Pill

The contraceptive pill is the most popular form of birth control. There are more than 30 different varieties of oral contraceptives, but they all function the same way. One pill is taken every day with the first 21 pills delivering combinations of synthetic estrogen and progesterone. This combination of hormones sends a false signal to the pituitary gland that the woman is pregnant, so there is no release of FSH to direct the ovaries to cause an ovum to mature. After 21 days, the hormones are no longer needed, so the woman either stops taking pills for seven days or takes "spacer pills," which contain no hormones, to keep her in the habit of taking a pill each day. During this period without the hormones, the woman menstruates as she normally would. If a woman forgets to take a dose of the pill, it is advised that she use another form of birth control until she begins her next round of the prescription.

Oral contraceptives are almost 99 percent effective in preventing pregnancy. The pill does not, however, protect against STIs. The pill may also have some side effects, especially when the woman first starts using it. These side effects include upset stomach,

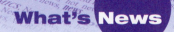

What's News

Research indicates that most people (66 percent) would like to see males take more responsibility for contraception. The news is that this may be close to reality. Drug companies worldwide are working on an oral male contraceptive. A low-cost, reversible, and long-acting form of a male hormonal contraceptive could become commercially available in the United States by 2011.

diarrhea, weight gain, and breast tenderness; some women may experience more severe side effects.

Contraceptive Patch

The contraceptive patch is worn on the lower abdomen or buttocks and releases a combination of progestin and estrogen that is absorbed into the bloodstream and prevents ovulation. The patch is replaced each week for three weeks. The fourth week, no patch is used, so the woman can menstruate. Levels of protection and the types of side effects are similar to those of the oral contraceptive. The patch requires a doctor's examination and prescription. It should be noted that the contraceptive patch delivers higher levels of progestin, and recent studies are showing that women using the patch are at greater risk for blood clots than women who use the contraceptive pill. A woman who may be considering the patch should consult her physician for the latest information.

Depo-Provera

Depo-Provera is a highly effective progestin injection given by a doctor every three months. Progestin is an artificial form of progesterone. This method works much like oral contraceptives. The progestin circulates in the bloodstream in amounts sufficiently high to mimic pregnancy and prevent ovulation. Depo-Provera requires a visit to the doctor's office for an examination and follow-up injections.

The possible side effects associated with Depo-Provera use include irregular bleeding, menstrual periods that are less frequent, and weight gain. After five years of use, menstrual periods may disappear altogether. If a woman decides to have a baby, she can discontinue the injections, although it takes a while for the body to completely rid itself of the progestin. Studies indicate that 93 percent of women who discontinue Depo-Provera can become pregnant within 18 months. The costs associated with this form of contraception range from $250 to $500 per year.

Lunelle

Lunelle is a once-a-month injection of an estrogen–progesterone formulation. The progesterone prevents the ovary from releasing an ovum, and the estrogen promotes a monthly menstrual period. If the injection is given within the first five days of a normal menstrual period, Lunelle provides immediate contraceptive effectiveness. Overall, this method of contraception is very effective. Less than 1 out of 100 women gets pregnant in a year using this method.

Like other hormonal methods of contraception, this product requires a doctor's visit and prescription. Side effects associated with Lunelle use include weight gain, nausea, possible changes in skin condition, and breast tenderness. The cost of using this method is slightly higher than that of Depo-Provera.

NuvaRing

NuvaRing is a contraceptive ring about two inches in diameter. The ring fits over the cervix and releases synthetic estrogen and progesterone for 21 days. The hormones help prevent ovulation and thicken the cervical mucus, making it difficult for sperm to enter the uterus. The ring has to be removed after three weeks and replaced after the fourth week. Theoretically, NuvaRing is 99.7 percent effective, but under actual use the effectiveness seems to be 92 percent. The cost of the ring is about $35 a month and requires a physician's prescription.

Emergency Contraception

Anyone engaging in sexual intercourse should consider all the potential outcomes. Couples should discuss possible risks and consequences and take the proper steps to protect against both unwanted pregnancies and STIs. Even with good communication, there may be occasions when proper contraception is not used or is not used properly. For example, the male partner may not withdraw before ejaculation using coitus interruptus, or there could be a tear in a condom. A far more traumatic situation would be when a woman is raped and has no opportunity to protect herself.

In these cases, one option is emergency contraception, also known as the "morning-after pill." This pill contains the same ingredients as regular birth control pills but at much higher doses. The doses are compressed into two separate tablets. The first tablet must be taken within 72 hours of unprotected intercourse. The second tablet is taken 12 hours later. The hormones in the tablets interrupt ovulation (if it has not occurred), fertilization, and implantation. Emergency contraception is not perfectly reliable, but it is effective about 75 percent of the time.

It is important to recognize that emergency contraception is not an "abortion pill." Because emergency contraception prevents ovulation and fertilization, a pregnancy never occurs. Emergency contraception is not recommended as a regular form of contraception. The morning after pill costs approximately $50 and is available from a registered pharmacist. The pill can be purchased without a prescription by any woman 17 years of age or older.

Male Contraceptives

There have been medical studies of male hormonal contraceptives (MHCs) that have demonstrated safety and effectiveness. The MHCs deliver hormones at levels that inhibit sperm production. The literature also reports the effectiveness of the "reversible inhibition of sperm under guidance" method. A large clinical trial of this method was conducted in India. It involves an injection of a gel into the vas deferens that disables sperm as they pass by during ejaculation.

As of this writing, none of the methods have been cleared for distribution in the United States. After you read this, use your health literacy skills and research the current information on male contraception. If you use Web sites to get some of your information, be sure that the information reported is from 2010 or later.

Sterilization

Sterilization is considered a permanent and highly effective method of birth control. In the United States, it is the most popular form of birth control among couples who have been married longer than 10 years and do not intend to have any more children. The decision to undergo sterilization must be weighed very carefully because the condition should be considered irreversible. Generally, male sterilization is the preferred method among couples for a number of reasons. Foremost is the fact that the procedure is much less expensive than female sterilization (approximately $900 vs. $3,000).

Female Sterilization

Female sterilization commonly involves some surgical procedure to block the oviduct so as to ensure that sperm and ovum do not meet. The woman still ovulates, and she continues to experience her menstrual period. The procedure is completed under general anesthesia using a **laparoscope**, a small tube containing a lens or camera where the surgeon can view the oviducts. Generally, an instrument is passed through the laparoscope to tie the

laparoscope
A slender tube containing a small camera and/or a surgical instrument that can be inserted into the abdomen

oviduct or seal it through electrocautery. Studies indicate that 2 to 6 percent of women in developed countries express interest in reversal, and complete reversal is not a guarantee, with data indicating that only 50 percent of procedures result in a pregnancy.

Male Sterilization

Male sterilization, or vasectomy, is performed under local anesthesia during an outpatient procedure. During the procedure, an incision is made on one side of the scrotum, and the physician locates the vas deferens. The vas deferens is then cut and tied off or cauterized to seal both ends. In some procedures, the tube is clipped. It is recommended that couples use alternate forms of contraception for the three months following the procedure. There are reversal procedures for vasectomies, but they are expensive, and the success rate is approximately 52 percent. However, the success rate is higher the closer the male is time-wise to his initial vasectomy procedure. Men thinking that they may want to father children following a vasectomy may want to consider freezing sperm before the procedure.

sexual identity
the inner sense that individuals have about their own sexual identity

pheromones
substances produced by animals that serve to attract a partner for reproductive purposes

Sexual Attraction

As males and females go through puberty, changes in their endocrine systems affect not only their reproductive systems but their nervous systems as well. It is during puberty that young people develop their sense of **sexual identity**. Sexual identity is the inner sense that you have about yourself as a sexual being, including your feelings of gender and attractiveness. The hormonal changes and the developing sense of sexual identity experienced by young people contribute to their growing interest in romantic relationships.

Physical Attractiveness

As humans, we are unique among animals in that our sexual attraction is not directly related to reproduction. Our genetic makeup and the social and psychological factors that have shaped our culture's sexual values place sexual behaviors in an entirely unique perspective. This is true for just about all human cultures. Sexual behaviors can take on numerous forms. For example, there are people who date one another without having sexual relations but enjoy the psychological comfort of their partnership. There are married couples who are romantically involved and have sex but do not want to have children.

There are many factors that make up sexual attraction. Perhaps the most dominant factor is physical appearance and what we perceive as attractive. Have you ever wondered why we find some people more attractive than others? Our own sexual psychology is one explanation, but there is actually a science that explains what we perceive to be beautiful. A mathematical formula explaining physical attractiveness was derived 800 years ago by an Italian mathematician, Leonardo Pisano, known now as Fibonacci. He created a formula, known as the Golden Ratio, used by scientists and artists to demonstrate balance and attractiveness in many aspects of nature. It is possible to use the measurements of an individual's facial features to mathematically calculate how closely he or she fits the ideal Golden Ratio calculations of approximately 1.6.

Did You Know...?

Pheromones are chemicals produced by animal organisms acting as sexual attractants in some species. Scientists are studying pheromones in humans to determine if there is a link between odors and sexual attraction. So far, no relationship has been proven, but there are companies already trying to sell "perfumes" labeled as pheromones.

WEB LINK
Golden Triangle

http://www.beautyanalysis.com

Go to this Web site and search some of the links. You will find information about standards of beauty and examples of the 1.6 ratio in nature.

SEARCH TERMS: golden triangle and beauty, beauty and the golden ratio, beauty and mathematics

The Human Sexual Response

Regardless of the source of arousal, men and women respond physiologically with a predictable set of responses. Renowned sex researchers William Masters and Virginia Johnson (1966) studied almost 700 male and female subjects ranging from young adults through elder adults. After recording more than 10,000 cases of sexual arousal and orgasms, they had data that allowed them to describe clearly what the sexual response is like for males and females across age-groups. One of the important findings was that the response was the same regardless of the subject's age.

The human sexual response involves two physiological mechanisms. **Vasocongestion** is a condition whereby more blood is flowing into genital tissue than is flowing out, and **myotonia** is a state of increasing muscle tension during sexual excitement. The response cycle has four major phases (Figure 7-10):

1. *Excitement phase.* As sexual stimulation increases, vasocongestion causes the sexual genitalia to become engorged with blood. For males, the penis becomes erect, and for females, the labia begin to swell, the clitoris enlarges, and the vagina moistens with lubrication. For elder adults, the response is not as complete as that of young adults. An elder male's erection is softer, and the elder female does not produce as much vaginal lubrication.

2. *Plateau phase.* All the changes that began in the excitement phase are enhanced during the plateau phase. In males, the penis becomes firmer, and the erection is more stable. The female's vagina expands, and lubrication intensifies.

3. *Orgasmic phase.* Depending on the person and the level of stimulation received, an **orgasm** will occur during the orgasmic phase. An orgasm is a burst of nervous stimulation and muscular contractions that follows the sexual tension of the plateau phase. It is characterized by pleasurable sensations and muscular contractions. In males, there is ejaculation of semen, consisting of sperm, prostate, and seminal fluid. Female orgasms are characterized by 5 to 20 seconds of muscle contractions in the uterus, pelvic floor, and anus. It appears that approximately 40 percent of women have reported ejaculation of fluid during orgasm. The actual source of the fluid has not been clearly identified, and while some women secrete the fluid so subtly that they don't notice it, about 6 percent are capable of ejaculating forcefully. Depending on the woman's physiology and level of continuous stimulation, she may have multiple orgasms. The orgasms may be a few seconds apart, or they may be 15 seconds or more apart.

4. *Resolution phase.* All the physiological changes that occurred through the first three phases are reversed because of the loss of vasocongestion. While some women may have multiple orgasms, men as a rule do not. Men enter a *refractory period* during which they will not respond to further stimulation for a period of time; some young males can be restimulated in a couple of minutes, while others may need hours.

Sexual Orientation

Sexual orientation is a lasting emotional, romantic, and/or sexual attraction to another person. Sexual orientation is most commonly **heterosexual** in nature, meaning that it is between a male and a female. Research shows, however, that sexual orientation actually

---

myotonia
involuntary muscle tension that occurs in males and females in response to sexual excitement

orgasm
a burst of nervous stimulation and muscular contractions that follows the sexual tension of the plateau phase

sexual orientation
a lasting emotional, romantic, or sexual attraction for another person

heterosexual
sexual attraction for someone of the opposite gender

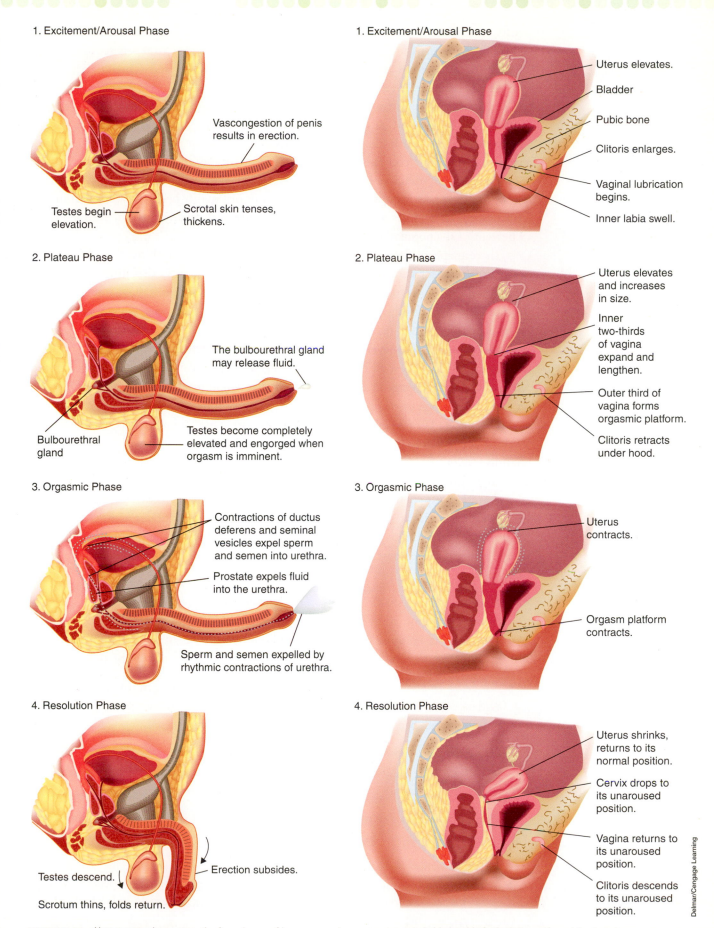

1. Excitement/Arousal Phase

Vascongestion of penis results in erection.

Testes begin elevation.

Scrotal skin tenses, thickens.

2. Plateau Phase

The bulbourethral gland may release fluid.

Bulbourethral gland

Testes become completely elevated and engorged when orgasm is imminent.

3. Orgasmic Phase

Contractions of ductus deferens and seminal vesicles expel sperm and semen into urethra.

Prostate expels fluid into the urethra.

Sperm and semen expelled by rhythmic contractions of urethra.

4. Resolution Phase

Testes descend.

Erection subsides.

Scrotum thins, folds return.

1. Excitement/Arousal Phase

Uterus elevates.

Bladder

Pubic bone

Clitoris enlarges.

Vaginal lubrication begins.

Inner labia swell.

2. Plateau Phase

Uterus elevates and increases in size.

Inner two-thirds of vagina expand and lengthen.

Outer third of vagina forms orgasmic platform.

Clitoris retracts under hood.

3. Orgasmic Phase

Uterus contracts.

Orgasm platform contracts.

4. Resolution Phase

Uterus shrinks, returns to its normal position.

Cervix drops to its unaroused position.

Vagina returns to its unaroused position.

Clitoris descends to its unaroused position.

Delmar/Cengage Learning

FIGURE 7-10 • Human sexual response: the four phases of human sexual response presented side by side for both the male and the female.

homosexual
sexual attraction for someone of the same gender

bisexual
sexual attraction for both genders

exists on a continuum from exclusively heterosexual to exclusively **homosexual**. Somewhere in the center of the sexual orientation continuum is **bisexual** orientation.

Sexual orientation is a condition that develops as males and females go through puberty. It is important to understand that sexual orientation is not simply a matter of choice, neither is it entirely dependent on the cultural norm. The truth is that males and females become aware of their sexual orientation long before they have any sexual experiences. The distribution of the various sexual orientations within the population has remained pretty constant over time. Sexual orientation exists on a continuum; it is not a question of exclusive heterosexuality, nor is it exclusively homosexuality. There are variations in the degree of sexual orientation, with bisexuality being the midpoint on the continuum. Individuals with an exclusively homosexual orientation make up less than 9 percent of the population.

There are people who have biases against homosexual relationships. These biases have been expressed for centuries, even to the point of passing laws declaring homosexual relations illegal. Laws, social pressures, and discrimination, however, have not eliminated homosexual relationships from the continuum of sexual behaviors. This is because no one "chooses" a sexual preference. Perhaps you can recall the first romantic attractions you had as a teen and never really understood why you felt that way or what you were really supposed to do with the feelings. If sexual preference *were* a choice, why would anyone choose to engage in a set of behaviors that would result in being rejected by society and becoming targets of prejudice?

There have been many well-intended efforts to "cure" homosexuals of their sexual preference. The truth is that such "cures" don't work. The American Psychological Association (APA) removed homosexuality from its list of psychological disorders in 1973. The APA also reports that any counseling should focus on helping individuals overcome the stress they experience when realizing and dealing with their same-sex feelings.

Available research shows that many misconceptions exist about same-sex orientation. Even though many people hold to these beliefs, inductive reasoning does not make them true. Here are some common myths, followed by information from the current literature:

- *Homosexuals attempt to "recruit" others to practice the same lifestyle.* Our sexual preference is determined by many factors. If an individual's orientation is heterosexual, he or she can no more be "recruited" to homosexuality than the heterosexual community can "recruit" homosexual individuals to a heterosexual orientation.

- *Just being around gay individuals can cause someone to become gay.* There is research evidence to indicate that this is not the case. It is no truer than believing that a gay individual can become "straight" by being around heterosexuals.

- *Gays are more likely to be child molesters.* This could not be further from the truth. In fact, gays are *less likely* than heterosexuals to be child molesters. It appears that heterosexual men are *twice as likely* to be child molesters as homosexual men.

- *Homosexuals cannot be good parents.* Research states just the opposite. Children raised by homosexual parents are no different than children raised by heterosexual parents.

- *Openly gay teachers, professors, or professionals are dangerous because they may influence young people close to them to become homosexuals.* This is extremely unlikely. Young people don't take on other personal traits of the professionals they associate with. Why would sexual orientation be an exception? The only thing that could result from this kind of relationship is that the professional person might be able to help a young person who is struggling with his or her sexual orientation.

- *Homosexuality is a lifestyle choice.* Same-sex orientation is a feeling, not just a lifestyle. Homosexuals can choose to eliminate their sexual behaviors, but they cannot change their feelings of attraction for the same sex. There are many individuals who attempt to be "straight" by getting married and having children, only to leave the heterosexual relationship years later when they accept their homosexuality.

Homosexual feelings are particularly difficult for young people. At the same time they are experiencing romantic relationships, they may encounter feelings toward someone of the same sex, all the time realizing that society accepts heterosexuality as the norm. They observe the heterosexual behavior of many of their peers. They are faced with the choice of being true to what they feel or trying to fit in to what is considered the culture's normal pattern of sexual partnering. This struggle leads to confusion and an attempt to deny the feelings and follow the norm. Many young people find it very difficult to cope with the pressures of being someone other than the person they feel they should be. Research has demonstrated a significant relationship between homosexuality and teen suicide. If someone you know is experiencing confusion and depression over these issues, he or she should be encouraged to seek help from a trained counselor.

BUILDING YOUR LIFETIME WELLNESS PLAN

No matter what your age, sexual health is an important wellness concern. This chapter only touches the surface of the issues related to sexual health. Reflect on the sexual health topics in this chapter that interest you and spend time elaborating on those topics as you develop your wellness plan. A good first step is to use your health literacy skills to investigate your chosen topics of sexuality. Your wellness plan for this chapter includes an opportunity to test your knowledge of sexuality and investigate topics that might interest you. The second wellness plan component puts you in the role of being a parent and asks you to describe topics you might discuss with children. There is also an exercise to help you learn more about the opposite sex. This exercise is designed to help enhance your understanding of gender issues related to sexuality. Your social and personal health can be enhanced with a level of understanding of those with whom you have a romantic interest.

●●● End-of-Chapter Activities

Opportunities for Application

1. The sexual anatomy and function is an important part of understanding and practicing sexual wellness. Review Figures 7-3, 7-5, and 7-6. Make a list of the major sexual structures in the male and female reproductive structures, then close the book and see if you can describe the important functions of each structure. Check your answers with the text after you complete the exercise and see how much you know.

2. Select eight types of contraceptives. Use the space here to list the contraceptives in order of *actual use* effectiveness from most effective through least effective. Explain the difference between actual use effectiveness and theoretical use effectiveness.

3. Reflect on the material you learned in this chapter. Given the topics that were covered, what topics that interest you were not covered or were covered insufficiently to suit you? Make a list of the three or four that were most important to you and research them using your health literacy skills. Prepare a one- to two-page report on each topic. Your report could include a one-paragraph introduction of each topic and the significance to your sexual education. The remainder of each report can be a bulleted list of significant pieces of information you uncovered.

Key Concepts

1. List and briefly describe the hormones that contribute to the development of male and female secondary sex characteristics.

2. Explain the mechanism that causes the penis to become erect.

3. List and describe the five major forms of birth control.

4. List and comment on five myths related to the cuase of homosexuality.

Answers to Personal Assessment: What Do You Know about Sex and Reproduction?

1. True

2. True

3. True

4. False. Statistically females begin developing secondary sex characteristics about 1.5 years sooner than males.

5. True

6. False. There is no bone in the male penis. Erection occurs because of accumulation of blood in the tissues within the penis.

7. True

8. True

9. False. The time of ovulation can vary from month to month and may be anytime between the twelfth and sixteenth day and be normal. It cannot be predicted.

10. False. The only birth control method that is 100 percent sure to prevent pregnancy is abstinence.

●●● References

Centers for Disease Control and Prevention. (2008). NCHS Health E-Stat: *Trends in Circumcision among newborns.* Retrieved May 20, 2010 from http://www.cdc.gov/nchs/ data/hestat/circumcisions/circumcisions.htm

Central Intelligence Agency. (2009). *The World Factbook 2009.* Washington DC: Author. Retrieved from https:// www.cia.gov/library/publications/the-world-factbook/ rankorder/2127rank.html?countryName=Mayotte &countryCode=mf&regionCode=af&rank =16#mf (March 2010).

Hatcher, R. A., Trussell, J., Stewart, F., Nelson, A., Cates, W. G., & Kowal, D. (2007). *Contraceptive technology* (19th rev. ed.). New York: Ardent Media.

Liandau, S.T., Schumm, L.P., Laumann, E.O., Levinson, W., O'Muircheartaigh, C., & Waite, L.J. (2007). A study of sexuality and health among older adults in the United States. *New England Journal of Medicine,* 357(8), 762–764.

Masters, W. H., Johnson, V. E., (1966). *The Human Sexual Response.* New York, NY: Bantam Books.

CHAPTER 8

The Physically Active Lifestyle

CHAPTER OBJECTIVES

When you finish this chapter, you should be able to:

- Explain the benefits of being physically active.
- List and describe the diseases associated with physical inactivity.
- Identify the various components of health-related physical activity.
- List and describe the major types of injury caused by physical activity.
- Develop a personal fitness plan.

KEY TERMS

aerobic capacity	dynamic stretching	hypokinetic diseases	static stretching
anaerobic activities	eccentric	isometric	target heart rate range
android fat	ergogenic aids	isotonic exercises	tendons
cardiorespiratory fitness	gynoid fat	muscular endurance	
concentric	health-related fitness	neurotransmitters	
cross training	hyponatremia	skill-related fitness	

●●● Introduction

Our bodies are created to move and participate in physical activity. Just like machines with moving parts, bodies function best when they are used regularly. Joints that go too long without moving can get "rusty" and be easily injured. To an extent, the more we demand of our bodies, the stronger and fitter they become.

A century ago, daily living required the performance of physically demanding tasks. There were no cars for transportation, and most labor had to be done by a person rather than by a machine. Most people engaged in a lot of physical activity just in accomplishing their daily tasks. Today, however, we often have to make a special effort to get enough physical activity to stay healthy and perform well. This chapter looks at what it means to be physically active, why it is important, and what you need to know to make smart decisions about physical activity.

PERSONAL ASSESSMENT
Physical Activity Quiz

Before reading this chapter, test how much you already know about physical activity. Read each statement and answer True or False. The answers are located at the end of the chapter.

1. Young adults in America are more physically active now than they were 25 years ago.
2. The most important type of health-related fitness is cardiorespiratory fitness.
3. The only way to be physically fit is to play some type of competitive sport.
4. In general, people who are physically active live longer than those who are inactive.
5. Young adults exercise more often than adults who are over the age of 55.
6. You can die of a heat-related illness such as heatstroke.
7. Research shows that being physically active may help you learn better.
8. You can develop and maintain good flexibility by stretching once or twice a week.
9. If you do strength training, you should exercise the same muscle group every day.
10. Research shows that regular physical activity may be just as effective as drugs or therapy for treating depression.

⬤⬤◯ The Benefits of Being Physically Active

There are so many benefits of being physically active that, as physician and founding director of the National Institute on Aging, Robert N. Butler said, "If exercise could be packed in a pill, it would be the single most widely prescribed and beneficial medicine in the nation (1985, p. 1)." Physical activity not only helps prevent chronic diseases such as heart disease and diabetes but also increases your level of energy (Figure 8-1). When you take part in physical activities that you enjoy, you're a triple winner! First, when you're doing the activity, you're having fun. Second, you gain extra energy to participate more fully in the other aspects of your life. Finally, you build habits that prevent chronic diseases. Being physically active on a regular basis has a multitude of benefits.

Physiological Benefits

Research has shown that people who engage in regular physical activity are much healthier physically than are those who are not regularly active. The Centers for Disease Control and Prevention (CDC) and the American College of Sports Medicine (ACSM) recommend that adults engage in at least 30 minutes of moderate-intensity physical activity on most—and preferably all—days. The surgeon general's report *Physical Activity and Health* (U.S. Department of Health and

WEB LINK
Physical Activity

You can find more detailed information about physical activity recommendations at the following Web sites:

- American College of Sports Medicine: **http://www.acsm.org**
- Centers for Disease Control: **http://www.cdc.gov** (click on "health promotion")
- President's Challenge: **http://www.presidentschallenge.org**

SEARCH TERMS: physical activity, physical activity guidelines

Human Services, 2002) noted that people who are usually inactive can improve their health by participating in even moderate levels of activity on a regular basis.

This physical activity does not have to be "exercise." It can be a part of play, games, sports, work, transportation, or recreation. The activity does not have to be strenuous in order to achieve health benefits, although generally the higher the level of activity, the greater the benefits.

Let's look at some of the specific benefits of exercise:

• *Improved function of the cardiorespiratory system.* During exercise, the cardiorespiratory system is forced to work harder to meet the body's oxygen demands, making the circulatory and respiratory systems stronger and more efficient. The heart muscle gets stronger and begins to pump more blood with each stroke. New capillaries are also formed, making circulation more efficient. As a result, the heart doesn't have to work as hard at rest or during lower levels of activity.

• *Increased basal metabolic rate (the rate at which the body burns calories while at rest).* More than two-thirds of your daily caloric intake is used to support basal metabolism. An individual who exercises regularly burns more calories when at rest than someone who doesn't exercise, so you benefit from exercise even when you're reading, watching television, or sleeping.

• *Increased muscle mass from strength training.* Strength training increases lean muscle mass in the body. Increasing muscle mass also increases the basal metabolic rate because it takes more calories to maintain muscle mass than fat. Low levels of body fat help prevent diseases such as **type 2 diabetes**.

• *Increased levels of high-density lipoproteins, the "good" cholesterol, and decreased levels of both low-density lipoproteins, the "bad" cholesterol, and triglycerides.* High levels of low-density lipoproteins and triglycerides are one of the six major risk factors for heart disease.

• *Reduced chance of hypertension.* Hypertension is abnormally high blood pressure, which is another risk factor for heart disease and stroke.

• *Decreased risk of colon cancer and possibly lower risks for breast and prostate cancer.* Colon cancer is the second-leading cause of cancer death for men and women combined. Prostate and breast cancers are the second-leading causes of cancer deaths for men and women individually.

• *Reduced risk of osteoporosis, a thinning of the bones.* Weight-bearing activities, such as running or walking, are necessary to reduce this risk.

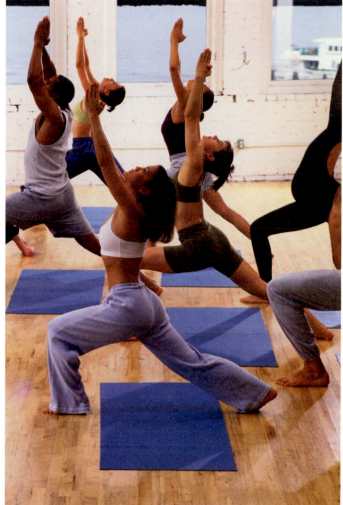

Courtesy of Photodisc

FIGURE 8-1 • One of the many healthful benefits of physical exercise is an increase in one's energy levels.

type 2 diabetes
a condition in which the body cannot transport enough glucose (sugar) to the cells to be converted into energy

Delmar/Cengage Learning

neurotransmitters
chemicals produced in the brain that allow transmission of impulses between nerve cells

TABLE 8-1 • Principal neurotransmitters produced through exercise.

Neurotransmitter	Activity
Serotonin	A moderating effect on mood, emotions, sexual arousal, and sleep
Norepinephrine	Influences arousal, learning, memory, and mood
Endorphins	Pain reducer

- *Improved immune function.* People who participate in regular, moderate physical activity have fewer colds and upper-respiratory infections that do inactive people.

- *Longer life span.* Many studies have found a high correlation between regular exercise and a longer life expectancy.

Psychological Benefits

In addition to the many physiological benefits, there are great mental and emotional benefits to be gained from physical activity. Doing something active that you enjoy is a great way to relieve stress. Even something as simple as going for a walk can be helpful in getting rid of anger and frustration.

Longer sessions of activities, between about 45 and 60 minutes, trigger physiological changes in the body that help improve mood. Although researchers have not yet determined exactly how exercise affects mood, studies show that people who are physically active feel less stressed, experience less anxiety, and are less likely to be depressed than are inactive people. There are several theories about how physical activity affects moods. One is that the rhythmic motion of the body during exercise stimulates an area of the brain associated with mood. Current research is showing that certain beneficial **neurotransmitters** are produced during regular bouts of exercise (Table 8-1).

Figure 8-2 is a photo of adults out hiking and demonstrates the advantage of participating in physical activities, providing opportunities for meeting new people, and doing fun things with friends. Participation may also increase creativity, and new evidence from brain-based research shows that physical activity helps us learn better!

Did You Know…?

Some studies show that regular physical activity can be just as effective as therapy or drug treatment in treating depression. If a person does not have any health insurance, talking to a therapist or taking a prescription drug may not be an option for him or her.

●●● Physical Fitness

What does it mean to be physically fit? There are two major types of physical fitness: health-related fitness and skill-related fitness. Before describing health-related fitness, let's take a look at skill-related fitness.

Skill-Related Fitness

skill-related fitness
the type of fitness required for participating in sports or other skill-related activities; includes such components as power, agility, coordination, speed, balance, and reaction time

Skill-related fitness includes power, agility, coordination, speed, balance, and reaction time. This type of fitness enables you to be successful in sport and motor skill performance. These skills are valuable at all ages—from a toddler just beginning to walk to an older adult who is working on maintaining his or her agility and coordination to accomplish tasks of daily living.

Most often, skill-related fitness is associated with athletic performance enhancement. Training centers that specialize in the development of athletes are becoming more common in the United States. These centers create training programs and regimens to improve performance in skill-related fitness specific to the sport or goal of the client. Many older adult recreation programs, the YMCA, and private recreation centers realize the need to address skill-related fitness components for the health and well-being of their clients. Learning new skills and participating in competitive sports can be both enjoyable and rewarding, adding to your sense of well-being at any age.

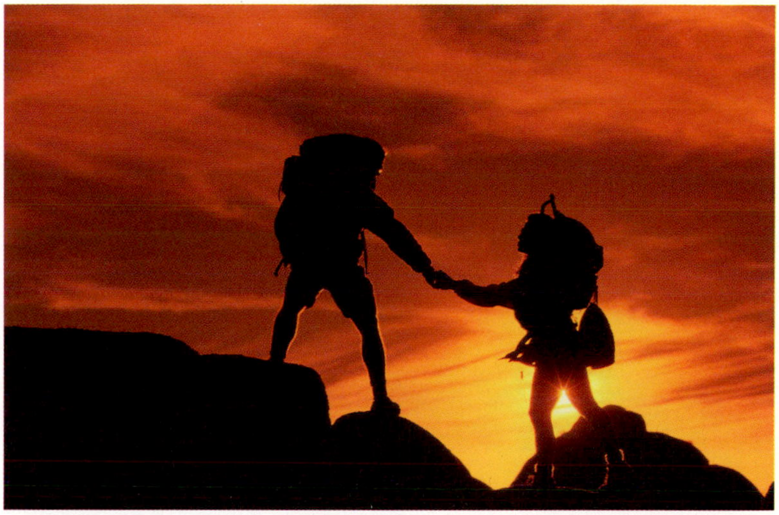

Health-Related Fitness

Health-related fitness is considered by medical experts to be the most important type of fitness. This form of physical fitness provides many of the physical benefits derived from exercise. Even mild physical activities help develop health-related fitness. Health-related fitness programs may contain five major components:

1. Cardiorespiratory endurance
2. Muscular strength
3. Muscular endurance
4. Flexibility
5. Body composition

FIGURE 8-2 • Socializing is a secondary benefit for these adults as they hike as part of their physical activity.

health-related fitness exercise activities that are specifically designed to provide health benefits to the participant

Cardiorespiratory Fitness

Cardiorespiratory fitness is the ability of the circulatory and respiratory systems to provide enough oxygen to sustain moderate levels of physical activity for long periods of time. It is often considered to be the most important component of health-related physical fitness. Cardiorespiratory fitness helps strengthen the heart muscle, improves circulation, and reduces the risk of heart disease. A strong heart, lungs, and circulatory system

cardiorespiratory fitness the ability of the respiratory and circulatory systems to deliver enough oxygen to sustain moderate levels of activity for long periods of time

What's News

New findings in brain-based research have shown that daily physical activity gives students an advantage for learning. Subjects who engaged in vigorous activities improved their short-term memory, creativity, and reaction times. In other studies, students performed activities that required movements that crossed an imaginary line down the center of the body. This activity seemed to help increase blood flow in all parts of the brain, making the brain more alert and ready to learn.

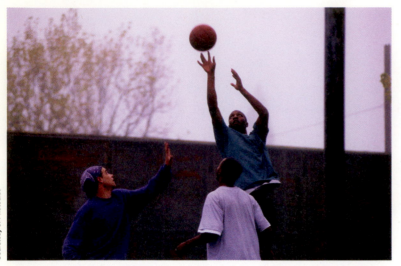

Courstesy of Photodisc

FIGURE 8-3 • Increasing your heart rate for a sustained period of time, as when playing basketball, is a good way to increase cardiorespiratory fitness.

aerobic activities
activities that require a continual supply of oxygen during the activity

anaerobic activities
activities that require short bursts of energy that cannot be sustained for long periods of time because the body cannot supply enough oxygen quickly enough to keep up with the demand

aerobic capacity
the maximum amount of oxygen that can be delivered to and used by the cells of the body during vigorous workouts

also help you perform physical activities. When you have good cardiorespiratory fitness, your heart and lungs function efficiently and don't have to work as hard during times of rest.

The best way to increase cardiorespiratory fitness is to participate in activities that increase your heart rate above your normal resting rate for a sustained period of time (Figure 8-3) and that involve the large-muscle groups of the body in continuous motion. Walking, running, cycling, and swimming are examples of these activities. Activities such as these that require a continual supply of oxygen are called **aerobic activities**. Activities that require short bursts of energy and that cannot be sustained for long periods of time are called **anaerobic activities**. Examples of anaerobic activities include sprinting, racquetball, and weightlifting. Anaerobic activities are not very effective for increasing cardiorespiratory fitness because they do not require sustained periods of exercise. Table 8-2 provides examples of both aerobic and anaerobic activities. It should be noted that, depending on the duration of the exercise, some sports we categorize as anaerobic could be aerobic as well. A recreational game of tennis would certainly be anaerobic, but a game of tennis played by two Wimbledon finalists would be more aerobic.

Aerobic Capacity

Aerobic capacity is the maximum amount of oxygen that can be delivered to and used by the cells of the body during vigorous workouts. If aerobic capacity is high, the heart, lungs, and circulatory system are able to deliver more oxygen to the body with fewer heartbeats per minute. Aerobic capacity can be measured by a treadmill test, in which you walk or run on a treadmill while heart rate and respiratory function measurements are taken. Aerobic capacity can also be estimated by field tests such as the Cooper Institute

TABLE 8-2 • Aerobic and anaerobic activities.

Aerobic Activities	Anaerobic Activities
Brisk walking	Weight training
Jogging/running	Push-ups and sit-ups
Swimming laps	Sprinting
Bicycling	Racquetball
Stair-climbing	Tennis
Cardiovascular equipment at the gym	Baseball
Aerobic dance/group exercise	Football
Water aerobics	Playing Frisbee

1.5-mile walk/run test, YMCA 3-minute step test, and the Two-minute Step-in-Place Test for Older Adults. More information on these tests can be found online.

Aerobic capacity can be improved by participating in regular aerobic activities. The heart rate must reach a certain level, known as the **target heart rate range**, to obtain improvements in aerobic capacity. The target heart rate range is a percentage of a person's predicted maximum heart rate. There are different ranges to aim for depending on the activity that you are doing and amount of time you plan to do it. It would not be healthy to operate at 80 percent of your target heart rate all of the time, but committing to even moderate activity for at least 30 minutes each day can make a big difference in how you feel and look and your overall cardiorespiratory health.

> **target heart rate range**
> the percentage of the predicted maximum heart rate that must be reached to obtain improvements in aerobic capacity

Components of a Cardiorespiratory Fitness Program

Developing cardiorespiratory fitness is important for everyone, not just athletes. Designing a program to increase your cardiorespiratory fitness is not difficult once you understand the four essential elements of the program. You can remember these elements by using the FITT acronym:

F = frequency

I = intensity

T = time

T = type of activity

Your fitness goals will determine how much emphasis to give to each component. Do you want to develop just enough cardiorespiratory fitness to receive health-related benefits? Or do you want to attain a high level of fitness so that you can participate in a competitive sport? These are questions you'll have to answer when developing a personal fitness plan for yourself. Whichever path you choose, it is important to incorporate the FITT principle for the most beneficial cardiovascular results.

Frequency. Frequency is the number of times each week that you engage in a physical activity. You can engage in mild or moderate levels of activity every day. For more strenuous activities, you may want to rest for a day or two during the week. At a minimum, for health-related fitness, you should engage in some type of aerobic activity at least three and up to five times a week.

If your goal is to achieve health-related fitness, you can choose low to moderate levels of activity, such as walking or cycling, and do them daily. To achieve a high level of fitness, you will need to work out at least five times a week at a higher level of intensity. As intensity and time increase, frequency may be decreased. Many aerobic fitness–related activities can also be enjoyable (Figure 8-4).

Intensity. Intensity is how much effort you expend during a typical workout. It is calculated using a formula based on your predicted maximum heart rate, which is 220 minus your age.

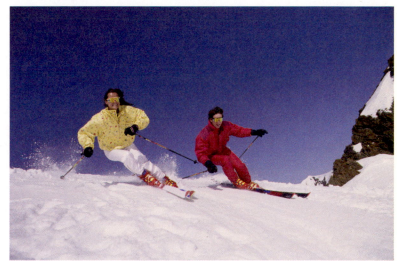

FIGURE 8-4 • Skiing is one example of a high-intensity workout.

Courtesy of Photodisc

The Karvonen Formula for Calculating Target Heart Rate Range

Predicted maximum heart rate is calculated by subtracting your age from 220. Resting heart rate is calculated by taking your pulse before getting out of bed in the morning. Exercise intensity is a percentage of 100%. In the following example, the target heart rate range is calculated for a 25-year-old with a resting heart rate of 70, and exercise intensity is calculated at 60% and 80%.

minus age	220 − 25 195	predicted maximum heart rate	
minus resting heart rate	− 70 125	125	
times percentage of exercise intensity	.60 75	.80 100	
plus resting heart rate	+ 70 145	to + 70 170	heartbeats per minute (target heart rate range)

Delmar/Cengage Learning

FIGURE 8-5 • The Karvonen formula can be used to calculate target heart rate.

For example, if you are 25 years old, your predicted maximum heart rate is 195. Taking a percentage of this predicted maximum heart rate gives an estimate of your target heart rate range, which is the level of physical activity necessary to increase your cardiorespiratory fitness. The Karvonen formula provides a more accurate way of calculating your target heart rate range. Figure 8-5 contains instructions on calculating your target heart rate range according to this formula.

If you are just beginning to participate in aerobic activity, starting at an intensity of 50 to 60 percent of your predicted maximum heart rate is usually about right. If you cannot carry on a normal conversation while working out at this level, you should decrease the intensity.

As your fitness increases, you should be able to work out at an intensity level of between 70 and 85 percent. Working out at intensity levels higher than 85 percent is not necessary unless you are training for a competitive activity or unless you want to achieve a very high level of cardiorespiratory fitness. Working out at intensity levels that are too high can make it difficult to participate in the activity long enough to achieve benefits and increases the risk of injury. It can also discourage you from regular participation in the activity because it will feel like too much work. Keep in mind that you can achieve the health-related benefits of physical activity at a moderate level of intensity.

Once you know your target heart rate range, how will you know if you are within that range while you are working out? There are several ways to monitor or measure your exercise intensity. One simple way is by taking your pulse. The benefit of this method is that it is fairly convenient, although you do need a watch with a second hand or a stopwatch. You can take your heart rate by locating your pulse at the carotid artery on the front side of your neck or your radial pulse at the wrist. After finding your pulse, you can count your heartbeats for a full minute or count for 10 seconds and multiply that by 6 (Figure 8-6).

There are two challenges with this method of measuring exercise intensity. One is that some people have difficulty locating and accurately counting their pulse, so the information ends up not being very reliable. The second challenge is physiological. If you choose to count your pulse for a full minute, your heart rate will slow down in response to your slowing down or stopping to take the pulse. This may not truly indicate the heart rate you were maintaining while exercising continuously.

For a more accurate and repetitive measurement, some exercisers are using heart rate monitors. These are devices that include both a strap that goes around your chest to monitor the heart rate and a wristwatch to give a digital readout to the exerciser. They can be expensive, although there is a wide price range, depending on the features and popularity of the brand. Heart rate monitors can be purchased online or at local sporting goods stores, health clubs, or even some department stores.

Another way to get an estimate of your exercise intensity is a method called rate of perceived exertion (RPE) developed by Gunnar Borg. Borg's RPE scale

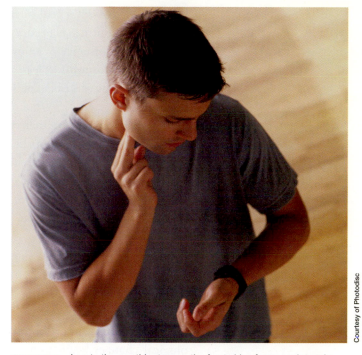

FIGURE 8-6 • Locate the carotid artery on the front side of your neck to take your pulse.

asks the exerciser to rate his or her level of exertion on a scale of 6 to 20 or using a modified scale of 1 to 10. Borg found that most people are quite accurate in assessing their level of exertion during exercise by correlating their stated levels of intensity with specific measures of heart rate during exercise treadmill testing. By simply asking yourself, "On a scale from 1 to 10, how hard do I think I am exercising?," you can get an estimate of your exercise intensity. If after asking yourself that question you answer "4," you can probably conclude that you are most likely below 50 percent of your heart rate maximum and that you had better speed up. Most people know when their exercise intensity is challenging and at a higher level, say at a level of 7, 8, or 9. The beauty of this method is that you don't have to slow what you are doing to take a pulse or look at a heart rate monitor. The downside is that psychological factors, mood states, environmental conditions, and other factors can affect your self-assessment of perceived exertion.

Time. Time (sometimes called duration) is the number of minutes you engage in an activity during a single point in time. According to recommendations made by the American College of Sports Medicine and the U.S. surgeon general, you should spend 20 to 60 minutes at a moderate level of intensity almost every day to gain health-related benefits. In most cases, as intensity increases, the length of time you need to spend performing the activity decreases. And the 20 to 60 minutes can be divided into several sessions throughout the day, as long as each session is at least 10 minutes long and allows you to reach your target heart rate range.

Type. To improve cardiorespiratory fitness, you must engage in an activity that is continuous in nature for a prolonged period of time. Using a combination of your larger muscle groups facilitates locomotor movement for activities that will sustain an elevated heart rate. Two important aspects of being able to improve your cardiorespiratory fitness are acknowledging your current level of fitness and selecting activities that you enjoy. Acknowledging your current level of fitness and choosing an appropriate level of participation is important for being able to stick with a cardiovascular fitness program. If you set a goal of running two miles (at a 10-minute-per-mile pace), three days a week, but it has been a while since you have run at all, you may not be able to complete that distance or enjoy doing it. It's important to select an activity that you can physically perform for at least 20 minutes in duration at the beginning of your fitness program so that you can experience the most amount of success with the least potential for injury.

Selecting an activity that you enjoy is a key to the success of your cardiorespiratory fitness program. If you don't like what you are doing, chances are you won't stick with it. Some people enjoy team activities, such as volleyball and basketball. Others enjoy activities they can do alone, such as running or bicycling. Even if you prefer team activities, you should find some activities you can do alone so that you can still exercise even when no one is available to join you.

Warm-Up and Cool-Down

Although they are not components of the FITT formula, proper warm-up and cool-down are important activities that give the body time to adjust to and recover from the demands of physical exercise. The ideal warm-up is a low-intensity activity that mimics the activity that you are about to perform. On initial movement of your body, physiological changes begin to occur. These changes prepare your body for the power and muscular efficiency to do the work that you will be asking your body to do. Some of the physiological changes include an increase in muscle and core body temperature, an increase in metabolic rate, the release of lubricating fluids to your joints, and the dilation of capillaries for better circulation. It's important that the warm-up is continuous for 5 to 10 minutes in duration. You can follow this with some gentle stretching through the full range of motion of your joints and muscles just to loosen up.

When you have completed your workout, take some time to cool down. A cool-down constitutes a gradual recovery from the more intense work your body has been performing, such as walking or jogging slowly for approximately five minutes following your more intense walk or jog. During workouts, much of the blood supply of the body is directed to the muscles. The cooling-down period allows for a gradual return of heart rate and blood pressure to near resting values, helping to redirect blood back to the rest of the body and reducing the potential for postexercise dizziness. A good time to do more substantial stretching is after this cooling-down period.

Muscular Strength

muscular strength
the amount of force a muscle is capable of exerting against a resistance with a single maximum effort

Muscular strength is the amount of force a muscle is capable of exerting against a resistance with a single maximum effort. You need muscular strength to perform simple everyday tasks, such as getting out of bed in the morning and getting in and out of a bathtub. You also need muscular strength to do household chores and home repairs or to lift a heavy box off the floor at the office.

The most common way to measure the strength of a muscle is to determine the maximum amount of weight it can move at one time. This is known as the one-repetition maximum. Muscular strength is increased by resistance training (also called strength training). Resistance can be provided by the weight of the body, elastic bands, or weights. In resistance training, the amount of weight is similar to intensity in cardiorespiratory fitness. If your primary goal is to achieve maximum muscular strength, your strength-training program should include heavy weights lifted 5 to 10 times. This exercise is usually repeated three times with rest in between.

Working a muscle group against an object that doesn't move is known as isometric exercise. Pushing against a wall is an example of an isometric exercise. Isometrics, however, do not provide strength throughout a range of motion, so they are not widely used.

Isotonic exercises are those in which the muscle group works against a movable heavy object and exercises a specific muscle through the muscle's range of motion. Push-ups, pull-ups, and lifting weights are examples of isotonic exercises. There are two types of muscular contractions that make up the motion involved in isotonic exercises: **concentric** and **eccentric** contractions. Muscles work in pairs. While one muscle contracts, the opposite muscle relaxes. To return to the position, the muscles change roles. The concentric phase of muscle contraction is the shortening phase of the primary working muscle. Envision a person performing a bicep curl. The arm is extended and located along the side of the thigh. As the palm is raised by bending at the elbow, you can see the bicep muscle in the upper arm starting to shorten or bulge. This is the concentric phase of muscle contraction. When the person returns the arm to the starting position, you will observe a lengthening or flattening of the bicep muscle. This is the eccentric phase of muscular contraction. The eccentric phase is still considered a contraction because muscle tension must be present so as not to drop the weight or damage the joint while lowering the weight. Muscles work in pairs. In this example, while the bicep is contracting or shortening, its partner (the triceps) is lengthening. This is important for muscle/joint support and stability as well as efficiency of movement.

You may have heard of **isometric** contractions. This type of exercise causes the muscle to work against an *immovable* object. An example would be to stand in a doorway and try to push the two sides of the door away from you. This type of strength training limits the development through a range of motion because the muscle is exercised in a static position.

The body is composed of many muscle groups. Each group must be exercised to develop strength throughout the body. But it is important not to overuse the muscles. The same muscle group should not be worked two days in a row because muscle tissue should be given at least 48 hours between workouts to repair itself. The American College of Sports Medicine recommends that weight training be performed as one set of 8 to 10 exercises, utilizing each of the major muscle groups, two to three times a week.

Muscular Endurance

Muscular endurance is the ability of a muscle to contract over and over again before becoming fatigued. We need muscular endurance for all types of daily activities, such as walking, climbing stairs, and participating in recreational sports.

Muscular endurance is measured by the number of times you can move a weight using a particular muscle. A practical example would be your ability to repeatedly carry bags of groceries from your car to where you live or the length of time you could continue to dig in your garden before your hands, arms, and other muscle groups would fatigue. These are known as repetitive movements or repetitions. If your goal is to increase muscular endurance, you will want to choose lighter weights and do more repetitions than when you are training to develop muscular strength. To increase muscular endurance, you have to continue the activity for a longer period of time.

Muscular endurance activities, as well as muscular strength activities, need recovery time so that the muscle groups involved have a chance to strengthen and repair. Most cardiovascular activities employ a certain amount of muscular endurance activities to facilitate the repetitive movements during the activity. While you can participate in

---

isotonic exercises
Exercises where the muscles move heavy weight through their range of motion

concentric
a muscle shortens as a result of moving a resistance

eccentric
a muscle lengthens in response to the release of weight held by a concentric contraction

isometric
muscle contraction without movement through a range of motion

muscular endurance
the ability of a muscle to contract repeatedly without becoming fatigued

cardiovascular activities on a daily basis, the intensity and type of activity you select will determine if your muscles need a day in between for rest. For example, if you go for a walk for 30 minutes at a moderate pace one day, most likely your body will be able to engage in a more intense cardiovascular activity like jogging or taking a kickboxing class the very next day, even though walking and jogging (or kickboxing) will involve some of the same muscle groups and range of motion. Listening to your body and paying attention to muscle soreness as well as levels of fatigue is a good indicator for activity selection and frequency.

Flexibility

Flexibility is the ability to move the joints of the body through a full range of motion, meaning the various directions that a joint can move. The joints throughout the body have different types and ranges of motion. Developing flexibility involves stretching the muscles and **tendons** that enfold each of the joints.

Flexibility is probably the most frequently overlooked component of health-related fitness. We are naturally flexible as infants and children, but flexibility begins to decline as we grow older, especially for people who don't regularly engage in activities that require stretching. Many back and joint problems are caused by lack of flexibility. Maintaining good flexibility can help you avoid injuries during work, play, and competitive sports.

When people think of improving their flexibility, they often think in terms of lower-body flexibility. Some people gauge their flexibility by whether they can "touch their toes." This type of flexibility specifically measures only one aspect of flexibility. While leg muscles need to remain supple, upper-body flexibility, such as the flexibility to scratch your back or reach over your head, is important too. Remember that flexibility is the ability to move all joints through a full range of motion without limitations or pain.

To be most effective, stretching exercises to maintain flexibility should be performed daily. The best time to stretch a muscle group is when it has been warmed up by exercise. Although it is good to stretch lightly before an activity, most stretching should be done at the end of a workout.

There are two main types of stretching exercises: **dynamic stretching** and **static stretching**. Dynamic stretching is slow and controlled movement through a range of motion. The muscle is stretched for 10 to 30 seconds to a point of mild discomfort and then returned to its original position. This process allows the muscle to relax and then stretch to a greater length than normal.

Static stretching involves slowly stretching a muscle to the end of its range of motion and then holding that position for an extended period of time (usually 15 to 30 seconds). This type of stretching is most effective in increasing flexibility. Perhaps you remember or heard about a jerky, bouncing type of stretching (ballistic stretching). Fitness experts no longer recommend this type of stretching because of the risk of injury to the muscles and tendons. Yoga has become a popular activity for static stretching, which is used in many of its postures (Figure 8-7). These postures are used to lengthen and strengthen muscles. Yoga originated in India and is both a mental and a physical activity that can help improve flexibility, posture, agility, and even mental health. Because there are many styles of yoga available, it is important to find out which of the styles works best for you.

Stretching before your workout should be dynamic, meaning a slow movement through the full range of motion around a particular joint. Think of your muscle as being like an elastic rubber band with memory. Your muscles want to be stretched and relaxed to the extent that they will be asked to perform. Static stretching should be performed at

flexibility
the ability to easily move the joints of the body through a full range of motion

tendons
dense connective tissues that attach muscle to bone

dynamic stretching
slow and controlled movement through a range of motion

static stretching
stretching a muscle to the end of its range of motion and holding that position for an extended period of time

the end of your workout for improvement in flexibility. Another popular activity used to both stretch and tone muscles is Pilates. Similar to Yoga, Pilates increases flexibility and agility but accomplishes this through resistance exercises that isolate certain muscle groups. Some Pilates exercises require that you use machines, but most exercises are done on a mat using resistance bands.

To optimize positive increase in flexibility, prevent injury, and have a successful workout, it is important to remember the following:

1. *Warm up*. Perform a cardiovascular warm-up for 5 to 10 minutes.

2. *Gently stretch*. Follow your warm-up by some gentle dynamic stretching.

3. *Perform your workout.*

4. *Cool down*. Follow up with a cardiovascular cool-down.

5. *Stretch*. Perform static stretching on a variety of muscle groups throughout your body, holding each position for 15 to 30 seconds.

Body Composition

Body composition is considered one of the five components of health-related fitness. Body composition is the relationship between fat-free mass, such as muscle, bone, and water, and fat tissue within the body. There are many factors that affect a person's body composition. For example, when you engage in cardiorespiratory fitness, depending on the level of intensity, your body uses primarily fat as a fuel, first from circulating fat in the bloodstream and later from fat stores in the body. This ultimately affects body composition. Muscular strength exercises increase muscle mass (fat-free mass). Nutrition and food choices affect body composition as well. As you can see, many things affect your body composition.

Body composition is an indicator of health because the amount of fat tissue in your body plays a role in physical functioning, such as the workload on your heart, lungs, circulatory system, and muscles. It's important to note that you need a certain amount of fat to ensure proper hormone regulation, protect internal organs, keep your skin healthy, and perform additional important physiological tasks.

Normal ranges for body fat vary by gender. For males, the approximate amount of body fat should be 15 to 18 percent and for females 18 to 24 percent. Females need a higher percentage of body fat to maintain hormone levels and ensure that the body is prepared to support a possible pregnancy.

There are several ways to measure body composition, with varying levels of convenience and reliability. Three of the most common methods are presented here, with more detail presented in chapter 10. The most accurate method is hydrostatic weighing. It is most commonly used in research settings and is considered the criterion method for assessing body fat percentages. This test is performed by weighing and then placing the person on a sling

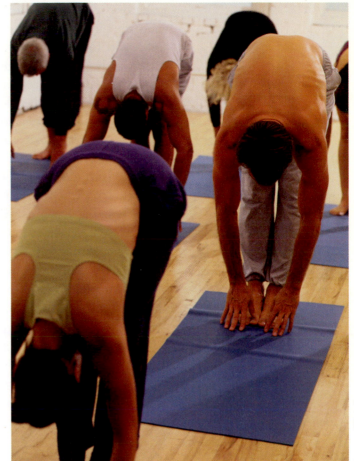

Courtesy of Photodisc

FIGURE 8-7 • Stretching is an important part of any workout.

body composition
the relationship between fat-free mass (muscle, bone, and water) and fat tissue within the body

attached to a special scale in a tank of warm water. The person submerges him- or herself under the surface of the water and exhales fully while the test administrator records his or her weight. The submerged weight and the body weight taken on land are used to calculate percent body fat. Some health and fitness facilities have the equipment and personnel to administer hydrostatic weighing. There are even companies that have a mobile hydrostatic weighing lab to make scheduled visits to health fitness facilities or community gatherings.

The second most reliable and one of the most widely used method for measuring body composition is skinfold caliper testing. This is a method of measuring skinfold thickness to determine percent body fat. The fat percentage value obtained by skinfold equations is typically within 4 percent of the value measured using hydrostatic weighing. The accuracy is dependent on the knowledge and skill of the health professional performing the test. The test administrator locates three to seven sites to "pinch" on the person to be tested. At precise locations and angles, the test administrator pulls a thickness of skin away from the muscle and measures using skinfold calipers.

The third method of assessing body composition is bioelectrical impedance analysis. This is a simple, noninvasive technique that assumes that tissues high in water content, such as muscle and bone, will conduct electrical current with less resistance than tissues with little water. Fat tissue will impede the flow of electrical current because it does not contain much water. The test is performed by sending a small electrical current through the body of the person being tested. This current is not detectable to the person being tested. While this test is quick and can be self-performed, it has a high level of error because it is dependent on the type of equipment, the equations used, and, most important, a person's state of hydration at the time of the test. There are standardized guidelines to be followed that can greatly increase the reliability of this test. Many health club facilities have this method of testing available for their members because of the ease of administration.

Research shows that as body fat increases above recommended levels, health risks also increase. Therefore, increasing muscle, decreasing body fat, or both are important aspects of being fit. Another consideration is body fat distribution. Researchers recognize that the pattern of body fat distribution is a predictor of certain health risks linked to obesity. **Android fat**, or trunk (abdominal) fat, creates an increased risk of hypertension, type 2 diabetes, coronary artery disease, and premature death as compared with individuals who display **gynoid fat** (fat distributed in the hips and thighs). Where you primarily deposit fat is genetically determined, but a person can decrease his or her overall amount of body fat to help combat the health risks associated with android or trunk obesity.

Nonperformance Health-Related Fitness

Along with the five components of health-related fitness, there are some additional components of fitness that are nonperformance related. Nonperformance components of fitness are those that relate to changes internally as a result of engaging in physical activity. The nonperformance components of fitness relate to internal biological systems that are influenced by regular participation in physical activity, such as metabolic fitness, morphological fitness, and bone integrity:

- *Metabolic fitness.* Metabolic systems and their adaptations in response to exercise includes variables predictive of the risk for diabetes and cardiovascular disease.

- *Morphological fitness.* Body composition factors that can be internally changed such as regional body fat distribution and body circumference are known as morphological fitness.

android fat
fat that has accumulated in the region of the trunk

gynoid fat
fat that tends to accumulate in the hips and thighs

- *Bone integrity*. Bone integrity relates to the level and state of bone mineral density in the body.

While these parameters are measurable, most people won't notice a metabolic fitness response, such as a positive change in their fat profile. These internal adaptations in response to habitual activity are the reasons why physically active individuals have a lower risk of premature development of **hypokinetic diseases** those diseases associated with physical inactivity such as type II diabetes, hypertension, and cardiovascular disease). Participation in activities that incorporate the five components of health-related fitness will also have a positive effect on the nonperformance-related measures of health as well.

> **hypokinetic diseases**
> diseases that are associated with prolonged periods of inactivity

●●● Avoiding Injury

Many people who begin fitness programs injure themselves and cannot continue. There is always some risk when participating in physical activities, and some activities have higher levels of risk than others. You can lower your risk of injury in several ways:

- Properly prepare your body for the activity.

- Learn how to perform the activity correctly.

- Practice proper safety precautions.

- Know your own limitations.

There are two main types of injury related to physical activity: overuse injuries and traumatic injuries.

Overuse Injuries

Overuse injuries involve the muscles and joints. Injuries are likely to occur when you try to do too much too quickly for too long. Perhaps you have experienced the aches and pains that can occur during normal walking after participating in a vigorous activity that you're not used to, such as running or playing basketball. Overuse injuries are not usually serious, but they can take a long time to heal, especially if you continue doing the same activity repetitively.

When you start a physical fitness program, it's easy to be overly enthusiastic and set your goals too high. As you push to accomplish these goals, your body doesn't have enough time to adapt, and you could suffer an overuse injury. The best way to prevent this type of injury is to start your workout program slowly and then gradually increase your activity level. Be sure that any increases in frequency, intensity, or time are added slowly. A good rule of thumb for progression of your exercise program is to increase either intensity or duration (but not both at the same time) by about 5 percent every one to two weeks, depending on your starting level of fitness.

If you feel pain in a joint or muscle when you exercise and believe that it may be an overuse injury, rest the painful area and avoid any activities that cause pain. Rest usually allows the body's tissues to repair themselves and prevents the need for further treatment. Once the pain is gone, you can resume activity. Just begin slowly and cut back again if the pain returns. If the pain continues, you may need to see a physician.

Good footwear, with good arch support and appropriate to the specific activity, is also critical for preventing overuse injuries. To find the best shoe for you, visit an athletic shoe store that sells a variety of brand names. There is no such thing as a "best" brand for a particular activity. The best shoe for you is the one that fits your particular foot and addresses your biomechanical and orthopedic needs.

Common types of injuries due to overuse include plantar fasciitis, shin splints, tendonitis, and runner's knee. Plantar fasciitis occurs when the plantar fascia, which are bands of tissue located on the bottom of the feet, become inflamed. This can result from repetitive weight-bearing activities, including running and walking. It can be prevented and alleviated by thorough stretching of the fascia before and after activities in addition to wearing shoes with good arch support.

Another common injury due to excessive weight-bearing activities is shin splints. Shin splints are often identifiable by pain and swelling at the outer side at the middle of the shin where there is soft tissue. While there is no treatment for shin splints, rest and icing of the affected area along with supportive shoes are the best ways to alleviate the symptoms.

Tendonitis is a common injury that is best described as an inflammation of the tendon. Tennis elbow is a classic example of this injury and is usually caused by overuse. Athletes and older adults are more prone to experiencing tendonitis, and the use of rest and ice to diminish swelling of the inflamed tendons are the most commonly used treatments to minimize the painful symptoms of tendonitis. In extreme cases, an injection of cortisone may be used to reduce the inflammation for a longer period of time.

Finally, runner's knee is a condition often detected by swelling and pain around the kneecap due to problems associated with the muscle, tendons, and ligaments in the knee. Just like the other injuries mentioned, the best way to reduce symptoms of runner's knee is to take a break from the activity causing the pain and find ways to build up the muscles around the kneecap that will reduce stress placed on the knee.

Traumatic Injuries

The second main category of injury is traumatic injury. These are usually sudden and unplanned. Examples of traumatic injuries include a sprained ankle, a strained knee, a broken arm, and a head injury. Traumatic injuries can be serious, even life threatening. It is best to try to prevent them rather than have to treat them once they occur. Effective prevention techniques include the following:

- Learning the proper skills needed to safely perform an activity

- Using caution while engaging in the activity

- Using appropriate safety equipment as needed

Safe cycling, for example, involves knowing how to properly ride a bicycle, following the rules of the road, watching out for cars or pedestrians that may not be paying attention to you, and wearing a helmet at all times (Figure 8-8). Wearing a helmet and safety pads also helps prevent serious injury while skateboarding or riding a scooter. Racquetball players should always wear protective eyewear. Eye injuries from a speeding ball can result in permanent loss of vision. Working out alone outdoors at night is a risk that you don't need to take. Find someone to go with you and always be aware of your surroundings. Be sure to wear reflective clothing so that you can be easily seen.

The treatment for a traumatic injury will depend on the nature of the injury. If you have a serious traumatic injury, such as a broken bone, you need to seek medical assistance immediately. For less serious injuries, like those overuse injuries previously mentioned, you may be able to do some initial treatment yourself. If you have a traumatic injury to soft tissue, such as a strain or sprain, using the RICE formula may help reduce swelling. RICE stands for the four components of the treatment:

R = rest

I = ice

C = compression

E = elevation

Apply ice in 10- to 20-minute intervals immediately after the injury. Place a towel or other cloth between the ice and the skin surface to avoid damage from the cold. Applying a compression wrap that is not too tight and elevating the injured area can also help keep the swelling down by helping to move the blood toward the heart. Traumatic injuries can often be serious, so it is best to consult medical personnel for proper treatment. Prompt treatment may prevent further damage to the injured part.

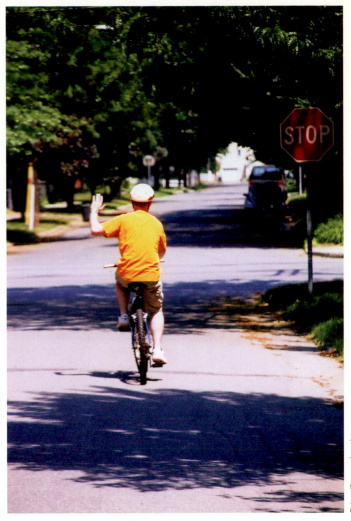

Delmar/Cengage Learning

FIGURE 8-8 • Always practice safe cycling to prevent traumatic injuries.

Safety Considerations

In addition to avoiding injury, there are other considerations to ensure your safety when you are participating in physical activities. For example, you should always wear reflective clothing if you exercise outdoors at night. Never exercise outdoors when lightning is present or in stormy weather. Be aware of hazardous conditions and use common sense to keep your fitness program healthy and enjoyable.

Hot Weather

You must take extra care when exercising in hot weather because your body may not be able to get rid of the extra heat it is generating. A combination of high humidity (the amount of moisture in the air) and high temperature presents an even more dangerous situation. Overheating and failing to take in enough fluids can result in heat exhaustion and heatstroke.

Heat exhaustion occurs when the body begins to overheat because of the loss of fluids. Heatstroke is even more serious. It occurs when the body is generating heat so rapidly that its cooling mechanism can't keep up with the demands on it. Heatstroke is a life-threatening emergency and can result in death very quickly. A person with suspected heatstroke needs immediate medical attention.

To prevent heat-related illnesses, avoid vigorous activity during the hottest part of the day or at times when both heat and humidity levels are high. Always get enough fluids to replace the amount you are losing. Drink at regular intervals; don't wait until you feel thirsty.

Cold Weather

Prolonged exposure to freezing or near-freezing temperatures can result in frostbite or hypothermia. Frostbite is an external freezing of the skin from prolonged exposure to cold temperatures. It can occur more rapidly if it is windy or if you get wet or damp. Fingers, toes, ears, and the facial area are particularly susceptible to frostbite. Keep these areas dry and protected from cold and wind. Frostbite should not be taken lightly. This condition can be serious and can result in the death of the injured tissues.

Hypothermia is a potentially fatal condition in which the body is losing heat faster than it can produce it. This imbalance results in an abnormally low core body temperature. If you are participating in a physical activity in cold and windy or wet conditions, wearing proper clothing is important. Choose layers of clothing and fabrics that will help "wick" the moisture away from your body. A great deal of heat escapes from the head, so always wear a hat. Pay particular attention to protecting the face, fingers, and toes. In extreme conditions, taking the day off from an outdoor activity may be a good idea.

Illness

Participating in physical activity during a mild illness, such as a cold, is usually okay if you feel like doing it. If you don't, it's a good idea to wait until you're feeling better. It is especially important to minimize physical activity if you have a fever, are being treated with prescription drugs, or feel weak, dizzy, or faint. If you do decide that you feel well enough to participate, you may want to decrease the intensity of the activity and not push yourself too hard.

Fluid Replacement

You can avoid many problems by drinking enough fluids to replace those that you are losing because of physical activity. The rule of thumb is to "drink before you're thirsty." By the time you feel thirsty, your body is already experiencing the effects of not having enough fluids.

A general guide is to drink at least eight ounces of water for every 30 minutes of activity and more if the weather is hot or humid. If your workout is less than 60 to 90 minutes long, water alone is sufficient to replace the fluids your body has lost. For intense exercise more than 60 to 90 minutes, a commercial energy replacement drink may help replace

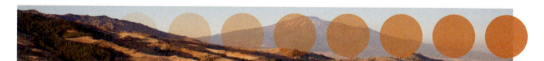

What's Your View?

According to an annual study sponsored by American Sports Data, Inc., people over the age of 55 exercise more often than people in any other age-group. Of people over the age of 55, 26 percent exercised at least 100 times in the past year, compared with only 18 percent of those 12 to 17, 20 percent of those 18 to 34, and 23 percent of those 35 to 54. Are you surprised? Why do you think such a small percentage of the population exercises, especially among younger adults? Perhaps younger adults think that if they are not overweight, there's no need to exercise. Maybe they think that they will have more time to exercise in the future than they do now. What other reasons do your friends and colleagues give for not exercising?

some of the electrolytes the body is losing and supply simple carbohydrates for energy. Inadequate fluid intake can cause your performance in an activity to suffer and affect how you may feel afterward. It can also contribute to serious problems such as heat exhaustion and heatstroke.

Nutritional Supplements

The use of nutritional supplements to enhance performance is a controversial subject. There is no quick, easy way to become stronger and fitter. Physical conditioning requires consistent, steady effort over a period of time and adherence to a nutritious eating plan. Many of the well-advertised supplements have little proof to support their claims. There have also been few studies conducted to determine how safe these supplements are. If it sounds too good to be true, it probably isn't true!

There are certain nutritional and pharmacological agents that some exercisers consume before, during, or after exercise in an effort to help fuel their bodies and/or to gain a performance advantage. These agents are referred to as **ergogenic aids**. There are a variety of products that provide no documented physiological advantage, such as bee pollen, brewer's yeast, or consumption of vitamins and minerals taken in higher-than-recommended

Did You Know...?

Jennifer Strange, a 28-year-old woman from Sacramento, California, died in 2007 after participating in a water-drinking contest through a radio station as a way to secure a Wii game console for her children. The coroner's report said that her death resulted from water intoxication, or **hyponatremia** (Figure 8-9).

hyponatremia
a result of a chemical imbalance of too much water and not enough electrolytes in the body

ergogenic aids
nutritional or pharmacological agents used by exercisers to help provide fuel and/or to gain a performance advantage

---

Is It Possible to Drink Too Much Water?

The answer is yes. While many people do not drink enough water, there are times when people overconsume water in the name of health. This condition is called hyponatremia, or water intoxication. Hyponatremia is a result of a chemical imbalance of too much water and not enough electrolytes in the body. Electrolytes are nutrients such as sodium, potassium, chloride, and calcium that are critical to organ function. Hyponatremia occurs most often when someone is participating in strenuous or long-endurance workouts and consumes extreme amounts of water in order to avoid potential dehydration. The strenuous exercise depletes the electrolyte levels, but since the person is consuming only pure water as replacement, this can cause a dangerous and potentially fatal chemical imbalance.

Oddly enough, the symptoms of hyponatremia mimic the symptoms of dehydration. Early signs may include nausea or muscle cramping, along with disorientation. Many people then drink even more water, thinking that they are dehydrated. This only makes the problem worse. Severe symptoms of hyponatremia include confusion, agitation, and seizures. Hyponatremia can be fatal if not treated.

If you are participating in long-endurance or high-intensity activities, you should replace lost body fluids with drinks that contain electrolytes, such as sports drinks, along with water. This will both hydrate you and protect the body's chemical balance. It will also ensure that you will feel good and perform well during the activity.

FIGURE 8-9 • Hyponatremia.

amounts. Other products, such as caffeine, have been shown to improve performance in endurance events. Caffeine and many other substances have been regulated by various amateur and professional sporting managerial groups (such as the International Olympic Committee) and deemed either illegal or permissible only in specified amounts.

There is some evidence that athletes who are training intensely may benefit from increasing their protein intake above the level recommended for a sedentary person. This protein increase should be in the form of food intake rather than supplements, as the interaction of nutrients plays an important role in the resulting usability of the protein. You cannot force the body to use protein it does not need. Intake of a balanced diet on a regular schedule is the best approach to fueling your workout.

● ● ● Developing a Personal Fitness Plan

There are two main steps in developing a personal fitness plan: (1) determining your goals and (2) designing a plan to achieve them. To get started, ask yourself these questions:

- What do I want to accomplish?

- What activities do I enjoy doing?

- What facilities and equipment will I need?

- Is there anything I'll need to buy?

- How much time do I have to devote to physical activities?

- How will I realistically schedule exercise into my day?

- What will help me stay motivated?

Designing Your Plan

When designing your fitness plan, keep in mind that there are various levels of physical activity. Some physical activities don't require much expenditure of energy, such as washing the car, raking leaves, and walking in the park but they are important in adding overall physical activity to your day and building on your health-related components of fitness. Unfortunately, many adults don't even get the minimal amount of physical activity that would fall into this category. Other physical activities may use a little more energy, although the energy required may not be constant. Activities that fall into this category include walking to school or doing errands, riding your bike to work or class, and playing softball. Then there are activities that consistently require a high expenditure of energy. Examples include hiking, biking, running, playing basketball, and swimming.

Even mild to moderate physical activities help develop health-related fitness. Participating in fast-moving, vigorous sports is not necessary. And some people have limitations that must be considered. For example, you may have a medical condition, such as asthma or diabetes, or you may have a physical challenge that makes it difficult to find an appropriate activity. Many activities can be adapted so that people of all abilities can participate and enjoy themselves. Wheelchair basketball and wheelchair tennis are examples of adapted activities. The Paralympics and Special Olympics are sport competitions

PERSONAL ACTIVITY PLAN

My Overall Goal:

My Plan to Achieve My Goal:

	Frequency	Intensity (if applicable)	Time	Type
Cardiorespiratory fitness	(Example: Four times per week)	(Example: 65%)	(Example: 30 minutes)	(Example: Walking)
Muscular strength				
Muscular endurance				
Flexibility				

Body composition: **Current body fat percentage:**

Body fat percentage goal:

People who will support me in my efforts:

How I'll reward myself for my progress:

Delmar/Cengage Learning

FIGURE 8-10 • Personal activity plan.

for people who have mental or physical challenges. Regardless of individual limitations, almost everyone can benefit from some type of physical activity. You can prepare a personal activity plan using a format like the one shown in Figure 8-10.

Increasing Your Chances of Success

Many people who start a personal fitness program don't stay with it very long. Starting any new routine can be difficult. It can be tempting to quit if you don't see immediate results or if you become overly sore or injured from doing too much too soon. Be patient—the results will come over time. With attention to a workable schedule or plan, you can create a method for success and a habit of regular physical activity. The first month is the most difficult. After that, you have developed a habit of physical activity, and it will become easier to maintain it. Beginning or enhancing a physically active

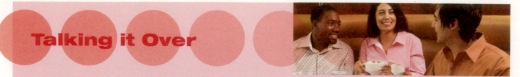

Talking it Over

What Keeps People Active?

Establishing a regular habit of physical activity is a key to good health. Ask some of your older friends or active, older family members if they were physically active as young adults. If they were, find out what activities they did during those times and how their activities in their younger years affected the physical activities they engage in today. If friends or family are not physically active, find out what keeps them from being physically active.

lifestyle will result in benefits for years to come. The habits you develop now are likely to determine how physically active you will be in the future. Many people who have been physically active all their lives remain active in their seventies, eighties, and beyond. You are laying the foundation for your future.

There are several things you can do to increase your chances of sticking with your fitness program and being successful. Following these suggestions can help you continue your fitness program and accomplish your goals without getting injured.

Start Out Slowly

Remember that your body needs time to adjust to new activity levels. Starting slowly also prevents overuse injuries. Depending on the type of activity, it will take your body about three to six weeks to adjust to your new activity level. Being patient and starting slowly increase your chances of avoiding injury and being able to continue your planned workout schedule.

Have Reasonable Expectations

It is also important to have reasonable expectations. It is *not* reasonable, for example, to think that you can run three miles seven days a week if you have not been exercising previously. The current condition of your body has developed over years. It will take time and consistent effort to make the changes you want. You will notice some immediate results or responses to your activity regimen, and additional results will occur after regular participation in your exercise program for a prolonged period of time.

Be Committed and Consistent

Success requires being committed to your program and not giving up easily. On some days, you will be excited and eager to work out. On other days, you may not feel very enthusiastic. When you don't feel like doing your planned activity, sometimes the only thing you can do is to follow the Nike slogan and "Just Do It." Sometimes, just getting started is the hardest part! The important thing is to do something active every day, even if only for a short period of time. Regular, consistent activity over time is the best way to achieve all the health-related benefits of physical activity.

Find an Activity Partner

Finding someone who has goals similar to yours and who wants to work out with you can make the difference in whether you continue with your fitness program or drop out. Knowing that someone is counting on you to show up makes it more likely that you will too. It's also more fun to work out with someone else. You should, however, have a plan for individual activities in case your workout partner can't join you. An alternative is important, too, if you participate in group activities. Have a backup plan in case the group is not available. Don't become dependent on others to make sure that you follow your plan.

Regularly Record Your Progress

Keeping track of the physical activities you engage in can help keep you motivated. Recording the time, distance, and number of days a week can help you determine if you are achieving your goals. Some people prefer simple systems, such as check marks if they work out. Others are willing to devote extra time to keeping more complicated records that give them a clearer picture of their status and improvement. Just getting into the habit of writing down your activities every day can help you maintain your commitment to your goals. Improvement is a great motivator. Review your activity journal periodically to see if you should make changes in your fitness plan.

Consider Cross Training

In recent years, **cross training** has become very popular. Cross training involves participating in two or more different activities to achieve cardiorespiratory fitness. It helps prevent the boredom of doing the same activity over and over. Cross training can also help avoid overuse injuries by giving the various muscle groups time to rest. One of the more popular types of cross training is triathlon-style training, which includes running, swimming, and bicycling. Even if you don't plan to compete in a triathlon, the combination of these activities can produce high levels of cardiorespiratory fitness and minimize the chances of boredom or injury.

cross training
participating in two or more different physical activities to achieve cardiorespiratory fitness

BUILDING YOUR LIFETIME WELLNESS PLAN

In this chapter, you learned about the benefits of physical activity and the ways to plan a program to increase your physical fitness. Exercise is one of the single most important things you can do to prevent disease and live a long, high-quality life. There is little doubt that physical activity is one of the best health-enhancing activities you can engage in. From exercise, you can gain a quality physical body, reduce stress, head off many diseases, and maintain healthy body composition. The important thing to remember is your motivation. *You* must make physical fitness an important part of your life.

●●● **End-of-Chapter Activities**

Opportunities for Application

1. Your neighbor has a teenage son, Seth, who wants to "get in shape" and has asked for your advice. His son is overweight, according to his doctor. Seth thinks that lifting heavy weights will tone him up and get him in shape. Explain how you would determine Seth's level of fitness. Discuss what you would advise Seth to do to get in shape. Provide supporting rationale for your exercise advice.

2. Your roommate is the volunteer coach of a soccer team made up of 15- to 16-year-old girls. She wants you to assist her in developing a conditioning program for her players. The two of you are committed to providing a safe, effective conditioning program for the players. Discuss some injury prevention strategies you would share with the team. Explain the conditioning program you would implement with the team. Provide supporting rationale for your program design.

3. One of your older relatives has not been exercising for a number of years and knows that you exercise quite often. He or she has asked your advice about how to get started on an exercise program. What advice would you give? What important considerations would you need to think about as you prepare your response?

Key Concepts

1. Describe the components of health-related fitness.

2. Identify the benefits of regular activity.

3. Explain factors that you (or someone else) should consider in designing an activity plan for improving general health.

Answers to Personal Assessment Quiz: Physical Activity Quiz

1. False. Twenty-five years ago, young adults were more physically active than they are now, and this contributes to the increase in overweight adults and young adults and the increased incidence of type 2 diabetes.

2. True

3. False. As demonstrated in this chapter, there are many ways to be active. From doing chores around the house to participating in both aerobic and anaerobic activities, there are numerous opportunities in our daily life to stay active.

4. True

5. False. Older adults, ages 55 and up, are one of the most physically active age-groups.

6. True

7. True

8. False. Although often overlooked in most exercise programs, exercises that incorporate stretching and flexibility should be done every day, especially for adults and older adults as their natural flexibility decreases.

9. False. Good strength training requires that you rotate muscle groups that are used. This helps prevent injuries caused by overuse and fatigue.

10. True

●●● References

American Sports Data Inc. (2006). *The superstudy of sports participation.* Retrieved from http://www.americansportsdata .com [November 2008].

Butler, R. (1985). Don't take it easy . . . exercise. *Age Page, (1)*1. National Institute on Aging.

U.S. Department of Health and Human Services. (2002). *Physical activity and health: A report of the surgeon general.* Atlanta: Author. Retrieved May 15, 2010 from http://aspe .hhs.gov/health/reports/physicalactivity

CHAPTER 9

Nutritional Wellness

CHAPTER OBJECTIVES

When you finish this chapter, you should be able to:

- List and discuss the major classifications of nutrients.
- Explain the relationship between foods and metabolism.
- Describe the significance of the essential amino acids.
- Discuss the significance of fats in the diet.
- Describe the difference between water-soluble and fat-soluble vitamins.
- Explain the rationale for the food pyramid.
- Describe how to read a food label.
- Explain how to handle food safely to prevent food-borne diseases.
- Describe nutritional needs of specific population subgroups.

KEY TERMS

alimentary canal
amino acids
antioxidant
basal metabolism
carbohydrates
complete protein
Daily Reference
   Values (DRVs)

disaccharides
essential amino acids
essential fatty acids
   (EFAs)
hydrogenation
incomplete proteins
ketosis
lipids

megadoses
milligram
monosaccharides
monounsaturated fats
nutrient density
osteoporosis
polysaccharides
polyunsaturated fats

Reference Daily Intakes (RDIs)
saturated fats
trans fat
unsaturated fats

●●● Introduction

Food is an important part of human existence. Of course, people need food to live. But food is more than a necessity; it also plays a very important social function. Food is often used to help celebrate special occasions. In fact, virtually every culture has special dishes to help celebrate holidays, marriages, family celebrations, and other important occasions. In many cultures, the special celebration meals are marked by foods that are hard to come by under normal eating conditions.

Your Eating Habits

Think about the foods you might eat on an average day and then answer the questions below as accurately as you can. Feedback is located at the end of the chapter.

1. How often do you eat breakfast?

   a. I don't eat breakfast.

   b. I eat breakfast some days.

   c. I eat breakfast most days.

   d. I eat breakfast every day.

2. On an average day, how many portions of fruit and vegetables do you eat?

   a. I don't eat fruit or vegetables.

   b. One or two portions

   c. Three or four portions

   d. More than four portions

3. On an average day, how many portions of meat do you eat?

   a. More than five portions

   b. Four or five portions

   c. Two or three portions

   d. One portion

4. How many portions of dairy products (milk, cheese, yogurt, or ice cream) do you eat on an average day?

   a. More than seven

   b. Six or seven portions

   c. Four or five portions

   d. Two or three portions

5. How many portions of pasta, bread, or grain products do you eat on an average day?

   a. None

   b. One portion

   c. Two or three portions

   d. Four or five portions

6. With respect to your physical condition, what would you say about your weight?

   a. I am significantly underweight.

   b. I am significantly overweight.

   c. I am gaining weight.

   d. My weight is about right.

7. If you had to choose one of the following snack foods to eat, which would you choose?

   a. Cheese puffs

   b. Apple pie

   c. Salted nuts

   d. Raw almonds

If you were asked to estimate the proportion of people in the United States who do not get enough food to eat, what would your estimate be? What is it that led you to that particular conclusion? In the United States, most people don't have to worry about starvation. Food is plentiful enough for all but a small portion of the population. A 2006 report on hunger in the United States reported that 25.3 million Americans, representing about 8 percent of the population, do not get enough food. For most people in the United States, the most serious nutrition problems are caused by too much rather than too little food. Most of us get plenty to eat. The key is to eat the correct amount of the type of food that is best for your health.

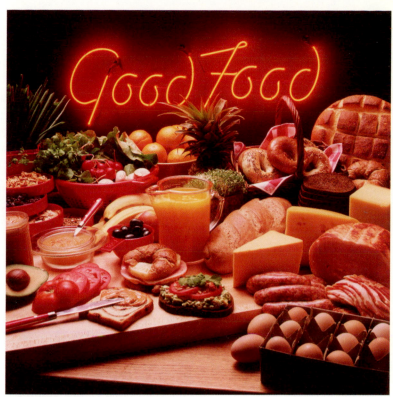

FIGURE 9-1 • Healthy nutrition comes from a variety of foods.

🟢🟢🟢 Nourishment

Most Americans take having sufficient food for granted, and they often satisfy hunger with foods they *like* to eat or foods that are *convenient* to eat instead of what foods are *best* to eat for meeting their nutritional needs. This is understandable because in the United States, we have numerous "feel-good" food products, most of which are packaged convenience foods, and high-fat foods from fast-food outlets. Eating what we like may be satisfying at the time, but poor eating habits over time can eventually result in negative health consequences. Our wellness goal should be to eat what is good for us while choosing from among the foods we like, such as those illustrated in Figure 9-1.

Being well nourished is not the same as being well fed. A person whose diet consists largely of fast-food and high-calorie snacks probably consumes enough food, but that person may not be well nourished. A person could have his or her hunger needs satisfied by eating fries and sugar-laden soft drinks all day, every day, but at what cost? The quality and quantity of nutrients would be extremely low. Moreover, consuming the same foods day after day would not provide the *range* of nutrients needed for optimal health. Being well nourished with a range of nutrients is important so that the body can function at its best. Most people are unaware of the science behind good nutrition. Knowing some of this science will help you develop your nutritional wellness plan.

Food Nutrients

Nutrients are the substances in food necessary for the body to function properly. There are six basic nutrients the body must have: carbohydrates, protein, fats, vitamins, minerals, and water. Although we eat to satisfy hunger, the real purpose of food is to supply the body with energy, with materials to build tissues, and with chemicals for regulating many body functions. Nutrients are extracted from foods during the digestive process, which

Super Size Me

Super Size Me was a documentary film produced in 2004 by Morgan Spurlock and Kathbur Pictures. The film chronicled the attempt of fast-food companies to "supersize" meal portions for just a little more cost. People would see the offer as a bargain to get more high-fat food portions for just a little more cost. The problem was that the customers were essentially unknowing of all the fat and calories they would get with their "bargain." The documentary and public pressure eventually forced food chains to give up the practice. You can view the entire film as a free download at http:// freedocumentaries.org (search for "Super Size Me").

alimentary canal
the tubular passage from the mouth to the rectum that functions in digestion, the absorption of food and water, and the elimination of waste

takes place in the stomach and small intestine as the food passes through the **alimentary canal** (also known as the gastrointestinal tract). Figure 9-2 illustrates the components of the digestive system.

Acids, enzymes, and other secretions in the alimentary canal break the food down into molecules that can be absorbed into bloodstream. The blood carries the molecules to the body's cells, where they are used to provide the energy, chemicals, and protein necessary for cell growth and functions. Nutrients come in many forms, and each serves a specific purpose in the body.

Carbohydrates

Carbohydrates are perhaps the single most important nutrient because they provide energy needed for all body functions, including sleep. Energy is needed for everything the body does, such as circulating blood, processing food, growing new cells, and repairing damaged cells. Energy is even necessary for thinking. The more active a person is, the more energy his or her body needs.

WEB LINK
Nutrition.gov

http://www.nutrition.gov

This is an excellent, searchable Web site with information on good nutrition practices, recent research, healthy food recipes, and more.

SEARCH TERMS: nutrition, nutrition information, good nutrition

The amount of energy needed to carry out the basic body functions, such as breathing, blood circulation, and cell growth and repair, when you are at complete rest (sleeping) is known as **basal metabolism**. As soon as you wake up and start moving, your metabolism increases because movement requires energy. When you exercise, your heart beats faster than normal, you breathe harder, and your muscles work harder, requiring extra energy. That's why someone who is actively exercising needs more energy sources than someone who is not active. Imagine the energy sources needed by a marathon runner! Your energy needs for your life span were highest during your teen years. Beginning in your twenties, your energy needs slowly decline throughout your life span (Table 9-1). The amount of energy needed to maintain basal metabolism gradually decreases with age as well. At a time in life when energy needs begin to decline, many people begin decreasing their level of physical activity, but they do not adjust their eating patterns. This is one reason why people tend to gain weight as they get older if they maintain the same eating patterns they had when they were younger.

carbohydrates
food substances that provide energy for the body

basal metabolism
the amount of energy needed to maintain body functions at rest

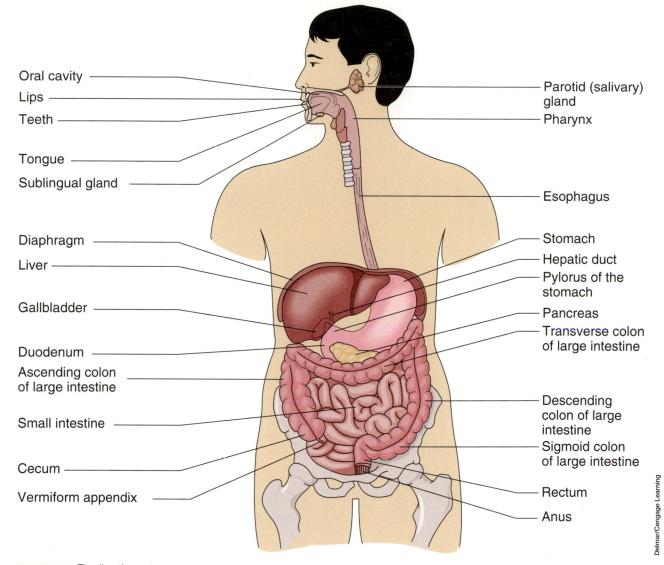

Oral cavity
Lips
Teeth
Tongue
Sublingual gland
Diaphragm
Liver
Gallbladder
Duodenum
Ascending colon of large intestine
Small intestine
Cecum
Vermiform appendix

Parotid (salivary) gland
Pharynx
Esophagus
Stomach
Hepatic duct
Pylorus of the stomach
Pancreas
Transverse colon of large intestine
Descending colon of large intestine
Sigmoid colon of large intestine
Rectum
Anus

Delmar/Cengage Learning

FIGURE 9-2 • The digestive system.

Energy is measured in calories. A **calorie** is a scientific measure of the amount of heat needed to raise the temperature of one kilogram (a little more than one quart) of water one degree Celsius (about 1.8 degrees Fahrenheit). This is why our bodies give off heat; more heat is generated during exercise and less heat during sleep. The number of calories a person should consume each day depends on how much energy is needed for that person to live and perform daily activities. This amount is determined by body weight, lean muscle mass, activity level, and age.

Carbohydrates come in three forms: monosaccharides, disaccharides, and polysaccharides. **Monosaccharides** are the simplest of sugars, existing in a form that requires no digestion. All other carbohydrates are broken down to monosaccharides during digestion. An example of a monosaccharide (simple sugar) is glucose. Glucose is the energy source provided through intravenous feeding during hospital stays. It can be delivered directly into the bloodstream so that the patient gets immediate energy. Monosaccharides provide a quick source of energy because they are rapidly processed by the body and absorbed into the bloodstream. Foods composed of simple carbohydrates are what you need if you are participating in an

calorie
a measure of the amount of energy needed to raise the temperature of one kilogram of water one degree Celsius; scientists burn foods to measure the number of calories they contain

monosaccharides
the simplest form of sugar that can be immediately absorbed into the bloodstream

TABLE 9-1 • Estimated calorie requirements for each gender and age group at three levels of physically activity.

Gender	Age (Years)	Activity Level		
		Sedentary	Moderately Active	Active
Female	14–18	1,800	2,000	2,400
	19–30	2,000	2,000–2,200	2,400
	31–50	1,800	2,000	2,200
	51+	1,600	1,800	2,000–2,200
Male	14–18	2,200	2,400–2,800	2,800–3,200
	19–30	2,400	2,600–2,800	3,000
	31–50	2,200	2,400–2,600	2,800–3,000
	51+	2,000	2,200–2,400	2,400–2,800

Adapted from: U.S. Department of Health and Human Services and U.S. Department of Agriculture (2005).

disaccharides
double sugar molecules that must be broken down to monosaccharides during digestion

polysaccharides
also known as "complex carbohydrates" because they are compounds of many monosaccharides

athletic event of short duration and requiring bursts of energy such as gymnastics, sprinting, golf, bowling, and so on.

Disaccharides contain pairs of monosaccharide molecules. They must undergo digestion and be broken down to monosaccharides before they can supply the body with energy. Examples of disaccharides are table sugar, known as sucrose, and fruit sugar, called fructose. This energy source would be useful in athletic events of longer duration because of the time needed for the body to make the conversion to monosaccharide. Another one of these sugars is lactose, found in milk and dairy products. Many people, particularly people from certain racial groups, are "lactose intolerant," meaning that they cannot break down lactose molecules. According to the National Institutes of Health, up to 80 percent of African Americans, 80 to 100 percent of American Indians, and 90 to 100 percent of Asian Americans are lactose intolerant (NIDDKD, 2006).

Polysaccharides are the starches we eat. They are water-insoluble molecules made up of numerous sugar compounds that take longer to digest than simple carbohydrates. The large molecules must be broken down into simple carbohydrates before their energy becomes available. For this reason, they release energy over longer periods of time. Beans, wheat bread, oatmeal, and tortillas are examples of complex carbohydrates. An athlete who is playing in a soccer match or running a marathon would benefit from a meal high in complex carbohydrates before the competition. Because complex carbohydrates take longer to convert to glucose, the athlete will have a constant supply of energy during the event.

The only animal product that contains significant amounts of carbohydrate is milk and milk products, such as cheese. Aside from skim milk, milk products also contain varying amounts of fat. Later in this chapter, you will learn more about the energy value of fat, but it should be noted that fat takes longer to become an energy source than do polysaccharides. Look at the fruits vegetables, milk products, and complex carbohydrates in

WEB LINK
Calorie Calculator

http://www.mayoclinic.com

Go to this Web site and enter "calorie calculator" in the search window. It will take you to a site where you can enter data to calculate your calorie needs per day. Retake the assessment a few more times entering different future ages for you. Compare the calorie needs you will have for future years.

SEARCH TERMS: calorie calculator

Figure 9-3 and see if you can identify the energy sources that are found in each of the foods.

Protein

Protein is the nutrient needed to build and repair tissue in the body and to build hormones and enzymes. Under conditions of starvation when carbohydrates and fat are unavailable to provide energy for the body, the body will convert protein to energy. The Recommended Dietary Allowance of protein for normal, healthy adults is about 0.36 grams of protein per pound of body weight. According to dietary recommendations, it is not difficult for the average person to meet his or her protein requirements. There is some protein in almost all the foods you eat, but animal products are especially high in protein. As food is digested, the protein compounds of the food are broken down into **amino acids**, the building blocks of protein. The amino acids are then recombined in the body to form the specific types of proteins needed for body tissues.

The human body needs approximately 20 amino acids. Many of these amino acids can be manufactured from foods we consume. Of the 20 amino acids, there are nine that the body cannot manufacture. These are known as **essential amino acids** because they *must* be present in the foods we eat. Foods that contain all nine of these amino acids are known as **complete protein** sources. Complete protein sources come from animal tissue, such as eggs, meats, cheese, milk, and fish. If you eat foods from plant sources, containing **incomplete proteins**, you can still get all the essential amino acids if the amino acids from the different foods are consumed in certain combinations, known as complementary proteins. Here are some examples of complementary protein combinations:

- Peanut butter and bread
- Soybeans and rice
- Beans and tortillas
- Tofu and rice

This does not mean that you need to concentrate on consuming complementary proteins. In general, a normal diet will capture the proteins you need. It would be wise, however, for a person to have a clear understanding of complementary proteins if he or she were interested in a vegetarian diet.

Individuals who are physically active or who participate in sports will need more protein than those who are less active. This is because sports injuries require tissue repair, and athletic training produces more muscle tissue. Because most Americans consume more protein than they normally need, there is no real reason for anyone, including a physically active person, to consume large amounts of protein or to take protein supplements. Some athletes involved in weightlifting or other strength sports mistakenly believe that if they eat more protein or take supplements, they can build

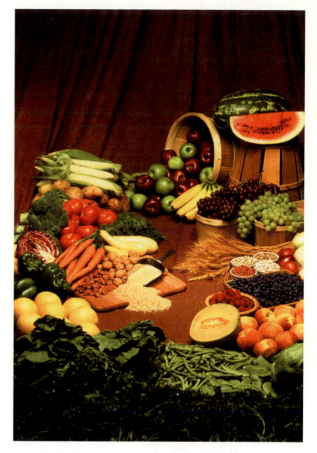

FIGURE 9-3 • Fruits, vegetables, grains, and milk products are good sources of carbohydrates. Courtesy of Agricultural Research Service, USDA.

protein
nutrient used by the body to build and repair tissue and to manufacture enzymes

amino acids
organic compounds that are the building blocks of protein

essential amino acids
the amino acids humans must get in their diet and that cannot be manufactured by the body

complete protein
protein source containing all nine essential amino acids

incomplete proteins
protein sources that do not contain all nine of the essential amino acids

more muscle tissue. The truth is that eating extra protein cannot cause an increase in muscles tissue. Muscle growth and strength come from training and an adequate diet, not from eating protein. Anyone who consumes large amounts of protein and little carbohydrates runs the risk of producing **ketosis**. Ketosis is an accumulation of acids in the bloodstream produced during metabolism of fat from the protein source. Long periods of ketosis can result in harm to the liver and kidneys.

Fats

Fats, also known as **lipids**, are greasy food materials that are concentrated sources of energy. A tablespoon of butter contains 100 calories, whereas a tablespoon of sugar has only 45 calories. Fats are usually the part of the meal that makes us feel full.

A small amount of fat in the diet is necessary for good nutrition. In addition to giving you energy, fats carry the fat-soluble vitamins through the body and help synthesize certain hormones. When stored in the body, fat helps cushion and support the organs. It is only when you consume too much dietary fat that health is threatened. The best recommendation is that you should receive *no more than 30 percent* of your total daily calories from fat sources. Not only is the amount of fat a concern, but so is the type of fat.

There are three major forms of fat in our diet: **saturated fats**, **monounsaturated fats**, and **polyunsaturated fats**. Saturated fats are found in animal fat sources. Butter, cream, cheese, fat on meat, palm oil, and lard are examples of saturated fats. These fats are firm at room temperature. Saturated fats are linked to coronary heart disease because they tend to raise the **cholesterol** level in the blood. The body needs some cholesterol to build cells and produce certain hormones (sex hormones are derived from cholesterol), but too much cholesterol can be harmful, especially to the circulatory system. You may have heard the expressions "bad cholesterol" and "good cholesterol." Bad cholesterol is low-density-lipoprotein (LDL) cholesterol. High levels of LDL can accumulate in the arteries and lead to heart disease and other health problems. Good cholesterol is high-density-lipoprotein (HDL) cholesterol. HDLs act as "cholesterol sponges" that help keep cholesterol from clinging to the walls of the arteries. It is desirable to have low levels of LDLs and high levels of HDLs. In addition to eating habits, the following wellness practices can have positive effects on cholesterol levels:

- Exercise tends to increase the level of HDL and lower the level of LDL.
- Nonsmokers have higher levels of HDL.
- Moderate sugar intake is better for HDL than high-sugar diets

The American Heart Association recommends that you consume no more than 300 milligrams of cholesterol each day. One egg contains approximately 215 milligrams. **Unsaturated fats** are found in plant oils. Some oils, such as corn oil and safflower oil, are polyunsaturated. Polyunsaturated fats are better for you than saturated fats because they do not significantly raise cholesterol levels. Even better are the monounsaturated fats, such as peanut oil, olive oil, and canola oil. These oils are actually called "heart healthy"

ketosis
buildup of ketone bodies, potentially poisonous by-products of fat metabolism

lipids
fatty compounds in foods that provide energy and transport certain vitamins

saturated fats
fats from animal sources that are firm at room temperature

monounsaturated fats
types of oils containing fats that contribute very little to the development of heart disease

polyunsaturated fats
fats that come from plant sources that are better for heart health than saturated fats

fats because they have a favorable effect on cholesterol levels. These fats are liquid at room temperature, unless they have had hydrogen added during processing to make them more solid. This process, known as **hydrogenation**, converts the unsaturated oils into **trans fat**. Examples of food products containing trans fats are margarine, commercially prepared pie crusts, baked goods, fried foods, and, to a lesser degree, butter. Research has shown that a number of health problems are associated with the consumption of trans fat. It appears that trans fat increases LDL levels and decreases HDL levels. Excess trans fat consumption by mothers has also been linked to low-birth-weight infants. Low birth weight is a leading risk factor for infant deaths during the first year of life. In January 2006, the U.S. Food and Drug Administration (FDA) required all packaged foods to be labeled with the amount of trans fat in the product.

Americans unknowingly consume large amounts of trans fat because it is in many processed foods, such as cookies, pie crust, processed cheese, and peanut butter (unless the peanut butter is naturally prepared, in which case the oil separates from the peanuts). It would be almost impossible to eliminate all trans fat from your diet. The best advice is to avoid eating large quantities of foods that contain hydrogenated or partially hydrogenated oils. Read your food labels and avoid oils that are "hydrogenated" or "partially hydrogenated."

Among the fats we need from our diet, **essential fatty acids (EFAs)** are probably the most important and most overlooked. EFAs are important because they are present in every cell of the body and are critical for normal growth and development.

Deficiencies in EFAs contribute to a number of health problems, including reduced growth rates, decreased immune function, and skin changes, such as dryness and scaliness. There are two forms of EFA: omega-3 fatty acids and omega-6 fatty acids. Omega-3 fatty acids are found in cold-water fish, such as salmon, tuna, mackerel, and flounder, but they also exist in nuts, vegetables, beans, and fruit. Omega-3 fatty acids are heart healthy. Omega-6 fatty acids are found in safflower, sunflower, and corn oils. Studies indicate that Americans eat 30 times more omega-6 fatty acids than omega-3 fatty acids. The reason is that we consume more foods fried in oils that contain omega-6 fatty acids (fries and potato chips) or made with omega-6 oils (cookies, pies, and packaged snack foods) than foods containing omega-3 fatty acids, such as fish, nuts, and vegetables.

Vitamins

Vitamins are compounds that are necessary in very small amounts to control a number of body processes. Contrary to popular belief, vitamins themselves do not give you energy. Rather, they enable the body to produce energy from the foods you eat. Select dietary vitamin requirements are expressed as **Reference Daily Intakes (RDIs)**. The

Did You Know...?

For a packaged food product to be labeled "low fat," it must, by law, contain no more than three grams of fat per serving.

cholesterol
a waxy, fatlike substance in the body an excess of which may contribute to heart disease

unsaturated fats
fats that come from vegetable oil sources

hydrogenation
the addition of hydrogen molecules to liquid fats to make them firm at room temperature

trans fats
liquid fats that have been intentionally enhanced with hydrogen to make them firm at room temperature or more suitable for frying

essential fatty acids (EFAs)
fats needed by the body that must be consumed in the diet because the human body cannot manufacture them

Reference Daily Intakes (RDIs)
the levels of a vitamin or mineral recommended to be included in the diet each day

What's News

The New York City Council has prohibited the use of trans fat in the city's restaurants beginning in 2007. Recognizing the health risks associated with trans fat, the New York City Board of Health recommended the trans fat ban to the city council.

RDIs for various nutrients have been set by the scientific and medical professionals according to research on humans and animals. There are no RDIs for fat, sodium, cholesterol, or carbohydrates. The recommendations for these and certain other foods are expressed as **Daily Reference Values (DRVs)**. The DRV for protein is determined by both age and gender. You should note that RDIs have a cushion built in to help ensure that sufficient amounts are consumed. For example, if you get 70 percent of the RDIs, you are likely to prevent deficiency symptoms. See Table 9-2 for a listing of nutrients and their corresponding RDIs and DRVs.

Although vitamins are important, they should not be overused. In fact, **megadoses** can be toxic (poisonous) if taken for long periods of time. For example, taking megadoses of vitamin A can lead to bone pain, decreased appetite, and hair loss. Excessive doses of vitamin C can lead to the development of kidney stones. The motto when taking vitamins is "if a little is good, a little is good enough." There is no need to take higher doses than the RDIs recommended.

Vitamins are classified according to whether they are water soluble or fat soluble. Water-soluble vitamins are easily destroyed by air, light, and cooking, so it is important to properly store and prepare the vegetables containing water-soluble vitamins. For example, one spear of raw broccoli contains 141 milligrams of vitamin C, but a cooked spear contains only about 110 milligrams. A **milligram** is a unit of metric weight that is one one-thousandth of a gram; 100 milligrams is equal to 0.0035 ounces—about the same weight as a pinch of salt. The more it cooks, the greater the vitamin C loss. Eating the vegetable raw can provide access to more vitamins, and they can also be retained if the broccoli is baked instead of boiled. One way to recover lost vitamins from cooked vegetables is to make soup from the cooking liquid.

Fat-soluble vitamins are not lost in cooking. When eaten, they are transported through the body by lipids in the bloodstream. Unlike water-soluble vitamins, which do not remain in the body, excess amounts of fat-soluble vitamins are stored in the liver and can be used later. This is why fat-soluble vitamin deficiencies are slower to appear than are water-soluble vitamin deficiencies. See Table 9-3 for a list of fat-soluble and water-soluble vitamins and their sources, functions, and deficiency problems.

Nutritionists used to believe that if people ate a balanced diet, vitamin supplements were unnecessary, but recent evidence indicates that this is not necessarily true. Taking a vitamin supplement has been shown to add health benefits, especially if you include an extra **antioxidant**, such as vitamin A, C, or E. For safety, just be sure you do not exceed the RDI for the day.

Facts and Myths about Vitamin Use

People have a general knowledge about vitamins, but they may hold certain misconceptions about accessing and using them correctly. Read each of the following statements and see if your working knowledge of vitamins is good:

- "Vitamins in food are better than vitamins from food supplements." Not true. The body recognizes vitamins as chemical elements for what they are able to do, not for where they come from. The chemical compositions of vitamins in foods and those in tablet form are the same.

Daily Reference Values (DRVs)
reference values of eight selected nutrients for a 2,000-calorie diet; the basis of nutrition labels

megadoses
doses that are much larger than what is recommended, approximately 5 to 10 times the RDI

milligram
a unit of metric weight that is one one-thousandth of a gram; 100 milligrams is equal to 0.0035 ounces—about the same weight as a pinch of salt

antioxidant
compound that interferes with the damaging effects of certain compounds in the body; may help lower LDL in the blood and prevent certain cancers

TABLE 9-2 • Reference daily intakes and daily reference values for a 2,000-calorie diet.

Nutrient	Reference Daily Intakes (RDIs)
Vitamin A	5,000 International Units (900 micrograms for men; 700 micrograms for women)
Vitamin B$_6$	2.0 milligrams
Vitamin B$_{12}$	6 micrograms
Vitamin C	75 milligrams
Thiamin	1.5 milligrams
Pantothenic acid	10 milligrams
Riboflavin	1.7 milligrams
Biotin	0.3 milligrams
Niacin	20 milligrams
Vitamin D	400 International Units
Vitamin E	22 International Units
Vitamin K	90 micrograms
Calcium	1.0 gram
Copper	900 micrograms
Folic acid	0.4 milligrams
Iodine	150 micrograms
Iron	18 milligrams
Magnesium	400 milligrams
Phosphorus	1.0 gram
Zinc	11 milligrams
Daily Reference Values (DRVs)	
Total carbohydrate	300 grams
Protein	50 grams
Fat	65 grams
Saturated fatty acids	20 grams
Cholesterol	300 milligrams
Fiber	25 grams
Sodium	2,400 milligrams
Potassium	3,500 milligrams

Delmar/Cengage Learning

TABLE 9-3 • Fat-soluble vitamins and water-soluble vitamins.

Name	Food Sources	Functions	Deficiency/Toxicity
Fat-soluble vitamins			
Vitamin A (retinol)	Animal Liver Whole milk Butter Cream Cod liver oil Plants Dark green leafy vegetables Deep yellow or orange fruit Fortified margarine	Maintenance of vision in dim light Maintenance of mucous membranes and healthy skin Growth and development of bones Reproduction Healthy immune system	Deficiency Night blindness Xerophthalmia Respiratory infections Bone growth ceases Toxicity Birth defects Bone pain Anorexia Enlargement of liver
Vitamin D (calciferol)	Animal Eggs Liver Fortified milk Fortified margarine Oily fish Plant None Sunlight	Regulation of absorption of calcium and phosphorus Building and maintenance of normal bones and teeth Prevention of tetany	Deficiency Rickets Osteomalacia Osteoporosis Poorly developed teeth and bones Muscle spasms Toxicity Kidney stones Calcification of soft tissues
Vitamin E (tocopherol)	Animal None Plant Green and leafy vegetables Margarines Salad dressing Wheat germ and wheat germ oils Vegetable oils Nuts	Antioxidant Considered essential for protection of cell structure, especially of red blood cells	Deficiency Destruction of red blood cells Toxicity none
Vitamin K	Animal Liver Milk Plant Green leafy vegetables Cabbage, broccoli	Blood clotting	Deficiency Prolonged blood clotting/ hemorrhaging Toxicity Hemolytic anemia Interferes with anticlotting medications
Water-soluble vitamins			
Thiamin (vitamin B₁)	Animal Lean pork Beef Liver Eggs Fish Plant Whole and enriched grains Legumes Brewer's yeast	Metabolism of carbohydrates and some amino acids Maintains normal appetite and functioning of nervous system	Deficiency Gastrointestinal tract, nervous system, and cardiovascular system problems Beriberi Toxicity None

TABLE 9-3 • Fat-soluble vitamins and water-soluble vitamins. (*continued*)

Name	Food Sources	Functions	Deficiency/Toxicity

Riboflavin (vitamin B_2)	Animal
	  Liver, kidney, heart
	  Milk
	  Cheese
	Plant
	  Green, leafy vegetables
	  Cereals
	  Enriched bread
		Aids release of energy from food
		Health of the mouth tissue
		Healthy eyes
			Deficiency
			  Cheilosis
			  Eye sensitivity
			  Dermatitis
			  Glossitis
			  Photophobia
			Toxicity
			  None

Niacin (nicotinic acid)	Animal
	  Milk
	  Eggs
	  Fish
	  Poultry
	Plant
	  Enriched breads and cereals
		Energy metabolism
		Healthy skin and nervous and
		  digestive systems
			Deficiency
			  Pellagra-dermatitis, dementia, diarrhea
			Toxicity
			  Vasodilation of blood vessels

Pyridoxine (vitamin B_6)	Animal
	  Pork
	  Fish
	  Poultry
	  Liver, kidney
	  Milk
	  Eggs
	Plant
	  Whole-grain cereals
	  Legumes
		Conversion of tryptophan to niacin
		Release of glucose from glycogen
		Protein metaboplism and synthesis
		  of nonessential amino acids
			Deficiency
			  Cheilosis
			  Glossitis
			  Dermatitis
			  Confusion
			  Depression
			  Irritability
			Toxicity
			  Depression
			  Nerve damage

Vitamin B_{12}	Animal
	  Seafood
	  Poultry
	  Liver, kidney
	  Muscle meats
	  Eggs
	  Milk
	  Cheese
	Plant
	  None
		Synthesis of red blood cells
		Maintenance of myelin sheaths
		Treatment of pernicious anemia
		Folate metabolism
			Deficiency
			  Degeneration of myelin sheaths
			  Pernicious anemia
			  Sore mouth and tongue
			  Anorexia
			  Neurological disorders
			Toxicity
			  None

Folate (folic acid)	Animal
	  Liver
	Plant
	  Leafy green vegetables
	  Spinach
	  Legumes
	  Seeds
	  Broccoli
	  Cereal fortified with folate
	  Fruit
		Synthesis of RBCs
		Synthesis of DNA
			Deficiency
			  Anemia
			  Glossitis
			  Neural tube defects such as
			    anencephaly and spina bifida
			Toxicity
			  Could mask a B_{12} deficiency

(continued)

TABLE 9-3 • Fat-soluble vitamins and water-soluble vitamins. (*continued*)

Name	Food Sources	Functions	Deficiency/Toxicity

Biotin	Animal
	  Milk
	  Live and kidney
	  Egg yolks
	Plant
	  Legumes
	  Brewer's yeast
	  Soy flour
	  Cereals
	  Fruit
		Coenzyme in carbohydrate and
		  amino acid metabolism
		Niacin synthesis from tryptophan
			Deficiency
			  Dermatitis
			  Nausea
			  Anorexia
			  Depression
			  Hair loss
			Toxicity
			  None

Pantothenic acid	Animal
	  Eggs
	  Liver
	  Salmon
	  Poultry
	Plant
	  Mushrooms
	  Cauliflower
	  Peanuts
	  Brewer's yeast
		Metabolism of carbohydrates, lipids,
		  and proteins
		Synthesis of fatty acids, cholesterol,
		  steroid hormones
			Deficiency
			  Rare: burning feet syndrome; vomiting;
			  fatigue
			Toxicity
			  None

Vitamin C (ascorbic acid)	Animal
	  None
	Plants
	  All citrus fruits
	  Broccoli
	  Melons
	  Strawberries
	  Tomatoes
	  Brussel sprouts
	  Potatoes
	  Cabbage
	  Green peppers
		Prevention of scurvy
		Formation of collagen
		Healing of wounds
		Release of stress hormones
		Absorption of iron
		Antioxidant
		Resistance to infection
			Deficiency
			  Scurvy
			  Muscle cramps
			  Ulcerated gums
			  Tendency to bruise easily
			Toxicity
			  Raised uric acid level
			  Hemolytic anemia
			  Kidney stones
			  Rebound scurvy

Delmar/Cengage Learning

WEB LINK
Antioxidants

http://medlineplus.gov

Go to this Web site and enter the search term "antioxidants." Doing so will take you to a number of sublinks with a lot of good scientific information on the sources and benefits of antioxidants.

SEARCH TERMS: antioxidants, benefits of antioxidants

- "Organically grown foods contain superior vitamins." Not true. It doesn't matter how the plants are grown. In fact, even if the plant is grown under very poor conditions and the fruits or vegetables are sparse or small, they will still contain vitamins and minerals.

- "Some vitamins may be harmful in large amounts." True. Anything can be harmful in large amounts. Niacin and vitamins A, B$_6$, D, and K may be particularly harmful.

- "Some vitamin supplements are better than others—you get what you pay for." Not true. Read the labels. If the product advertises a certain percentage of the RDI, you can rely on the nutrients being available. According to FDA policies, the label must accurately reflect the product being sold.

- "If one daily vitamin is good for you, two would be better." Not true. Taking mega-doses is not a good practice.

- "Some people require more vitamins to be healthy." Not true. Remember that vitamins are needed in very small amounts to be useful. More vitamins will not make you healthier.

Minerals

Minerals are elements that are found in the earth. Our bodies need them in small amounts, but we cannot manufacture them. They must come from our food or from diet supplements. Most of the minerals in your diet come from plant sources. Foods from animal sources indirectly supply small amounts of minerals. Much like vitamins, the RDIs for minerals vary according to age and gender.

The most common mineral in the human body is calcium, but although calcium is the most abundant mineral in the human body, it makes up only 2 percent of one's body weight. Calcium has several important functions in the body. More than 99 percent of total body calcium is stored in the bones and teeth, where it is used as support material. The remaining 1 percent is found throughout the body in blood, muscle, and the fluid between cells. The presence of this unbound calcium is needed for muscle contraction, blood vessel contraction and expansion, the secretion of hormones and enzymes, and sending messages through the nervous system. A constant level of calcium is maintained in body fluid and tissues so that these vital body processes function efficiently. Generally, we need about 1,000 milligrams of calcium per day to replace the calcium lost as a result of metabolism and help retain bone strength. A woman who is pregnant or over age 50 needs about 1,100 milligrams a day.

What's News

Osteoporosis

The U.S. surgeon general has warned that by 2020, half of all Americans older than 50 will be at risk for fractures from osteoporosis and low bone mass if no immediate action is taken by people at risk, doctors, health care systems, and policymakers. The warning appeared in the report *Bone Health and Osteoporosis: A Report of the Surgeon General* (U.S. Department of Health and Human Services, 2004).

The report states that 10 million Americans currently over the age of 50 have osteoporosis, the most common bone disease, while another 34 million are at risk for developing osteoporosis. And each year, roughly 1.5 million people suffer a bone fracture related to osteoporosis.

We have been taught to believe that milk and dairy products are good sources of calcium. While this is true, it is important to understand that not everyone is going to drink milk. There are some people who cannot digest milk properly (lactose intolerant) and should not drink it; there are some people who just don't like milk. There are alternative sources of calcium. Calcium can also be found in other food products, including dark green leafy vegetables, such as kale, spinach, and collard greens, and in dried beans and legumes. Another option would be to drink beverages such as fruit juices that are fortified with calcium. A third alternative might be to take calcium supplements. Regardless of the calcium source, it is also important to understand that in order to absorb and use calcium, the body needs to have a sufficient supply of vitamin D, which is why you will see "fortified with vitamin D" on milk containers.

osteoporosis
a condition where the bones get weak and brittle because of a lack of calcium

Osteoporosis is a condition of the bones caused by inadequate amounts of calcium during a person's life. Without adequate exercise, calcium, and vitamin D, the bones of an elderly person become brittle with age, resulting in deformities of the spine and fractures. More information on osteoporosis is presented in chapter 14.

There are two classifications of minerals. Major minerals are those needed in amounts greater than 100 milligrams per day. Trace minerals are those needed in amounts less than 100 milligrams per day. See Tables 9-4 and 9-5 for a list of major minerals and trace minerals people need and their specific functions.

Phytonutrients

Scientists are constantly testing foods to determine the quantity and quality of nutrients. They also study the effects of food on human health and performance. Researchers initially learned that food provided energy, material for tissue growth, and materials to regulate body processes. Now they are learning that there are specific elements in food that contribute to specific health conditions. These elements, which have been referred to as phytonutrients or phytochemicals (*phyto*, from Greek, meaning "plant"), are organic components of plants that scientists have isolated as being beneficial to human health. Unlike traditional nutrients (protein, fat, vitamins, and minerals), phytonutrients are not "essential" for life. As scientists uncover more and more benefits of phytonutrients, it may be that phytonutrients will someday be classified as essential nutrients. Fruits, vegetables, grains, legumes, nuts, and teas are excellent sources of phytonutrients.

Phytonutrients are health protective in many ways. Some of the major functions that have been identified:

- Enhancing the body's immune response

- Serving as antioxidants, which are chemicals in the body that tend to prevent cancer growth

- Causing cancer cells to die

- Repairing DNA damage to cells

For example, in one research study, people who consumed diets very high in collard greens or spinach (sources of one phytonutrient, lutein) were found to have a 46 percent less risk for macular degeneration, a serious eye disorder. Another phytonutrient, flavonoid, found in dark chocolate, has been linked to reducing heart disease among elderly Dutch men.

TABLE 9-4 • Major Minerals.

Name	Food Sources	Functions	Deficiency/Toxicity
Calcium (Ca^{++})	Milk, cheese Sardines Salmon Some dark green, leafy vegetables	Development of bones and teeth Transmission of nerve impulses Blood clotting Normal heart action Normal muscle activity	Deficiency Osteoporosis Osteomalacia Rickets Tetany Retarded growth Poor tooth and bone formation
Phosphorus (P^{-})	Milk, cheese Lean meat Poultry Fish Whole grain cereals Legumes Nuts	Development of bones and teeth Maintenance of normal acid-base balance of the blood Constituent of all body cells Necessary for effectiveness of some vitamins Metabolism of carbohydrates, fats, and proteins	Deficiency Poor tooth and bone formation Weakness Anorexia General malaise
Potassium (K^{+})	Oranges, bananas Dried fruits Vegetables Legumes Milk Cereals Meat	Contraction of muscles Maintenance of fluid balance Transmission of nerve impulses Osmosis Regular heart rhythm Cell metabolism	Deficiency Hypokalemia Muscle weakness Confusion Abnormal heartbeat Toxicity Hyperkalemia
Sodium (Na^{+})	Table salt Beef, eggs Poultry Milk, cheese	Maintenance of fluid balance Transmission of nerve impulses Osmosis Acid-base balance Regulation of muscle and nerve irritability	Deficiency Nausea Exhaustion Muscle cramps Toxicity Increase in blood pressure Edema
Chloride (Cl^{-})	Table salt Eggs Seafood Milk	Gastric acidity Regulation of osmotic pressure Osmosis Fluid balance Acid-base balance Formation of hydrochloric acid	Deficiency Imbalance in gastric acidity Imbalance in blood pH Nausea Exhaustion
Magnesium (Mg^{++})	Green, leafy vegetables Whole grains Avocados Nuts Milk Legumes Bananas	Synthesis of ATP Transmission of nerve impulses Activation of metabolic enzymes Constituent of bones, muscles, and red blood cells Necessary for healthy muscles and nerves	Deficiency Normally unknown Mental, emotional, and muscle disorders
Sulfur (S)	Eggs Poultry Fish	Maintenance of protein structure For building hair, nails, and all body tissues Constituent of all body cells	Unknown

Courtesy of *Nutrition and Diet Therapy* 9th Edition by Ruth A. Roth, 2007. Clifton Park, NY: Delmar/Cengage Learning

TABLE 9-5 • Trace minerals.

Name	Food Sources	Functions	Deficiency/Toxicity

Iron (Fe^+)	Muscle meats
	Poultry
	Shellfish
	Liver
	Legumes
	Dried fruits
	Whole grain or enriched breads and cereals
	Dark green and leafy vegetables
	Molasses
		Transports oxygen and carbon dioxide
		Component of hemoglobin and myoglobin
		Component of cellular enzymes essential for energy production
			Deficiency
			  Iron deficiency anemia characterized by weakness, dizziness, loss of weight, and pallor
			Toxicity
			  Hemochromatosis (genetic)
			  Can be fatal to children
			  May contribute to heart disease
			  Injure liver

Iodine (I^-)	Iodized salt
	Seafood
		Regulation of basal metabolic rate	Deficiency
			  Goiter
			  Cretinism
			  Myxedema

Zinc (Zn^+)	Seafood, especially oysters
	Liver
	Eggs
	Milk
	Wheat bran
	Legumes
		Formation of collagen
		Component of insulin
		Component of many vital enzymes
		Wound healing
		Taste acuity
		Essential for growth
		Immune reactions
			Deficiency
			  Dwarfism, hypogonadism, anemia
			  Skin changes
			  Loss of appetite
			  Impaired wound healing
			  Decreased taste acuity

Selenium (Se^-)	Seafood
	Kidney
	Liver
	Muscle meats
	Grains
		Constituent of most body tissue
		Needed for fat metabolism
		Antioxidant functions
			Deficiency
			  Unclear, but related to
			    Keshan disease
			    Muscle weakness
			Toxicity
			  Vomiting
			  Loss of hair and nails
			  Skin lesions

Copper (Cu^+)	Liver
	Shellfish, oysters
	Legumes
	Nuts
	Whole grains
		Essential for formation of hemoglobin and red blood cells
		Component of enzymes
		Wound healing
		Needed metabolically for the release of energy
			Deficiency
			  Anemia
			  Bone disease
			  Disturbed growth and metabolism
			Toxicity
			  Vomiting; diarrhea
			  Wilson's Disease
			  (Genetic)

Manganese (Mn^+)	Whole grains
	Nuts
	Fruits
	Tea
		Component of enzymes
		Bone formation
		Metabolic processes
			Deficiency
			  Unknown
			Toxicity
			  Possible brain disease

Courtesy of *Nutrition and Diet Therapy* 9th Edition by Ruth A. Roth, 2007. Clifton Park, NY: Delmar/Cengage Learning

(continued)

TABLE 9-5 • Trace minerals. (*continued*)

Name	Food Sources	Functions	Deficiency/Toxicity

Fluoride (F⁻)	Fluoridated water
	Seafood
		Increases resistance to tooth decay
		Component of bones and teeth
			Deficiency
			  Tooth decay
			    Possibly osteoporosis
			Toxicity
			  Discoloration of teeth (mottling)

Chromium (Cr)	Meat
	Vegetable oil
	Whole grain cereal and nuts
	Yeast
		Associated with glucose and lipid metabolism	Deficiency
			  Possibly disturbances of glucose
			    metabolism

Molybdenum (Mo)	Dark green, leafy vegetables
	Liver
	Cereal
	Legumes
		Enzyme functioning
		Metabolism
			Deficiency
			  Unknown
			Toxicity
			  Inhibition of copper absorption

Dietary Fiber

Fiber is the indigestible plant material in food. It cannot be digested because it is composed of cellulose, a product that cannot be absorbed into the human bloodstream. Studies indicate that the average American consumes about half the recommended amount of fiber each day. Complex carbohydrates are high in fiber. Although fiber is not a nutrient, it is an important component of the diet and has many health benefits. In addition to helping move waste materials through the digestive tract, fiber gives a feeling of fullness after a meal without adding calories. This benefit is important to weight management and reducing the chance of obesity. A high-fiber diet helps prevent weight gain and promotes weight loss. It also is believed to slow fat absorption. Research confirms that fiber is helpful in preventing diabetes, cancer, and heart disease. Fiber is also important for proper bowel function, helping reduce constipation and disorders of the colon.

If you don't eat much whole-wheat bread or consume several servings of fruits and vegetables each day, you are probably not getting enough fiber. If you feel that your diet is low in fiber and you want to increase your fiber intake, it is best to do it gradually while drinking plenty of water with meals. Consuming too much fiber in a short period of time can cause intestinal discomfort. Whole grains, cereals, fruits, and vegetables contain fiber; milk and meat products do not.

Choosing to get fiber from whole-grain sources brings with it numerous other dietary benefits. Grains are important sources of many nutrients, several B vitamins (thiamin, riboflavin, niacin, and folate), and minerals (iron, magnesium, and selenium). Dietary fiber from whole grains, as part of an overall healthy diet, helps reduce blood cholesterol levels and may lower the risk of heart disease.

Water

Water has no direct nutritional value (i.e., it lacks carbohydrates, vitamins, protein, and so on), but it is essential to our survival because the body is composed of 60 percent water. Water must continually be replaced because the body cannot store water. Depending on conditions, a person can live up to one week without water. Because water contains

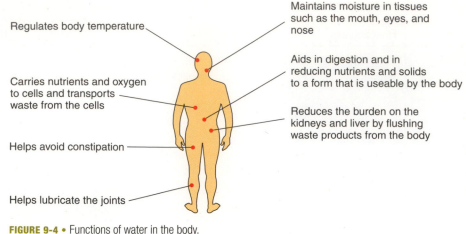

Regulates body temperature

Maintains moisture in tissues such as the mouth, eyes, and nose

Carries nutrients and oxygen to cells and transports waste from the cells

Aids in digestion and in reducing nutrients and solids to a form that is useable by the body

Reduces the burden on the kidneys and liver by flushing waste products from the body

Helps avoid constipation

Helps lubricate the joints

Delmar/Cengage Learning

FIGURE 9-4 • Functions of water in the body.

Did You Know…?

Eighty percent of the earth's surface is water. Ninety-seven percent of the earth's water is ocean water. Two percent of the earth's water is frozen and unusable. How much of the earth's water is suitable for drinking? One percent!

no calories, it does not require digestion. In fact, your body will burn about 50 calories as it processes 16 ounces of water. Water serves many purposes in the body (Figure 9-4).

Under normal conditions, water is lost through breathing, sweating, loss of urine, and other body functions. Replacement can come from drinking water or other beverages, eating foods high in fluid content such as soups, and consuming fruits and vegetables. Generally, food accounts for 20 percent of water intake. The other 80 percent comes from beverage consumption—about eight cups. The body loses more water during periods of exercise, hot weather, or illness, and under these circumstances the water needs to be replaced. Sport drinks are often used by athletes to replace fluids and minerals, but water can do about the same thing. It is recommended that if you are an athlete, you drink only water before exercise, alternate water and a sport drink during the event, and use sport drinks immediately

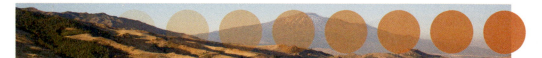

What's Your View?

Water Fluoridation

Some communities have chosen to add fluoride to the town's water supply in an effort to help prevent tooth decay. While this practice has the endorsement of the American Dental Association, there are many medical experts who do not approve of the practice. These opponents site lack of definitive studies supporting the value of fluoridation and demonstrating its safety over time. Some opponents express concern about the appropriateness of infusing an entire community with a chemical intended to reduce a dental condition not considered to be life threatening. What is your position on this practice? If you are unclear, do some research to gather information to develop your own opinion. Write your findings in an essay or your health journal.

following the workout or event. There is no exact science as to the precise amount of water one needs to consume since there is individual variability. If you consume enough fluid that you don't feel thirsty and produce between one and two quarts of colorless or slightly yellow urine a day, your fluid intake is sufficient.

The current wisdom seems to be that everyone should consume at least eight, eight-ounce glasses of water every day. This recommendation is without scientific verification. Karen Bellenir (2009) summarized the sources and the weaknesses of this assertion in her *Scientific American* article. It appears the recommendation came from a 1945 report from the Food and Nutrition Board. According to Bellenir, a number of researchers have come to the same conclusion; that the recommendation is without scientific merit. In 2004, the Food and Nutrition Board revised the recommendation, citing that people following a healthy diet get plenty of water from numerous dietary sources, such as milk, tea, coffee, juice, soda, fruits, vegetables. People can meet their daily hydration needs by letting thirst be their guide.

Planning to Eat Well

Knowing about nutrients and what they do for the body is a proper first step in developing good eating habits, but the information must be applied to food planning and eating behavior if wellness is to occur. Applying the information means making healthy choices about what you eat and when you eat it. In the United States, most people have so many foods available to them that the greatest challenge may be eating foods that are good for them while choosing from among the foods they enjoy. For example, when you eat a meal, it not absolutely necessary to be drinking anything with the food, but, more important, high-calorie soft drinks are no more useful to the meal than plain water. If you look around, you will see many people in who are "overfed." In fact, overweight and obesity are becoming major health problems because these conditions contribute to a variety of serious diseases and conditions, specifically heart disease, cancer, and diabetes. Perhaps there was no other time in your life when you attempted to examine the content of the foods you eat. If this is the case, now may be a good time to look closer at the science of foods and determine how you can put the information to work for nutritional wellness.

nutrient density
how many nutritional elements are present in a given amount of food

Nutrient Values in Food

Scientists have investigated the nutritional value of food in the laboratory. In the United States, it is the Agricultural Research Service (ARS) of U.S. Department of Agriculture (USDA). Researchers analyze virtually all types of foods to determine the energy, carbohydrate, protein, fat, vitamin, and mineral content of just about any food material. The ARS has a searchable database where someone can obtain information on all the nutrients contained in any type of food, including commercially packaged foods (see the following "Web Link"). If you ever have any questions about the nutrient content of foods, you can search the database to get the information you need.

When nutritionists talk about foods and health, they are concerned about the **nutrient density** of the food compared to the amount of energy produced by the food. Nutrient-dense foods contain numerous vitamins, minerals, proteins, and fiber, while

WEB LINK
Food Nutrients

http://www.nal.usda.gov

Go to this Web site and enter the search term "nutrient database." When you get to the database page, there is a search screen where you can enter the type of food for which you want information. The searchable database will show foods related to your search term in the database and ask you to select the exact food and portion size. Select your portion size, and you will find a table with all the nutritional information on the food.

SEARCH TERMS: nutrient tables, USDA Nutrition Tables, food nutrients

energy-dense foods contain a lot of energy but little in the way of nutrients. Let's consider a few examples. Imagine you are using bread for a sandwich. One option might be to use white bread, containing 160 calories and containing about .8 milligrams of vitamin E and no fiber. On the other hand, choosing whole-wheat bread will give you about the same amount of calories and slightly more than 1.0 milligram of vitamin E and six grams of fiber. A can of soda with your sandwich contains about 120 calories and no nutrients other than the energy from the sugar. The equivalent amount of apple juice will have about the same number of calories but will contain vitamin C, niacin, riboflavin, vitamin B_6, calcium, potassium, and iron. Energy foods that lack nutrients are known as "empty-calorie foods." Soft drinks, candy, and alcoholic beverages are good examples of empty-calorie foods. People are familiar with the energy content of nondiet soft drinks but are unaware that alcohol contains calories. There is more information about this topic in chapter 12.

The Food Guide Pyramid

The Food Guide Pyramid was developed in 1984 to make it easier for consumers to select the right types and amounts of foods to stay healthy. The pyramid categorized food into five major food groups and presented the number of daily recommended servings from each major food group. A revision of the pyramid was released in 1996 in order to expand the meaning of the pyramid and make it easier for consumers to understand it. The last version, released in 2005, reflects new discoveries about how food contributes to wellness, and the model was branded as My Pyramid. The model is computerized and accessible online so that people could develop a nutritional plan based on their personal needs. My Pyramid is illustrated in Figure 9-5; go to the My Pyramid Web site and explore the inside of the pyramid to find the basic information on food groups as they pertain to your age, gender, and activity level.

The specific nutritional needs of a person on a 2,000-calorie diet are presented in Table 9-2. If you follow the guidelines in the food pyramid, you can be assured that your nutritional needs will be met. Even if you don't follow the guide every day, you can make good wellness decisions by keeping the basic principles in mind. For example, if you are in doubt about what to eat when you're hungry, choose vegetables, fruits, or grains.

Reading Food Labels

The USDA and the FDA require that most packaged foods (meat and poultry are excluded) be clearly labeled with nutritional information for the consumer. The nutrient information required by law includes what makes up a serving size, the number of servings per container, and the number of calories per serving. Labeling requirements were modified by federal law in January 2006 to include the amount of trans fat in the food product. Look at the typical food labels shown in Figure 9-6. Note that all the values listed on the label are *per serving*. This fact is important; a person who doesn't know this might eat a whole package of food, thinking that the total calories listed are for the entire package! In addition, the label must contain the amounts per serving for each of the following nutrients:

- Fats: total calories and the amounts of saturated fats, cholesterol, and trans fat

- Sodium

- Total carbohydrates

WEB LINK

My Pyramid

http://www.mypyramid.gov

Go to this Web site and select the link for "My Pyramid Plan." When you get to that page, you can enter your personal information to determine your nutritional needs. You will also find other links to help you develop your nutritional wellness plan.

SEARCH TERMS: food groups, food pyramid, nutrition food groups

- Dietary fiber
- Sugars
- Protein
- Vitamin A
- Vitamin C
- Calcium
- Iron

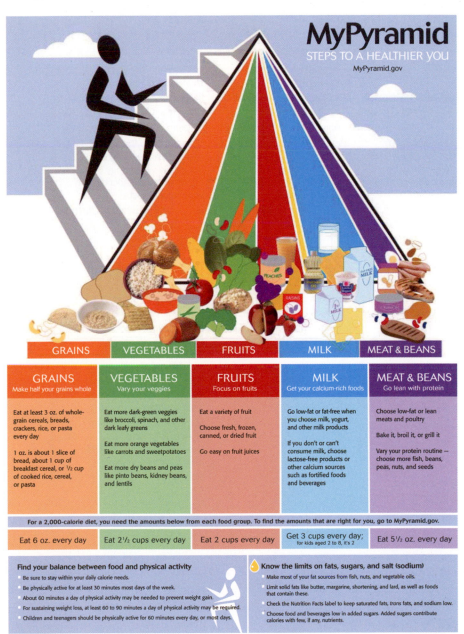

FIGURE 9-5 • The food pyramid. Courtesy of the U.S. Department of Agriculture, www.mypyramid.gov.

Potato Chips
Nutrition Facts
Serving Size: 1oz.
(28g/About 19 Chips)
Servings Per Container: 6

Amount Per Serving

Calories 150

Calories from Fat 90

% Daily Value*

Total Fat 10g	**15%**
Saturated Fat 2.5g	**13%**
Cholesterol 0mg	**0%**
Sodium 340mg	**14%**
Total Carbohydrate 15g	**5%**
Dietary Fiber 1g	**4%**
Sugars 1g	
Protein 2g	

Vitamin A 0% • Vitamin C 10%
Calcium 0% • Iron 2%

*Percent Daily Values are based on a 2,000 calorie diet. Your daily values may be higher or lower depending on your calorie needs:

	Calories	2,000	2,500
Total Fat	Less than	65g	80g
Sat Fat	Less than	20g	25g
Cholesterol	Less than	300mg	300mg
Sodium	Less than	2,400mg	2,400mg
Total Carbohydrate		300g	375g
Dietary Fiber		25g	30g

Calories per gram:
Fat 9 • Carbohydrate 4 • Protein 4

Ingredients: Potatoes, Vegetable Oil (Contains one or more of the following: Canola, Corn, Cottonseed, or Partially Hydrogenated Canola, Soybean or Sunflower Oil), Salt.

Pretzels
Nutrition Facts
Serving Size: 7 Pretzels
(30g)
Servings Per Container: 9.4

Amount Per Serving

Calories 120

Calories from Fat 10

% Daily Value*

Total Fat 1g	**2%**
Saturated Fat 0g	**0%**
Cholesterol 0mg	**0%**
Sodium 360mg	**15%**
Total Carbohydrate 24g	**8%**
Dietary Fiber 1g	**4%**
Sugars 1g	
Protein 3g	

Vitamin A 0% • Vitamin C 0%
Calcium 0% • Iron 2%

*Percent Daily Values are based on a 2,000 calorie diet. Your daily values may be higher or lower depending on your calorie needs:

	Calories	2,000	2,500
Total Fat	Less than	65g	80g
Sat Fat	Less than	20g	25g
Cholesterol	Less than	300mg	300mg
Sodium	Less than	2,400mg	2,400mg
Total Carbohydrate		300g	375g
Dietary Fiber		25g	30g

Calories per gram:
Fat 9 • Carbohydrate 4 • Protein 4

Ingredients: Unbleached Wheat Flour, Water, Corn Syrup, Partially Hydrogenated Vegetable Oil (Soybean), Yeast, Salt, Bicarbonates and Carbonates of Sodium.

Wheat Snack Crackers
Nutrition Facts
Serving Size: 25 Cracker
(30g)
Servings Per Container: 7

Amount Per Serving

Calories 150

Calories from Fat 70

% Daily Value*

Total Fat 7g	**11%**
Saturated Fat 2g	**10%**
Cholesterol 0mg	**0%**
Sodium 310mg	**13%**
Total Carbohydrate 16g	**5%**
Dietary Fiber 1g	**4%**
Sugars 2g	
Protein 3g	

Vitamin A 0% • Vitamin C 0%
Calcium 0% • Iron 4%

*Percent Daily Values are based on a 2,000 calorie diet. Your daily values may be higher or lower depending on your calorie needs:

	Calories	2,000	2,500
Total Fat	Less than	65g	80g
Sat Fat	Less than	20g	25g
Cholesterol	Less than	300mg	300mg
Sodium	Less than	2,400mg	2,400mg
Total Carbohydrate		300g	375g
Dietary Fiber		25g	30g

Calories per gram:
Fat 9 • Carbohydrate 4 • Protein 4

Ingredients: Enriched Flour, Partially Hydrogenated Soybean and/or Cottonseed Oil, Dehydrated Potatoes, Steamed Crushed Wheat, Sugar, Salt, Natural and Artificial Flavors, Corn Syrup, Monosodium Glutamate, Dehydrated Cheddar Cheese, Dextrose, Nonfat Dry Milk, Artificial Color (Yellow 5, Yellow 6).

Delmar/Cengage Learning

FIGURE 9-6 • Sample food labels.

When you shop for packaged foods, it is a good idea to compare nutrients among products and brands to ensure that you are getting the nutrients you want and need for the price you are willing to pay. The products may be labeled as the same meal or product, but the quantity and quality of the ingredients may vary. When you read a product's "Ingredients" label, remember that the ingredients are listed in order according to volume, so the first ingredient is the most abundant by weight. Look carefully and compare products if the first ingredients are "water" and/ or "sugar."

Vegetarianism

People who choose to eat foods only from plant sources are known as vegetarians. These individuals follow a **vegetarian** diet for a variety of reasons. Some people object to killing animals; some are concerned about all the land needed to raise meat sources compared with the amount of land needed for vegetarian sources. Some people eat plants and vegetables to avoid the fat in meat. There are many personal reasons influencing one's choice to be vegetarian, and there are some people choosing to follow "mostly vegetarian" diets.

How much protein do we need? The USDA Recommended Dietary Allowance recommends that one consumes 0.8 grams of protein for every kilogram of body weight (or about 0.36 grams of protein per pound). This recommendation includes a generous safety factor for most people. If planned correctly, a vegetarian diet can provide the amount of protein needed, be very nutritious, and help reduce obesity, heart disease, and some cancers. Although most vegetarians avoid eating all types of meat, there are three forms of vegetarians:

1. *Lacto-ovo vegetarians* eat plants, dairy products (cheese, milk, yogurt, and so on) and eggs but consume no meat, poultry, or fish.

2. *Lacto-vegetarians* use dairy products with their plant foods but eat no meat, poultry, fish, or eggs.

3. *Vegans* avoid all animal products. Vegans consume plant foods only.

If you have any interest in vegetarian eating, be sure to research the topic well before you begin. Vegetarian diets are not perfect. For example, a strict vegan diet tends to be very low in calcium and iron. For good nutrition, it is important that you plan your menus correctly to ensure that you get all the nutrients you need for proper growth and wellness. It will take some planning on your part.

vegetarian
the practice of consuming foods only from plant sources, except eggs or dairy products in some instances

WEB LINK
Vegetarianism
http://medlineplus.gov
Go to this Web site and enter the search term "vegetarianism." Doing so will take you to a number of sublinks with a lot of good scientific information on the vegetarian diet.

SEARCH TERMS: vegetarianism, vegetarian health

Eating Safely

We sometimes take the safety of our food for granted. Although we have many laws and procedures in place to protect our foods, we still need to be careful to handle foods correctly and safely. Even with inspections, packaging, and refrigeration, improper handling of food can cause serious illnesses and even death. Each year, approximately 325,000 people are hospitalized with a diagnosis of food poisoning, and approximately 5,000 of those people will die. The three most significant food-borne illnesses are the following:

• *Campylobacter* is a bacterial pathogen that causes fever, diarrhea, and abdominal cramps. These bacteria live in the intestines of healthy birds, and most raw poultry meat has *Campylobacter* on it. Eating undercooked chicken or other food that has been contaminated with juices dripping from raw chicken is the most frequent source of this infection.

• *Salmonella* is also a bacterium that is widespread in the intestines of birds, reptiles, and mammals. It can spread to humans via a variety of different foods of animal origin. The illness it causes, salmonellosis, typically includes fever, diarrhea, and abdominal cramps.

- *E. coli O157:H7* is a bacterial pathogen that may be found in cattle and other similar animals. Human illness typically follows consumption of food or water that has been contaminated with microscopic amounts of cow dung. The illness that this pathogen causes is often a severe and bloody diarrhea and painful abdominal cramps without much fever.

There are two ways in which contaminated food can do damage to the body:

1. Organisms invade food products and alter the food by releasing toxic (poisonous) chemicals. These organisms can grow inside improperly prepared or damaged cans. See chapter 13 for more information about organisms that contribute to food poisoning. Meanwhile, *never* purchase or eat food in a can that appears to be bulging. The bulge is caused by gasses produced by the organism's toxins.

2. Organisms enter the body and cause illness, using foods as a means of transport.

Organisms that cause illnesses can be present in the air, on food preparation surfaces, or on the hands of the food preparer. There are some important basic rules you should follow to prevent food-borne illnesses:

- When you shop, try to purchase frozen and refrigerated items last. If you buy refrigerated items first, they have more time to be exposed to warm temperatures that could encourage the growth of disease-causing organisms.

- Refrigerate foods within two hours or less after cooking because cold temperatures will help keep harmful bacteria from growing and multiplying.

- Read labels. Don't buy foods that have passed their expiration date. Expired foods are likely to spoil quickly.

- Always wash your hands before handling food, especially after using the bathroom or changing diapers. Your hands contact germs on surfaces all day long. If you get sick from your food, it is most likely because of the germs you had on your hands.

- Keep raw meat, poultry, or seafood and their juices away from ready-to-eat foods.

- If you choose to marinate meat, do it in the refrigerator. Doing it at room temperature encourages bacteria growth.

- Be careful when preparing foods on cutting boards, especially wooden boards. Germs can get caught in the cut marks and become transferred to your food. You can occasionally sanitize the board with one teaspoon of bleach in one quart of water and thoroughly wash it with soap and hot water after each use.

- Do not thaw meats at room temperature. The outside of the meat will thaw first and become a place for bacteria to multiply. Defrost food in the refrigerator overnight.

- Cook meats thoroughly. Doing so will ensure that the disease-causing organisms are destroyed all the way through the food.

Handle and prepare foods on a clean surface, such as the one shown in Figure 9-7, and be sure not to contaminate foods that you may serve in the raw state with blood or fluids from meats that have not been cooked.

The Diversity of Nutritional Needs and Practices

There is a wide range of nutritional needs and practices. Very often we look at our eating habits and preferences through the lens of our own upbringing. We have favorite foods, favorite combinations of foods, and favorite settings where we enjoy the food experiences. Our culture and family history tend to shape these personal preferences. But it is a big world out there, and food choices play different roles for various individuals. Furthermore, all people do not have the same nutritional needs, and those needs vary according to gender, culture, and age.

Diverse Nutritional Needs

Americans are now enjoying the foods from other cultures. Restaurants are appearing that specialize in meals from Mexico, Japan, China, Indonesia, India, Greece, Italy, and so on. Of note is the fact that you can now go to local grocery stores and find that there are aisles in the stores specifically labeled as "Ethnic Foods." You can purchase and learn to prepare your favorite ethnic dishes at home. Different cultures have varying characteristics of their foods. In the American population, there are many people with diverse nutritional requirements. The diversity of food needs and desires make food preparation much like a symphony, bringing many elements together for a pleasant experience.

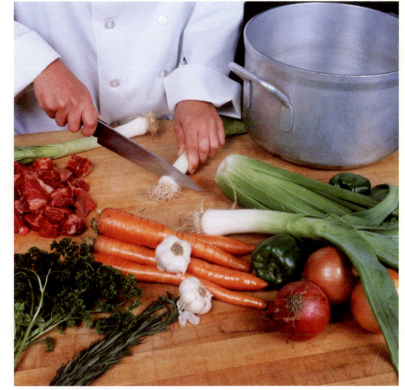

Courtesy of Photodisc

FIGURE 9-7 • Safe food preparation.

Eating Healthy with Ethnic Foods

Whether eating out or preparing the dishes at home, you can get very healthy meals by making the choices that fit best with your wellness plan. Ethnic dishes are no exception. Seeking out ways to eat healthy is the key. Let's look at some of the various cultures and examine some of the food choices available for a healthy diet.

Chinese foods tend to be lower in fat content. Foods tend to be stir-fried or steamed and include lots of vegetables. Chinese foods include monosodium glutamate (MSG) as a flavor enhancer similar to salt. A person with a history of high blood pressure can order dishes in restaurants without MSG as a seasoning. Chinese menu dishes may have names such as "jum" (poached), "kao" (roasted), and "shu" (barbecue). The cooking styles are heart friendly. You may find some Japanese food prepared "tempura" style, meaning that the seafood or vegetables are dipped in a light batter and deep-fried. The meals come with steamed rice, but you can increase fiber with little added calories by choosing fried brown rice. The Asian diet also includes tea. Green tea is very high in antioxidants.

Mexican cuisine is generally high in fat content. Many foods like refried beans are cooked in lard, and many dishes could include beef and cheese. The Mexican culture does not see skinny people as healthy, so their meals generally will not be low calorie. There

Did You Know…?

Salsa has passed ketchup as the number one condiment of choice in the United States.

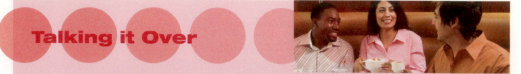

Talking it Over

Family Food History

Our food choices and preferences are often related to the family in which we are raised, and our family's preferences are based on the preferences of the family in which they were raised. These preferences are part of our family histories. Talk with your family members and friends just to see what food preferences and recipes have been handed down from generation to generation. See if you can find out where the food preferences originated as they may relate to the racial or cultural background of your family. In your health journal, summarize what you learned about the following topics:

- What are some "generational" recipes you learned about?
- How do the foods/recipes match up against the nutrition standards of today?
- To what extent will you continue the food practices/recipes?

---

are things one can do to consume Mexican food that meets wellness goals. Chips are an appetizer in a Mexican restaurant. They are high in carbohydrates and, because they are cooked in fat, may have a reasonably high fat content. If you dip the chips in salsa instead of queso (cheese dip), they will be healthier. Meals generally come with refried beans, but you can keep the protein of the beans and make it healthier if you substitute whole beans or, better yet, whole black beans.

Mediterranean foods include unprocessed ingredients and fresh as well as dried fruits and vegetables. The diet includes cheese and olives in many forms. They cook foods and dip breads in olive oil and serve wine with their meals, and sweets are made with honey rather than refined sugar. As a result, those who live in the Mediterranean region have the lowest recorded rates of chronic diseases and the highest life expectancy in the world.

Special Nutritional Needs among Elder Adults

People who are aged have different nutritional needs than they did when they were younger. The physiological changes of aging have a significant effect on the amounts and kinds of nutrients needed. Elderly people are less active, so they need fewer calories. The change in their metabolism makes it more difficult to absorb vitamins efficiently. Their limited physical activity has an effect on their body composition: they lose muscle mass and have a greater percentage of body fat. Their nutrient needs stay the same or possibly increase, so it becomes very important that they remain nourished while keeping the calorie count down. For example, older adults should be encouraged to seek low-fat sources of protein. Elders do not feel thirsty like their younger counterparts, yet they require a higher level of hydration to prevent constipation and dehydration.

Older adults need at least eight eight-ounce glasses of fluid each day. However, research indicates that elder adults are often dehydrated. Data from one investigation revealed that 37 percent of older adults studied did not meet the recommendation for water consumption (Mentes, 2006). Since elderly individuals do not feel thirsty, it is important for them to get their hydration from foods such as soups and juices.

Because they don't need extra calories, elders should be encouraged to consume nutrient-dense food sources, and they should be encouraged to consume high-fiber foods.

Older adults need to be concerned about food safety. Their senses become affected by the aging process; as a result, they are not as likely to smell food that has spoiled, clearly see changes on the food surface, or taste food that has gone bad. If they do eat something that has spoiled, they face a greater threat for serious illness because their bodies have less effective immune systems and their stomachs produce less stomach acid to help eliminate harmful bacteria. Elderly people should be encouraged to practice safe food handling if they prepare their own meals: keep food preparation surfaces clean, don't cross contaminate foods, and cook foods thoroughly. These practices may have been something they did routinely as younger adults, but with aging comes some level of forgetfulness.

Nutritional Needs of Infants

Babies grow quickly. At no other time in the infant's life will he or she double in size in a five-month period of time. By the time a baby is one year old, he or she will be three times larger than at birth. The growth rate is rapid, so proper nutrition is very important. For the first four to six months of the baby's life, he or she should have only breast milk or iron-fortified formula. The baby neither needs nor is able to digest any other form of food. The mother will make the decision whether she will breast-feed or formula-feed her baby. Pediatricians recommend breast feeding for a number of reasons:

- Breast milk is the perfect food for a newborn. The mother's human milk has the precise nutritional composition of proteins, fat, vitamins, and minerals the infant needs.

- Breast milk is easily digested.

- The mother's breast milk also includes substances that help build the baby's immune system. Breast-fed infants are sick less often that formula-fed babies; studies even suggest that they are healthier in adulthood.

- Breast feeding meets the emotional needs of the baby. It is a bonding time for mother and baby.

- Breast-fed babies have fewer bowel movements, and the stool is light in color and does not have a heavy odor.

- Breast milk is free, and no one has to go to the store for formula.

Busy work schedules and other personal reasons may lead the mother to prefer formula feeding. Formula feeding is certainly good nutrition for the infant. Nutritionists have done a good job of duplicating mother's milk, but the formula is not exact. If formula is the desired feeding method, the formula chosen should be fortified with iron.

It is not uncommon for infants to "spit up" a small amount after eating or during burping, but a baby should not vomit after feeding. Vomiting, if it does occur, can be due to overfeeding, but vomiting after every feeding may be an indication of a digestive problem, allergy, or other problem that needs medical attention.

Childhood Nutrition

Children do not have nutritional needs that vary significantly from the nutritional needs of adults. In fact, the USDA's *Dietary Guidelines for Americans 2005* encourages the same nutritional needs for Americans over the age of two. Caloric needs may vary, but the

WEB LINK
Body Mass Index for Children and Teens
http://www.cdc.gov
Visit the CDC Web site. Enter "Children's Body Mass Index" in the search feature. At the next page you can use the BMI calculator, and link to additional information regarding BMI for adults and children.

SEARCH TERMS: body mass index, BMI for children

nutrients remain constant. Toddlers and young children benefit from adult supervision for their food choice. Adults should have some knowledge of the nutritional value of foods and see that youngsters are fed appropriately. Adults have the opportunity to set a child's eating patterns for life if they choose carefully and encourage children to eat healthy. Children get hungry, and they want to eat. The adult can provide a nutritious snack, such as raw vegetables or fruit, or give the child what is fast but not necessarily healthy, such as a candy bar. Children can grow to appreciate and enjoy healthy foods if such foods are made available.

As children grow into their teen years, their caloric needs will reach their peak. Depending on a teen's exercise habits, the need for calories can be offset by activity, but by the time they graduate from high school, they will need fewer calories each decade for the rest of their lives. There is a need to modify eating habits as people get older. To help young people develop sound eating habits, parents should encourage three things:

- Make smart choices from every food group for each meal during the day.

- Find your balance between food and physical activity.

- Get the most nutrition out of your calories (i.e., nutrient density).

Nutritional Needs for Exercise

An athlete's diet does not have to be anything special if he or she is already following good nutritional practices. The athlete may want to give special attention to the nutritional needs of his or her specific event and tailor the diet to supply the specific carbohydrate needs for that event. For example, a marathon runner's meals 24 hours prior to the race should include more complex carbohydrates. To get the most out of workouts or training programs, an athlete needs to attend to four basic nutritional practices:

1. Eat a full breakfast. Energy from the foods consumed the night before is likely to have dissipated overnight. If you participate in an early morning workout, try to eat an hour before the workout. If you don't have this much time, eat a smaller meal and supplement it with a sport drink.

2. Schedule your meals. You should eat your large meals about three hours before exercising. Depending on the type of training program, be sure to choose your food sources to fit your training schedule (e.g., if you are doing endurance training, include complex carbohydrates in your meal). Snacks before workouts are okay if they come from simple carbohydrate sources.

3. Don't skip meals. Some people think it is best to work out on an empty stomach. This is not a good idea. Skipping meals will deprive you of the energy needed for training or events. If you feel light-headed, dizzy, or weak during your workout, you probably are skipping meals or not getting enough to eat when you do eat.

4. Eat after you finish your workout. Muscles will recover more quickly and regenerate energy stores if you eat within two hours of your workout or athletic contest.

Remember, too, that special muscle building supplements are not necessary for good athletic performance.

BUILDING YOUR LIFETIME WELLNESS PLAN

Eating well is one of the best and easiest things you can do for yourself. You eat several times a day, and every time you eat, you get to make decisions about what you eat and how much food you consume. This behavior can have both positive and negative effects on your health, depending on the choices you make. As you develop your nutritional wellness plan for nutrition, there are a few essential things you may keep in mind:

- Develop a basic working knowledge of the food nutrients. Understand what specific nutrients do for you and what quantities are necessary for good health. This knowledge will enable you to understand food labels and to make healthy decisions when you select what foods you will eat.

- Identify nutrients, such as trans fat, cholesterol, and sugar, that in excess may be harmful to your health. Learn what foods contain large amounts of these nutrients and plan ways to avoid consuming large quantities of them.

- Make an effort to develop good eating patterns at each meal. This does not mean planning every meal on paper. It does mean remembering to follow the food pyramid when making food choices and not eating in excess.

- Use the safe food-handling practices discussed in this chapter whenever you are preparing food.

End-of-Chapter Activities

Opportunities for Application

1. Visit the grocery store or look at some of the foods in your cupboard at home. You will need to look at products that are very similar, such as different cereals or canned vegetables. Read the labels and compare food values. Use the information you have about food labels to draw conclusions regarding the nutritional value of the various foods. You may want to take the activity a step further and find out how much the products you compared cost. Paying more for each serving of a product does not necessarily mean it's more nutritious. Keep track of your findings in a table and place them in your health folio.

2. Keep track of all the things you eat and drink for a day. Do the best you can to estimate the portion sizes. Develop a worksheet containing a table on which you list all the foods and their serving sizes in the left-side column. Across the top row, list the following nutrients as the column headings and create a table for vitamins:

Foods and portion size	Calories	Vitamin A	Vitamin B_1	Vitamin B_2	Vitamin B_3	Vitamin B_6	Vitamin B_{12}	Vitamin C	Vitamin D	Vitamin E

Do the same for minerals:

Foods and portion size	Calcium	Potassium	Iron	Zinc	Phosphorus	Sodium	Chloride	Magnesium	Iodine

Research the foods you ate on the food tables at the USDA Web site at http://www.usda.gov/wps/portal/!ut/p/_s.7_0_A/7_0_1OB?navtype=SU&navid=FOOD_NUTRITION and place check marks in the appropriate boxes (or you can record the amount of each nutrient if you prefer). You will be able to determine how dense your nutritional intake was by how many boxes you filled in.

3. Go to the Web site for the FDA at http://www.cgsan.fda.gov/label.html. Go to "Label Claims" and search "Nutrient Content Claims." Find out the legal conditions for labeling a product as "free," "low," or "reduced." See how this information affects the products you buy. Use your health literacy skills to learn more about other claims in labeling, such as "fresh" and "organic," and search further to find out the meaning of other terms used in product labeling. Knowing these terms will help you become a more informed consumer.

Key Concepts

1. How many calories do you need each day? Do the math and find out. Fill in the calculations here.

   a. Calculate your basal metabolism. Determine how much you weigh. Each day, you need about 10 calories per pound of body weight. Enter the number of calories. _____

   b. Calculate the number of calories you need for normal activities. That would be three calories per pound. Enter the total for daily activities.

   _____

   c. Calculate the number of calories you need for *each half hour* of exercise. Perform an Internet search using "exercise calorie expenditure" as your search term. The search will lead you to a table of exercises and calories according to weight. Be sure to adjust the calories based on the number of minutes you exercise.

   Enter the total exercise calories for a typical day.

   _____

   Total all three solutions. _____

   Look at the total calories you calculated. Compare this to your caloric needs in Table 9-1 or some other source. Do the calories you take in match the number of calories expended? What can you do to adjust your calorie needs? Does your exercise pattern match what you used to calculate exercise calories?

2. List and explain food preparation behaviors needed to prevent food borne illness.

3. List and explain five things you would suggest or do for your grandparents to help them with their nutritional needs.

Answers to Personal Assessment Quiz: Your Eating Habits

1. d. Studies show that people who eat breakfast every day are healthier than those who do not.

2. d. Try to eat four or more portions per day; the equivalent of four and a half cups.

3. d. You need only one portion of meat a day—five and a half ounces—but you can eat a couple of smaller portion sizes and spread it out. Two serving would be okay if you choose meat sources that are lean.

4. d. You need only the equivalent of three cups of milk per day unless you are lactose intolerant.

5. d. Grain products are good if not overconsumed. Whole grain is best.

6. d. Your weight should be within an acceptable range. Check the BMI charts established by the Centers for Disease Control.

7. d. Raw almonds are fat healthy and can help protect against heart disease.

●●● References

Bellenir, K. (June, 2009). Fact or fiction? You must drink 8 glasses of water daily. *Scientific American.* Retrieved March 20, 2010 from http://www.scientificamerican.com/article.cfm?id=eight-glasses-water-per-day&page=2.

Mentes, J. (2006). Oral hydration in older adults. *American Journal of Nursing, 106,*(6), 40–49.

National Institutes of Health. (2004). *Bone Health and Osteoporosis: Report of the Surgeon General.* Bethesda, MD: National Institutes of Health.

National Institute of Diabetes and Digestive and Kidney Diseases. (2006). *Lactose Intolerance.* NIH publication 06-2751. Retrieved May 27, 2010, from http://digestive.niddk.nih.gov/ddiseases/pubs/lactoseintolerance/lactoseintolerance.pdf

U.S. Department of Health and Human Services. (2004). *Bone health and osteoporosis: A report of the surgeon general.* Rockville, MD: Author.

U.S. Department of Health and Human Services and U.S. Department of Agriculture. (2005). *Dietary Guidelines for Americans,* 6th Edition, Washington, DC: U.S. Government Printing Office.

CHAPTER 10

A Healthy Approach to Weight Management

CHAPTER OBJECTIVES

When you finish this chapter, you should be able to:

- Discuss the historical and social perceptions regarding weight.
- Identify the factors that affect body image.
- Describe the relationship of overweight and obesity to health.
- Explain how overweight or obesity can have a negative impact on health.
- Identify the four main factors that affect weight management.
- Describe healthy techniques and strategies to manage weight.
- Describe three types of eating disorders and identify the factors that contribute to them.
- Develop a personal plan for healthy weight management.

KEY TERMS

android fat pattern	body composition	essential body fat	pedometer
anorexia athletica	body mass index (BMI)	gynoid fat pattern	purging
anorexia nervosa	bulimia nervosa	ketosis	storage fat
bariatric	disordered eating	mindful eating	weight bias
binge-eating disorder	patterns	muscle dysmorphia	

● ● ● Introduction

Today's society places a great deal of emphasis on how people look. For females, "thin is in," while for males, the focus is on being muscular and "built." Even the hiring process, promotions, and job success have been associated with appearance. Most people want to fit in and be the "right" size and weight. We often compare ourselves with the size and weight of friends or the people we see on television and in the movies. Often it is assumed that thinness or muscularity brings happiness. There is a barrage of information

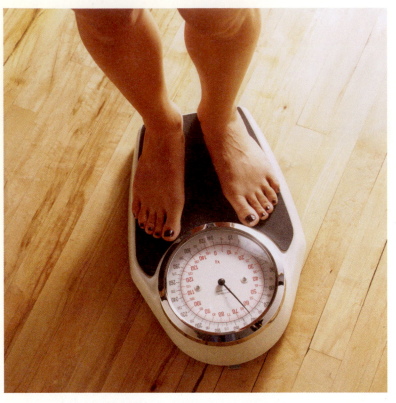

Courtesy of Photodisc

FIGURE 10-1 • Healthy weight management should be approached as a component of total health and a balanced lifestyle in cooperation with medical assessment and advice.

citing the prevalence of obesity in the United States, coupled with reality television shows promoting weight loss. While weight loss and weight management can be healthy endeavors, weight management needs to be addressed in the realm of total health and a balanced lifestyle in cooperation with medical assessment and advice (Figure 10-1). So how do you know what is healthy for *you*?

Americans seem to be obsessed with diet, exercise, nutrition, and weight loss. Yet the majority of Americans weigh more than is considered healthy. Medical professionals are encouraging Americans to eat better, exercise more, and lose weight. At the same time, unhealthy eating patterns are on the rise. How can you make sense of all this confusing information and create a healthy weight management plan that works best for you? In this chapter, you will have the opportunity to learn some of the information and skills you need to make healthy choices about managing your weight.

American Views about Weight

For much of American history, it was desirable to be overweight. Attractive women were "round and plump." Extra weight on men was an indication that they were successful and wealthy. It was not until the 1890s that these cultural ideals began to change as women pushed for broader roles outside their home, roles that valued women's intelligence and nondomestic skills and talents. For the first time, weight became a matter of public concern and discussion. As the culturally ideal figure became thinner, disgust for those who had excess body weight began to appear. Restricting food intake for the specific purpose of losing weight became popular. The word *diet*, which had previously referred simply to the food that a person consumed, now began to be associated with weight loss.

A curious thing has happened over the past 100 years. While the focus on weight control has increased, Americans have gotten fatter. We now weigh more on average than at any other time in our history, and that includes our children. The result is that what we want to weigh and what we actually weigh are moving in opposite directions. What are some of the causes of this phenomenon?

Many things contribute to this weight increase. Overweight and obesity are usually created by an energy imbalance over a prolonged period of time. The weight we carry is a combination of genetics, metabolism, behavior, environment, culture, and socioeconomic status. While genetics cannot be controlled, other factors, such as behavior and environment, can. These areas are the focus of the *U.S. Surgeon General's Call to Action to Prevent and Decrease Overweight and Obesity*. (U.S. Department of Health and Human Services, 2001). Our lifestyles have changed over the past 25 years. More Americans eat out as a result of the availability of fast-food choices and freedom from work and personal responsibilities.

PERSONAL ASSESSMENT
Weight Management Quiz

Before reading this chapter, see how much you already know about weight management. Read the questions below and on a separate sheet of paper answer True or False. Then check your answers at the end of the chapter.

1. About 25 percent of all Americans weigh more than is considered healthy.

2. The American cultural "ideal" for women is much thinner than it was 100 years ago.

3. Eliminating 500 calories a day from your diet will lead to a weight loss of two pounds per week.

4. Fat deposited around the abdomen ("apple" shape) is more dangerous to your health than fat deposited in the hips and thighs ("pear" shape).

5. Obesity can increase the risk of diabetes and coronary heart disease.

6. Certain diets and exercises can result in "spot reducing" (losing weight in a specific region of the body).

7. Approximately 25 to 35 percent of college-aged women practice bingeing and purging as weight management techniques.

8. For safe and healthy weight loss, most experts recommend losing no more than two pounds per week.

9. About 50 percent of all people who diet are successful in losing weight and maintaining their new weight.

10. Images of extreme thinness in women promoted by the advertising and entertainment industries may be a factor in the rise in eating disorders.

The idea that "more is better" is a societal notion that transfers to food. The portion sizes in restaurants are larger than they were in the past. Even the size of a bagel has doubled in the past 25 years. These trends encourage Americans to consume two to three times more than a single-portion size really should be. This phenomenon is seen as more value for the dollar, providing a large amount of food when busy schedules (and poor planning) may lead a person to consume only one meal a day.

Another contributor to rising body weight is the increased use of technology. Fewer people are engaged in manual labor and are more sedentary, and more people work at a computer or with other mechanized, time-saving devices. It is not uncommon for adult physical activity to be limited to walking around the house in preparation for work, walking to the car, walking into the office, and then reversing that process at the end of the day. As mentioned in chapter 8, this sedentary lifestyle contributes to too few calories burned throughout the day, not to mention the negative effects it can have on overall health and well-being. While change is good in some respects, the cost of change and the rapidity of change have not allowed the American public to "catch up" in terms of health, balance, and weight management.

Did You Know…?

Today, the average woman in the United States wears a dress size of 12 to 14. Yet the typical store mannequin is a size 6, and many models and actresses claim to wear a size 4 or smaller.

Influences on Ideas about Weight

The **media** represent a powerful influence on our ideals about weight. We are constantly bombarded by advertisements, magazine articles, television programs, and movies that suggest that if we are a certain size, weigh a certain amount, or look a certain way, we will be successful and happy. The message is that what you look like determines how successful you will be and the extent to which you will be liked. In reality, this is not true. Although your appearance may contribute to your success in school, business, or interpersonal relationships, it is not the most important factor in determining your value and quality of life. Most places of employment or school settings value and reward work ethic and interpersonal skills, such as honest and responsive communication. When these skills are emphasized and encouraged, a person can experience feelings of worth and success that can be internally motivating. Placing value and focusing on these types of personal attributes puts physical attributes in perspective for many.

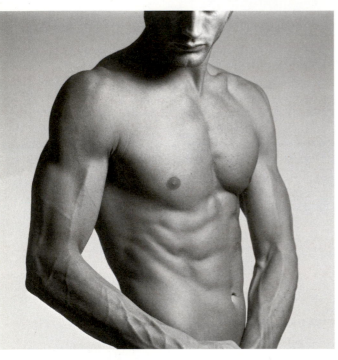

Courtesy of Photodisc

FIGURE 10-2 • This is an example of the media's portrayal of the "fit" male; however, as you read on through this chapter, you will realize that it can be unhealthy and unrealistic to compare ourselves to others.

The media have created ideal images of men and women as part of a sales strategy to sell more material. The masculine ideal is portrayed as strong, powerful, and muscular. Figure 10-2 shows a man with a very muscular physique. Often the media suggest that this might be the norm for each male when in reality it is rare to have this much muscle mass and definition. The feminine ideal is tall, very thin, and strikingly beautiful. In real life, one's appearance is much more diverse than that. If everyone fit these ideal images and looked the same, life would not seem as interesting.

Advertisements try to appeal to our emotions and create needs. For example, if we don't look like the people in the ads, we may feel the need to buy the products and services offered in order to look like the ideal. What the ads don't tell us is that the ideal doesn't really exist. They show people made to look their best with the help of makeup artists, hairstylists, clothing consultants, lighting experts, physical trainers, and even cosmetic surgery to totally change their looks. The desired images may even be computer generated, electronically edited, or airbrushed to achieve a certain effect. But to us, they

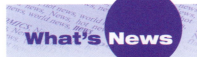

What's News

Researchers studied a group of women to assess their perceptions of their perceived body image, their actual body size and their ideal body size (Potti, et.al 2009). What they found was that the women tended to underestimate their actual body size. The underestimations were more likely to be reported by overweight and obese women, and African American and Hispanic women.

look like the "real thing." Most of us don't have the time, the money, or even the desire to invest that much to create a temporary image.

You can become a more critical viewer of the many media messages you are exposed to each day. The next time you see an advertisement, remind yourself that the "perfect" person you see has been created in order to persuade you to buy something. Ask yourself, "What are they trying to sell me?" Being aware of the motives of advertising can help you make conscious decisions about whether to accept what is being promoted. This awareness can help you develop a more realistic and healthy view of yourself.

Exploring Body Image

Body image is the way you see yourself when you look in the mirror or when you picture yourself in your mind. Body image is influenced by your beliefs about your appearance, such as how you feel about your height, shape, and weight. Some people have an image of themselves that is very close to reality. But many people have a distorted body image and don't see themselves as they really are. This is especially true for girls and women. It would be impossible to predict how this woman in Figure 10-3 feels about her body. Research indicates that body image is linked to our larger, or "global," self-esteem, and for some, how they feel about their body overshadows their overall assessment of themselves.

In many instances, women who are actually underweight classify themselves in the overweight category. In other words, they see themselves very differently from the way they actually look. People who have a negative body image often feel ashamed, self-conscious, and uncomfortable about the way their bodies look or move. This can affect the way they feel about themselves and the way they relate to other people.

Many factors contribute to your body image: past experiences, family, friends, and the influence of the media. You may have been teased about your weight or the shape of your body in the past. Or you may compare yourself to others or to unrealistic media images. A poor body image can lead to an obsession with weight and body shape. Most of us know someone who is constantly counting calories, fat grams, or trying a new fad diet. Constant worry and obsession about weight wastes valuable time and energy that can be devoted to achieving more important goals. Moreover, people don't stay with the regimen to lose the weight, nor are they able to control their ideal weight if they do reach their goal.

The first steps toward achieving a positive body image are recognizing and respecting the natural shape of your body and appreciating the many ways your body works for you. People who have a positive body image feel comfortable and confident in their bodies and refuse to spend an unreasonable amount of time worrying about their appearance. They also avoid engaging in

body image
the way you see yourself when you look in the mirror or when you picture yourself in your mind

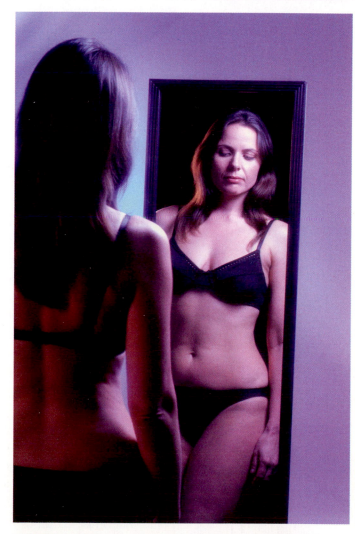

Courtesy of Photodisc

FIGURE 10-3 • Many women compare their bodies to those portrayed in the media.

negative self-talk, especially about their bodies. Talking negatively about your body is easy to do, as many of us are in the habit of checking the mirror for that hair out of place or spot on our clothes before we leave home. This habit has trained us to look in the mirror for flaws rather than what's beautiful about our bodies. Many of us, especially women, are very critical while trying on clothes in the dressing room of a store. It's important to remember that people come in many different sizes and shapes and that no one style or design could possibly fit us all, regardless of a particular size on the tag. Try attributing a style that doesn't fit your body as a design flaw, not your body's flaw.

This idea of negative body image is not exclusive to females. There is an increased prevalence of males focusing on body image. The American Psychiatric Association has identified diagnostic criteria for a type of disorder called **muscle dysmorphia**, which characterizes the behaviors of males who are preoccupied with body image. Males who are excessively preoccupied with muscularity or fitness, have a distorted body image, and abuse sports supplements and/or anabolic steroids are classified as exhibiting muscle dysmorphia. In Figure 10-4, the National Eating Disorders Association outlines a list of helpful ideas for both males and females to create a positive body image, and Figure 10-5 suggests nine things that men can do to maintain or develop a healthy outlook on body image.

muscle dysmorphia
a male's excessive preoccupation with a very muscular body image

How Much Should I Weigh?

You will hear many different recommendations about how much you should weigh. Some of the oldest methods for estimating "ideal weight" are based on the relationship of weight to height. Others are based on the increased likelihood for specific health problems if you weigh more than a certain amount. The simplest way to define your **ideal body weight** is the weight at which you feel strong and energetic and are able to lead a healthy, normal life. While formulas, charts, and expert recommendations can help guide you in determining exactly how much you should weigh, your ideal body weight is the weight at which *you* are healthy and feel good.

ideal body weight
the weight at which you feel strong and energetic and lead a healthy life

There is no one ideal number or weight at which a body is most healthy. Most people's weight fluctuates periodically for one reason or another; for example, it may drop if you are dehydrated or increase during holidays. Determining a weight range

1. Begin treating your body—the way it is—with respect and kindness.
2. Create a list of all the things your body is able to do.
3. When you wake up in the morning, thank your body for resting and preparing you to enjoy the day.
4. Put a sign on each of your mirrors that reminds you, "I'm beautiful, inside and out."
5. Don't let your weight or shape keep you from doing activities you enjoy.
6. Wear comfortable clothes that you like and that feel good to you.
7. Find a way of getting regular physical activity that you enjoy.
8. Surround yourself with people and things that make you feel good about yourself and your abilities.
9. Keep a list of at least 10 things that you like about yourself without mentioning anything about your appearance.
10. When you go to bed at night, thank your body for all that it helped you accomplish that day.

FIGURE 10-4 • Ten steps toward a positive body image. Adapted from: National Eating Disorders Association (2005a).

1. Develop the qualities in yourself that you like which are not related to your physical appearance.
2. Be analytical and critical of advertisements that emphasize the "bodybuilding" message.
3. Remember that your body, no matter what the size or shape it is, has nothing to do with your identity as a man.
4. Surround yourself with people who are not overly concerned with weight or appearance.
5. Assertively correct people who comment on your physical appearance— either positively or negatively.
6. Demonstrate a respect for other men who possess body types or personality traits that do not meet our cultural standard for masculinity.
7. Avoid negative self-talk about your physical appearance.
8. Focus the things your body can do to help you participate fully in your daily activities.
9. Focus on mastering your life goals and objectives, not simply on your bodyweight and/or appearance.

FIGURE 10-5 • Enhancing male body image. Adapted from: *Enhancing Male Body Image.* National Eating Disorders Association (2005b).

that is within healthy parameters is beneficial. It helps us create some leeway to eating and energy balance and is more realistic with how life really unfolds. People who have lost weight and are able to keep it off report that understanding their weight range and making modifications when they are over or under their weight range enables them to continue to maintain a healthy weight. This is a testament to healthy, balanced eating and exercise habits that are lifelong.

It is important to remember that "healthy weight" doesn't mean the current societal ideals about thinness or muscularity. It is natural to have a great deal of diversity among people. Every *body* is different. Discovering your own healthy weight is part of developing your individuality as a human being.

Defining Overweight and Obesity

Guidelines to describe different levels of excess weight have been developed to help people determine if they are at increased risk for health problems. **Overweight** is a term to describe body weight that is too high in relation to age, gender, and height. **Obese** is a term to describe an excessively high amount of body fat in relation to lean body mass, generally 20 percent over the ideal weight for the person's age, gender, and height.

The United States leads the world in the percentage of its population that is overweight or obese. National and state-level data have been acquired through the National Health and Nutrition Examination Survey (NHANES) and Behavioral Risk Factor Surveillance system indicating the continued increase in obesity among American adults. The Centers for Disease Control (CDC, 2006a, 2006b) reported data indicating that approximately 60 percent of all adults in the United States were overweight, 24 percent were obese, and 3.0 percent were extremely obese. Rates for minority women were higher than the national average for women. While 26 percent of all adult women were obese, 39 percent of African American women and 36 percent of Hispanic women were obese.

overweight
a term to describe body weight that is too high in relation to height

obese
a term used to describe an excessively high amount of body fat in relation to lean body mass

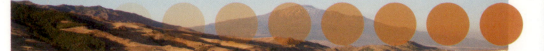

What's Your View?

Recently, as the problem of overweight and obesity among children and teenagers has increased, some schools have started sending "weight alert" letters to parents of children when a health examination reveals that the child or teenager is overweight or obese. Some school districts have even proposed adding this information to report cards. Some parents have been offended by these letters. They believe that weight is a personal issue and not something that schools should report. Schools respond that if a school health examination reveals vision or hearing problems, the parents are contacted. They question why a weight problem should be any different. They suggest that overweight and obesity are major health concerns and that parents should be warned of the potential dangers. What do you think?

Additionally, increases in health care charges have been associated with physical inactivity, overweight, and obesity. Original research conducted for the CDC revealed that 23 percent of health plan health care charges and 27 percent of national health care charges were associated with physical inactivity, overweight, and obesity.

Of growing concern is the rising number of overweight and obese children and teenagers. Older children and teenagers who are overweight are at increased risk for becoming overweight or obese adults. Results from the NHANES in 2004 revealed that approximately 14 percent of children and adolescents were overweight. The percentage of overweight adolescents (12 to 19 years of age) increased from 5 percent in 1988 to 17 percent in 2004.

Body Composition

The assessment of overweight or obesity can be determined by comparing height to weight, though a better indicator is comparing fat-free body lean mass (muscle, bone, and water) to fat mass, typically referred to as percent body fat. The relationship of lean mass to fat is known as **body composition**. Body composition is a better indicator of the body's health than using only weight. Imagine a young college athlete. This athlete is highly trained, is 5 feet 8 inches tall, weighs 140 pounds, and has a body fat composition of 18 percent. This athlete trains hard, burn calories, eats well, and has little difficulty maintaining the appropriate body composition. Imagine this same person 20 years later, still 5 feet 8 inches tall, not training or eating for competition, and weighing 142 pounds, but body composition has changed. The percent body fat is now 26 percent. Can you visualize the differences between the two body types? You can see why people say, "I weigh only two pounds more than I did in college, but my waist is two inches larger."

Body composition is the relationship between fat-free mass (muscle, bone, and water) and fat tissue in the body. Determining your body composition requires learning what percent of your body weight is fat weight and what percent is fat-free mass or lean body weight. While most would agree that a low amount of body fat is desirable, the body needs a certain amount of fat tissue to function properly. This is known as **essential body fat**. It is the minimum amount of body fat needed by the body to metabolize certain vitamins (A, D, E, and K), provide insulation, cushion body organs, and maintain

body composition
the relationship between fat-free mass (muscle, bone, and water) and fat tissue in the body

essential body fat
the amount of fat necessary for use by the body to provide insulation, cushion body organs, and maintain normal bodily functions

normal bodily functions. Essential body fat requirements are estimated to be about 3 to 7 percent in males and about 12 percent in females. Females need a higher percentage to support proper levels of hormones and to support pregnancy should it occur.

Additional body fat is known as **storage fat**, which results when excess food calories are stored by the body. Because of the differences in the amount of essential body fat, ideal body composition varies between males and female. For males, the approximate percentage of total body fat should be 12 to 15 percent. For females, the approximate percentage of total body fat should be 18 to 21 percent. This range may vary with age but is a healthy range that one can strive to maintain at any age.

Weight gain usually occurs when someone consistently consumes more calories than the body uses. The way in which this extra weight is distributed tends to differ between males and females. Most males store extra body fat in what is called an "apple" pattern, or **android fat pattern**. This means that it is concentrated around the middle of the body in the abdominal area. In contrast, most females store extra body fat in the hips and thighs in what is called a "pear" pattern, or **gynoid fat pattern**. Although females are quick to complain about the tendency to acquire this pear shape, it is not as dangerous to health as storing extra body fat in an apple pattern. The extra fat concentrated in the abdominal area has been linked to an increased risk of heart disease. Figure 10-6 shows the common areas that men and women are likely to carry excess weight.

Did You Know…?

It takes 3,500 extra calories to create one pound of storage fat. Conversely, to remove one pound of storage fat, it requires the expenditure of 3,500 calories (or the combination of exercise and reduction of food consumption).

storage fat
body fat as a result of excess calories stored by the body

android fat pattern
accumulation of excess fat around the abdominal area, characteristic of male weight gain pattern

gynoid fat pattern
accumulation of excess fat in the hips and thighs, characteristic of female weight gain

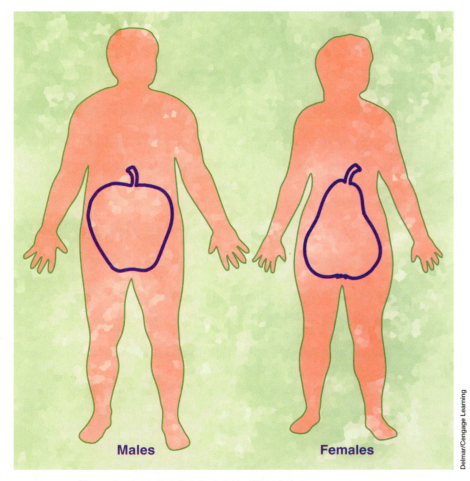

Males   **Females**

Delmar/Cengage Learning

FIGURE 10-6 • Men and women store their body fat in different places.

Calculate your body mass index (BMI):

1. Multiply your weight in pounds by 703.

2. Divide the result by your height in inches.

3. Divide that result by your height in inches again.

FIGURE 10-7 • Method for calculating body mass index.

Calculate your waist-to-hip ratio:

1. Measure waist circumference in inches.

2. Measure hip circumference in inches.

3. Divide waist circumference by hip circumference.

FIGURE 10-8 • Method for calculating the waist-to-hip ratio.

Assessing Body Composition

There are many ways to determine how much body weight is lean mass and how much is fat tissue. Traditional height–weight charts have been used for many years to suggest "ideal weights." But they cannot accurately estimate body composition. A better indicator is the **body mass index (BMI)**, which measures the relationship (or ratio) of weight to height using a mathematical formula. BMI is more closely correlated to percentage of body fat than any other sophisticated height–weight measures, such as hydrostatic weighing or electrical impedance. It has become the most common standard for assessing overweight and obesity because it is reasonably accurate and easy to use. See Figure 10-7 for instructions on how to calculate your own BMI.

One of the disadvantages of BMI is that it is not a good body fat indicator for highly muscular people. Highly muscular people may weigh more for their height because muscle tissue has a higher density than fat. Their actual percent body fat would indicate that they are lean or within a normal healthy range. According to health experts, a BMI of 18.5 to 25.0 represents a weight at which a person is unlikely to experience health problems due to excessive weight. If BMI falls below 18.5, there is a risk that weight is too low to be healthy. If BMI is above 25.0, there is an increased risk for health problems related to excess weight. People who have a BMI of 25 to 29.9 are classified as being overweight. People who have a BMI of 30 or above are classified as obese according to government guidelines. Notice the range of acceptable BMI. This provides evidence that there is no one single "ideal weight" for an individual.

Another mathematical formula used to predict health risks associated with body fat is the calculation of the waist-to-hip ratio. A ratio of 1.0 or higher indicates a higher level of risk for health problems for both men and women. Ideal ratios are .90 or lower for men and .80 or lower for women. See Figure 10-8 for instructions on calculating the waist-to-hip ratio.

body mass index (BMI)
a commonly used measure of the relationship (or ratio) of weight to height expressed in a mathematical formula

WEB LINK
Body Fat Calculation

http://www.about.com

At this Web site, enter "fitness evaluations and assessment" in the search bar. At the assessment page, you will be able to access a number of body composition assessment techniques, including electrical impedance, fat calipers, and hydrostatic weighing.

SEARCH TERMS: body composition, body fat assessment, body fat measurement

A third method for determining body fat is the skinfold caliper "pinch" test. A skinfold caliper (Figure 10-9) is used to measure skinfold at designated points on the body. To ensure accuracy, it is important that the test be done by someone who is well trained and experienced. The results are then correlated with standardized body fat measures to estimate the actual percentage of body fat.

Weight and Health

While obsession with weight is not healthy, it is true that excess weight can contribute to serious health problems. The CDC (2010) reported that obesity is responsible for an estimated 112,000 premature deaths each year, second only to the number of deaths related to smoking. The risks for heart disease, stroke, diabetes, and certain types of cancer are all higher in adults who are overweight. The more overweight a person is, the greater his or her chances are for having weight-related health problems.

Disadvantages of Being Overweight

The medical research is definitive: there is no health value in being overweight. Excess body fat taxes many of the body systems. Too much weight places a strain on the respiratory and cardiovasular systems and stresses the weight-bearing joints in the body. The American Medical Association (2004) estimates that 400,000 Americans die each year from obesity-related conditions. Following is a summary of some of the medical evidence:

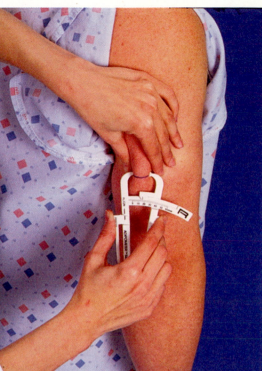

FIGURE 10-9 • Measuring triceps skinfold.

Delmar/Cengage Learning

- Overweight people are twice as likely to develop type 2 diabetes as people who are not overweight. Among people diagnosed with type 2 diabetes, 67 percent have a BMI ≥ 27, and 46 percent have a BMI ≥ 30.

- Overweight individuals are more likely to have high blood pressure, a major risk factor for heart disease and stroke.

- Overweight people, especially males, are prone to sleep apnea, a condition whereby the person periodically stops breathing during his or her sleep. Sleep apnea is related to heart failure. Interestingly, people with sleep apnea who lose weight are known to exhibit less sleep apnea.

- There are a number of cancers associated with being overweight. In women, these conditions include cancer of the uterus, gallbladder, cervix, ovary, breast, and colon. Overweight men are at greater risk for developing cancer of the colon, rectum, and prostate.

- Extra weight appears to increase the risk of osteoarthritis by placing extra pressure on the joints and wearing away the cartilage that normally protects the joints.

WEB LINK

Relationship of Overweight and Obesity to Health

For more information about the relationship of overweight and obesity to health, see the following Web sites: Office of the Surgeon General at **http://www.surgeongeneral.gov** (search for "overweight and obesity") and National Heart, Lung, and Blood Institute at **http://rover.nhlbi.nih.gov** (search for "Obesity Education Initiative Website").

What's News

According to a study conducted by Steven Blair, former director of research at the Cooper Institute for Aerobics Research in Dallas, Texas, previous studies linking obesity and death from heart disease and other major killers may have missed the important influence of exercise (2006). Blair's study followed more than 30,000 men and women for 10 years. The results showed that obese people who exercise enough to be fit have *half* the death rate of those who are slender but not fit. Blair says that people who are both thin and active are more accepted by society. But in terms of lowering health risk for heart disease and diabetes, his study shows that it is a low fitness level rather than excess weight that is the most important risk factor.

Factors Influencing Body Weight

It isn't fully understood why some people struggle so much to maintain a healthy weight and why others maintain a healthy weight without even thinking about it. It appears that there are a number of factors that influence whether a person will become overweight or obese. A complex interaction of these factors accounts for individual differences in body weight. Let's look at how these factors affect body weight.

Genetics/Heredity

Have you ever noticed how family members often have similar body types and shapes? One reason may be that family members have similar eating and exercise patterns. But experts in weight management have consistently documented that genetics influences body shape, size, and weight. Everyone has a genetic predisposition for their level of **metabolism**. For example, your genetic heritage can affect your metabolic rate, or the speed at which your body burns energy. Some people have a higher metabolism and burn energy (calories) at a higher rate than others. These are the kinds of people we hold in awe when we say, "Wow, you are so lucky you can eat anything you want and never gain weight." People with high metabolic rates burn more food than those with slower metabolism. For example, men naturally have higher rates of metabolism than women. Teens have higher metabolic rates than adults. Adults have higher metabolic rates than elder adults. People's caloric needs in general are the highest during their late teen years. After age 30, you can expect your caloric needs to drop 5 percent per decade for the rest of your life. Suppose that two people start at the same weight. Even if they eat exactly the same foods and exercise exactly the same amount, it is unlikely that they will have the same weight at the end of a year.

Not everyone can achieve the same weight goals regardless of their efforts. This does not mean that if you have a genetic predisposition for gaining weight or being too thin, you can't do anything about it. It simply means that you will have to put forth more effort to achieve and maintain a healthy weight.

metabolism
the process of converting food into energy for the body; also includes converting body fat to energy if other energy sources are not available

WEB LINK
Metabolism

http://www.webmd.com

This Web site has a wealth of information about metabolism. Enter "metabolism" in the search bar, and you will find numerous other links to related topics.

SEARCH TERMS: metabolism, basal metabolism, energy expenditure

Food Intake

There's no denying it: what you put into your mouth plays a big role in your body size and weight. In many instances, it is not how much you eat but rather the caloric density of how much you eat (review chapter 9). All things considered, however, the fact remains that 3,500 extra calories will convert to one pound of body fat. A general guideline is that we gain weight when we take in more calories than we burn. It may be helpful to assess your eating habits in order to provide a baseline to understand your caloric intake:

- *What kind of foods do you eat?* Do you eat mostly fruits and vegetables or mostly hamburgers, fries, sweets, and pizza? There's nothing wrong with eating any of these items, but a steady diet of foods like these can add too many calories and too much fat to your diet, especially if you aren't burning calories with physical activity. This makes it hard for you to manage your weight and get enough of the nutrients your body needs to function well. Figure 10-10 offers some healthy alternatives to many of the high-calorie snacks that are available. Remember also that alcohol contains empty calories. If you drink, you may want to conduct an Internet search to get a sense of how many calories are in the various alcoholic drinks and drink mixers.

- *When do you eat?* Do you eat most of your calories early or later in the day? Several studies indicate that eating the majority of your calories early in the day, while your body is most active, helps to avoid weight gain. Consuming a high number of calories in the evening may make it easier for your body to store the excess calories as fat. Remember that when you are sleeping, you are burning the least amount of energy. Excess calories in the evening may be converted to fat.

- *Where do you eat?* It's easy to consume a lot of calories very quickly if you're not paying attention to what you're eating. Avoid eating while you are doing something else, such as driving or watching television. Make eating a special occasion and concentrate on enjoying your food.

- *Why do you eat?* The best reason to eat is because your body lets you know it's hungry. But often, we eat for other reasons. A particular food may look good, everyone else is eating something, or we rely on the clock rather than our hunger to tell us to eat. Research indicates that overweight individuals eat according to the clock regardless of whether they are hungry or not. Normal-weight people eat when they are hungry. We may use food to respond to our emotions. People under stress will eat more than those who are not stressed. If we develop the habit of using food to make us feel better or as a reward, we may eat much more than we need for healthy body functioning.

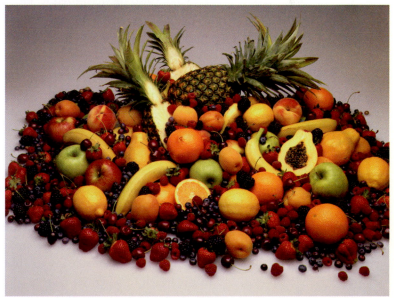

Courtesy of Photodisc

FIGURE 10-10 • Fresh fruit is a great snack option when on the go or between meals.

Physical Activity

Your level of physical activity plays a big role in healthy weight management. People who are consistently active burn more calories, even when they are at rest. You don't necessarily have to exercise or work out vigorously—even moderate activity burns calories. Whenever you have a choice, *choose to move*. For example, take the stairs instead of the elevator. Walk instead of driving in the car or riding on the bus. Don't waste your time trying to get the closest parking space. Parking a little farther away is not a bad thing unless the weather prevents doing so. Physical activity alone won't keep your weight at a healthy level, but it is certainly a key part of an effective weight management plan. You'll also feel better and have more energy if you're physically active. Refer to chapter 8 to recall the many health benefits of physical activity.

Psychological Factors

Many people use food as a coping mechanism under conditions of stress. Think back to when you were a small child. Perhaps there were times when you were offered special foods when you were upset about something, such as getting candy as a "reward" for behaving well at the doctor's office. Foods eventually become associated with comfort. If this happened to you, can you remember what those foods were? When you feel a certain way now, do you use food to make yourself feel better? Eating because you are bored, lonely, sad, nervous, or frustrated instead of because you are truly hungry can add calories quickly. And eating is usually not an effective way to solve the problem that's causing the stress in the first place. When you are stressed or emotionally upset, instead of eating, think of ways that you can make yourself feel better without using food, such as going for a walk or talking to a friend.

weight bias
negative attitudes and stereotypes that have a detrimental effect on interpersonal relationships

Those individuals who are overweight, especially those who are obese, are subject to **weight bias**. Overweight or obese individuals are not viewed favorably among many in our society. As a result, they can be mistreated in a number of ways. They can be verbally teased about their size: they may be recipients of negative comments and may be made fun of by way of comments, jokes, and so on. Some overweight people, especially children, can be bullied or physically attacked by others who may not accept them. They may also be victimized when others exclude them from social events and activities, being ignored, and having people look away when they pass them in public. There are a number of scientific studies that demonstrate the existence of weight bias. The condition exists in health care facilities, academic institutions, and employment settings.

Research indicates that weight bias produces negative psychological effects on the overweight individuals who are recipients of these bias behaviors. Children and adults who are recipients of weight bias show depression, anxiety, low self-esteem, poor body images, and suicidal thoughts. The reduction of weight bias resides with the transformation of societal views of overweight and obesity and in the ability of the overweight person to develop a comfort level with his or her body image.

In the long run, however, the American concern over body weight transcends the issues related to diseases and body image. It really should be about each individual's concern for his or her well-being and the well-being of those around them. It is unfortunate that people suddenly become concerned about their weight only after being overweight takes on a prominent role in their lives, such as when we need to "look good" for that trip to the beach or when we go to a special social occasion. The best strategy is to be motivated enough to ensure that our eating and exercise habits do not create abusive caloric overload that puts us in a serious weight gain situation.

●●● Weight Management Strategies

It is apparent many people in America struggle with their weight. There are many reasons why this is so, but, sadly, it is the reality. Reasons become only excuses for allowing the conditions to exist. In order to successfully address overweight and obesity, we must first create a cultural value that welcomes something other than having more than 50 percent of society being overweight. Until that time, we will continue with the following menu of strategies available to the populace to help them fight the "battle of the bulge."

Dieting

How often do you hear someone say, "I can't eat *that*. I'm on a diet"? **Dieting** has become a national obsession in the United States. A study by the Calorie Control Council (2005) indicated that 33 percent of Americans were on a diet, a 35 percent increase from the council's 2000 study. For adolescent and young adult females, the percentage of dieters was even higher. Although American males are not as obsessed with dieting as American females, a substantial number of males eat an unbalanced diet in order to achieve a certain body size or shape. The dietary restrictions are often so severe that people do not regularly get enough of the nutrients their bodies need. Without proper nutrition, physical and mental performance can suffer.

The biggest problem with dieting for weight loss is that *dieting usually doesn't work*—at least not over the long term—because it is a short-term solution for something that needs to be maintained throughout a lifetime. Several studies have shown about 95 percent of people who lose weight by dieting regain all the pounds they lost (and sometimes more) within a year of "going off" the diet. Some experts believe that this weight loss and gain (known as the "yo-yo effect") can lead to changes in the body's metabolism that make it even more difficult to manage weight effectively.

Despite the thousands of weight loss books and products sold, the long-term success rate for dieting is quite low. That's one reason why there is always a new **fad diet** on the market. You may or may not have heard of the "7 Day All You Can Eat Diet," the "Atkins Diet," the "Cabbage Soup Diet," or the "Lemonade Diet". According to the people who make these things up, they do take the weight off. People who fail with one diet continue their search for the magic pill, plan, or formula to solve their weight problems. Most fad diets overemphasize one particular food or type of food and generally contradict the guidelines of balanced nutrition. At best, they are ineffective; at worst, they can be dangerous to one's health. Only after it has depleted energy from carbohydrate sources will the body turn to body fat reserves. Using fat reserves for energy results in the production of ketones, a process known as **ketosis**. Ketones are not necessarily bad, as the heart and kidneys would rather use ketones as an energy source. Ketosis over a long period of time can lead to death in severe cases. Other harmful effects of caloric deprivation include low blood sugar, sensitivity to cold, heart rate irregularity, dehydration, diarrhea, headaches, and fatigue.

When we "go on a diet," the assumption is that that we will also eventually "go off a diet." Attaining and maintaining a healthy weight takes time. There are no quick, easy, and safe ways to lose weight. Healthfully

dieting
temporary patterns of eating that restrict calories for the purpose of losing weight

fad diet
an eating regimen that overemphasizes one particular food or type of food and contradicts the guidelines of good nutrition

ketosis
the body's process of converting body fat to ketones

Did You Know...?
In 2005, Americans spent more than $46 billion a year on dieting and diet-related products. That's about the same amount the U.S. federal government spends on *education* each year. Do you think this money is being spent wisely? In your opinion, what is the best way to direct this money so that the health of Americans is improved?

managing weight requires the formation of new habits. You can make eating healthy a new way of life. While it may take longer to achieve the results you want, you are much more likely to keep the weight off permanently.

Fad Exercise Plans

Exercise is a well-respected method of balancing calorie intake and managing weight. If someone is serious about establishing a healthy weight management plan, exercise is a must. You will read more about exercising in a healthy manner later in this chapter. There are exercise misconceptions of which you should be aware. First, you cannot sweat your way to weight management. A good weight management program addresses the issue of balancing caloric intake with caloric expenditure. Sweating (e.g., using a sauna, rubber suit, or sweat clothes) does nothing more than eliminate water from the body. There will be a temporary weight loss because the water has been eliminated. But then the individual must rehydrate by drinking water or run the risk of illness due to dehydration. When one sweats, one does not metabolize glycogen or fat.

Don't be misled by exercise gimmicks. There isn't any exercise equipment that is best for weight loss. Any exercise will do. You can walk, jog, swim, lift weights, play tennis, and so on. The key is to *move*, and you don't have to do it rapidly. Movement at a steady pace over 20 minutes a day will burn calories. The notion of exercising only certain body parts to "reduce the fat" in only those parts doesn't really work either. If someone weight trains a particular muscle group *while engaging* in a weight management program of diet and exercise, he or she will lose fat but gain muscle mass in the exercised area.

●●● Healthy Techniques and Strategies to Manage Weight

If dieting doesn't work, then what *can* you do to manage your weight? First, weight management must be approached as a long-term commitment. You must also be willing to change some lifestyle and eating habits. Here are some suggestions to increase your chances for success.

Keep Your Weight in Perspective

Managing your weight is an important goal to have that will help keep you healthier throughout your lifetime. However, it is not the only thing that is necessary. A better approach is to focus on your overall health and well-being, not just your weight. Often, when people start an exercise program, they plan to work out at a time that they may need for sleep or connecting with their families. This strategy is not unlike dieting in that if the program robs you of other healthful things in your life, you will not stick with it. Creating a plan that fits in with your commitments and responsibilities will help you adopt habits in order to maintain an equal energy balance. One idea is to schedule activity breaks into your day or use your lunchtime to exercise. Working activity into your day, such as taking the stairs or parking farther away, have additional health benefits that can increase the amount of calories you burn each day. It is suggested that each adult walk 10,000 steps each day, so wearing a **pedometer** is a practical way of assessing your daily activity level.

pedometer
a personal calculator worn by someone to measure the steps taken during a given time period

Exercise

Exercise should be an integral part of any weight management program. Recall from chapter 8 that there are numerous benefits associated with an exercise program but that it is essential to incorporate exercise as a complement to a well-balanced, nutritious eating program. As mentioned previously, the form of exercise is not important. Choose something you enjoy (Figure 10-11). Simply performing household chores and tasks and using the stairs instead of the elevator can help burn calories.

The amount of calories expended during activity will depend on the weight of the participant, the type of activity, the duration of the activity, and the speed at which the activity is performed. Table 10-1 lists a variety of activities. The data in the cells represent the number of calories burned during 30 minutes of that particular exercise for an individual weighing the amount presented at the top of the columns. If you conduct an Internet search, you may find a number of sites that will help you calculate caloric expenditure for other activities in which you might have an interest.

Listen to Your Body

A good technique for healthy weight management is learning to listen to your body. This means eating when you are truly hungry and stopping when you are comfortably full. Every day you are bombarded by cues to eat, what kind of foods to eat, how often to eat, and how much to eat. Food is readily available at home, in vending

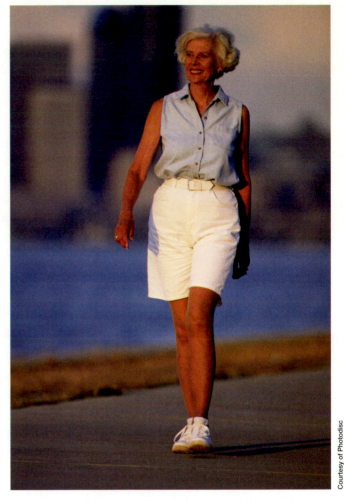

Courtesy of Photodisc

FIGURE 10-11 • Choosing exercise activities that you enjoy can help you successfully incorporate exercise into your weight management program.

TABLE 10-1 • Caloric expenditures according to weight and 30-minute activity.

Activity	Weight (pounds)					
	100	120	160	180	220	240
Housework	90	108	144	162	198	216
Bowling	55	66	88	99	121	132
Walking (three miles per hour)	80	96	128	144	176	192
Jogging (12 minutes per mile)	185	222	296	333	407	444
Golf (no cart)	100	120	160	180	220	240
Snow skiing (downhill)	130	156	208	234	286	312
Tennis	160	192	256	288	352	384
Grocery shopping	60	72	96	108	132	144
Weight training (90 seconds between sets)	255	306	408	459	561	612

Delmar/Cengage Learning

machines, at fast-food restaurants, and at convenience stores. Sometimes people eat because they are bored, stressed, lonely, or restless. It takes some effort to recognize true hunger signals from your body. It also takes some discipline to refuse to eat "just because you want to." We tend to forget that the only reason we need to eat is to "stay alive."

The same is true for learning to stop eating when you are satisfied. The saying "my eyes were bigger than my stomach" is often shared after someone has piled his or her plate too high and became too full to eat all the food. It takes your brain about 20 minutes to register that you have eaten. Have you ever started eating and gotten interrupted, only to find that you feel satisfied and not interested in finishing your meal? Being aware of food portion sizes and taking time to enjoy the food by taking smaller bites and chewing your food more slowly as you eat will help your body give you the cues to let you know that it is satisfied.

We live in a fast-paced society. We often eat in a hurry and are not aware that we just consumed a burger, an order of fries, and a large soft drink in five minutes! Doing so can make you feel full and sluggish. This results in digestive issues that may cause discomfort and lethargy for completing additional tasks. The effect on your blood sugar levels and your body's ability to adapt to the challenges of no food versus a lot of food can create havoc within your physiologic systems. Listen to your body to eat at regular intervals and eat a moderate amount slowly rather than suffer from the effects of overeating.

Eat Breakfast

Although it is tempting to skip breakfast, studies indicate that people who are successful at losing weight and maintaining the weight loss eat breakfast regularly. The word *breakfast* is a term describing "breaking the fast" after having slept or being away from nutrients for a period of time. If you don't eat breakfast, your body's metabolism slows to conserve energy for what you might ask it to do throughout the day. Your brain relies only on glucose for fuel; it cannot utilize fats or proteins. This slowing down of metabolism and lack of blood sugar caused by not eating breakfast can make you feel lethargic, give you a headache, and limit your body's willingness to expend calories. If your body has incoming calories, it is more likely to let go or give up calories. Think of eating a nutritious breakfast as a catalyst for burning calories for the day and for giving you the energy you need to start your day.

A Diverse Diet

Eating a wide variety of foods helps ensure that your body has all the nutrients it needs to perform at its best. While you should try to get most of your calories from foods that are healthy for you, such as fruits and vegetables, don't fall into the trap of labeling foods as "good" or "bad." Fast food is not "bad food." While fast foods tend to be high in fat and calories, it is food nonetheless because it contains carbohydrate, protein, fats, vitamins, minerals, and so on. A well-balanced weight management plan can include all types of food as long the foods are varied and consumed in moderation. When you indulge in fast food, choose the lowest-fat foods you can find on the menu or share your meal with someone. By all means, avoid "supersizing" your meal.

Pay Attention to Portion Sizes

American portions are much larger than portions in other countries. We have options to "supersize" our meals or choosing the two-for-one "value" meals. Foods that are high in calories and/or fat are often packaged with several servings in a single container. For example, potato chip bags are notorious for having more than one serving in a single bag. You think that you are consuming "one bag of chips" when in reality it is two or three servings. Check food labels to make sure that you are eating the serving size that is best for you. Restaurants often serve very large portions. You can't necessarily check a food label, although many restaurants will provide the caloric content of their food if you ask. As of this writing, Congress is considering the passage of the LEAN (Labeling Education and Nutrition) Act. If passed the legislation will require all chain restaurants with 20 or more outlets to publicly display the caloric content of foods on their menus. Good techniques to avoid overeating are to share a meal with a friend or to eat half of what you're served and ask for a container to take the remainder home. You'll save on calories and money for a future meal.

Check your sodas and sport drinks for serving size amounts as well. Research indicates a strong positive relationship between the consumption of sugar-sweetened beverages (e.g., regular sodas and fruit punches) and the risk of diabetes. Schulze et al. (2004) reported that increasing one's consumption of sugary soft drinks significantly increases the risk for both weight gain and type 2 diabetes. Remember that soda is considered an "empty-calories" food with little if any nutritional value. The simple sugars in the soda can erode teeth, add hidden calories, and often contribute to dehydration. If a person drinks caffeinated soft drinks throughout the day, he or she most likely is not drinking the requisite amount of water his or her body needs to function properly. When thinking about nutrition choices, it's important to remember that you don't have to eat or drink the amount that is available or served if you are no longer hungry. In fact, you do not have to drink soda or some other soft drink; water is fine with a meal.

Practice Mindful Eating

Mindful eating means paying attention to the food you are eating and enjoying its tastes, smells, and textures. Mindful eating can help you learn to recognize your body's cues for when to start and stop eating. Too often, we eat while we are doing something else and don't pay attention to the amount we are consuming. For example, people who watch television while they eat often consume much more than they intended. It's easy to go through most of a bag of potato chips or cookies without being aware of how much you have eaten. Preparing a simple meal and setting aside time to savor the meal can be one of the first steps to mindful eating (Figure 10-12).

mindful eating
paying attention to the food you are eating and enjoying its tastes, smells, and textures

Medical Interventions for Weight Control

When all these measures are unsuccessful, it might be important to seek medical attention through the use of prescription drugs, or a last

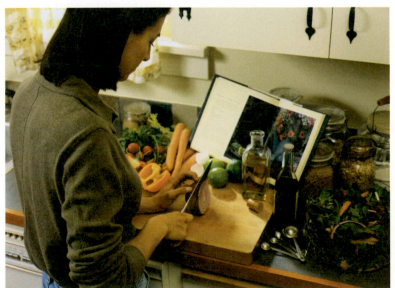

Courtesy of Photodisc

FIGURE 10-12 • Setting aside time to prepare food can be an enjoyable and healthy part of daily routine.

Bariatric
surgical interventions specific to obesity treatment

eating disorders
problems related to food, weight, and body image that are harmful to physical or psychological health

anorexia nervosa
an eating disorder in which a person does not eat enough food for the body to function at a healthy level or to maintain a healthy weight (can result in death by starvation)

resort might include surgery. While drugs may help an obese person lose up to 10 percent of his or her weight, there are many negative side effects of weight loss drugs, resulting in the U.S. Food and Drug Administration (FDA) pulling some of these drugs off the market. One example of this was Redux, otherwise known as fen-phen. Repeated tests showed that Redux, used over a long period of time, caused damage to heart valves.

When lifestyle changes and drugs are still ineffective, a doctor may recommend surgery. The medical community generally reserves **bariatric** surgical interventions, such as gastric bypass or gastric banding, for the obese patient, commonly someone with a BMI of 40 or higher. Gastric banding is becoming more common because it is less invasive and can be reversed. During gastric banding, a surgeon places a band around the upper part of the stomach where the stomach connects to the esophagus. This reduces the amount of food a person needs to feel full. Gastric bypass, on the other hand, is irreversible and more invasive; however, the results are often more dramatic. Problems associated with bypass surgery include nausea and vomiting because the remaining stomach is very small and can process only a very small amount of food or liquid at a time.

● ● ● Understanding Eating Disorders

Eating disorders are problems related to food, weight, and body image that are harmful to physical or psychological health. There are several types of eating disorders, but they all cause significant health problems. Eating disorders are much more common in females than in males. About 90 percent of eating disorders occur in females, and even though there has been an increase in males who report having an eating disorder, only about 10 percent of disorders occur in males. These percentages translate to as many as 10 million females and 1 million males who are struggling with an eating disorder in some form.

Identifying eating disorders early and getting proper treatment are the keys to preventing serious health problems and even death. Without treatment, up to 20 percent of people who have serious eating disorders die. Of those who receive treatment, only about 2 to 3 percent die. Let's take a look at the major eating disorders in the United States today.

Anorexia Nervosa

Anorexia nervosa is perhaps the most common and serious of all the eating disorders because of the high rates of death associated with it. People who have **anorexia nervosa** do not eat enough to maintain body function at a healthy level. Their weight may fall to 85 percent or less of what is expected for their age and height. In spite of dramatic weight loss and extreme thinness, anorexics view themselves as "fat" and continue to deny themselves enough food.

Anorexia nervosa is most common in adolescent and young adult females. Research suggests that about 1 percent of female adolescents have anorexia. Although this disease is considered to be psychosocial in nature, there are recent studies that suggest that genetics may predispose individuals to the disease. Without treatment, persons with anorexia gradually starve themselves to death. Of all the psychiatric disorders, anorexia has the highest rate of mortality.

Successful treatment focuses on restoring the weight loss; providing psychotherapy to treat the distortion of body image, low self-esteem, and relationship difficulties; and sustaining long-term recovery. Anorexia requires treatment from medical personnel for both physical and psychological issues. Early treatment for anorexia focuses on restoring body weight so that the person doesn't die. Resolving underlying psychological issues is also a part of the treatment plan. It is not unusual for full recovery from anorexia nervosa to take at least five years.

Bulimia Nervosa

Bulimia nervosa is an eating disorder in which a person eats a great deal of food and then vomits or uses other methods, such as laxatives or overexercising, to avoid gaining weight. This effort to rid the body of food that has been consumed is called **purging**. It is estimated that somewhere between 1 and 3 percent of the female population in the United States meets the criteria for bulimia. It is estimated that 25 to 35 percent of college-aged women engage in bingeing and purging as methods for weight management and that approximately one-third of athletes practice detrimental behaviors, such as self-induced vomiting, bingeing, and taking laxatives, diuretics, and diet pills. In contrast to those with anorexia, most people with bulimia have normal or near normal body weight so other people may not realize they have an eating disorder. This can result in treatment being delayed or not occurring at all.

Bulimics describe themselves as feeling out of control while eating and unable to stop themselves. Since they believe that their self-worth depends on their being thin, they become caught in the cycle of overeating and then purging to get rid of the food they consumed to avoid gaining weight. Psychologically, bulimics often report feeling depressed, lonely, ashamed, and unworthy, although these conditions may not be obvious to other people. It appears that psychological distress contributes to the development of bulimia in the first place rather than being a result of the disorder.

About half of all cases of bulimia nervosa appear to have a genetic component. With proper treatment, most bulimics are able to recover and return to a more normal pattern of eating. Successful treatment often includes the use of antidepressant drugs and psychotherapy. In contrast to anorexia nervosa, the primary focus of treatment is directed toward resolving psychological issues.

Binge-Eating Disorder

Binge-eating disorder is when a person eats large amounts of food frequently and repeatedly. They describe themselves as feeling out of control and unable to stop eating during binges. Since they feel guilty and ashamed of these binges, they often eat in secret so that no one can see how much food they are consuming. In contrast to persons with bulimia, binge eaters do not regularly vomit, overexercise, or abuse laxatives. They usually have a long history of unsuccessful dieting and tend to be obese. It is estimated that about 1 percent of females in the United States have a binge-eating disorder. About 30 percent of women who seek treatment to lose weight admit to being

bulimia nervosa
an eating disorder in which a person eats a great deal of food and then vomits or uses other methods, such as laxatives or overexercising, to avoid gaining weight from the overeating

purging
removing undesirable substances; in the case of bulimia nervosa, refers to vomiting or using laxatives or exercise to remove excessive amounts of food consumed

binge-eating disorder
a condition in which a person eats large amounts of food frequently and repeatedly

binge eaters. Our society tends to consider binge eating more abnormal and inappropriate for women than for men. Men also seem to experience less guilt related to their binge-eating behavior.

Disordered Eating Patterns

disordered eating patterns
occasions when dieting, food restriction, fear of becoming overweight, and body image dissatisfaction interfere with normal daily life

anorexia athletica
a disorder that is most often common in competitive athletes and that occurs when someone starts compulsive exercising and does so in an amount of time or at an intensity that is beyond normal

Disordered eating patterns occur when concerns about dieting, food restriction, fear of becoming overweight, and dissatisfaction with body image interfere with normal daily life. Disordered eating patterns may lead to the development of an eating disorder, although this does not occur in all cases. More commonly, the person becomes so focused on dieting, food, weight, and body image that other important goals and activities are cast aside. Often this focus is coupled with behaviors such as compulsive exercise or periodic purging. If you find yourself giving dieting, food, weight, and body image a great deal of your attention, you may want to think about ways to find a better balance in your life. If you are unable to do this on your own, you should consider seeking professional assistance. There's so much more to life than eating!

The diagnosis of anorexia and/or bulimia, binge-eating disorder, **anorexia athletica**, and muscle dysmorphia are based on strict criteria set by the fourth edition of the *Diagnostic and Statistical Manual of Mental Disorders* (American Psychiatric Association, 1994). There are also many people who fall into a category called "eating disorders not otherwise specified." These people display some but not all of the clinical diagnostic criteria and often exhibit severe harmful behaviors that are going undiagnosed or underdiagnosed. If you or someone you know is struggling with these types of behaviors, seek help from a qualified professional who can help you work through issues surrounding your choice to treat your body in this manner.

●●● Creating a Healthy Weight Management Plan

You may decide to apply what you have learned in this book to create a personal weight management program. The first step is to be sure that you are motivated to move forward and determine realistic goals. What do you want to accomplish? Do you want to gain weight, lose weight, or maintain your current weight by eating a healthier diet?

The next step is to identify ways to help you make slow, steady progress toward your goals. Each person will have a different plan. When losing weight, some people prefer to increase their physical activity to burn up extra calories. Others would rather eat less to decrease the number of calories they consume, though the best approach is a combination of the two. Still others may need to learn to recognize their body's hunger signals and how to limit eating to only those times when they are truly hungry. A combination of these actions may result in a plan that is just right for you. It helps to be patient with yourself as you try to adopt new habits. Remember that truly successful weight management requires a plan that you can stick to over an extended period of time or, better yet, for a lifetime.

Increase Your Chances of Success

It's important to develop a weight management plan that you can maintain for the rest of your life. If you embark on a program to address your body composition, it is a imperative that you develop your program so that it is eventually self-sustaining.

Weight management is not something you should be redoing every two to three years. The following actions will increase your chances of success in managing your weight.

Have Realistic Expectations

Many people start their weight management program with unrealistic expectations about losing weight. They think that if they just eat less, they will be able to lose weight at a rapid pace—such as five pounds a week or more. Losing five pounds in a week, without increasing activity level, would require consuming 17,500 calories less than your body needs! That's a reduction of about 2,500 calories a day, more than many people normally eat in a day. Cutting too many calories leaves too few calories to carry on normal bodily functions, not to mention the effect it produces on your metabolic set point. Your body's metabolism slows down because it thinks that food is scarce, and it responds by trying to protect its fat stores. Rapid weight loss is unhealthy and makes it difficult to maintain the weight loss. Weight management experts believe that a loss of approximately one to two pounds per week is the most that should be attempted. Thus, if you're thinking about trying a fad diet to lose 10 pounds for some big event next weekend, think again. There is no healthy way to do that. Instead, focus on progressing slowly over a longer period of time.

Be Committed and Be Consistent

Once you have created a healthy weight management plan, the best way to ensure success is to be committed to the plan and consistent in following through with your intentions. Small changes, carried out consistently, can make a big difference. For example, if you have decided to reduce the amount of sweets you eat, simply eliminating 250 calories per day (about the number of calories in a chocolate bar) will result in lowering your caloric intake by about 1,750 calories a week. This is the same as half a pound. Maintained consistently, this one behavior can add up to a loss of more than 25 pounds in a year.

Find a Support Buddy

A positive way to help you stay committed to your weight management plan is to find someone who is willing to support you in your efforts. This might be someone who is trying to lose weight as well, or it might be someone who cares about you and is willing

What's News

A research team from the California Institute of Technology has uncovered some interesting information to explain why some dieters are more successful than others at staying with their weight loss regimen (Hare, Camerer, and Rangel, 2009). They had a group of self-indentified dieters go through a series of photo comparisons of various foods, and measured certain brainwave activity. Their experiment revealed 19 subjects who demonstrated significant dietary self-control. They also identified 18 volunteers who exhibited very little self-control. The results help explain why some people can stick with their goals and some people can't succeed.

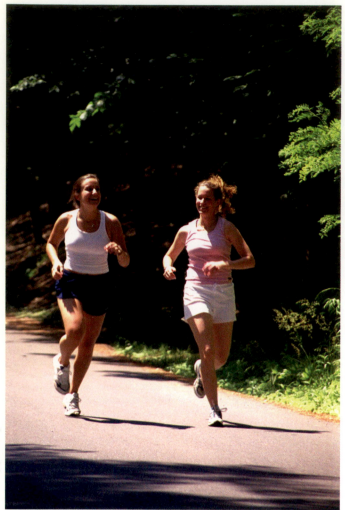

Delmar/Cengage Learning

FIGURE 10-13 • Finding someone who is willing to support your weight management plan is a smart way to keep you motivated and focused on achieving your goals.

to help motivate you to stay on track. Do you have a family member or close friend who could support you? You may want to ask more than one person. Different people may be able to offer different kinds of support. For example, a family member might be willing to cook meals that are healthier and less fattening. Your best friend might encourage you by reminding you of your goals and doing little things to let you know how important you are. Maybe there's a classmate or work colleague who exercises regularly who will agree to work out with you (Figure 10-13). Having several sources of support to keep you focused on your goals can help you avoid the temptation to quit before you see the results.

Do you have friends, work colleagues, or members of your family who would be willing to support you in your weight management efforts? Perhaps they may want to join you. Talk to them about your plans and tell them what you want to accomplish. What kinds of actions would make you feel supported? Make a list of these actions and then ask those you select if they would be willing to do some of those things. Be sure they understand that helping you doesn't mean nagging, trying to make you feel guilty about eating, or making fun of you to make you stick to your plan. You might discover that other people you know are interested in joining your efforts and that you can achieve success together.

Record Your Progress Regularly

Keeping track of your progress in a weight management journal can help keep you motivated and focused on attaining your goals. Recording the times you eat, the foods you eat, and how you are feeling at the time you eat can help you identify your eating patterns and understand what is working and what isn't in your weight management plan. It can also help you stay committed to your goals. Reviewing your journal can also help you see if your plan is helping you achieve your goals. You may discover that something is not working for you and that you need to try something new. It may take some time, but eventually you'll discover a plan that works. Don't be discouraged if you don't lose weight, especially if you are exercising. Remember that exercise may build muscle mass and that muscle tissue weighs more than fat. In addition to using a scale to measure progress, you might also measure your waist or changes in muscle strength.

BUILDING YOUR LIFETIME WELLNESS PLAN

Maintaining a healthy weight is one of the most important things you can do to achieve maximum wellness. This is especially important given the fact that overweight and obesity are risk factors associated with a number of disease conditions, such as heart disease, some cancers, and diabetes. Weight management is also something over which you have personal control, and it is something you can do without spending a lot of money to accomplish your goals. This chapter provided information that you can apply to develop a successful, lifelong weight management plan:

- Determine a healthy weight and appropriate body image for *you*.

- Explore the different personal and/or environmental factors that affect your weight. Learn which ones might be problems for you and steps that you can take to control them.

- Stay informed about why maintaining a healthy weight is important for achieving a high level of wellness. Learn about the diseases and conditions that can be prevented by avoiding excess weight.

- Learn to recognize the signs of eating disorders. Be prepared to help both yourself and others who may suffer from these conditions.

- Create a personal weight management plan that you can live with permanently.

●●● End-of-Chapter Activities

Opportunities for Application

1. Conduct research and compare and contrast the weight range of models and movie stars with average males and females in a similar age-group.

2. Research the various techniques for assessing body composition—height/weight, BMI, hydrostatic weighing, fat calipers, and electrical impedance. Create a table that includes method, scientific basis, advantages, disadvantages, and accuracy.

3. Calculate your BMI using a calculator on the Web or following Figure 10-7 and calculate your waist-to-hip ratio following Figure 10-8. On the basis of these calculations, assess your current body weight.

Key Concepts

1. Describe the current state of overweight and obesity in the United States. List some key factors that have contributed to this situation.

2. Discuss the influence of the media on body image.

3. List and discuss key disadvantages of being overweight or obese in the United States.

4. Describe the differences between anorexia nervosa, bulimia nervosa, binge-eating disorder, and disordered eating.

Answers to Personal Assessment Quiz: Weight Management Quiz

1. False. Studies show that closer to 60 percent of Americans weigh more than what is considered healthy.

2. True

3. False. Removing 500 calories a day from your diet might help an individual lose one pound per week.

4. True

5. True

6. False. Body type/shape, genetics, and body mass greatly influence one's weight, so it is unrealistic and could be potentially unhealthy for all people of the same height to weigh the same amount. There is no exact healthy weight; rather, there is a healthy range.

7. True

8. True

9. False. Only about 5 percent of individuals who lose weight from dieting are able to keep the weight off. Ninety-five percent gain the weight back or gain more weight back.

10. True

●●● References

American Medical Association. (October 2004). *National Summit on Obesity: Executive Summary and Key Recommendations*. Retrieved March 20, 2010 from: http://www.ama-assn.org/ama1/pub/upload/mm/433/exec_sum.pdf

American Psychiatric Association. (1994). *Diagnostic and statistical manual of mental disorders* (4th ed.). Washington, DC: Author.

Blair, S.N., Haskell, W.L., (2006). Objectively measured physical activity and mortality in older adults. *JAMA, 296,* 216–218.

Calorie Control Council. (December 15, 2005). Press release: *Health-Conscious Trends for Weight Loss in 2006: Small Changes Are "In"*. Retrieved March 20, 2010 from: http://www.caloriecontrol.org/pressrelease/health-conscious-trends-for-weight-loss-in-2006-small-changes-are-in

Centers for Disease Control. (2006a). *Overweight and obesity: An overview*. Retrieved from http://www.cdc.gov/nccdphp/dnpa/obesity/contributing_factors.htm

Centers for Disease Control. (2006b). State-specific prevalence of obesity among adults—United States, 2005. *Morbidity and Mortality Weekly Report, 55*(36).

Hare, T.A., Camerer, C.F., Rangel, A. (2009). Self-control in decision-making involves modulation of the vmPFC valuation system. *Science, 324*(5927), 646–648.

National Center for Health Statistics. (2004). *National Health and Nutrition Examination Survey, 2002–2004*. Retrieved March 15, 2010 from: http://www.cdc.gov/nchs/nhanes/nhanes2003–2004/nhanes03_04.htm

National Eating Disorders Association. (2005a). *Ten Steps to a Positive Body Image*. Retrieved March 18, 2010 from: http://www.nationaleatingdisorders.org/nedaDir/files/documents/handouts/TenSteps.pdf

National Eating Disorders Association. (2005b). *Enhancing Male Body Image*. Retrieved March 18, 2010 from: http://www.nationaleatingdisorders.org/nedaDir/files/documents/handouts/MalesEnh.pdf

Potti, S., Milli, M., Jeronis, S., Gaughan, J.P., & Rose, M. (2009). Self-perceptions of body size in women at an inner-city family-planning clinic. *American Journal of Obstetrics and Gynecology, 200*(5), e65–e66.

Schulze, M., Manson, J., Ludwig, D., Colditz, G., Stampfer, M., Willett, W., et al. (2004). Sugar-sweetened beverages, weight gain, and incidence of type 2 diabetes in young and middle-aged women. *Journal of the American Medical Association 292*(8), 927–934.

U.S. Department of Health and Human Services. (2001). *The surgeon general's call to action to prevent and decrease overweight and obesity*. Rockville, MD: Author.

U.S. Department of Health and Human Services. (2010). *The Surgeon General's Vision for a Healthy and Fit Nation*. Rockville, MD: U.S. Department of Health and Human Services, Office of the Surgeon General. Retrieved March 16, 2010 from: http://www.surgeongeneral.gov/library/obesityvision/obesityvision2010.pdf

CHAPTER 11

Tobacco

CHAPTER OBJECTIVES

When you finish this chapter, you should be able to:

- Describe the structure and function of the respiratory system.
- Describe the structures and functions of the circulatory system.
- Explain how tobacco products harm the body.
- List and describe the diseases associated with tobacco use.

- Explain why it is hard for people who smoke to quit.
- List ways you can help someone quit smoking.
- Explain why there is no such thing as a safe cigarette.

KEY TERMS

acute bronchitis
alkaloid
alveoli
bronchi
bronchiectasis
bronchioles

cilia
dose related
emphysema
environmental
    tobacco
    smoke

exhaled mainstream
    smoke
hemoglobin
leukoplakia
mainstream smoke
periodontal tissue

sidestream smoke
smokeless tobacco
trachea

●●● Introduction

Everyone knows cigarette smoking is harmful to one's health, but people may not realize that according to medical research, tobacco use is also *the number one* most preventable cause of illness and death in the United States. The impact of tobacco use on the morbidity and mortality costs to society is staggering. More than $75.5 billion of the total U.S. health care costs each year are attributable directly to tobacco use. In addition to health care costs, the costs of smoking-related fires, health care for low-birth-weight babies, and lost productivity due to smoking effects are estimated at $92 billion per year, bringing a conservative estimate of the economic burden of smoking to more than $167 billion per year.

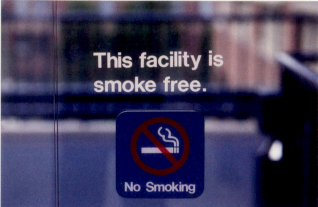

Courtesy of Photodisc

FIGURE 11-1 • The use of tobacco products is the number one most preventable cause of disease and death in the United States. Choosing to abstain from the use of tobacco products will have a significantly positive impact on your health and wellness.

If you have chosen not to use tobacco products, you have made a decision that will help you live a longer and more productive life (Figure 11-1). Making a decision to be tobacco free at any point of your life is a good wellness decision. In fact, medical evidence indicates that there is increased life expectancy for all the time a person is tobacco free—even if he or she chooses to quit smoking after many years of smoking behavior. For example, one year after quitting, the excess rate of heart disease is reduced by half. After 15 years of abstinence, the risk for heart disease becomes similar to that of people who have never smoked.

This chapter contains information to help reinforce your motives not to use tobacco. If you have thought about starting to smoke, the information and activities presented in this chapter will help you strengthen your commitment to wellness by not smoking. If you are a tobacco user, it is hoped that the information will motivate you to do all you can to become tobacco free.

PERSONAL ASSESSMENT
Smoking Quiz

Indicate which of the items you think are true and which of the items you believe are false. You can check your answers against the correct answers at the end of the chapter.

1. More than 5 million smokers age 18 years or younger who are currently alive will die from smoking-related diseases.

2. The younger a person is when he or she starts smoking, the greater the risk of lung cancer.

3. Cigarette smoking kills more people each year than automobile crashes, drug use, and HIV infections.

4. Nicotine is the only psychoactive, addictive drug in tobacco smoke.

5. Research indicates that nicotine is addictive in ways similar to those of heroin, cocaine, and alcohol.

6. Smoking raises the level of cholesterol in the blood.

7. Studies have shown that early signs of the blood vessel damage that could cause heart attack or stroke can be found in young adults who smoke.

8. Smokers suffer from shortness of breath almost three times as much as teens who do not smoke.

9. Cigarette smoking has a negative effect on sexual and reproductive health.

10. Smoking increases one's risk of developing osteoporosis.

⬤⬤⬤ The Respiratory System

The respiratory system is directly affected by tobacco smoke because most smokers inhale smoke directly into the lungs. It makes sense, then, that much of the harm inflicted by cigarette smoke occurs in the mouth, throat, and lungs. Before you learn how smoking tobacco harms the respiratory system, it may be helpful to review the parts of the respiratory system and how breathing occurs. Refer to Figure 11-2 as you read about this important body system.

The **trachea** is the main airway that extends from the throat to the lungs. The trachea is made of **cartilage**, a firm material that keeps the airway open for the passage of air from outside the body. The trachea branches off into two main sections that enter into each lung. These branches are known as **bronchi**. As the bronchi enter the lungs, they divide into smaller and smaller branches. The smallest of these branches are known as **bronchioles**, and at the end of the smallest bronchioles are the **alveoli**. The alveoli have the appearance of microscopic grape clusters. Like tiny balloons, they fill with air when we inhale. The bronchioles consist of thin layers of tissue that are wrapped with **capillaries**, and it is here that oxygen and carbon dioxide are exchanged in the lungs.

Breathing

The purpose of breathing, also called **respiration**, is to allow air to enter the lungs so that blood circulating in the capillaries of the alveoli can give up carbon dioxide and pick up oxygen for transport to the body tissues. Breathing is controlled by special

trachea
the airway that extends from the throat to the lungs

cartilage
a firm but elastic material that keeps the trachea open for the passage of air

bronchi
the branches of the airway that enter the lungs

bronchioles
the very ends of the bronchial tree

alveoli
structures at the ends of the bronchioles that inflate with air when we breathe

capillaries
the smallest of blood vessels, where oxygen and nutrients are exchanged for carbon dioxide and waste at the cell level

respiration
the exchange of oxygen and carbon dioxide in the lungs

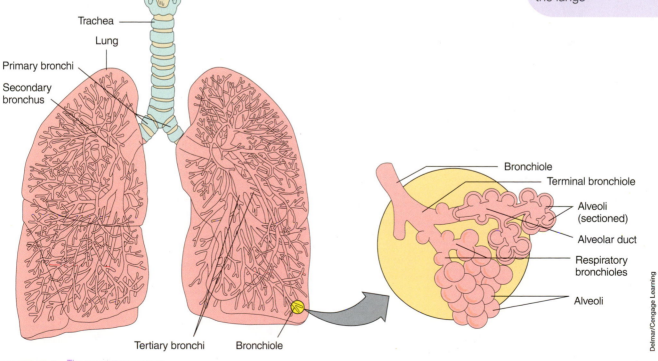

FIGURE 11-2 • The respiratory system.

Delmar/Cengage Learning

nerve centers in the brain stem regulating the rate and depth of breathing according to needs of the body. The physical act of breathing is related to the action of the **diaphragm**, a large muscle that sits just above the abdomen at the base of the chest (Figure 11-3). Although breathing seems automatic and continuous to most of us, it is a complex process that is controlled by a detection system in the nervous system. When the amount of carbon dioxide reaches a certain level in the bloodstream, the nervous system triggers the breathing mechanism. This starts with the diaphragm lowering toward the stomach as it contracts. This movement increases the volume in the chest cavity, and, as the volume increases, the pressure in the lungs decreases, creating a situation in which the air pressure inside the lungs is lower than the air pressure outside the body. This difference in pressure causes air to rush into the lungs. If the airways are clear, the air travels all the way to the alveoli, which then expand. When oxygen in the air gets to the alveoli, oxygen crosses the alveolar membrane and binds with hemoglobin in the red blood cells; simultaneously, carbon dioxide is given up by the bloodstream into the lungs. When the diaphragm relaxes, the volume in the chest cavity decreases, and air is forced out of the lungs.

The *respiration rate* is determined by the number of breaths taken per minute. The approximate respiration rate for adults is between 12 and

diaphragm
a muscle just above the abdomen that supports breathing

Did You Know...?

If you were to take all the alveoli out of your lungs, slice them in half, and lay them out flat, they would cover the area of a tennis court.

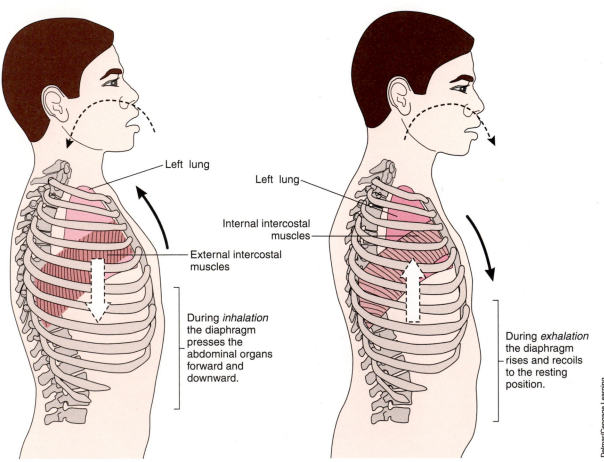

Left lung

External intercostal muscles

During *inhalation* the diaphragm presses the abdominal organs forward and downward.

Left lung

Internal intercostal muscles

During *exhalation* the diaphragm rises and recoils to the resting position.

Delmar/Cengage Learning

FIGURE 11-3 • The process of respiration.

20 breaths per minute. The variability arises from differences in gender and physical condition. The respiratory rate for infants and children is higher. Respiration rates increase with exercise, fever, illness, and other medical conditions. The increased respiration rate occurs because the oxygen demand of the body increases. Respiration rates at rest may be lower among well-trained athletes or those people who practice yoga.

Respiratory Defenses

Have you ever noticed how many tiny particles are floating in the air? They are easy to see when a stream of natural light enters through a window. The air we breathe contains a variety of particles, organisms, and chemicals that are continually inhaled into the lungs. The body has amazing defense mechanisms that work together to prevent germs and chemicals from harming the lungs and airways. For example, the hairs in the nose filter particles in the air and prevent them from going into the airway. Any foreign particles that get into the airway are removed by specialized cells called **cilia** that line the trachea. Cilia are microscopic cells that contain minute hairlike extensions that sweep dust, chemical residue, and mucus up from the airways to the throat. When the material is moved to the base of the throat, it triggers a reflex that clears the throat or creates a cough to allow the material to be removed from the airway. When we get throat or airway infections, our bodies produce more mucus to capture infectious materials so that they can be removed from the body before reaching the lungs.

> **cilia**
> microscopic hairlike projections on certain cells that line the airways and sweep mucus and debris up the airway to the throat

Tobacco

Tobacco is a tall leafy plant that is grown throughout the world. One species, *Nicotiana tabacum*, known as common tobacco, is the main source of commercial tobacco used in producing cigarettes and smokeless tobacco in the United States. Most species of tobacco are believed to be native to the Western Hemisphere. The product is native to South America, Mexico, and the West Indies but is also farmed commercially in this country. Tobacco is grown, harvested, and cured by the farmers who grow it, and it is handled in a manner that produces the unique qualities of the tobacco required by the commercial manufacturer. Tobacco is usually cured in one of two ways. Tobacco that is air cured ends up as chewing tobacco or snuff; fire-cured tobacco is very dry and is used to manufacture cigarettes. After tobacco is cured, the grower keeps it in storage for up to three years, depending on the type of tobacco. Once it is ready for sale, the tobacco is graded according to specific characteristics.

Tobacco naturally contains many of the chemicals that produce the effects on the body as the tobacco product is used; however, there are some chemicals and carcinogens that are formed when the tobacco is cured or burned when it is smoked. The effects of tobacco use are similar regardless of whether the tobacco is smoked, snorted, or placed in the mouth as chewing tobacco or snuff. This means that there is no safe way to use tobacco. The product is addictive, poisonous, and cancer producing.

Why People Smoke

Approximately 21 percent of Americans over age 18 were smokers in 2006 (Figure 11-4). Anglos are more likely to be smokers than any other racial group, followed by African Americans and Hispanics, respectively. Males are more likely to be smokers than females.

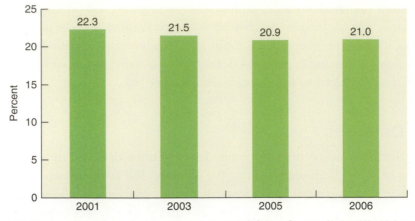

FIGURE 11-4 • Percentage of adult smokers in the United States. Courtesy National Health Interview Survey (2008)

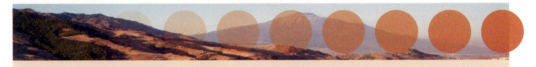

What's Your View?

Why do you think people start to smoke and continue to smoke? After all, just about everyone knows that smoking is a harmful, expensive habit. These facts make it hard to imagine why anyone would want to smoke in the first place. There are actually many reasons why people use tobacco products, and the reasons can be complex. Try answering the following two questions using only a few words:

1. Why do young people start smoking?

2. Why do adults smoke?

Typical answers to the first question include "to be cool," "because my friends smoke," "because I'll appear older," and "because I want to." Teens are *not* likely to include "for good health" or "because I'm addicted" as reasons to start smoking. On the other hand, common answers to the second question include "it's a habit," "I'm addicted," "to control my weight," "I can't stop," or "to calm my nerves." Why do young people and adults have different reasons for smoking? Why don't adults smoke to be cool? The answers lie in the needs that are satisfied by smoking. Youth want to be recognized and are concerned about how they are viewed among their peers. Some use smoking as a way to satisfy a need for recognition. Older adults are more confident in their image, but they find themselves smoking because they are addicted.

Although the overall percentage of smokers represents a 4 percent decline since 1997, the number of people who continue to smoke and those who take up the habit represent a major health concern.

Statistics show that 90 percent of all smokers begin smoking before age 19. Soon after they start, the addictive nature of tobacco takes over and becomes the main reason for smoking. Tobacco contains a highly addictive chemical called **nicotine**. The addictive nature of tobacco is what makes cigarette smoking a high-risk behavior. Young adults who think they can smoke now and quit later are likely to regret their decision to start smoking because they find themselves as older adults with an expensive, unhealthy habit that is difficult to give up.

Nicotine

Nicotine is the ingredient in cigarettes that gives the user the "feel-good" feeling that comes from cigarette smoking, but it is also a toxic poison. Sixty milligrams of nicotine, about the amount found in three or four cigarettes, entering the bloodstream at the same time, would be enough to kill an adult. Nicotine is a liquid **alkaloid** and is in the class of compounds that also include caffeine. Each cigarette smoked yields about one milligram of nicotine into the bloodstream. The nicotine is readily absorbed through the tissues in the mouth, throat, and alveoli. The nicotine circulates in the bloodstream and almost immediately goes to the brain. In addition to providing the euphoric effect, it is also responsible for the withdrawal characteristics that occur when nicotine administration is shut off. Evidence indicates that some people who smoke have a greater genetic predisposition to nicotine addiction than other tobacco users.

Nicotine's effect on the body goes beyond the euphoric feeling that comes from smoking tobacco. Nicotine causes an elevation of cholesterol levels in the blood, increasing the likelihood of heart attack or stroke. There are other chemicals in cigarette smoke that cause additional health effects, such as cancer and emphysema (to be discussed in chapter 14). The greatest health threat resulting from nicotine exposure is drug addiction. When a tobacco user is exposed to nicotine for a period of time, addiction occurs as the body adjusts to the effects of nicotine. Over time, the body's nervous system requires more nicotine to achieve the "drug effect." The nicotine in cigarette smoke is an addicting drug, and the addictive effects of the drug are **dose related**. Simply stated, the more tobacco smoke consumed, the greater the exposure to nicotine and the higher the level of addiction. This addiction can become a difficult barrier to the smoker's desire and ability to quit smoking. When the body is deprived of nicotine, a nervous system response to the absence of nicotine causes a considerable amount of discomfort that can be relieved only with nicotine administration. This explains why many people have a hard time quitting tobacco use.

nicotine
an addictive chemical stimulant found in tobacco

alkaloid
an organic compound containing carbon, hydrogen, and nitrogen

Did You Know…?

Nicotine is the most widely used addictive drug in the United States. It is consumed by more than 60 million people who use tobacco products.

dose related
drug effects increase as the frequency and quantity of a drug increases

What's News

In 2007, some Harvard researchers concluded that the amount of nicotine that smokers typically inhale per cigarette rose 11 percent from 1998 to 2005. The findings were derived from information submitted to the Massachusetts Department of Public Health by major cigarette manufacturers and analyzed by the Harvard research team (Connolly, et al., 2007). The amount of nicotine in tobacco increased an average of 1.6 percent per year regardless of brand.

●●● Effects of Tobacco Smoke

The first time a person tries to smoke a cigarette, he or she is likely to cough heavily because the body is trying to eliminate the irritating foreign substances that are entering the airway and lungs. In fact, smokers have to train and discipline themselves to tolerate smoke in the throat and lungs. If beginning smokers paid attention their body's reaction to the cigarette smoke and quit smoking before they got addicted, they could prevent many health problems.

Without question, the greatest threat to the human respiratory system is cigarette smoke. This smoke is not simply gray air but rather a vapor that contains more than 4,000 known chemical substances, 60 of which are known to cause cancer. Particulate matter (solid and liquid) makes up about 21 percent of the smoke, and gases make up the rest. Some of these substances are poisonous or otherwise harmful to the cells in the mouth, airway, and lungs. Other substances in smoke are addictive or cause birth defects and cancer. Some of the known substances in cigarette smoke are presented in Table 11-1.

As the smoke is inhaled, the chemicals are deposited on the tissues of the mouth, throat, and airways. Over time, the constant assault of these chemicals harms these tissues. Because the damage caused by cigarette smoking is dose related, the earlier a person begins smoking, the more cigarettes smoked, and the deeper the smoke is inhaled, the greater the harmful effects will be.

TABLE 11-1 • Selected chemicals in cigarette smoke.

Chemical	Uses	Health Effect
1-aminonaphalene	Weed control	Causes cancer
Acetaldehyde	Glues and resins	Increases the absorption of other hazardous chemicals into the lungs
Acetone	Used in solvents	Irritates the throat, nose, and eyes; long-term exposure can cause liver and kidney damage
Benzene	Solvents, pesticides, and gasoline	Causes leukemia and other cancers
Chromium	Metal plating, wood treatments, and preservatives	Causes lung cancer
Formaldehyde	Manufacture of particleboard; used as a lab preservative	Causes nasal cancer; damages lungs, skin, and digestive system
Hydroquinone	Paints, varnishes, and motor fuel	Eye damage, skin irritation, and central nervous system effects
Lead	Metal alloys (once used in paint)	Damages brain, nervous tissue, and reproductive system
Isoprene	Rubber manufacturing	Suspected carcinogen; causes irritation of the skin, eyes, and respiratory system
Nicotine	Highly controlled insecticide	Causes growth retardation, depresses the central nervous system, and is toxic to fetuses
Tolune	Solvents, oils, and resins	Causes fatigue, confusion, and memory loss; linked to permanent brain damage

Harm to the Respiratory System

Because tobacco smoke is inhaled through the mouth and makes its way to the lungs, it stands to reason that the primary effects of smoking are on the structures of the respiratory system. Some of the effects, such as bronchitis, can occur within a relatively short period of time; other conditions, such as lung cancer, appear after many years of smoking. All things considered, the harm to the respiratory system occurs in a fairly well defined pattern as described in the following sections. Keep in mind that hot cigarette smoke enters a body that has a lower temperature than the smoke; thus, smoke will cling to the cooler body tissues. It is a fact that smokers exhale less smoke than they inhale. The deeper a smoker inhales, the more tissue surface there is for the smoke to cling to. Some smokers hold their breath when they inhale smoke into their lungs to in order to get a better "dosage" of tobacco's stimulating drug effect.

Bronchitis

Bronchitis is a condition in which the airways of the lungs (bronchi) become inflamed. Inflammation can come from a variety of sources, such as infection, asthma, fumes, and so on. **Acute bronchitis** generally results from an infection caused by a virus or bacteria. Acute bronchitis is characterized by chest pain, persistent productive cough, and fever. It lasts for a defined period of time and can be treated with antibiotics and rest. The condition can become **chronic bronchitis**, meaning that it persists for a long time. Chronic bronchitis is caused by long-term exposure to chemicals, pollution, and/or tobacco smoke. Chronic bronchitis is characterized by heavy coughing and production of excess mucus. Have you ever heard the term *smoker's cough*? This is a cough that often occurs in the morning and is characteristic of chronic bronchitis. The smoker has accumulated smoke residue and mucus in the lungs while sleeping. The early cough is needed to purge the accumulated material. Chronic bronchitis does not respond well to antibiotic treatment and paves the way for other, more serious medical conditions.

bronchitis
Inflammation of the major airways in the lungs (bronchi)

acute bronchitis
inflammation of the bronchi (airways) by microorganisms

chronic bronchitis
bronchitis characterized by a productive cough that continues for at least three months

Bronchiectasis

The constant irritation from chronic bronchitis can lead to a condition known as **bronchiectasis**, in which the airways become scarred, swollen, and filled with mucus. Chronic bronchitis is the body's effort to remove the chemicals and residue of the tobacco smoke from the lungs. The smallest airways get swollen and damaged by the constant pressure of the coughing and the inability of the lungs to easily expel the chemicals and residue. The result is that even though the smoker can inhale air as the chest cavity expands, exhaling is difficult because the airways close quickly, trapping air and chemical irritants in the alveoli. The chemicals eventually create a destructive effect on the air sacs, paving the way for emphysema.

bronchiectasis
a condition in which the airways of the lungs become scarred, swollen, and filled with mucus

Emphysema

Bronchiectasis can lead to **emphysema**, a word that comes from the Greek word *emphysan*, meaning "to inflate." The irritants and air trapped as a result of bronchiectasis cause the tiny alveoli to overinflate. The increased pressure due to overinflation and trapped chemicals from the smoke eventually cause the alveoli to tear. Once they are torn, the alveoli cannot be

emphysema
a condition in which the alveoli tear because of overinflation

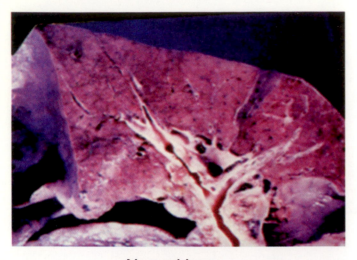

Normal lung

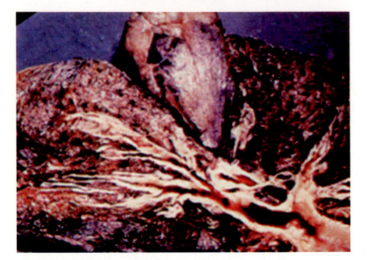

Emphysema

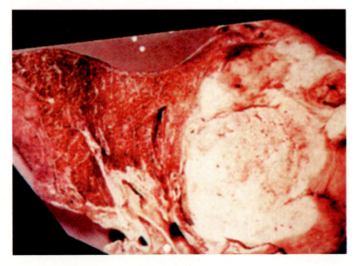

Cancer

repaired and no longer function properly in the exchange of oxygen and carbon dioxide. This condition, known as emphysema, is almost exclusively a smoker's disease. If the individual with emphysema continues to smoke, the alveoli will continue to tear, eventually causing death when the lungs can no longer transfer the needed oxygen into the body. Interestingly, the person with emphysema has no trouble inhaling, but he or she experiences a great deal of difficulty completely *exhaling*. When the individual with this condition loses a significant amount of lung functioning, he or she must be permanently fixed to an oxygen source. Figure 11-5 shows photographs of both a normal lung and a lung with emphysema. Note the blackness from the cigarette smoke and the lack of tissue density in the emphysema lung.

Lung Cancer

The tar in cigarette smoke is actually the solid matter in the smoke that contains about 63 chemical substances known to cause cancer. Tar is what gives smoke its gray color and what makes tobacco a **carcinogen**, a cancer-causing substance. Five cigarettes contain about half a teaspoon of tar. It is a sticky, brown smelly liquid that clings to hair, skin, clothes, and the tissues of the airways. The manner in which tobacco smoke contributes to lung cancer has been well known for many years. With years of smoking, the smoke entering the lungs delivers so much tar that the cilia in the airways become paralyzed and can no longer sweep out the smoke materials, chemicals, and mucus. Without the help of cilia, the chemicals, especially tar, remain trapped on the lung tissue and cause alterations in the genetic makeup of lung cells to the point that they become cancerous. Figure 11-6 shows a picture of a cancerous lung. The white tissue on the right side of the photo is the cancer.

Needless to say, lung cancer is a very serious condition and is closely linked to cigarette smoking. Research indicates there is a 20-year time lag that exists between smoking initiation and the occurrence of lung cancer. Notice in the cancerous lung in Figure 11-6 that the cancer formed deep in the lung tissue. Because the cancer develops deep in the lungs, by the time the smoker notices any symptoms, the cancer is likely to have spread to other parts of the body. For this reason, most lung cancer patients do not survive the disease. Data indicate that 90 percent of all lung cancer patients were smokers. If the patient is fortunate to get his or her condition diagnosed early enough, the best treatment is surgery,

What's News

According to the National Center for Health Statistics, since 1998, lung cancer has been the number one cause of cancer death among women. In fact, the lung cancer death rates for women steadily increased since 1950, when such cancer statistics were first reported. As more and more women took up smoking, the lung cancer death rate for women has risen from approximately 5 per 100,000 women in 1950 to 40 per 100,000 in 2006, the most recent year for which statistics are available. Beginning in 2005, however, the lung cancer death rates have dropped slightly. An interesting fact about female lung cancer is that the incidence of this type of cancer is highest among white women. Currently, the percentage of the population smoking cigarettes is getting lower. Perhaps this will be a contributing factor as the lung cancer rates continue to drop.

but the chances for survival are not good. Only 16 percent of lung cancer cases are diagnosed in this early stage, and even then only 50 percent of those patients will survive. Despite the medical advances over the past 40 years, the five-year survival rate for lung cancer patients has climbed from 10 to 15 percent.

carcinogen
a substance that causes cancer

Effect of Smoking on the Circulatory System

The circulatory system contains a four-chambered heart that pumps the nearly six quarts of blood around the body (Figure 11-7). Arteries are the largest of the blood vessels and carry blood from the heart. The arteries branch off, becoming smaller and smaller to eventually become capillaries, blood vessels so small that red blood cells may have to pass through the capillaries in single file. It is through the walls of the capillaries that the exchange of oxygen and carbon dioxide takes place. Veins carry blood back to the heart. Circulation actually has three distinct components. *Systemic circulation* is the movement of blood around the body. *Pulmonary circulation* is movement of the blood to and from the lungs, where oxygen and carbon dioxide are exchanged. *Coronary circulation* is the circulation of blood within the heart muscle, not the circulation of blood through the chambers.

The chemicals from tobacco smoke enter the circulatory system through the alveoli into the pulmonary capillaries. Among these chemicals is nicotine. Because nicotine is a stimulant drug, its effect on the body occurs after the chemical is absorbed into the pulmonary capillaries or, in the case of smokeless tobacco, into the capillaries through the mucous membranes of the mouth. Other chemicals in smoke cause the body's capillaries to constrict (get smaller). The combination of rapid heartbeat and narrowed blood vessels produces high blood pressure because the heart has to pump harder to move the blood through smaller blood vessels. Chemicals in cigarette smoke also cause a change in the blood chemistry. The red blood cells become "sticky," and the blood cholesterol rises, increasing the likelihood of fatty deposits on the walls of the blood vessels. Combined, all these conditions increase the risk of heart attack and stroke. This situation is dose related—more cigarettes mean more adverse conditions. A smoker faces three times the risk of having a heart attack than a nonsmoker.

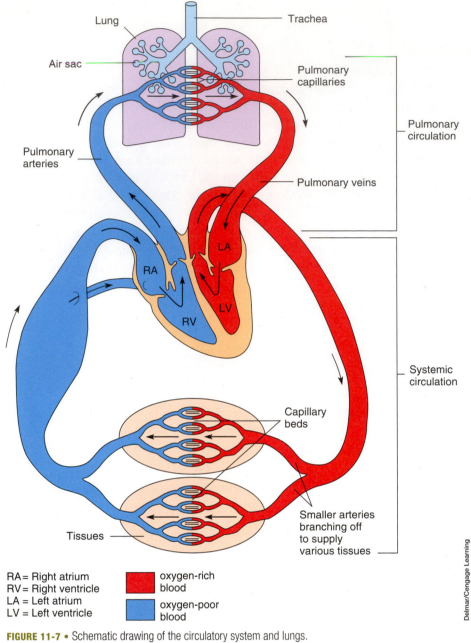

Lung

Trachea

Air sac

Pulmonary
capillaries

Pulmonary
circulation

Pulmonary
arteries

Pulmonary veins

LA

RA

LV

RV

Systemic
circulation

Capillary
beds

Smaller arteries
branching off
to supply
various tissues

Tissues

RA= Right atrium
RV= Right ventricle
LA = Left atrium
LV = Left ventricle

oxygen-rich
blood

oxygen-poor
blood

Delmar/Cengage Learning

FIGURE 11-7 • Schematic drawing of the circulatory system and lungs.

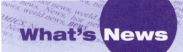

What's News

Research indicates that smoking increases a woman's risk of heart disease
more so than a man's. In one study, smoking increased a woman's risk of
having a heart attack 57 percent more than a man's. In general, women—
especially younger women—have a lower risk of heart disease than men of
similar age. Smoking seems to cancel out this natural protection.

Cigarette smoke contains **carbon monoxide**, a colorless, odorless gas that enters the bloodstream through the lungs. This poisonous gas is also a major ingredient of automobile exhaust. If enough carbon monoxide enters the bloodstream, it can cause death because it interferes with the blood's ability to transport oxygen to the body's cells. When red blood cells pass through the capillaries in the alveoli, **hemoglobin** in the red blood cells normally acts as an oxygen magnet, picking it up and carrying it throughout the body. But if both carbon monoxide and oxygen molecules are present, hemoglobin is more likely to attract the carbon monoxide. Smokers are unable to transport a full load of oxygen because so much of their hemoglobin is tied up with carbon monoxide. This process helps explain why smokers get winded so quickly and tire more easily than nonsmokers.

carbon monoxide
a colorless, odorless, poisonous gas

hemoglobin
an iron-rich compound in the red blood cell that carries oxygen

Effects on Appearance

Most people are concerned about their appearance. They keep themselves well groomed, use beauty and bath products, and spend money on cosmetic dentistry, plastic surgery, and the latest clothing styles. Unfortunately, cigarette smoking can quickly negate some of these behaviors by affecting one's appearance in negative ways. Research indicates that nonsmokers tend to perceive smokers as unattractive because of tobacco's effect on a personal appearance. Tobacco smoke will affect the following:

- *Breath*. Cigarette smoke dries out the mucous membranes of the mouth and throat. This drying encourages the growth of bacteria that cause odors. Smoke also clings to the mouth and airways and causes smelly tobacco breath. Mint-flavored gum does not mask it well, especially if the person has smoked for a long time; menthol-flavored cigarettes don't help either.

- *Hair and clothes*. Smoke clings to most anything it comes in contact with—hair, skin, clothes, furniture, car, and anything else in the environment. There is a reason for this. Cigarette smoke has a positive chemical charge, whereas items in the environment have negative charges. The two charges create an attraction, and the smoke clings long after the smoker has put out a cigarette.

- *Teeth*. Smoking eventually damages tooth enamel, and the chemicals in tobacco smoke contribute to gum disease. The gums are more prone to accumulate plaque and bacteria, leading to periodontal disease. This condition not only contributes to foul breath odor but also can eventually result in tooth loss and possibly heart disease (as you will see in chapter 14).

- *Skin*. Young people who smoke cigarettes may not notice the wrinkle effects until they get older, but studies show that cigarette smokers have more wrinkles in their skin than nonsmokers. The skin ages because nicotine prevents a good blood flow to the skin cells. The skin of nonsmokers stays younger longer (Figure 11-8).

WEB LINK
Women and Smoking
http://www.cdc.gov/tobacco/index.htm

At this Web site, click on "Surgeon General's Reports." From there, you can go to the 2001 report on women and smoking.

SEARCH TERMS: smoking and women, women and tobacco.

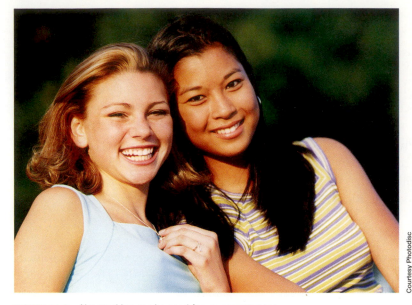

Courtesy Photodisc

FIGURE 11-8 • Not smoking can be good for your appearance.

Smoking's Effect on Others

Tobacco smoking has been taking place for centuries. It wasn't until the 1964 *Surgeon General's Report on Smoking* that the medically harmful effects of smoking were illuminated. Since then, medical and social research has confirmed tobacco smoke's harmful effects. There is little doubt that cigarette smoking harms the smoker. Evidence is accumulating now that cigarette smoking also is harmful to the environment, to nonsmoking individuals who spend time around smokers, and to developing fetuses.

Environmental Tobacco Smoke

Did you know that it's possible to have your health negatively affected by smoke even if you never light a cigarette yourself? Medical data indicate that both exhaled smoke and smoke from the burning end of a cigarette are harmful to the health of nonsmokers who are in the area. When smokers take a drag on a cigarette, they inhale **mainstream smoke**. Mainstream smoke is filtered by the tobacco and the filter on the cigarette. Once exhaled, it is called **exhaled mainstream smoke** and contributes to **environmental tobacco smoke**. Commonly referred to as secondhand smoke, environmental tobacco smoke is inhaled by anyone who is near a smoker or in a smoky environment. The smoke that comes from the burning end of a cigarette between puffs or from a cigarette sitting in an ashtray is known as **sidestream smoke**. Other sources of harm are the contaminants that diffuse through cigarette paper into the environment and contribute to the chemical composition of secondhand smoke.

Environmental tobacco smoke (ETS) contributes to a variety of ear, nose, and throat infections among nonsmokers. Children exposed to ETS have higher rates of bronchitis and asthma than do children not exposed to ETS. More important, ETS ranks third as a major preventable cause of death. Only direct smoking and alcohol abuse rank higher as preventable causes of death. It is estimated that ETS is responsible for approximately 3,000 lung cancer deaths among nonsmokers each year. In June 2002, a group of scientists in the World

mainstream smoke
smoke that comes directly to the smoker from the cigarette

exhaled mainstream smoke
smoke that is exhaled by the smoker

environmental tobacco smoke
smoke that people breathe when they are in a smoky environment; also called secondhand smoke

sidestream smoke
smoke that comes from the burning end of a cigarette

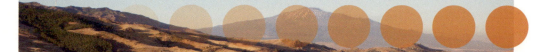

What's Your View?

Nonsmoking Laws

Clean-indoor-air laws and policies that restrict smoking to designated areas have been enacted in 49 states and the District of Columbia. These laws vary from restricting smoking to certain sections of restaurants and civic buildings to banning smoking in all public places, such as government buildings, schools, elevators, and retail stores. The purpose of the laws is to protect nonsmokers from the harmful effects of secondhand smoke. Some people think that such laws take away from the freedom of smokers. How do you feel about this kind of restriction? Should smokers be forced to give up something they want to do so that nonsmokers can have a smoke-free environment?

What's News

The U.S. Department of Health and Human Services (2006), in *Health Consequences of Involuntary Exposure to Tobacco Smoke*, cites research indicating that there is no safe level of exposure to secondhand tobacco smoke.

Health Organization reviewed 50 research studies and concluded that secondhand smoke is linked to cancer. Information on the harmful effects of ETS has prompted many local and state governments to pass laws to ensure smoke-free environments for nonsmokers.

Women and Smoking

Each year, lung cancer kills about 70,000 women in the United States. Lung cancer, once rare among women, has long since surpassed breast cancer as the leading cause of female cancer death in the United States, now accounting for 25 percent of all cancer deaths among women. Surveys have indicated that many women do not know this fact. Moreover, lung cancer is only one of numerous serious disease risks faced by women who smoke. Figure 11-9 summarizes some of the findings presented in the *Report on Smoking and Women* (National Center for Chronic Disease Prevention and Health Promotion, 2001).

Smoking during Pregnancy

Smoking during pregnancy is not a good idea. In fact, smoking harms every phase of reproduction. Studies show that smoking has a negative effect on male sperm production, but males manufacture so many sperm that it does not have a major effect on a man's ability to contribute to conception. Studies reveal that female smokers have more

1. Lung cancer is now the leading cause of cancer death among U.S. women; it surpassed breast cancer in 1987.
2. Smoking during pregnancy remains a major public health problem despite increased knowledge of the adverse health effects of smoking during pregnancy.
3. Cigarette smoking plays a major role in the mortality of U.S. women.
4. About 90 percent of all lung cancer deaths among U.S. women smokers are attributable to smoking.
5. The totality of the evidence does not support an association between smoking and risk for breast cancer.
6. Smoking is a major cause of coronary heart disease among women. For women younger than 50 years, the majority of coronary heart disease is attributable to smoking.
7. Women who smoke have increased risks for conception delay.
8. The risk for perinatal mortality—both stillbirth and neonatal deaths—and the risk for sudden infant death syndrome are increased among the offspring of women who smoke during pregnancy.
9. Postmenopausal women who currently smoke have lower bone density than do women who do not smoke.
10. Limited but consistent data suggest that women smokers have more facial wrinkling than do nonsmokers.

Delmar/Cengage Learning

FIGURE 11-9 • The effects of smoking on women.

difficulty becoming pregnant and have a higher risk of never becoming pregnant. Women who smoke during pregnancy have a greater chance of complications with pregnancy, premature birth, low-birth-weight infants, stillbirth, and infant mortality. Remember that cigarette smoke contains thousands of chemicals that enter the bloodstream of the smoker. A woman who smokes during pregnancy will deliver these chemicals through her bloodstream, through the placenta, and into the bloodstream of her fetus. These chemicals can produce harmful effects both before and after birth, such as the following:

1. Smoking women are likely to deliver before their scheduled due date.

2. Fetuses born to smoking mothers are likely to be low-birth-weight babies (those who weigh less than 5.5 pounds at birth). Low-birth-weight babies are at risk of dying before their first birthday.

3. Children born to smoking mothers are at greater risk for birth defects than are children of nonsmokers.

Low birth weight is a leading cause of infant deaths. More than 300,000 infants die each year in the United States. Babies born to smoking women have less muscle mass and are fatter than babies born to nonsmokers. Nicotine causes the blood vessels to constrict in the umbilical cord and womb. This decreases the amount of oxygen to the unborn baby and reduces the amount of blood in the baby's system. These factors can lead to low birth weight. Pregnant smokers eat more than pregnant nonsmokers, yet their babies weigh less. If a woman stops smoking before the third trimester (the last three months), her baby is more likely to be close to normal weight.

Even if a woman does not smoke during her pregnancy, her fetus can still be harmed by the smoking of others. Secondhand smoke is an environmental hazard and can adversely affect fetal development and elevate the risk for low birth weight. In addition to not smoking themselves, pregnant women should avoid exposure to ETS.

Statistically, there is a greater likelihood that children born to mothers who smoked during their pregnancy are more likely to be smokers themselves. Buka, Shenassa, and Niaura (2003) compared the smoking and nonsmoking behaviors of pregnant mothers to the smoking behaviors of their children over a 29-year period. There were 1,248 subjects in the study. Offspring of mothers who smoked up to one pack of cigarettes a day during pregnancy were 20 percent more likely to be tobacco addicted at some time during the study. Children of mothers who smoked a pack a day or more during their pregnancy were 60 percent more likely to become addicted to tobacco. This means that smoking during pregnancy can have behavioral effects on the child over time, and it appears that these effects are dose related and not related to other factors, such as socioeconomic status.

Sudden Infant Death Syndrome

Sudden infant death syndrome (SIDS) involves the sudden, unexplained death of an infant under one year of age. For every 100,000 births, there approximately 50 deaths due to SIDS. Although studies have identified certain risk factors for SIDS, such as putting infants to bed on their stomachs, there has been little understanding of the syndrome's exact biological causes. A 2006 study reported in the *Journal of the American Medical Association* indicated that the condition occurs in babies with abnormal development in part of the brain stem. Exposure to tobacco smoke, before and after birth, appears to be a significant risk factor. Babies exposed to secondhand smoke after birth have double the risk of SIDS. Babies whose mothers smoke before and after birth are three to four times more likely to die from SIDS.

The death rate from SIDS has fallen by more than half since the "Back to Sleep" campaign began in the 1990s. This campaign reminds parents that babies should lie on their backs while sleeping. Research also indicates that babies are less likely to die from SIDS if they are breast fed.

Environmental Damage

Cigarette smoking can do great harm to the environment. Most of this damage results from fires caused by mishandling cigarettes. The tobacco in cigarettes is designed to

What's News

As of July 2011, all 50 states will require the sale of "fire safe" cigarettes. Fire safe cigarettes are manufactured with special paper that have special "speed bumps" built into the paper that extinguish the cigarette if it is not smoked continually. Since cigarette-ignited fires are the major cause of home fire deaths, the new cigarettes have the potential to save up to 900 lives a year.

Did You Know ...?

The worst industrial disaster in U.S. history took place in April 1947 at a ship loading dock in Texas City, Texas. A careless smoker cast a cigarette butt into the hold of a ship fully loaded with ammonium nitrate. The ammonium nitrate exploded, and the explosion damaged 90 percent of the buildings in the nearby city, killed almost 600 people, and hospitalized more than 4,000 people. The cost of the disaster was more than $4 billion.

smolder as it burns, so when a cigarette is carelessly discarded or accidentally dropped into a cushion, it can smolder, unnoticed, until the smoker has left the area. When it does erupt into a blaze, there may be no one available to put it out. Even worse, people may be sleeping in the home and not be able to escape the fire in time. According to the American Cancer Society (2007), more people die from cigarette-caused fires (about three people every day) than from fires started by any other single cause.

Smoking also contributes litter to the environment. Take a look at the areas outside of nonsmoking buildings or at the pavement and gutters near a bus stop. Most likely, they are littered with cigarette butts. Not only is this litter unsightly, but the cellulose filters on the cigarettes present health problems to animals or small children who may eat them.

The Economics of Smoking

Smoking costs money. The costs built into every pack of cigarettes include the cost of manufacturing and distributing the cigarettes, profit for the seller, and taxes paid by the consumer. The federal government imposes a tax of about 40 cents on each pack of cigarettes. Each state has the capacity to collect a tax on each pack of cigarettes according to its own desires. As of January 1, 2006, Rhode Island has the highest tax at $3.46 per pack, New York's tax on a pack of cigarettes was $2.75; Virginia was the lowest at 30 cents per pack. The taxes on cigarettes serve to bring revenues to the state and federal government, but they also have an effect on tobacco use. As taxes go up, cigarette sales drop, and the people who quit smoking or smoke less don't require as much health care and miss fewer days of work. Data show, however, that as tobacco use goes down, state tobacco revenues keep increasing. It is estimated that for every 10-cent increase in cigarette tax, we save $7 on health care and loss of work time because the increase causes many people to quit smoking.

The amount of money spent on tobacco products is huge and results in large profits for the tobacco companies. Americans spend approximately 77 billion dollars on cigarettes. As one example, Philip Morris, a subsidiary of Altria reported a profit on tobacco sales of $5.3 billion in 2009 (Altria, 2010). Did you ever think about what goes on behind the scenes to encourage people to purchase cigarettes? An advertising agency gets paid a lot of money to create advertising campaigns encouraging people to buy certain products or services. Advertising agencies are responsible for virtually all the commercials we see on television. You probably already know there are no commercials for tobacco products. If you don't know why this is, the following example can help put this in perspective.

Imagine that you own an advertising agency, and a customer asks you to develop an advertising program to help sell a product. When you ask the customer to provide information about the product, you learn the following.

- It is taken by mouth but has no nutritional value whatsoever.

- Once it gets into the body, it robs the body of oxygen.

- It is addictive.

- People who use it die sooner than people who don't.

- It kills almost 450,000 people a year.

- The product costs about $12 a pound.

As the owner of the advertising agency, how would you feel about accepting money to promote such a product? Do you think you could create an advertising message to motivate someone to buy this product? Clearly, advertising this product would not be an easy task. It is difficult to "sell" tobacco products using health-promoting messages. What messages have you seen in tobacco ads that try to make tobacco use appealing? Can you understand why many tobacco companies are now trying to increase tobacco sales in underdeveloped countries?

⬤⬤⬤ Low-Tar, Low-Nicotine Cigarettes

There are companies that advertise low-tar and low-nicotine cigarettes. Are these cigarettes safe for the user? The answer is no. It seems as if low-nicotine cigarettes would be less addictive than high-nicotine cigarettes, but they aren't. Research shows that smokers who are addicted require certain levels of nicotine. If regular smokers attempt to switch to low-tar and low-nicotine cigarettes, they end up inhaling more deeply, smoking faster, and consuming more cigarettes than when they smoke regular cigarettes. Moreover, research on cigarette smoking now shows that people who smoke the so-called low-tar cigarettes often inhale the same level of cancer-causing tar as people who smoke regular cigarettes and are just as likely to suffer the negative health effects of smoking as those who smoke regular cigarettes. Even low-tar cigarettes contain tar and other chemicals. If the companies were to eliminate all tar, they would be eliminating the smoke, and then cigarettes would not be pleasing to smokers. The truth is there just isn't any level of tar that is safe.

> **Did You Know ...?**
>
> After decades of research on the effects of tobacco products, it is clear that there is no safe tobacco product. In fact, the intended outcome of tobacco use by its very nature is unhealthy. The use of any tobacco product—including all brands of cigarettes, cigars, pipes, and spit tobaccos; "mentholated," "low tar," "naturally grown," or "additive free"—can cause cancer and other adverse health effects.

⬤⬤⬤ Bidi Cigarettes

Bidis are hand-rolled cigarettes from India that have no filter. They are made with tobacco from the Southeast Asia region. The cigarettes have been used by young people because they are sweetly flavored with strawberry, chocolate, cherry, and mango (because the tobacco from that region is harsh), and they are less expensive than American cigarettes. Bidi cigarettes should not be viewed as a natural substitute for cigarettes that is safe and trendy. Despite their sweet flavor and colorful packaging, bidis represent a greater health risk than American cigarettes.

1. Research on bidis indicates that, ounce for ounce, bidis contain much higher levels of the toxic elements than do American cigarettes.

2. The tobacco in bidis contains 8 percent nicotine (compared with 1 percent in regular cigarettes), making them more addicting and more harmful to the circulatory system.

3. Bidis contain no filter, so the burning product releases three to five times more tar and nicotine than regular cigarettes.

4. The tobacco does not burn well, and the user has to "drag" more strongly to keep the bidi lit. In the process, pieces of tobacco and paper are inhaled into the throat and lungs.

●●● Smoking Cessation

You have already learned that smoking is the most preventable cause of death and disability in the United States today. If you or someone you know is a smoker, this section will provide information that may help with smoking cessation decisions. The Centers for Disease Control and Prevention reported that in 2008, 46 million adults (20.6 percent of the population over age 18) in the United States were current smokers: roughly 23 percent of men and 18 percent of women (Dube, et al., 2009). Approximately 70 percent of these smokers said that they wanted to quit. Recall the exercise earlier in this chapter where you compared the reasons for smoking between teens and adults; teens have psychological reasons for starting to smoke, and adults have an addiction that keeps them doing something they would rather stop. Individual reasons for smoking cessation generally relate to medical concerns. Giving up smoking is not easy. Writer and humorist Mark Twain is attributed with saying, "To cease smoking is the easiest thing I ever did. I ought to know because I've done it a thousand times." Indeed, there are many adults who give up smoking, only to resume it again because the habit is so powerful.

In order for someone to give up smoking, they must begin with a strong motivation to do so. There are motivators that work for everyone. Smokers will come to their decision for their own unique reason. For some people, health is the main reason, while for others, it may be the cost of the cigarettes that drives them to quit. Some people may quit because there are antismoking ordinances that prohibit smoking in the community and/or the workplace, and still others quit because their family members worry about them and encourage them to stop. Depending on the person's level of addiction, he or she will go through a specific sequence of feelings during a withdrawal period (Table 11-2).

Benefits of Quitting

Anyone who takes the time to think about it will conclude that there are far more benefits to quitting than there are for continuing to smoke. Smoking harms nearly every organ in the body. Tobacco products can exacerbate in some way almost any disease condition of the body. It seems every year that the list of diseases confirmed to have a link to cigarette smoking grows. The 2004 *Surgeon General's Report on Smoking and Health* listed abdominal aortic aneurysm, acute myeloid leukemia, cataract, cervical cancer, kidney cancer, pancreatic cancer, pneumonia, periodontitis, and stomach cancer as the latest additions to the list. Aside from

---

WEB LINK

Smoking Cessation

http://www.cancer.org/docroot/home/index.asp?level=0

At this Web site, under the "Find It Fast" link, click on "Guide to Quitting Smoking." You will find a lot of information to help with smoking cessation, including a self-test to help determine the level of smoking addiction and how to approach cessation. You may also want to visit **http://www.quitnet.com**. Quitnet is a large online support program to help you quit.

SEARCH TERMS: smoking cessation, quitting smoking

Did You Know ...?

Twelve hours after quitting, the carbon monoxide level in the ex-smoker's blood returns to normal levels. Five to 15 years after quitting, an ex-smoker's stroke risk is reduced to that of a non-smoker.

TABLE 11-2 • Smoking withdrawal symptoms and remedies.

Symptom	Cause	Duration	Remedy
1. Irritability	Craving for nicotine	Two to four weeks	Walks, hot baths, relaxation techniques (e.g., soft music, stretching)
2. Tired/lack of energy	Absence of the stimulating effect of nicotine	Two to four weeks	Take a nap if you're tired; don't push yourself
3. Trouble sleeping	Altered brain waves and sleep patterns; adjustment to no nicotine	One week	Avoid caffeine (e.g., coffee or sodas), especially in the evening
4. Cough, dry throat, mucus	Your body is getting rid of mucus from your airways	A few days	Drink a lot of water or juice but not soft drinks, as they are high in calories
5. Dizzy feeling	Your body is getting more oxygen	One or two days	Stand up slowly
6. Poor concentration	Your body needs time to get used to being without the constant stimulation (boost) from nicotine	A few weeks	Take relaxation breaks
7. Tightness in chest	Sore muscles from coughing or tense muscles from nicotine cravings	A few weeks	Deep breathing
8. Hunger	You can confuse craving for cigarettes with hunger; your mouth is getting used to having nothing to do	Two to four weeks	Drink water and eat low-calorie snacks: raw vegetables, pretzels, popcorn, fruit
9. Craving a cigarette	Withdrawal from the highly addictive drug nicotine	Cravings occur most often in the first few days and gradually subside; some people may have occasional cravings for months	Hang on—craving will last only a few minutes; try another activity—have a drink of water, take a walk, or call a friend

Source: Adapted from Canadian Lung Association (2009).

the health benefits, there are benefits to your bank account. Cigarettes are approximately $4 per pack. A pack-a-day smoker can expect to spend about $1,400 a year on cigarettes, perhaps more for health care. There are benefits to lifestyle and image; the nonsmoker is perceived as healthier and cleaner than the smoker. With more and more businesses and community buildings being smoke free, the nonsmoker does not have to be one of the social outcasts who have to go to a designated smoking area outside the building. There are some benefits that improve personal attributes. Food tastes better, clothing and household items no longer smell of smoke, the smoker will no longer be a smoking role model for younger people, and physical activity will not leave the individual short of breath and without stamina.

Quitting Readiness

Everyone arrives at their level of quit readiness in their own way. It is not as though the smoker just says, "I quit." There are a number of psychological and physical battles the smoker must work through in order to be ready to quit. To get to that level, the individual may go through specific stages of change. Psychological researchers James Prochaska and Carlo DiClemente (1992) developed a transtheoretical model that included stages of change describing how people with addictive behaviors deal with behavior change. This model fits very well with smoking cessation. According to their behavioral research, not all smokers are alike in how they quit, but they appear to go through distinct stages:

- *Precontemplation.* In this stage, the smoker has not yet acknowledged there is a problem behavior; that is, the smoker may know that smoking is unhealthy but has not come to grips with the seriousness of situation.

- *Contemplation.* The smoker may realize that there is a problem by virtue of the personal consequences of his or her behavior but does not see the problem as serious enough to be addressed at this point in time. During this stage, the smoker may think about the process he or she will use to quit and the specific quit strategies that will work into his or her plan. He or she may also develop an awareness of new information that will move him or her toward action.

- *Preparation/determination.* In this stage, the individual clearly realizes that "I have to do something about this." The smoker may begin to gather information to help him or her with the final move toward changing the behavior. The smoker will also accumulate cognitions to help him or her stay motivated to move forward.

- *Action.* At this point, the smoker will have all the cognitions and motivations to put quitting into action. It is not as simple as "giving up smoking" for most quitters, as they need to move toward other behaviors to replace the one they are giving up.

- *Maintenance.* During the maintenance stage, the ex-smoker will use all of his or her motivational tools to stay the course. Success may well depend on his or her ability to find successful substitutions for the old behavior.

- *Relapse.* It is not uncommon for the ex-smoker to relapse and go back to smoking again. Sometimes relapse is short lived, and the smoker returns to abstinence quickly, but sometimes the ex-smoker will go back to smoking for months or years. If he or she relapses for a longer period of time, he or she will then go back through the previous stages to give up smoking once again. In fact, people may fluctuate among stages through this whole process.

Helping Someone Quit Smoking

Do you know someone who wants to quit smoking—maybe a parent, relative, neighbor, or friend? There are things you can do to help, but first you must understand that smoking plays a significant role in the life of the smoker. It is a strong habit, both physically and psychologically, and can be very difficult to give up. It takes courage to even reach the decision to quit smoking. Quitting successfully also requires *continual motivation* to not smoke. This is where you can help by acting as a member of the ex-smoker's **social support network** and helping him or her stay focused on success and on the factors that triggered his or her desire to quit smoking. Triggers may have included a doctor's order, knowledge of a smoking friend who died or became

social support network
a network of family, friends, and acquaintances who encourage, support, and provide positive feedback

very ill because of smoking, the desire for wellness, the need to set an example for children, or the high monetary costs of smoking. The closer your relationship to the ex-smoker, the greater the opportunity you have to reinforce his or her motives for not smoking.

When someone you care about announces his or her intention to quit smoking, you can do more than just say, "That's nice" or "Congratulations!" You can help reinforce the person's motives, strengthen his or her resolve, and even strengthen your relationship with him or her by doing some of the following:

1. Ask the person to tell you how he or she feels about not smoking. Talking about feelings helps the quitter develop nonsmoking attitudes and strengthens his or her motivation to stay off tobacco.

2. If the person complains about how difficult it is to give up smoking, tell him or her how proud you are of the decision and that you are confident that he or she can succeed.

3. Don't let the person get away with saying that he or she is going to start up again. Be encouraging; don't say "go ahead—I didn't think you could do it" in an effort to shame them into continuing. There are several things you can say to help the person over the hump:
   - Let the person know that he or she seems healthier since quitting smoking.
   - Remind the person that every day makes a difference. Celebrate abstinence a day at a time.
   - Tell that person how much better off he or she will be after working through it.
   - Ask the person to retell you the things that motivated him or her to quit in the first place.
   - Encourage the person to talk about the sense of pride and accomplishment he or she will feel after completely quitting.
   - Remind the person of the money that will be saved and encourage him or her to put the money into a savings account to set aside money for something special.

Perhaps you can think of other ideas. The key is that you remain involved with the ex-smoker and do all you can to help keep the focus on the positive reasons for not using tobacco. The more you get him or her to verbalize their commitment and admire his or her courage and strength, the greater will be the likelihood for success.

Keep in mind that it is common for people who are trying to quit smoking to slip. Most smokers don't become completely abstinent until they have tried six or seven times. If they made the decision to quit, rest assured that they really wanted to stop, but the habit is very strong, and nicotine is one of the most addicting substances known to science. Make sure your friend knows you are there for him or her. You can't make them quit, nor can you fix it if they give up. All you can do is offer help if they ask for it.

WEB LINK
Help with Smoking Cessation

http://www.lungusa.org

If you or someone you know is contemplating smoking cessation, visit this Web site.

From the home page, click the "Stop Smoking" link. The link will take you to a number of pages with good smoking cessation strategies, questions, and answers.

SEARCH TERMS: smoking cessation, quitting smoking

Ex-smokers may need new behaviors to fill the time formerly occupied by smoking. You can help by inviting them to exercise with you, share a hobby, listen to music, take a walk, play video games, or even just get coffee or a drink and talk. Watching television is not a good idea because it lets them sit too quietly and be in a situation that may leave them feeling the urge to light up. They will benefit from being involved in some type of activity.

Smokeless Tobacco

Smokeless tobacco comes in two basic forms: chewing tobacco made of leaf tobacco, or "plugs," and powdered tobacco, known as "snuff." The leaf form is chewed and formed into a wad that rests between the check and gum and mixes with saliva. The chemicals from the tobacco are absorbed into the bloodstream through the cells lining the cheek and gum.

Overall, about 3 percent of the U.S. population uses smokeless tobacco. Usage is higher among males (6 percent) than females (.04 percent). Only about 8 percent of young people use **smokeless tobacco**, and its use has declined since the early 1990s. The decline in smokeless tobacco use and the high level of social disapproval of this behavior indicates that there is little support among young adults to use smokeless tobacco. This is good news because smokeless tobacco is not a safe alternative to cigarettes. Smokeless tobacco contains chemicals that are highly addictive and 28 known substances that contribute to cancer and heart disease. The immediate and short-term effects of using smokeless tobacco are dose related and include the following:

> **smokeless tobacco**
> tobacco that is not smoked but is used orally, such as snuff or chewing tobacco

- Increased heart rate caused by nicotine's presence in the bloodstream releasing adrenaline. The heartbeat may also be irregular.

- Increased blood pressure caused by nicotine in the bloodstream.

- Constricted blood vessels: nicotine constricts the blood vessels, slowing down the circulation of oxygen-rich blood to the organs and increasing the possibility of heart attack or stroke.

- Discoloration of teeth: the products in smokeless tobacco *permanently* stain teeth.

- Halitosis: Bad breath caused by chewing tobacco is socially unacceptable and offensive.

- Tooth decay: Smokeless tobacco contains high quantities of sugar. This sugar mixes with the plaque on the teeth, forming acids that eat away at the tooth's enamel and causing cavities.

> ### Did You Know ...?
>
> Smokeless tobacco use is not as popular as it was years ago, but it is still being used by a lot of people. In 2005, the smokeless tobacco industry sold 116,200,000 pounds of smokeless tobacco. The corporations spent $218,663,983 on advertising and recovered $1,765,423,249 in sales.

Long-term health conditions associated with the use of smokeless tobacco include the following:

- *Tooth abrasion*. Grit and sand particles in smokeless tobacco can scratch teeth and wear away the tooth enamel.

- *Gum recession*. When someone uses smokeless tobacco of any kind, the tobacco is typically held in the same spot in the mouth. The nicotine and other chemicals enter the capillaries in the skin. Retaining the tobacco in this same spot over time can result in permanent damage to **periodontal tissue** (the supporting tissue around the tooth root). The injured gums can pull away from the teeth and eventually lead to inflamed gums and tooth loss.

- *Oral cancer.* Cancer of the mouth (including the lip, tongue, and cheek) is one of the 10 most common cancers in the world. The risk of mouth cancer is four times greater for the smokeless tobacco user than it is for the nonuser. The cancer is most likely to occur in the spot where the tobacco rests in the mouth. Tobacco and its irritating juices are left in contact with gums, cheeks, and lips for long periods of time.

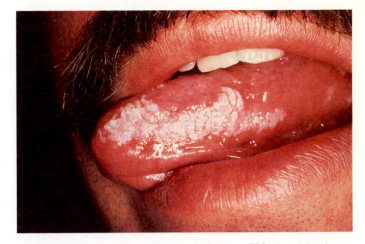

FIGURE 11-10 • Leukoplakia on the tongue. (Courtesy CDC; photo taken by Sol Silverman Jr., DDS)

This long-term contact can eventually result in a condition called **leukoplakia**. Leukoplakia sores appear either as smooth white patches or as leathery-looking wrinkled skin around the tongue and/or gum line (Figure 11-10). Leukoplakia results in cancer in 3 to 5 percent of all cases. Oral cancer treatments can disfigure patients because a lot of bone and tissue must be removed from the patient's face. Oral cancer is especially dangerous because it can spread quickly to the brain.

- *Throat cancer.* The risk of cancer of the throat is up to 50 times greater for the person who chews tobacco. The longer smokeless tobacco is used, the greater the risk.

periodontal tissue
supporting tissue around the tooth root

leukoplakia
a precancerous sore that develops after prolonged exposure to tobacco

BUILDING YOUR LIFETIME WELLNESS PLAN

A wellness plan for tobacco cessation is very simple: don't use tobacco products, and if you are already using them, quit. Cigarette smoking is the number one most *preventable* cause of illness and death in the United States because it is a *voluntary* behavior using a highly toxic substance that poses a very high risk to health. Young people may not believe that they are being harmed by smoking, but young adults who smoke are setting themselves up for a life of addiction and many future health problems. An older adult who is smoking has already incurred some physical damage to his or her body, but quitting can reverse some of the damage that has already taken place. It appears

that no matter when a person gives up smoking, there are health benefits to be derived. Develop your wellness plan to include a goal related to tobacco use—for you or for your relationship with others. You might want to select from the following list or create your own:

- Define and clarify your wellness goals to include abstaining from tobacco use as a wellness practice.
- Use your health literacy skills to learn more about the dangers of tobacco use.
- Support someone you know who is trying to quit.

●●● End-of-Chapter Activities

Opportunities for Application

1. Review Table 11-1. Select five of the chemicals listed in the table and research them in more detail. Prepare a bulleted summary for each of the chemicals pertaining to the health effects of the chemicals and make note of the sources where you obtained your information. You can use this summary to explain to other people why cigarette smoking is harmful to health.

2. In your opinion, what is the worst thing about tobacco use? Use your writing skills to prepare a personal statement describing social, physical, and psychological reasons why smoking is harmful.

3. Calculate the cost of cigarette smoking. Determine how much a pack of cigarettes costs in your community. You may also find out how much a carton costs and extrapolate the cost of cigarettes per pack. You can calculate the dollar amounts for one pack a day, a pack and a half a day, and so on. Determine how much cigarette smoking would cost for a year. Given the amount of money spent, what could the individual do with the money saved if he or she quit smoking? List some ideas.

Key Concepts

1. Explain what is meant by the statement, "There is no such thing as a safe cigarette."

2. Some people believe that smokeless tobacco is a safe alternative to cigarette smoking. Explain why this statement is false.

3. List some of the health problems facing women smokers.

4. List and explain the stages-of-change model as it applies to cigarette smoking cessation.

Answers to Personal Assessment: Smoking Quiz

Each of the statements is true.

●●● **References**

Altria. (2010). *Altria reports 2009 full-year results.* Retrieved May 24, 2010, from http://investor.altria.com/phoenix.zhtml?c=80855&p=irol-newsArticle&ID=1380055

American Cancer Society. (2007). *Cancer facts and figures 2007.* Atlanta: Author.

Buka, S. L., Shenassa, E. D., & Niaura, R. (2003). Elevated risk of tobacco dependence among offspring of mothers who smoked during pregnancy: A 30-year prospective study. *American Journal of Psychiatry, 160*(11), 1978–1984.

Canadian Lung Association. (2009). *Withdrawal Symptoms and How to Cope.* Retrieved January 12, 2010 from http://www.lung.ca/protect-protegez/tobacco-tabagisme/quitting-cesser/withdrawal-sevrage_e.php

Connolly, G.N., Alpert, H.R, Wayne, G.F., & Koh, H. (2007). *"Trends in Smoke Nicotine Yield and Relationship to Design Characteristics Among Popular US Cigarette Brands 1997–2005."* A Report of the Tobacco Research Program Division of Public Health Practice, Harvard School of Public Health. Retrieved March 20, 2010 from: http://www.medicalnewstoday.com/articles/61210.php

Dube, S.R., Asman, K., Malaarcher, A., Carabollo, R. (November 13, 2009). Cigarette smoking among adults and trends in smoking cessation—United States, 2008. *MMWR Weekly, 85*(44), 1227–1232.

National Center for Chronic Disease Prevention and Health Promotion. (2001). *Women and smoking: A report of the Surgeon General.* Rockville, MD: U.S. Department of Health and Human Services.

National Center for Chronic Disease Prevention and Health Promotion. (2004). *The health consequences of smoking: A report of the Surgeon General.* Dept. of Health and Human Services, Centers for Disease Control and Prevention. Washington, DC: Superintendent of Documents.

Paterson, D. S., et al. (2006). Multiple serotonergic brainstem abnormalities in sudden infant death syndrome. *JAMA, 296,* 2124–2132.

Prochaska, J. O., & DiClemente, C. C. (1992). Stages of change in the modification of problem behavior. In M. Hersen, R. Eisler, & P. M. Miller (Eds.), *Progress in behavior modification* (Vol. 28, pp. 184–214). Sycamore, IL: Sycamore Publishing.

U.S. Department of Health and Human Services. (2006). *The health consequences of involuntary exposure to tobacco smoke: A report of the surgeon general—Executive summary.* Pittsburgh, PA: Author.

World Health Organization. (2007). *Protection from exposure to second-hand tobacco smoke: Policy implications.* Retrieved January 16, 2010, from http://whqlibdoc.who.int/publications/2007/9789241563413_eng.pdf

CHAPTER 12

Alcohol and Other Drugs

CHAPTER OBJECTIVES

When you finish this chapter, you should be able to:

- Discuss factors that contribute to substance abuse.
- Explain why ethyl alcohol is considered an addictive drug.
- Describe both the negative and the positive health effects of moderate alcohol consumption.
- Explain the meaning of binge drinking and why it is harmful.

- Discuss the health effects of alcohol use and abuse.
- Explain the difference between over-the-counter, prescription, and illicit drugs.
- Identify the risks, dangers, and social implications associated with drug abuse.
- Describe the categories of abused drugs and give examples for each category.

KEY TERMS

alcohol dehydrogenase (ADH)
binge drinking
blood alcohol concentration
   (BAC)
cardiomyopathy
dopamine

drug abuse
drug dependence
fermentation
fetal alcohol
   syndrome (FAS)
hypothermia

inpatient
medicine
neurotransmitter
outpatient
over-the-counter
   (OTC) medications

prescription drug
   abuse
prescription medicines
proof
tolerance
withdrawal

●●● Introduction

It seems that the use of various chemical products to modify mood or behavior is an acceptable social behavior in the United States. The use of products such as caffeinated drinks and alcoholic beverages are part of our normal social activities. On the other hand, products such as the nonmedical use of prescription drugs, marijuana, cocaine, and other mind-altering materials are frowned on, as is alcohol abuse. We have been aware of this paradox for many years and have struggled with attempts to put our use of legal and illegal drugs in proper perspective. For example, there were social groups at the turn of the twentieth century who lobbied to make alcohol an illegal substance. In response, the federal government passed legislation in 1920 to prohibit the sale and use of alcoholic beverages in the United States. The legislation resulted in illegal alcohol use and the expansion of criminal organizations that sold alcohol illegally. Public pressure to remove the ban, coupled with the costs of combating the illegal activity, led to the law's being rescinded in 1933. Thus, alcohol continues to be a legal drug in the United States.

Significant efforts to combat drug abuse in the United States began in the 1970s at a time when many middle-class young people began turning to recreational drug use. Since then, we have spent billions of dollars to dissuade people from illicit drug use, but drug abuse and the effect it has on the community continue to be significant social problems. The magnitude of the problem is so great that we attempt to engage many of our social institutions (i.e., families, churches, schools, and community organizations) to help ameliorate the problem. Moreover, we invest additional billions of dollars to stop drug trafficking and to rehabilitate addicted users. Illicit drugs aren't the only substances that pose harm to society and to the individuals who use the drugs.

We often overlook the fact that alcohol is a drug. Because it is a "legal" drug, we fail to notice alcohol abuse and the effect it has on our lives. Our culture tends to look at alcohol consumption with a certain amount of ambivalence. In one sense, we view alcohol consumption as a normal social activity and laugh at the party drunk, yet we are horrified at the family of four who are killed by a drunk driver. Although alcoholic beverages are consumed in varying amounts by most adults, people tend to overlook the fact that alcohol abuse, similar to drug abuse, poses many personal and social problems.

As an adult, you have probably put alcohol and drug use in perspective. It is hoped that your perspective does not include the misuse or abuse of these chemical substances.

PERSONAL ASSESSMENT
Facts about Substance Abuse

Read each of the statements below and write down whether you think each one is true or false. You can find all the answers at the end of the chapter.

1. There are no calories in alcoholic beverages.

2. Liquor consumed with soda will affect the body more quickly than liquor consumed with a mixer such as orange juice.

3. Eating while consuming alcoholic beverages will slow the absorption of alcohol.

4. Coffee and a cold shower will sober up a person who is drunk.

5. A person cannot become an alcoholic by drinking only wine.

6. Most of the alcohol consumed is absorbed into the body through the stomach.

7. The average age for starting drug use in the United States is 18.

8. A person cannot become addicted to marijuana.

9. The drug most likely to be associated with emergency room admissions is cocaine.

10. Most prison inmates have used drugs at some time in their lives.

If you have chosen a wellness lifestyle that does not include the abusive use of alcohol or drugs, you may find information in this chapter that will reinforce your attitudes and perhaps assist you with helping someone else make good choices in this regard. If you have not made such a choice or if you are seeking more information to help clarify the role you expect these substances to play in your life, you will likely find information in this chapter to help you gain clarification.

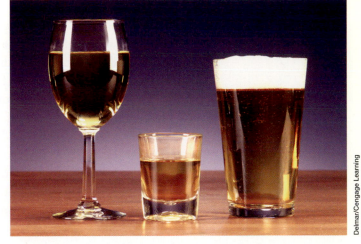

FIGURE 12-1 • Each of these drinks contains approximately the same amount of alcohol.

Delmar/Cengage Learning

Beverage Alcohol

Beverage alcohol is a by-product of **fermentation**, a process whereby sugars from fruits or grains are allowed to sit without oxygen in the presence of yeast. The yeast uses the sugar as a food source and produces ethyl alcohol as a by-product. The fermentation process varies depending on whether the manufacturer of the alcoholic beverage intends to produce wine, beer, or liquor. The various forms of alcoholic beverages contain comparatively different levels of alcohol. In general, 12 ounces of beer, 6 ounces of wine, and 1.5 ounces of liquor each contain approximately half an ounce of absolute alcohol (Figure 12-1). The alcohol content of beer ranges from 4 to 6 percent. The percentage of alcohol in wine varies (11 to 14 percent) and is stated on the product label. The alcohol in liquor results from a process known as distillation, in which the alcohol is removed from fermented products such as barley, corn, or potatoes and then mixed with other ingredients. Liquor products express the amount of alcohol as **proof**. Proof is stated on the label of the product and reflects twice the amount of alcohol. For example, 86-proof bourbon is 43 percent alcohol.

fermentation
the process of converting sugars into ethyl alcohol and carbon dioxide

proof
the measure of the amount of alcohol in a liquor; a 90-proof liquor is 45 percent alcohol

Alcohol as a Food Source

Beverage alcohol is known as ethanol or ethyl alcohol. It is the only form of alcohol fit for human consumption. Although ethyl alcohol contains calories, it has no nutritional value. When alcohol is consumed, the body metabolizes the alcohol as an energy source. Ethanol is an example of empty calories, that is, energy with no other nutritive value. In fact, food calories are metabolized by the body *after* the alcohol calories. Thus, if the energy needs of the body are met by the alcohol calories, the unused food calories are stored as fat in the body. People interested in managing their weight would be wise to reflect on the amount of alcohol they consume if they do drink.

Did You Know...?

In your science classes, you may have used *denatured ethyl alcohol* in the alcohol burners. This is the same alcohol that comes from the sugar fermentation process, but it cannot be consumed. Denatured ethyl alcohol contains chemicals added during production, making it unfit for human consumption.

Alcohol the Drug

Alcohol is a depressant drug. It causes central nervous system impulses to travel more slowly, creating a sedating effect on the individual. This results in many body functions slowing down. Believe it or not, more than 100 years ago, doctors used alcohol as anesthesia for surgical procedures. This practice was risky and is no longer followed because the amount of alcohol needed to mask pain is extremely close to the amount of alcohol capable of causing death. If enough alcohol is administered, the brain centers controlling respiration and heart rate are affected and begin to shut down. It is unsafe to drink more than one drink per hour because of the amount of alcohol that accumulates in the body.

The body protects itself from overconsumption of alcohol by triggering a vomiting response to remove alcohol from the stomach, but this response usually occurs after a good deal of the alcohol has entered the bloodstream. Some people believe that vomiting during a drinking episode is a result of drinkers "mixing their liquors," but this is not the case. Vomiting is a clear sign that the amount of alcohol consumed is reaching a dangerous level.

The most common reason people drink alcohol is to achieve a "drug effect." The problem is, as with other depressant drugs, that the body builds up a **drug tolerance** to the effects of alcohol. In order to feel the desired drug effect at each drinking episode, a person must consume larger amounts of alcohol. The stronger the effect desired, the more the person needs to consume. It is common for heavy drinkers to feel a sense of discomfort, including nausea, when they do not have alcohol in their bloodstream. As with all abused depressant drugs, this discomfort is a symptom of withdrawal.

drug tolerance
physical change in the body that causes one to adapt to the effects of a drug, causing the person to use more of the drug to get the same effect

Drinking Behaviors

Each person has to decide the role, if any, that alcohol will play in his or her life. Many people choose not to drink any alcohol, some choose to drink occasionally, and others choose to drink at unhealthy levels. All behaviors related to alcohol consumption can be viewed as a continuum, ranging from abstinence to alcohol dependence (Figure 12-2). Definitions of consumption should be used with caution, however, because there are factors other than the amount of alcohol that influence consumption patterns, such as how the individual responds to alcohol, the length of time over which consumption takes place, the type of drinks consumed, and the body size and gender of the drinker. In addition, since the behaviors are on a continuum, gray areas exist between categories.

Anyone choosing to consume alcoholic beverages has a social and personal obligation to drink in a responsible manner. Many years of research confirms that moderate alcohol consumption as described in the following section is characteristic of responsible drinking behavior. There are also attitudes and skills that contribute to responsible drinking behaviors, including the following:

- *Decision-making skills*. By the time people reach the age of 21, the legal age for drinking throughout the United States, they should be able to make responsible decisions regarding alcohol consumption. They should also have the communication skills needed to express their values and turn down invitations to drink if they have decided that doing so is in their best interest.

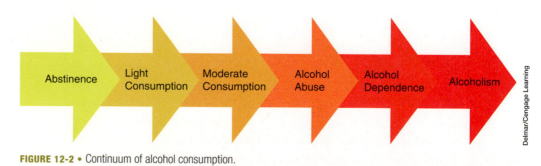

FIGURE 12-2 • Continuum of alcohol consumption.

- *The ability to say no.* Individuals should be able to confidently communicate that they don't drink or don't want any additional drinks during a particular drinking episode.

- *Acceptance of abstainers.* Anyone who makes the decision to drink alcohol should never force drinks on those individuals who choose not to drink. If someone chooses to abstain, for whatever reason, their decision should be respected by others and not challenged.

- *Practice safe behaviors.* In the event that you choose to drink or are around people who are drinking, take the time to protect yourself by practicing safe behaviors. Figure 12-3 lists some safety tips you may want to consider.

Alcohol consumption patterns and the knowledge and attitudes that support individual behaviors vary from person to person. In the following sections, we examine the various segments of the alcohol continuum. You will be able to see where you are on the continuum; it is hoped that you fall on the responsible side of the continuum. If not, you may want to address your alcohol consumption attitudes and behaviors in your wellness plan.

Abstinence

Data from the 2008 *National Survey on Drug Use and Health* (Substance Abuse and Mental Health Services Administration, 2009) reveal that slightly more than 48 percent

There may be a time when you choose to drink or gather with friends who are drinking. Here are some tips for safe drinking.

- Drink only if it is your choice. You have responsibility for your own health, and you don't have to drink alcohol.

- If you choose to drink, drink moderately; never have more than three drinks in one drinking episode.

- Don't drink more than one alcoholic beverage per hour.

- Don't engage in "drinking games" or drinking challenges.

- Consider drinking nonalcoholic "look-alikes." It helps keep "alcohol pushers" away.

- Be aware of drinking roles. If you go to a party and choose to be the designated driver, remember you have the responsibility to be the designated nondrinker. Remember that not being the designated driver does not mean you should be the designated drunk.

- Never ride in a vehicle with a driver who has been drinking.

- Always drink responsibly if you choose to drink.

Delmar/Cengage Learning

FIGURE 12-3 • There will be a time when you choose to drink or gather with friends who are drinking. Here are some tips for safe drinking.

of the people over the age of 12 in the United States do not consume alcoholic beverages. People who make the choice to abstain from alcohol consumption may do so for a variety of reasons:

- They simply do not like the taste of alcoholic beverages.

- They do not care for the drug effects that come from alcohol.

- They are concerned about their health and well-being and recognize that alcohol consumption can be unhealthy.

- They may be taking prescription medications that react negatively to the presence of alcohol.

- They may have family members or friends who were alcohol dependent.

- They hold religious beliefs advocating abstinence as a way of keeping the body pure and healthy.

- They have decided that the cost of alcohol, a nonfood substance, is more than the product is worth.

- They want to be positive role models and present good examples of healthy habits for family, friends, and children.

Light Consumption

There are people who do not abstain from alcohol use but drink very lightly. They may have a glass of wine with a meal, for example, or one drink at a social event where alcohol is being served. Light consumption is no more than one drink a day, three or fewer times a week.

Moderate Consumption

The moderate drinker consumes no more than one or two drinks a day—one drink for a woman, two drinks for a man. Three drinks on a single occasion represent the *upper* limit of moderate alcohol consumption. It is important to remember that both the number of drinks and the distribution of drinks over time are important in defining moderate consumption. For example, people who do not drink all week so that they can have more than three drinks per episode during the weekend would *not* qualify as moderate drinkers.

According to medical research, alcohol consumption within moderate levels does not pose a health threat; in fact, consumption may be beneficial. For example, men who drink alcohol moderately three or more days per week have a reduced risk of heart attack compared with men who drink less frequently. Men who drink less than one drink a day reportedly have similar risk reduction compared to those who drink three. It also appears women who drink moderately benefit from stronger bones than women who don't.

Alcohol Abuse

Alcohol abuse occurs if the upper limit of moderate consumption is exceeded during any single drinking episode. Drinking beyond this limit on a continual basis can lead to physical problems (liver damage, cardiovascular problems, and accidents) and social troubles (drinking-and-driving offenses, public intoxication, and relationship problems). Research indicates the following:

- There are more than 300 alcohol-poisoning deaths in the United States each year.

- Approximately every 31 minutes, a person is killed in an alcohol-related traffic accident.

- Seventy-six percent of traffic fatalities between midnight and 3:00 a.m. are alcohol related.

- The alcohol abuse costs to society are almost twice as high as are the costs associated with all other forms of drug abuse.

Women appear to be more vulnerable to the adverse health effects of alcohol than men, including organ damage. This trait may be due in part to the fact that women absorb and metabolize alcohol slightly more slowly than men do. Data point to the fact that women become addicted more easily than men. Today, young women start drinking at a younger age and drinking more than women of similar ages in the 1960s.

Binge Drinking

A form of alcohol abuse and a significant drinking problem among some college students and adults is the practice of **binge drinking** (Figure 12-4). By definition, binge drinkers consume five or more alcoholic drinks in any single drinking episode. Although these drinkers don't drink every day, when they do consume alcoholic beverages, they drink to excess. Binge drinking has been seen in youths as young as 13 years of age, but the highest rates of binge drinking are reportedly among young adults ages 18 to 25, and males are more likely to binge drink than are females. Many students see alcohol

> ### Did You Know...?
>
> In the late 1800s, a British physician, Francis E. Anstie, proposed a rule for safe drinking that became known as Anstie's Limit of Safe Drinking, a rule that still defines the upper limit of moderate consumption. He stated that it was safe for a man to consume no more than 1.5 ounces of absolute alcohol a day. As mentioned previously, 12 ounces of beer, 1.5 ounces of liquor, or 6 ounces of wine each contain half an ounce of ethyl alcohol.

> **binge drinking**
> drinking consisting of five or more alcoholic drinks on a single drinking occasion for males and four or more drinks for females

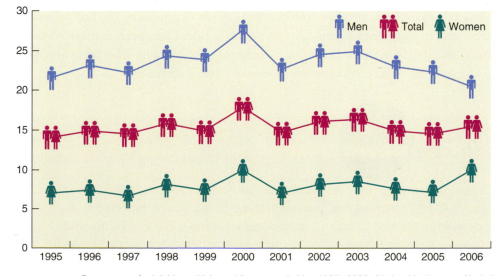

FIGURE 12-4 • Percentage of adult binge drinkers, 18 years and older, 1995–2006. (National Institute on Alcohol Abuse and Alcoholism, 2009)

consumption as part of the college experience. If they believe this is true, the important thing to remember is that alcohol can be part of a college student's life (or any other adult for that matter), but we should not lose sight of subscribing to a mandate for consuming alcohol in a responsible manner. Recent data indicate that binge drinking is not as prevalent as it was a few years ago. Perhaps more people are choosing to drink responsibly.

The most serious consequence of binge drinking is alcohol poisoning. Alcohol poisoning is a severe and potentially fatal overdose of alcohol. It occurs when too much alcohol is consumed over a short period of time. Problems arise as the depressing nature of alcohol deprives the brain of oxygen and causes a slowing of the heart rate, breathing, and suppression of the gag reflex. Signs of alcohol poisoning include the following:

- Confusion/stupor

- Vomiting

- Unconsciousness

- Breathing slowly (fewer than eight breaths a minute or 10 or more seconds between two breaths)

- Pale/blue, cold, clammy skin

A person showing any of these signs needs immediate medical help because these symptoms indicate a dangerous level of alcohol in the bloodstream. A common misconception is that vomiting means that the body has rid itself of alcohol. Vomiting is a sign that an overdose of alcohol has occurred. Although much of the alcohol may have already entered the bloodstream, vomiting is the body's response to purging alcohol from the stomach. Vomiting must be seen as an indication of concern because a person whose gag reflex is suppressed because of the effects of alcohol poisoning may choke on their vomit. Any person vomiting or showing any of the other symptoms of alcohol poisoning should not be left to "sleep it off," nor should other attempts, such as giving the person coffee or a cold shower, be made to help the person sober up. A passed-out drunk should not be left alone; he or she may very well be close to death. Call 911 and request medical attention immediately.

Binge drinking leads to other problems in addition to poisoning the body. Possible consequences of binge drinking include automobile accidents, property damage, physical or sexual assault of others, or becoming a victim of sexual assault. The dependence on binge drinking may also predispose the drinker to alcohol addiction.

What's News

Drinking at an early age can lead to later alcohol dependence. A study by Grucza (2008) reported that one out of three subjects who reported that they started drinking at age 17 or younger were more likely to be alcohol dependent, whereas one out of 10 people who started drinking after age 21 reported alcohol dependency. This effect was more than twice as likely to occur among females than males.

Alcohol Dependence

If you were asked to define alcohol dependence, the word *alcoholism* may come to mind. In fact, these terms are used interchangeably, although current terminology among treatment specialists is *alcohol dependence*. Health professionals have a number of definitions for alcoholism and alcohol dependence. Simply put, alcohol dependence is a level of alcohol consumption marked by continued alcohol abuse. At exactly what point abuse turns to dependence is not easy to explain, but the National Institute on Alcohol Abuse and Alcoholism (2000) describes alcohol dependence as a disease with four main characteristics:

- A craving to drink alcohol

- The inability to control drinking behavior once it begins

- Withdrawal symptoms (nausea and anxiety) after drinking stops

- Tolerance, which means having to drink more and more in order to get "high"

Currently, about one of every 14 adults, or about 18 million Americans, is an alcohol abuser or is alcohol dependent. These individuals may be binge drinkers or people who consume alcohol beyond the limits of moderate consumption as described previously. Data indicate that 72 percent of the adult population in the United States drinks responsibly. Among this group, less than one person in 100 develops some form of alcohol-related disorder. Conversely, 10 percent of the adult population consumes alcohol in excess. Individuals in the latter group have a 50 percent probability of developing alcohol disorders (NIAAA, 2006).

Causes of Alcohol Dependence

It appears that personality, social, and genetic factors all contribute to the development of alcoholism, with estimates that almost 60 percent of the risk for developing alcoholism is genetic in origin. This does not mean alcohol dependence is inherited; rather, it means that genetics can influence how an individual is likely to respond to alcohol. Anyone with a family member who is an alcoholic would be well advised to avoid alcohol use altogether.

Treatment of Alcohol Dependence

Almost 700,000 people in the United States receive treatment for alcoholism every year. Just as there are various forms of alcoholism and causes of alcoholism, there are various ways of treating alcoholism. The first step in all treatment programs is to separate the patient from alcohol and rid the abuser's body of the physical need for alcohol. The most acceptable way to do this is through treatment in a medical facility. During hospital treatment, this step can be completed on either an **inpatient** or an **outpatient** basis. Various drug therapies, such as Topiramate, Naltrexone, and Acamprosate, are emerging to help with addiction treatment by preventing relapse. Counseling is an important and necessary aspect of treating alcohol dependence that is carried out by licensed therapists in hospitals or by private counselors. Once the individual is beyond his or her medical intervention, he or she may continue with private counseling sessions or support groups, such as Alcoholics Anonymous (AA), an international fellowship of men and women who at one time had drinking problems of their own. The AA program is a nonprofessional program and is led by peers. There are no age or education requirements, and membership is open to anyone who wants to do something about his or her drinking problem, and commit to provide support for other people who are trying to escape their dependence on alcohol.

inpatient
referring to treatment programs that take place while the patient stays in a hospital or other health care setting

outpatient
referring to treatment programs given to patients who do not stay in a health care setting

Prevention of Alcohol Dependence

The best way to prevent alcoholism is to avoid using alcohol. After all, a person cannot get addicted to a drug they never used. Abstinence would be an important consideration for anyone who has relatives with drinking problems. Someday there may be a simple blood test to screen for a genetic predisposition for alcoholism. This type of screening could be performed on infants and the information used to help parents counsel the child to avoid alcohol as an adult. The second-best preventive measure is to provide information about responsible alcohol consumption so that abstinence or responsible-use patterns can be incorporated into personal wellness plans.

Effects of Alcohol Consumption on Health

Research about alcohol consumption reveals good news and bad news. As a chemical compound and depressive drug, alcohol produces numerous effects on body tissues, especially the brain and the central nervous system. Alcohol has an effect on the liver since that is the organ where alcohol metabolism takes place. The effects of alcohol are dose related, meaning that the effects become more pronounced as the amount of alcohol consumed increases.

Medical evidence appears to support the notion that light to moderate alcohol consumption does not produce negative effects on one's health. This information must be cautiously interpreted, however. In general, medical research supports the protective effect of alcohol, but one must also take into account the genetic, physiological, and social factors related to the individual. To the contrary, it is evident that there are some people who suffer negative effects on their health when they consume alcohol beyond moderate levels. Alcohol is a chemical irritant and carcinogen and, when consumed in an abusive manner, is estimated to contribute to about 4 percent of cancer cases. Some people have been advised by their doctors to stop drinking. Some individuals choose to follow certain medical recommendations coming from the National Institute on Alcohol Abuse and Alcoholism (2000) to stay away from alcohol. These recommendations include women who are pregnant, nursing, or trying to conceive; people who plan to drive or engage in other behaviors requiring attention or skill, such as airline pilots and surgeons; people taking medication, including over-the-counter medications; recovering alcoholics; and persons under the age of 21. Diabetics should refrain from alcohol use because alcohol raises blood sugar levels.

Alcohol Metabolism

Metabolism is the process of converting food substances into energy for use by the body. Although alcohol is not a food per se, it is metabolized in the body to produce energy. The first step is having the alcohol absorbed into the bloodstream. Alcohol absorption begins as soon as it reaches the stomach, although most of the absorption takes place in the small intestine. Once alcohol enters the bloodstream, it is carried to the liver, where it is metabolized by an enzyme, **alcohol dehydrogenase (ADH)**. Alcohol metabolism, regulated by ADH, produces carbon dioxide and water as end products. If the alcohol were not removed, it would create a toxic environment for the body's tissues and organs, and the increase in alcohol concentration would lead to death.

Individuals respond differently in the way they metabolize alcohol. The rate of alcohol metabolism is fixed for every person according to the drinker's genetic makeup. In general, this rate is approximately half an ounce of absolute alcohol (one drink) per

alcohol dehydrogenase (ADH)
an enzyme in the liver responsible for alcohol metabolism

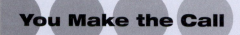

You Make the Call

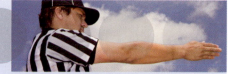

Scientists continue to study biological conditions in individuals that can predict a predisposition for alcoholism. In one study of adolescent males, a particular brain wave exhibited by sons of alcoholics as a response to a stimulus predicted alcoholism *and* drug addiction. If information such as this is valid, it could lead to the possibility of testing people to determine their predisposition for addiction. How would you feel about the possibility of testing school-age children for a predisposition to addiction?

hour. Because alcohol is consumed and absorbed in the stomach and small intestine at a rate faster than the rate of metabolism, some alcohol will continue to circulate in the blood, causing the drug effect. It is this effect that gives the drinker a relaxed feeling at low doses and an anesthetic effect at high doses. If a drinker consumes more than one drink per hour, the amount of alcohol that is not metabolized raises the level of alcohol circulating in the blood and the magnitude of its sedating effect. Too much alcohol consumed in a short period of time can lead to alcohol poisoning.

Nothing can increase the rate of alcohol metabolism and reduce drunkenness. Some people believe that exercising ("Let them walk it off"), drinking lots of coffee, or taking a cold shower will sober up a drunk. None of these techniques work. If a person is extremely intoxicated and not responsive, he or she should not be left to sleep it off. (see the previous section on alcohol poisoning, p. 326). The best way to treat drunkenness is to not drink too much in the first place.

Body Structures Affected by Alcohol

Alcohol circulating in the bloodstream affects a number of body structures. It slows down the brain and nerve activity. Muscular coordination is disrupted, reaction time is increased, speech is slurred, and concentration and decision making are impaired. People under the influence of alcohol tend to do unreasonable things that they probably wouldn't do were they not intoxicated.

Alcohol's effects on the circulatory system are reportedly good and bad. The type of effect is related to the amount of alcohol consumed. Research indicates that alcohol consumed in low doses is beneficial; in high doses, it creates harmful effects. One 12-year study of 38,077 male health professionals (Makamural, et al., 2003) found that those men who drank approximately one alcoholic drink three or more days a week had a reduced risk of heart attack compared with men who drank less frequently. On the other hand, heavy consumption leads to a **cardiomyopathy**, a condition characterized by an enlarged heart muscle resulting in a weak pump and ultimately leading to congestive heart failure. Studies report that 20 to 50 percent of all cardiomyopathy cases are directly attributable to alcohol consumption.

Sometimes a condition perceived as being a beneficial effect of alcohol can actually be a negative effect. For example, a common belief is that alcohol is good for warming a person up in cold weather. Alcohol causes the blood vessels in the circulatory system to dilate (open), causing the drinker's skin to *feel* warm. Just the opposite is

cardiomyopathy
an enlarged but weak heart muscle

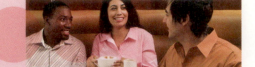

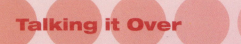

Talking it Over

Should Physicians Encourage Their Patients to Consume Alcohol to Protect Their Health?

- Talk to your friends or family members to get their views on the medical value of alcohol use.
- If you were a physician, would you counsel patients to consume alcohol?
- Compare your opinions with the people you talk to about this topic. Do their views match yours?

After talking it over, did any part of your opinion change? If so, explain.

---

hypothermia
loss of body heat due to exposure to extreme cold

true. When blood vessels dilate, the body *loses* heat, so drinking alcohol in cold weather increases the risk of **hypothermia**, a condition that can be life threatening. A person can tell when he or she is experiencing hypothermia as soon as he or she begins to shiver. Survival time is dependent on the temperature of the environment, the length of exposure, the type of clothing the person is wearing, and the body composition of the person. If a person's body core temperature drops from the normal 98.6 degrees to below 80 degrees Fahrenheit, the risk of dying increases.

One of alcohol's beneficial effects on the circulatory system is its influence on fat deposits in the bloodstream. Evidence indicates *light* alcohol consumption can help reduce these fat deposits, thus decreasing the risk of heart disease. (More information about heart disease is presented in chapter 14.) The bad news is that high doses of alcohol over time can negatively affect the circulatory system by contributing to cardiomyopathy. Consistently high alcohol consumption also contributes to high blood pressure, a risk factor for cardiovascular disease.

Did You Know...?

Women appear to be more susceptible to alcohol-caused cardiomyopathy than men. Research indicates that alcoholic women are significantly more likely to develop cardiomyopathy while consuming less alcohol over a shorter period of time than male counterparts.

Fetal Alcohol Spectrum Disorders

Fetal Alcohol Spectrum Disorders (FASD) is an umbrella term describing the range of effects that can occur in a child whose mother drank alcohol during pregnancy. These effects can include physical, mental, and behavioral problems; learning disabilities; or a combination of these conditions with possible lifelong implications. Among these conditions is the more common and most serious condition known as fetal alcohol syndrome.

Fetal Alcohol Syndrome

fetal alcohol syndrome (FAS)
a characteristic set of birth defects that can occur among babies whose mothers drank alcohol during their pregnancies

Fetal alcohol syndrome (FAS) is a syndrome characterized by birth defects in babies born to women who drink alcohol in excess during their pregnancies. Each year, there are as many as 12,000 cases of FAS and as many as 48,000 cases of a milder form of the syndrome, known as fetal alcohol effects. The effects on the child are dose related, meaning that the more the mother drinks, the more numerous and serious the effects are likely to be.

There is reasonably good evidence that 30 to 45 percent of women who consume six or more alcoholic beverages a day during their pregnancies will give birth to a child with FAS. Of all forms of birth defects, FAS is the easiest to prevent. In fact, it is 100 percent preventable because the syndrome never appears in babies born to women who do not drink during their pregnancies.

The birth defects associated with FAS can affect the baby in three ways:

- *How the child looks.* Examples of FAS characteristics include low birth weight, small head circumference, and abnormalities of the face, such as flattened cheekbones and small eye openings.

- *How the child's brain and nervous system develops.* The child may have learning difficulties or epilepsy, a disease characterized by abnormal electrical activity in the brain.

- *How the child grows and develops.* The child with FAS doesn't develop at the same rate as other children. The child may exhibit social withdrawal, poor coordination, lack of imagination, and poor social skills.

The research data are clear. The best thing a woman can do for her unborn baby is to avoid any alcohol use during her pregnancy. It appears that there is no level of safe drinking for a pregnant woman.

> **WEB LINK**
> ## Fetal Alcohol Syndrome
> ### http://www.cdc.gov
> At this Web site, click on "diseases and conditions." This page will give you a link to "fetal alcohol syndrome." This will take you to a page with current information on FAS and FASD.
>
> **SEARCH TERMS:** fetal alcohol syndrome, fetal alcohol spectrum disorders

Alcohol and the Law

Alcohol use is controlled by laws and regulations because of alcohol's potential harm to the drinker and others in the community. The legal drinking age has been set at 21 because of the potential harm to teens resulting from alcohol consumption. Remember, alcohol is a drug, and, as such, it has a potential for addiction, overdose, and a wide array of social problems associated with drinking and driving.

Blood Alcohol Concentration

When alcohol enters the body, it is quickly absorbed into the bloodstream, resulting in a level of alcohol in the blood known as the **blood alcohol concentration (BAC)**. Sometimes the BAC is expressed as blood alcohol level or blood alcohol percentage. The level of BAC in the body following a drinking occasion depends on four conditions:

> **blood alcohol concentration (BAC)**
> the percent of ethyl alcohol present in the bloodstream after drinking alcoholic beverages

1. *Body size.* A large person has a greater volume of blood and water in which to disperse the alcohol.

2. *Amount of body fat.* Alcohol does not penetrate fat tissue well.

3. *Amount of food in the stomach.* Food in the stomach, especially fats and starches, can slow alcohol absorption. Conversely, a BAC level is likely to be higher if alcohol is consumed on an empty stomach.

4. *Amount of alcohol consumed in a particular time frame.* The longer it takes an individual to consume the alcoholic beverage, the less likely the BAC level will

rise because the body will have time to metabolize the alcohol. Depending on body size and gender, a grown person will metabolize approximately one alcoholic beverage an hour. You can see why a person's BAC level would reach an unsafe level if he or she were to consume four to five drinks in a two-hour period.

As BAC increases, so does alcohol's sedating effect on the body. Furthermore, alcohol will remove inhibitions of some personality disorders, such as exposing the "belligerent drunk." The same number of drinks will result in different BAC levels for men and women, but the same BAC level will produce the same types of effects on the nervous systems of both sexes. Examples are the following:

- At a BAC of 0.02, light to moderate drinkers begin to feel some effects.

- At a BAC of 0.08, there is definite impairment of muscle coordination and driving skills; this is the level at which intoxication is legally defined. The person may have difficulty balancing and will probably have slurred speech.

- At a BAC of 0.12, vomiting usually occurs.

- At a BAC of 0.40, most people lose consciousness; some die.

- At a BAC of 0.50 (at only one-half of 1 percent), coma or death will occur.

Tables 12-1 and 12-2 show the effects and legal implications of various alcohol levels on men and women.

TABLE 12-1 • Blood alcohol levels for men.

Body weight (pounds)	100	120	140	160	180	200	220	240	
Number of Drinks*	Approximate Blood Alcohol Concentration (Percent)								Effect
1	0.04	0.03	0.03	0.02	0.02	0.02	0.02	0.02	Alcohol effect
2	0.08	0.06	0.05	0.05	0.04	0.04	0.03	0.03	
3	0.11	0.09	0.08	0.07	0.06	0.06	0.05	0.05	Driving skills affected
4	0.15	0.12	0.11	0.09	0.08	0.08	0.07	0.06	
5	0.19	0.16	0.13	0.12	0.11	0.09	0.09	0.08	
6	0.23	0.19	0.16	0.14	0.13	0.11	0.10	0.09	Legally intoxicated
7	0.26	0.22	0.19	0.16	0.15	0.13	0.12	0.11	
8	0.30	0.25	0.21	0.19	0.17	0.15	0.14	0.13	
9	0.34	0.28	0.24	0.21	0.19	0.17	0.15	0.14	
10	0.38	0.31	0.27	0.23	0.21	0.19	0.17	0.16	Criminal penalties

Note: Subtract 0.01% for each 45 minutes of drinking.

*One drink = 1.25 oz. of 80-proof liquor, 12 oz. of beer, 5 oz. of wine.

Delmar/Cengage Learning

TABLE 12–2 • Blood alcohol levels for women.

Body weight (pounds)	90	100	120	140	160	180	200	240	
Number of Drinks*	Approximate Blood Alcohol Concentration (Percent)								Effect
1	0.05	0.05	0.04	0.03	0.03	0.02	0.02	0.02	Alcohol effect
2	0.10	0.09	0.08	0.07	0.06	0.05	0.05	0.04	Driving skills affected
3	0.15	0.14	0.11	*0.10	0.09	0.08	0.07	0.06	
4	0.20	0.18	0.15	0.13	0.11	0.10	0.09	0.08	
5	0.25	0.23	0.19	0.16	0.14	0.13	0.11	0.10	
6	0.30	0.27	0.23	0.19	0.17	0.15	0.14	0.12	Legally intoxicated
7	0.35	0.32	0.27	0.23	0.20	0.18	0.16	0.14	
8	0.40	0.36	0.30	0.26	0.23	0.20	0.18	0.17	
9	0.45	0.41	0.34	0.29	0.26	0.23	0.20	0.19	Criminal penalties
10	0.51	0.45	0.38	0.32	0.28	0.25	0.23	0.21	

Delmar/Cengage Learning

Note: Subtract 0.01% for each 45 minutes of drinking.

*One drink = 1.25 oz. of 80-proof liquor, 12 oz. of beer, 5 oz. of wine.

Because of all the research on the effects of BAC on behavior, judgment, and driving skill, all 50 states, the District of Columbia, and Puerto Rico have laws establishing the legal limit for alcohol intoxication at 0.08. Moreover, all states and the District of Columbia have established very low BAC levels of .01 to .02 for underage drivers. These laws are known as per se statutes, meaning that any detectable level of alcohol expressed by underage drivers can lead to immediate suspension of a driver's license.

●●● Drug Use

A **medicine** is any substance used to treat an ailment or illness. Medicines have been used by virtually all civilizations throughout recorded history. The number of medications available today is constantly changing. In the United States, there are currently more than 4,000 prescription medications available to the consumer or medical community. Approximately 30 percent of these medicines come from naturally occurring products.

Medications are available to the public in one of two forms. **Prescription medicines**, also called drugs, must be prescribed by a trained, licensed medical practitioner to ensure that the drugs fit the medical condition for which they are being taken and that the dosage matches the age, size, and physical condition of the intended user. **Over-the-counter (OTC) medications** do not require a doctor's prescription. No prescription is needed for OTC medications because they are considered "safe drugs," but the potential

medicine
a chemical substance used to treat an ailment or illness

prescription medicines
medicines that must be prescribed by a trained physician to ensure that they fit the medical condition for which they are being taken

Did You Know...?

According to the National Highway Traffic Safety Administration (2009), the highest percentage of drivers involved in fatal crashes who had BAC levels of .08 or higher was for drivers 21–24 years of age. In 2008, this represented 1,829 deaths. In that same time period, 57 percent of the fatalities among drivers who had been drinking had BAC levels above 15.

over-the-counter (OTC) medications
medicines that do not require a doctor's prescription

for harm varies from product to product. Users of OTC products must remember that the medications should always be used according to the directions on the label to ensure safety (Figure 12-5).

Scientists have developed and tested drugs and medicines to determine the most effective dosages and means of delivering drugs to the troubled area of the body as timely and as safely as possible. Drugs are formulated and tested to be effective and safe for children, adults, and elder adults if used correctly. Each of these three age-groups may require a different dosage to produce a safe effect. Drugs come in different forms, depending on the purpose of the medication. Have you ever wondered why some drugs come as tablets and others as capsules? The drugs have been designed and tested to ensure the most efficient mechanism for getting the drug into the body. For example, uncoated tablets dissolve in the stomach and are absorbed directly through the stomach lining, coated tablets dissolve later in the stomach or small intestine, and capsules dissolve and release their medication only after they reach the small intestine.

Drugs need to be taken exactly as they are intended. It is extremely important to read label directions carefully, especially with OTC medications, to make sure the medicine is used correctly. When medicines are prescribed by your health care provider, you should discuss the proper use of the medication with your pharmacist or doctor. Although medicines are safe and effective if used correctly, there can be harmful consequences if they are misused. For example, not taking the entire prescription of antibiotic medication to cure an infection can result in a return of the infection. Not only could the infection recur, but it is possible for the bacteria causing the infection to mutate and develop a resistance to the antibiotic. This is precisely why there are now bacteria that are unaffected by antibiotics, making it very difficult to treat infections. Patients should also be aware of the possible side effects of medications they are taking and which side effects are serious enough to require medical attention. Doctors monitor all drugs that a patient may be using in order to avoid problems caused by medication interactions.

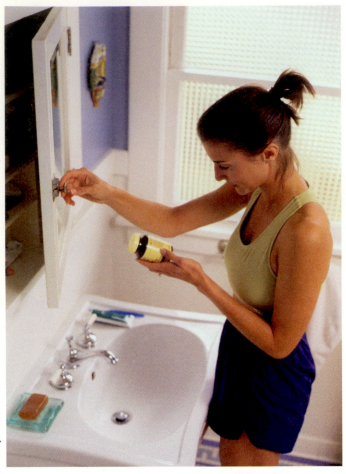

Courtesy of Photodisc

FIGURE 12-5 • For both over-the-counter medications and prescription medicines, always follow the directions on the label to ensure safety.

Misuses of Medicines

Drugs and medicines should be used only according to directions or as prescribed and only by the person for whom the drugs are intended (Figure 12-6). Unused medications should be destroyed when they are no longer needed or if they have passed their expiration date. All drugs, including OTC drugs, should be kept away from children and discarded when they expire. There are times when someone misuses prescription drugs. A prescription drug is considered to be *misused* if it is taken in any of the following ways:

- Taking more of a drug than has been prescribed or continuing to use it when a qualified health care provider indicates that it is no longer needed

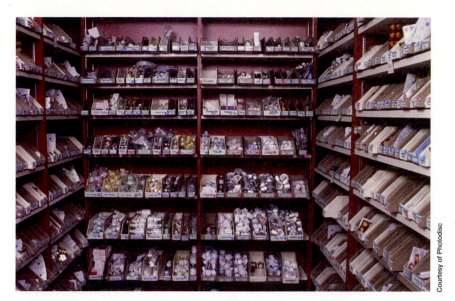

Courtesy of Photodisc

FIGURE 12-6 • Pharmacists carefully control and distribute prescription drugs.

- Using a drug to treat a medical condition other than that for which the drug was intended

- Using a medication that is prescribed for someone else

Drug misuse is not uncommon among elder adults. The elderly use prescription medications approximately three times more frequently than people in the general population. Studies show, however, that elder adults have the poorest record for following medication directions correctly.

Prescription drug abuse occurs when a prescription medicine is used for something other than the drug's intended purpose, that is, to obtain a drug "high." The most commonly abused forms of prescription drugs are painkillers and antidepressants. Abusing drugs of any kind in any form is a risky practice. Drugs are tested on animal and human subjects to determine how effective the drug is. Along the way, scientists calculate the drug's *effective dose* (ED, or the number of subjects getting an effective response to the drug) against the drug's *lethal dose* (LD, or the amount of the drug needed to produce death). An ED_{50} means that at a particular dose, 50 percent of the sample will experience the desired drug effect, and an LD_{60} means that at a particular dose, 60 percent of the sample will die. Each drug has an ED/LD ratio. A drug with an ED/LD ratio of 49 would be highly therapeutic but not very lethal (ED_{98}/LD_2).

prescription drug abuse
the use of a medical drug product for nonmedical reasons

●●● Drug Abuse

There are times when people intentionally seek out chemical or drug substances in order to achieve an altered mental state by engaging in **drug abuse**. These chemical substances can be drugs that were produced for legitimate medical use (amphetamines, sedatives, or morphine), substances that have no medical value (alcohol, LSD, heroin, or PCP), or chemicals that were designed for other purposes but that are sought out for their nervous system effects (aerosol paint, butane, or paint thinner). While drug abuse may be a behavior that serves to produce an altered state for the user, abuse brings with it social and/or physical risks to wellness.

drug abuse
the intentional use of chemical substances to achieve an altered mental state

Reasons Why People Abuse Drugs

People misuse and abuse drugs for a variety of reasons, and the reasons vary from drug to drug and from person to person. Our culture places heavy emphasis on the use of drugs and medicines to cure all sorts of physical and mental problems. Have you noticed the number of television and magazine advertisements for prescription drugs? It stands to reason that illicit drug use is influenced by our cultural belief that anything wrong with a person can be corrected with medicinal drugs. As a result, some people see drug use as a type of "self-medication" for the normal everyday "pains" they have to go through. Researchers have uncovered other reasons for drug use.

Curiosity

Some people want to try illicit drugs just to see what they are like. This type of experimentation involves a great deal of risk, however, because many addicts began by "just trying" drugs. There is no way to know in advance if someone is highly susceptible to drug addiction. For some people, "just trying" drugs is the first step toward using other drugs. The novice user enjoys the initial feeling of the drug and feels safe because he or she hasn't had any problems with the trial period and may begin using other drugs to experience different sensations.

Emotional Pressures

Some people use drugs in an attempt to relieve emotional problems, such as stress, depression, anger, rejection, and/or boredom. Using drugs to relieve problems is a bad strategy because when the effects of the drugs are gone, the emotional problems are still there. Even worse, drug use eventually creates another set of problems.

Companionship

Everyone enjoys and desires companionship. Some individuals feel lonely and left out of social groups. In an attempt to gain friendship and feel accepted, these individuals will end up "befriended" by drug users. Although this may be an occasion to gain friends, in truth, any friendship is very shallow. Drug abusers often extend friendships to encourage drug use among the people they know. According to the U.S. Center for Substance Abuse Prevention, the circle of drug-using friends often becomes the group of clients the drug abusers sell drugs to so that they can afford to purchase their own drugs.

Perception of Social Norms

Some people believe that "everyone else" is using drugs, and they don't want to be left out, so they begin to try drugs as well. Social psychologists refer to this as "reaction to perceived norms," that is, people responding to what they see around them that they perceive as the social norm. Their mantra becomes, "Well, if so and so and so and so are doing it, then everyone must be doing it." In truth, "so and so and so and so" may not be doing it at all, and, according to published studies, most young people and adults *don't* use illegal drugs.

drug dependence
a need for a drug that results in a continuous use of the drug

Drug Dependence

Drug dependence is a phenomenon that is likely to occur during a period of drug abuse. A user becomes dependent when he or she develops a need for a drug because of mental or physical changes that make it difficult for users to control or stop their drug use. Drug dependence is commonly referred to as "addiction." There are two types of drug dependence:

1. *Psychological dependence.* A particular drug is constantly on the user's mind, and he or she feels an overwhelming need to use the drug. The drug becomes such an important part of daily activities that the abuser habitually uses the drug to fill what would be an otherwise empty space. For example, you may have noticed that some people consume large amounts of particular soft drinks because they enjoy the taste and/or convenience, but certainly they do so because of psychological preferences, not physical needs. Drugs like LSD, mescaline, and marijuana have a potential for psychological dependence.

2. *Physical dependence.* Physical dependence develops when abusers use drugs like heroin, morphine, cocaine, and methamphetamine. These drugs produce effects that create tolerance over a period of time. The drug's pharmacology causes a person to need more of the drug over time in order to obtain the drug effect. As tolerance develops, the user needs more of the drug to get the drug effect, in turn leading to more tolerance. The abuser's body develops a physical need for the drug in order to avoid the discomfort of withdrawing from it. Not all drugs produce physical dependence, but they may still be abused because of their perceived effects or as a result of the user's psychological dependence.

The Science of Addiction

Studies on drug abuse and addiction have been going on for almost 30 years, and researchers have learned much about the mechanism of addiction. There are numerous drugs being abused, and each drug has its unique way of changing the brain, but many drugs also share critical common characteristics. For example, virtually every drug of abuse, including nicotine, marijuana, cocaine, heroin, and methamphetamine, will elevate levels of the neurotransmitter **dopamine** in the brain pathways that control the experience of pleasure.

dopamine
a neurotransmitter in the brain

In testimony to a Senate committee on the judiciary, Dr. Alan I. Leshner (2001), director of the National Institute on Drug Abuse, stated, "Prolonged use of these drugs eventually changes the brain in fundamental and long-lasting ways, explaining why people cannot just quit on their own, why treatment is essential. In effect, drugs of abuse take over, or 'highjack' the brain's normal pleasure and motivational systems, moving drug use to the highest priority in the individual's motivational hierarchy, which override all other motivations and drives. These brain changes, then, are responsible for the compulsion to seek and use drugs that we have come to define as addiction. Moreover, these brain and behavioral changes persist long after the individual has stopped using drugs." This explains why addicted users have such a difficult time becoming and staying abstinent.

Withdrawal

When drug abusers stop using drugs on which they have become physically dependent, they may go through a process of withdrawal. **Withdrawal** involves feelings of mental and physical discomfort ranging from mild to severe. The intensity and amount of discomfort varies according to the type of drug the person being using, the amount of the drug being used, and the length of time the drug was used before it was discontinued.

withdrawal
feelings of discomfort that occur when the body is deprived of a drug to which it is addicted

Many long-term drug users are no longer seeking a high when they use drugs; rather, they are using drugs to avoid the discomfort of withdrawal. Withdrawal symptoms are not the same for all drugs. The general withdrawal symptoms for three drugs—alcohol, cocaine, and marijuana—are presented in Table 12-3. Severe cases of withdrawal require medical attention.

TABLE 12-3 • Withdrawal symptoms of selected drugs.

	Drug		
	Alcohol	**Cocaine**	**Marijuana**
Symptoms	Sweating or rapid pulse; increased hand tremor; insomnia; physical agitation; anxiety; hallucinations or illusions	Agitation; depression; intense craving for the drug; anxiety; angry outbursts; shaking; irritability; disturbed sleep	Irritability; anxiety; physical tension; decreases in appetite and mood
Notes	Symptoms are determined by the level of chemical dependence; symptoms begin to appear as soon as 5 to 10 hours after the last drink	Psychological dependence is very high	Symptoms of marijuana withdrawal among chronic users first appear within 24 hours; marijuana withdrawal is most pronounced for the first 10 days

Delmar/Cengage Learning

TABLE 12-4 • Commonly abused drugs.

Substances: Category and Name	Examples of *Commercial* and Street Names	DEA Schedule*/ How Administered**	*Intoxication* Effects/Potential Health Consequences
Cannabinoids			euphoria, slowed thinking and reaction time, confusion, impaired balance and coordination/cough, frequent respiratory infections; impaired memory and learning; increased heart rate, anxiety; panic attacks; tolerance, addiction
hashish	boom, chronic, gangster, hash, hash oil, hemp	I/swallowed, smoked	
marijuana	blunt, dope, ganja, grass, herb, joints, Mary Jane, pot, reefer, sinsemilla, skunk, weed	I/swallowed, smoked	
Depressants			reduced anxiety; feeling of well-being; lowered inhibitions; slowed pulse and breathing; lowered blood pressure; poor concentration/fatigue; confusion; impaired coordination, memory, judgment; addiction; respiratory depression and arrest; death
barbiturates	*Amytal, Nembutal, Seconal, Phenobarbital:* barbs, reds, red birds, phennies, tooies, yellows, yellow jackets	II, III, V/injected, swallowed	*Also, for barbiturates—sedation, drowsiness/depression,* unusual excitement, fever, irritability, poor judgment, slurred speech, dizziness, life-threatening withdrawal
benzodiazepines (other than flunitrazepam)	*Ativan, Halcion, Librium, Valium, Xanax:* candy, downers, sleeping pills, tranks	IV/swallowed, injected	*for benzodiazepines—sedation, drowsiness/dizziness*

TABLE 12-4 • Commonly abused drugs. (*continued*)

Substances: Category and Name	Examples of *Commercial* and Street Names	DEA Schedule*/ How Administered**	*Intoxication* Effects/Potential Health Consequences
flunitrazepam***	*Rohypnol:* forget-me pill, Mexican Valium, R2, Roche, roofies, roofinol, rope, rophies	IV/swallowed, snorted	*for flunitrazepam*—visual and gastrointestinal disturbances, urinary retention, memory loss for the time under the drug's effects
GHB***	*gamma-hydroxybutyrate:* G, Georgia home boy, grievous bodily harm, liquid ecstasy	I/swallowed	*for GHB*—drowsiness, nausea/vomiting, headache, loss of consciousness, loss of reflexes, seizures, coma, death
methaqualone	*Quaalude, Sopor, Parest:* ludes, mandrex, quad, quay	I/injected, swallowed	*for methaqualone—euphoria*/depression, poor reflexes, slurred speech, coma
Dissociative Anesthetics			*increased heart rate and blood pressure, impaired motor function*/memory loss; numbness; nausea/vomiting *Also, for ketamine—at high doses, delirium, depression, respiratory depression and arrest*
ketamine	*Ketalar SV:* cat Valiums, K, Special K, vitamin K	III/injected, snorted, smoked	
PCP and analogs	*phencyclidine;* angel dust, boat, hog, love boat, peace pill	I, II/injected, swallowed, smoked	*for PCP and analogs—possible decrease in blood pressure and heart rate, panic, aggression, violence*/loss of appetite, depression
Hallucinogens			*altered states of perception and feeling; nausea; persisting perception disorder (flashbacks)*
LSD	*lysergic acid diethylamide:* acid, blotter, boomers, cubes, microdot, yellow sunshines	I/swallowed, absorbed through mouth tissues	*Also, for LSD and mescaline—increased body temperature, heart rate, blood pressure; loss of appetite, sleeplessness, numbness, weakness, tremors*
mescaline	buttons, cactus, mesc, peyote	I/swallowed, smoked	*for LSD—persistent mental disorders* *for psilocybin—nervousness, paranoia*
psilocybin	magic mushroom, purple passion, shrooms	I/swallowed	
Oploids and Morphine Derivatives			*pain relief, euphoria, drowsiness*/nausea, constipation, confusion, sedation, respiratory depression and arrest, tolerance, addiction, unconsciousness, coma, death
codeine	*Empirin with Codeine, Fiorinal with Codeine, Robitussin A-C, Tylenol with Codeine:* Captain Cody, schoolboy; (with glutethimide) doors & fours, loads, pancakes and syrup	II, III, IV, V/injected, swallowed	

(continued)

TABLE 12-4 • Commonly abused drugs. (*continued*)

Substances: Category and Name	Examples of *Commercial and Street Names*	DEA Schedule*/ How Administered**	*Intoxication* Effects/Potential Health Consequences
fentanyl and fentanyl analogs	*Actiq, Duragesic, Sublimaze:* Apache, China girl, China white, dance fever, friend, goodfella, jackpot, murder 8, TNT, Tango and Cash	I, II/injected, smoked, snorted	*Also, for codeine—less analgesia, sedation, and respiratory depression than morphine for heroin—staggering gait*
heroin	*diacetyl-morphine:* brown sugar, dope, H, horse, junk, skag, skunk, smack, white horse	I/injected, smoked, snorted	
morphine	*Roxanol, Duramorph:* M, Miss Emma, monkey, white stuff	II, III/injected, swallowed, smoked	
opium	*laudanum, paregoric:* big O, black stuff, block, gum, hop	II, III, V/swallowed, smoked	
oxycodone HCL	*Oxycontin:* Oxy, O.C., killer	II/swallowed, snorted, injected	
hydrocodone bitartrate, acetaminophen	*Vicodin:* vike, Watson-387	II/swallowed	
Stimulants			
amphetamine	*Biphetamine, Dexedrine:* bennies, black beauties, crosses, hearts, LA turnaround, speed, truck drivers, uppers	II/injected, swallowed, smoked, snorted	*increased heart rate, blood pressure, metabolism; feelings of exhilaration, energy, increased mental alertness/rapid or irregular heart beat; reduced appetite, weight loss, heart failure, nervousness, insomnia*
cocaine	*Cocaine hydrochloride:* blow bump, C, candy, Charlie, coke, crack, flake, rock, snow, toot	II/injected, smoked, snorted	*Also, for amphetamine—rapid breathing/tremor, loss of coordination; Irritability, anxiousness, restlessness, delirium, panic, paranoia, impulsive behavior, aggressiveness, tolerance, addiction, psychosis*
MDMA (methylenedioxy-methamphetamine)	Adam, clarity, ecstasy, Eve, lover's speed, peace, STP, X, XTC	I/swallowed	*for cocaine—increased temperature/chest pain, respiratory failure, nausea, abdominal pain, strokes, seizures, headaches, malnutrition, panic attacks*
methamphetamine	*Desoxyn:* chalk, crank, crystal, fire, glass, go fast, ice, meth, speed	II/injected, swallowed, smoked, snorted	*for MDMA—mild hallucinogenic effects, increased tactile sensitivity, empathic feelings/impaired memory and learning, hyperthermia, cardiac toxicity, renal failure, liver toxicity*
methylphenidate (safe and effective for treatment of ADHD)	*Ritalin:* JIF, MPH, R-ball, Skippy, the smart drug, vitamin R	II/injected, swallowed, snorted	*for methamphetamine—aggression, violence, psychotic behavior/memory loss, cardiac and neurological damage; impaired memory and learning, tolerance, addiction*

TABLE 12-4 • Commonly abused drugs. (*continued*)

Substances: Category and Name	Examples of *Commercial* and Street Names	DEA Schedule*/ How Administered**	*Intoxication* Effects/Potential Health Consequences
nicotine	cigarettes, cigars, smokeless tobacco, snuff, spit tobacco, bidis, chew	not scheduled/ smoked, snorted, taken in snuff and spit tobacco	*for nicotine*—additional effects attributable to tobacco exposure; adverse pregnancy outcomes; chronic lung disease, cardiovascular disease, stroke, cancer, tolerance, addiction
Other Compounds			
anabolic steroids	*Anadrol, Oxandrin, Durabolin, Depo-Testosterone Equipoise:* roids, juice	III/injected, swallowed, applied to skin	*no intoxication effects*/hypertension, blood clotting and cholesterol changes, liver cysts and cancer, kidney cancer, hostility and aggression, acne; in adolescents, premature stoppage of growth; in males, prostate cancer, reduced sperm production, shrunken testicles, breast enlargement; in females, menstrual irregularities, development of beard and other masculine characteristics
Dextromethorphan (DXM)	*Found in some cough and cold medications; Robotripping, Robo, Triple C*	not scheduled/swallowed	*Dissociative effects, distorted visual-perceptions to complete dissociative effects*/for effects at higher doses see 'dissociative anesthetics'
inhalants	*Solvents (paint thinners, gasoline, glues), gases (butane, propane, aerosol propellants, nitrous oxide), nitrites (isoamyl, isobutyl, cyclohexyl):* laughing gas, poppers, snappers, whippets	not scheduled/inhaled through nose or mouth	*stimulation, loss of inhibition; headache; nausea or vomiting; slurred speech, loss of motor coordination;wheezing*/unconsciousness, cramps, weight loss, muscle weakness, depression, memory impairment, damage to cardiovascular and nervous systems, sudden death

Source: National Institute on Drug Abuse, information retrieved from http://www.nida.nih.gov/, updated January 3, 2008.

*Schedule I and II drugs have a high potential for abuse. They require greater storage security and have a quota on manufacturing, among other restrictions. Schedule I drugs are available for research only and have no approved medical use; Schedule II drugs are available only by prescription (unrefillable) and require a form for ordering. Schedule III and IV drugs are available by prescription, may have five refills in 6 months, and may be ordered orally. Some Schedule V drugs are available over the counter.

**Taking drugs by injection can increase the risk of infection through needle contamination with staphylococci, HIV, hepatitis, and other organisms.

***Associated with sexual assaults.

Commonly Abused Drugs

At this point in your life, you know that drug abuse is a significant health problem in the United States. Furthermore, you have probably already established your position on drug abuse. In that regard, we will not go into a great deal of detail for the various categories of drugs. You may refer to Table 12-4 for a summary of these drugs and use the Web sites listed in the following "Web Link" to get the latest information on commonly abused drugs.

Drug abuse is a condition affecting all of society. Much of substance abuse deterrence activity has been directed toward preventing drug abuse among the nation's youth. But all segments of society are vulnerable to drug-taking behaviors, especially college learners, because they are people who are for the most part living independently from family influences (Figure 12-7). You can use the information from Table 12-4 or the "Web Links" section to become informed about abused drugs, but there are four drugs in particular that deserve significant attention because of the serious risks they pose to college learners.

Rohypnol

Rohypnol is the trade name for a chemical compound, flunitrazepam, commonly known as the "date rape drug." The drug is a very powerful central nervous system depressant manufactured as a short-term treatment for insomnia. Rohypnol is legal in South America and Europe, but the drug cannot be manufactured in the United States, nor is it approved for sale. Because this drug is odorless and tasteless, it can be placed in the drink of an intended sexual assault victim. In this case, the individual to be affected by the drug does not take it intentionally; thus, abuse occurs when someone places a tablet in the drink of an unsuspected victim. Once consumed, Rohypnol causes a slowing of psychomotor performance, muscle relaxation, decreased blood pressure, sleepiness, and/or amnesia. The impaired party becomes so heavily sedated that the perpetrator(s) can perform sexual acts on the helpless victim. Moreover, the victim may awaken 10 to 12 hours later and have no clear recollection of what happened.

The actual incidence rate of Rohypnol-induced sexual assaults is difficult to track because victims are embarrassed to report the incident or do not have a clear enough recollection of events to describe the situation to legal authorities. The use of this date rape drug has declined somewhat since 1999 because the Drug Enforcement Agency is intercepting the drug as smugglers attempt to bring it across the border. In addition, the manufacturer now produces the tablet so that if it is dissolved in liquid, the liquid turns blue. This telltale sign can be masked if perpetrators serve blue tropical drinks. Furthermore, some of the original noncolored tablets are still in circulation.

The advice is simple for anyone who wants to avoid becoming a victim of Rohypnol intoxication. Whenever you are at a social gathering where beverages of any kind are available, *always* get your own drink, and never let your drink sit on table while you go do something else. Take your drink with you when you go talk with someone, use the bathroom, get something to eat, and so on.

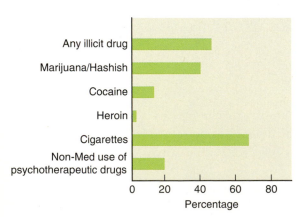
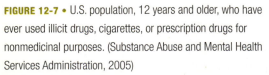

FIGURE 12-7 • U.S. population, 12 years and older, who have ever used illicit drugs, cigarettes, or prescription drugs for nonmedicinal purposes. (Substance Abuse and Mental Health Services Administration, 2005)

Methamphetamine

Methamphetamine is a derivative of amphetamine and has limited medical uses for the treatment of narcolepsy (a sleep disorder) and attention-deficit/hyperactivity disorder. The doses of methamphetamine used to treat these two disorders are much lower than those typically taken by abusers.

Methamphetamine is an addictive stimulant drug that strongly activates certain systems in the brain. The central nervous system actions that result from taking even small amounts of methamphetamine include increased wakefulness, increased physical activity, decreased appetite, increased respiration, hyperthermia, and euphoria. Other central nervous system effects include irritability, insomnia, confusion, tremors, convulsions, anxiety, paranoia, and aggressiveness. Because prescription use is carefully controlled, methamphetamine is not readily available, so it is made in illegal laboratories and has a high potential for abuse and addiction.

Although statistics indicate methamphetamine use slightly declined in recent years among noninstitutionalized (e.g., prisoners and mental health patients) respondents, the number of users is still quite high, with 850,000 people aged 12 and older admitting in 2008 that they used the drug during the past year. (SAMHSA, 2009).

Methamphetamine is taken orally, by snorting the powder, by needle injection, or by smoking. Abusers often become addicted quickly, needing higher doses that are administered more often. Frequent use may lead to irritability, anxiety, insomnia, confusion, tremors, convulsions, cardiovascular collapse, and death.

The health effects of "meth" are well documented. Methamphetamine releases high levels of the **neurotransmitter** dopamine, which stimulates brain cells, enhancing mood and body movement. Methamphetamine also appears to have a neurotoxic effect, damaging brain cells. Over time, the user may develop a tremorlike disorder similar to Parkinson's disease. The National Institute on Drug Abuse reports almost 20 years of animal research confirming that meth damages nerve endings, which do not repair themselves. The drug causes increased heart rate and blood pressure and can cause irreversible damage to blood vessels in the brain, producing strokes. Long-term effects may include paranoia, aggressiveness, extreme anorexia, memory loss, visual and auditory hallucinations, delusions, and severe dental problems. Methamphetamine can cause damage to the brain that is detectable months after long-term use of the drug. Methamphetamine use leads to brain damage similar to effects caused by Alzheimer's disease, stroke, and epilepsy.

Methamphetamine addiction is very difficult to treat because of the highly addictive nature of the drug. The methamphetamine user goes through a great deal of discomfort during withdrawal of the drug. Trying to treat the user on an outpatient basis (not hospitalized) is difficult because the user spends much of his or her time in an environment laden with numerous cues that rekindle the individual's craving for the drug. It is one thing to help the user withdraw from meth use; the most challenging phase of treatment is to restructure the social, emotional, and cognitive elements associated with the methamphetamine craving.

neurotransmitter
a chemical in the body that regulates the movement of impulses among nerve cells

Did You Know...?

Methamphetamine is harmful not only to the meth user but to the environment. Meth is manufactured in illegal laboratories. For every pound of methamphetamine manufactured in these laboratories, there are five to seven pounds of waste dumped into community landfills and sewers.

Cocaine

Cocaine is a powerfully addictive stimulant drug. The powdered form of cocaine can be snorted or dissolved in water and injected with a syringe. "Crack cocaine" is cocaine that has not been processed to create the powdered form. Crack is found as a rock crystal that can be heated and its vapors smoked. The term *crack* refers to the crackling sound one hears when the drug is heated. Cocaine's effects appear almost immediately after single dose and disappear within a few minutes or hours, depending on how the drug was

What's News

A 2009 study revealed that adolescents who use cocaine or ecstacy may be more likely to develop "reinforcing effects," making them more vulnerable to developing addiction.

Did You Know…?

According to the Drug Abuse Warning Network (SAMHSA, 2008), emergency room reports related to drug misuse or abuse indicate that cocaine has been associated with more emergency visits than any other drug, including alcohol. Among 958,164 emergency rooms visits for treatment of illicit drug abuse, 548,608, cases involved cocaine (57 percent).

administered. Taken in small amounts (up to 100 milligrams), cocaine usually makes the user feel euphoric, energetic, talkative, and mentally alert, especially to the sensations of sight, sound, and touch.

The physical effects of cocaine on the body include constricted blood vessels, dilated pupils, and increased body temperature, heart rate, and blood pressure. The user's nervous system is hyperstimulated. The initial high is dependent on the method of administration. If crack is smoked, the high is quick and intense but diminishes quickly. Users who look for the intense high find themselves quickly addicted to the drug. Some users of cocaine report feelings of restlessness, irritability, and anxiety. There are many users who use the drug very frequently in order to avoid the uncomfortable feelings that set in when the drug is not present.

The health effects of cocaine are numerous and depend to some extent on the method of administration. Regularly snorting cocaine, for example, can lead to a reduced sense of smell, nosebleeds, problems with swallowing, hoarseness, and a chronically runny nose. Ingesting cocaine can cause severe bowel gangrene due to reduced blood flow in the intestines. People who inject cocaine can experience severe allergic reactions and, as with all forms of injected drug use, increase their risk for contracting HIV and other blood-borne diseases.

It is not uncommon for cocaine users to develop a tolerance for the drug. Some users will frequently increase their doses to intensify and prolong the euphoric effects. People who have recently stopped abusing stimulant drugs such as cocaine generally experience a condition known as "abstinence syndrome" characterized by low energy, irritability, restlessness, an inability to feel pleasure, and problems with concentration. Anxiety and panic attacks also are sometimes associated with cocaine abstinence.

Marijuana

Marijuana is by far the most commonly abused illicit drug in the United States. The principal chemical ingredient in marijuana is THC (delta-9-tetrahydrocannabinol). When someone smokes marijuana, THC rapidly passes from the lungs into the bloodstream, which carries the chemical to organs throughout the body, including the brain. In the brain, THC connects to specific sites called *cannabinoid receptors* on nerve cells, influencing the activity of those cells. Some brain areas have many cannabinoid receptors; others have few or none. Many cannabinoid receptors are found in the parts of the brain that influence pleasure, memory, thought, concentration, sensory and time perception, and coordinated movement. The effects may last from one to three hours.

Marijuana use contributes to a number of health effects. The short-term effects of marijuana can include problems with short-term memory and learning, distorted perception, difficulty in thinking and problem solving, loss of coordination, increased heart rate, and diminished reaction time. Some of marijuana's adverse health effects occur because THC impairs the immune system's ability to fight disease. In laboratory experiments that exposed animal and human cells to THC or other marijuana ingredients, the normal disease-preventing reactions of many of the key types of immune cells were inhibited. Marijuana use may compromise the circulatory system. One study indicated that a user's risk of heart attack more than quadruples in the first hour after smoking marijuana. This is likely due to the influence of the marijuana chemicals on the heart and blood vessels. Regular marijuana smoking apparently produces effects on the lungs similar to the effects from tobacco smoking.

In addition to the addictive nature of marijuana, research asserts that early exposure to marijuana can increase the likelihood of a lifetime of subsequent drug problems. A recent study examined the marijuana habits of more than 300 fraternal and identical twin pairs. The pairs differed on whether they used marijuana before the age of 17, and the results indicated that the twin who used marijuana during his or her younger years was more likely to report elevated rates of other drug use and drug problems later in life when compared with the twin who did not use marijuana before age 17.

Marijuana Treatment

There is not much literature on the success of treating marijuana abuse. The problem with getting this information is that people are generally not treated for marijuana abuse alone. Treatment data indicate that, in 2002, marijuana was the primary drug of abuse in about 15 percent (289,532) of all admissions to treatment facilities in the United States. When users present themselves for rehabilitation, they generally are using marijuana in combination with other drugs. According to research at the National Institute on Drug Abuse (2005), interventions that treat the whole person, not just the drug dependence, are most successful. The most successful interventions include intense counseling sessions, including group and individual counseling. The success rate is not very good. It appears that only 25 to 40 percent of clients are abstinent at follow-up (six months to one year later). Scientists are testing cannabinoid antagonists (medications that block the receptor sites for THC) on animals. Perhaps in the years to come, there may be a medication to treat marijuana dependence.

Social Costs of Drug Abuse

There are many costs and harmful consequences associated with drug abuse. According to the White House Office of National Drug Control Policy (2007), the total economic cost of drug abuse in the United States is estimated at nearly $200 billion. Approximately

WEB LINK

National Institute for Drug Abuse in Spanish

http://www.drugabuse.gov/NIDAHome.html

At this Web site, you will see a link for materials "En Español." If you have family, friends, or neighbors who are Spanish speaking, the link may be useful.

SEARCH TERMS: drug trafficking, drug penalties, drug laws

40 percent of this total comes from the abusers and their families. It is no wonder that drug abuse also contributes to poverty, dysfunctional neighborhoods, homelessness, gang activities, drug trafficking, and the disruption of family systems. Drug users, both males and females, are often involved in domestic violence and divorce.

In 2005, American hospitals managed a total of 108 million emergency room visits, and the Substance Abuse and Mental Health Services Administration (2008) estimates that 1,449,154 emergency room visits were associated with drug misuse or abuse. Those emergency room visits are characterized as follows:

- Thirty-one percent involved illicit drugs only.

- Twenty-seven percent involved pharmaceuticals only.

- Seven percent involved alcohol only in patients under the age of 21.

- Fourteen percent involved illicit drugs with alcohol.

- Ten percent involved alcohol with pharmaceuticals.

- Eight percent involved illicit drugs with pharmaceuticals.

- Four percent involved illicit drugs with pharmaceuticals and alcohol.

WEB LINK
Drug Stories

http://www.drugstory.org/index.asp

At this Web site, you will find good information about drug abuse topics. Of special interest is a section where there are true personal stories from ex-drug users and family members about problems with all categories of drug abuse. Another good site, especially if you are or will be a parent, is **http://www.drugfree.org.**

SEARCH TERMS: stories of drug abuse, drug effects, drug categories, drug information for parents

Human Costs of Drug Abuse

Research indicates that drug abusers have a shorter life expectancy than do people who are not drug abusers. Approximately 20,000 people die every year from causes related to illicit drug use. Drug abusers expose themselves to the risks of overdose, poisoning, liver damage, and accidental death. Nonphysical consequences include job loss, ended friendships, and legal punishment, such as imprisonment. Risks increase even more if the user is selling drugs to support his or her drug habit; the illegal drug market is laden with violence.

The risks and consequences of various drugs are well documented. Although there are many physical and psychological problems related to drug abuse, the real tragedy lies in the users' loss of personal control and failure to achieve life goals. The preoccupation with drugs takes people away from the really important tasks of managing their adult lives and preparing for retirement. Generally, a person who continues using illegal drugs will experience one of three outcomes:

1. They may outgrow or overcome their need for drugs and get on with their lives.

2. They may be sent to jail.

3. They may suffer serious illness or die while using drugs (overdose, accidents, or homicide).

Drug Testing

Drug abuse is such a social concern that some employers use drug testing to ensure that their employees are not drug users. Airlines, hospitals, law enforcement agencies, and

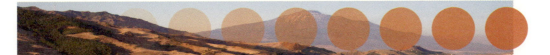

What's Your View?

Imagine that you are applying for a job, and the employer asks you to submit to a drug test.

- How would you feel about being asked to take such a test in order to get a job?

- What circumstances would be legitimate reasons for employers to require drug testing?

- Do you feel that companies should be permitted to make drug screening a condition for employment?

- Do you believe that employers should have the right to randomly test employees after they have been employed?

other organizations where drug use by employees may put the public at risk have adopted this strategy. Some companies may implement drug testing to avoid hiring employees who may bring drug problems with them.

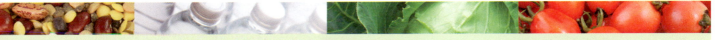

BUILDING YOUR WELLNESS PLAN

Virtually every adult will make a decision regarding beverage alcohol. Some people choose to consume alcohol; some choose to abstain from consumption. Not everyone needs to drink, nor will everyone who chooses to drink become an alcoholic. By now, you probably have made your decision, and it is hoped that you have accumulated information to support your decision. Perhaps you are still contemplating whether you want to drink. It is hoped that the material in this chapter will help you reach a good wellness decision. Here are a few key things you may want to take with you:

- It is okay to abstain. You can abstain without starting, and you can stop after you have started. The key is to be safe.

- Be informed. It does not matter if you are an abstainer or a user; good information can help you defend your decision and protect your well-being.

- Respect the decisions of others—to a point. If, for example, you choose to use alcohol and a friend wishes to abstain, give your friend support for his or her decision, but if your friend gets to the point of abusing drugs or alcohol, don't be afraid to advocate for a wellness lifestyle.

- Develop a set of values that you will be able to transmit to family or friends. This is especially true if you have a family of your own. You have a responsibility to protect your children.

Opportunities for Application

1. Imagine you have a close friend who is beginning to abuse drugs or alcohol. Prepare a letter to him or her expressing your concern and include some information about the kind of drug he or she is involved with and the potential negative effects of continuing with the drug taking.

2. Go on the Internet and find three sites that you would give as referrals to a friend whom you perceive as having a drug addiction. Record the names of the sites, their URLs, and a brief summary of the information presented.

3. Imagine that alcohol and marijuana were about to be introduced to Isovania (a fictitious country in eastern Europe, isolated because of its mountainous terrain, and having a democratic government). What advice would you give the government regarding the introduction of these two substances into the country?

Key Concepts

1. Prepare a list of the three most dangerous drugs and justify why each drug is on your list.

2. Explain why alcohol is a drug and discuss its potential for abuse and addiction.

3. Imagine that a child, yours or a friend's, comes to you and poses one of the following questions:

"Which is worse, smoking marijuana or tobacco?"

"Which is worse, using marijuana or alcohol?"

Prepare responses to each of the questions and include scientific evidence in your response.

Answers to Personal Assessment: Facts about Substance Abuse

Facts about Substance Abuse

1. False. Each gram of pure alcohol contains seven calories.

2. True

3. True. Especially if the foods eaten are high in fat content.

4. False. Doing so only results in a wide awake drunk.

5. False. Alcohol dependence does not favor a particular beverage.

6. False. Seventy-eight percent of the alcohol is absorbed in the small intestine.

7. False. The answer would be true if alcohol were not included. Doing so lowers the age.

8. False. Recent experiments on laboratory animals demonstrated that addiction can occur.

9. True. Alcohol is second.

10. True. In fact, 70 percent of all inmates were using drugs before they went to prison.

●●● References

Grucza, R. (2008). Drinking at an early age can lead to later alcohol *dependence*. Retrieved June 2, 2008, from http://www.brighsurf.com/news/headlines/38162/Drinking_at_an_early_age_can_lead_to_later_alcohol_dependence

Leshner, A. I. (2001). *Treatment, education and prevention: Adding to the arsenal in the war on drugs.* Retrieved January 6, 2007, from http://www.nida.nih.gov/Testimony/3-14-01Testimony.html

Makamural, K.J., Conigrave, K.M., Mittleman, M.A., Camargo, C.A., Stampfer, M.J., Willett, W.C.,

Rimm, E.B. (2003). Roles of drinking pattern and type of alcohol consumed in coronary heart disease in men. *The New England Journal of Medicine, 348,* 109–118.

National Highway Traffic Safety Administration. (2009). *Traffic Safety Facts, 2008 Data: Alcohol-Impaired Driving.* Washington, DC: NHTSA's National Center for Statistics and Analysis [DOT HS 811 155].

National Institute on Alcohol Abuse and Alcoholism. (2006). *U.S. Adult Drinking Patterns.* Retrieved May 17, 2010 from http://www.niaaa.nih.gov/NR/rdonlyres/E170A639-B684-41A6-8EB6-1237AF74E56C/0/DrinkingPatterns.pdf

National Institute on Alcohol Abuse and Alcoholism. (2000). *10th special report to the U.S. Congress on alcohol and health*. Washington, DC: U.S. Department of Health and Human Services.

National Institute on Alcohol Abuse and Alcoholism. (2009). Percentage of adults who reported binge drinking by state and gender, BRFSS, 1984–2008. Retrieved March 20, 2010 from http://www.niaaa.nih.gov/Resources/DatabaseResources/QuickFacts/Adults/brfss03.htm

National Institute on Drug Abuse. (2005). *Research report: Marijuana abuse* (Publication No. 05-3859). Rockville, MD: National Institutes of Health.

Substance Abuse and Mental Health Services Administration (SAMHSA), Office of Applied Studies. (2008). *Drug Abuse Warning Network, 2006: National Estimates of Drug-Related Emergency Department Visits*. DAWN Series D-30, DHHS Publication No. (SMA) 08-4339, Rockville, MD.

Substance Abuse and Mental Health Services Administration (SAMHSA). (2009). *Results from the 2008 National Survey on Drug Use and Health: National Findings* (Office of Applied Studies, NSDUH Series H-36, HHS Publication No. SMA 09-4434). Rockville, MD.

White House Office of National Drug Control Policy. (2007). *Office of National Drug Control policy*. Retrieved from http://www.whitehousedrugpolicy.gov/index.html

CHAPTER 13

Infectious Diseases

CHAPTER OBJECTIVES

When you finish this chapter, you should be able to:

- Explain why most infectious diseases are not as dangerous as they once were.
- State the causes of infectious diseases.
- Describe the chain of infection.
- Discuss ways of preventing infectious diseases.
- Describe the five stages of the disease process.
- List the most common infectious diseases among college students, their causes, and specific ways to prevent them.
- Explain the meaning and significance of bioterrorism.

KEY TERMS

bacterial meningitis
botulism
Campylobacter
cauterization
cryosurgery
endotoxins
Escherichia coli
exotoxins
fomites
infectious diseases
opportunistic
   infections
pathogenic organisms
replication
salmonellosis
scabies
secondary infection
self-imposed
   quarantine

●●● Introduction

It is hoped that as you read this chapter, you are in a state of optimal health. It would be nice if everyone always stayed healthy and well, but the reality is that humans share the ecosystem with organisms that can make us ill. Recall that **infectious diseases**, though less life threatening than they were at the start of the twentieth century, are still with us. Despite years of medical advances, **pathogenic organisms** can still make us ill. Some infectious diseases are dealt with by our immune system, with the body healing naturally, but some infections require medical attention (Figure 13-1), and others may last a lifetime; still other diseases can result in death. This chapter is about infectious diseases, how they affect your health, and how you can prevent illnesses that are caused by contagious organisms.

infectious diseases
diseases that are caused by some form of pathogenic organism

pathogenic organisms
also called pathogens, living organisms that can cause disease by invading the body's tissues and multiplying; commonly referred to as germs

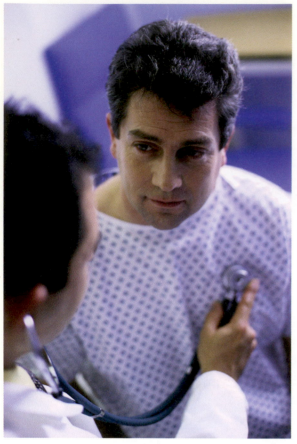

Courtesy of Photodisc

FIGURE 13-1 • Infectious diseases are caused by pathogenic organisms that may require medical attention when the body's immune system is unable to handle the disease naturally.

●●● History of Infectious Diseases

Infectious diseases were the leading causes of death throughout history through the early 1900s. In chapter 1, you learned that the major causes of death in the United States at the beginning of the twentieth century were tuberculosis, pneumonia, diarrhea, and intestinal and stomach diseases. Back then, not many children lived to see adulthood, and most adults died by the time they were 45 years old. It is hard to believe that during the Spanish-American War in 1898, only 968 U.S. soldiers died of battle injuries. The other 5,438 deaths during that war were the result of infectious diseases (Figure 13-2).

Medical research has contributed much to our knowledge of infectious diseases. The health habits we routinely practice now, such as hand washing and bathing, were not viewed in the same way 200 years ago. The value of these practices was largely unknown at the time because we did not have a complete understanding of "germs." Once we understood that certain organisms led to diseases, we were able to emphasize the importance of good hygiene practices. These practices, combined with improved medical procedures and medications, have greatly reduced death and illness caused by bacterial and viral infections. By the mid-1940s, chronic diseases replaced infectious diseases as the number one cause of death, and the human life span was greatly increased. Do infectious diseases still kill people? Yes, but far fewer than 100 years ago.

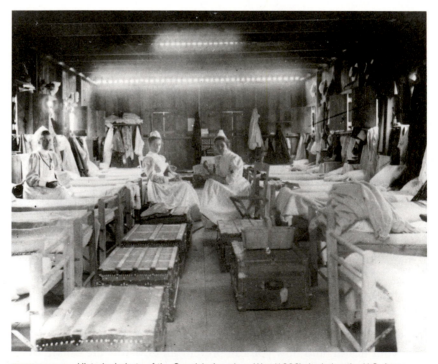

FIGURE 13-2 • Historical photo of the Spanish-American War (1898) depicting the U.S. Army Sternberg General Hospital, Camp Thomas, Cickamauga, Georgia, "Dormitory C." Photo courtesy of the U.S. Army Center for Military History

PERSONAL ASSESSMENT
Personal Habits

Read each of the statements below and record your answers. Briefly explain your reasons for doing or not doing each of the behaviors. An interpretation of your answers is located at the end of the chapter. Do you:

1. Know which immunizations you have had and when you had them? List the immunizations and the dates they were given.

2. Wash your hands often and especially before you eat?

3. Share grooming products (razor, makeup, hairbrush, comb, and so on) with others?

4. Cover your nose and mouth when you sneeze and cough?

5. Share food, eating utensils, straws, or drinks with others?

6. Wear clean socks and clothes?

7. Get regular medical checkups? Give the date of your last checkup.

8. Avoid coming into contact with the blood or body fluids of another person without wearing protection?

9. Know how to safely handle and store food?

10. Take care of your body by eating a balanced diet, getting exercise, and getting plenty of rest?

TABLE 13-1 • Types of pathogens.

Pathogen	Description	Common Diseases	Treatment
Viruses	Smallest units of living material; requires host cells to reproduce	Common cold, measles, mumps, chickenpox, influenza, herpes, human immunodeficiency virus	No cure; drugs and medications to relieve symptoms. Vaccines help prevent the diseases.
Bacteria	One-celled microorganisms	Tetanus, strep throat, food poisoning, tuberculosis, pneumonia, syphilis, gonorrhea	Antibiotics. There are about 150 antibiotics available; certain antibiotics are cures for specific bacterial infections.
Fungi	Plantlike pathogens such as molds and yeasts	Athlete's foot, vaginal yeast infection, athletic itch, ringworm	Various antifungal medications
Protozoa	One-celled microscopic animal-like organisms	Dysentery, giardiasis, malaria, vaginal infection	Various medications designed to kill the organism
Multicellular parasites	Organisms composed of numerous cells that use humans or animals as hosts	Scabies, tapeworm, hookworm	Various lotions and medications designed to kill the organism

Delmar/Cengage Learning

●●● Causes of Infectious Diseases

The organisms that cause infectious diseases come in a variety of forms and sizes. You have probably heard about bacteria or viruses, but you may not know that there are many other organisms such as fungi and parasites that can also cause illness. Each pathogenic organism potentially causes a specific disease. Table 13-1 describes the various types of

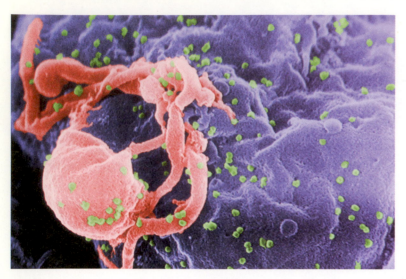

FIGURE 13-3 • Scanning electron micrograph of HIV-1 virus on a lymphocyte.
Courtesy of CDC; photo by C. Goldsmith, P. Feorino, E. L. Palmer, and W. R. McManus

pathogens, some common diseases, and treatments. More detail is presented in the following sections.

Viruses

Viruses are the smallest of all life forms, so small that they can be seen only with very powerful electron microscopes (Figure 13-3). Viruses need host cells in order to survive and reproduce. These organisms can affect animals, plants, or bacteria. In humans, when a virus enters the body, it will seek out a specific type of cell and attach itself to that host cell. For example, the human rhinovirus is the cause of the common cold. There are more than 100 variations of the rhinovirus, and it is believed that the virus is constantly mutating. This is why we are able to get repeated colds year after year. Here's how the cold virus infects the upper respiratory system:

1. A virus particle enters the body because you touched a contaminated surface and brought your fingers to your mouth and/or nose or inhaled droplets with viruses from the air.

2. The virus attaches to cells lining the back of your nose and throat, where temperature and moisture are just right for **replication**.

3. The virus enters the host cell and quickly produces new viruses using the genetic material from the host cell.

4. The infected host cell breaks, sending new virus particles to infect the upper respiratory tract. Because you have lost some cells that line your throat and sinuses, fluid is able to flow into your nasal passages, giving you a runny nose.

5. Viruses in the fluid that drips down the back of your throat also attack cells lining your throat, causing your throat to feel sore. The pathogen does not go deep into the lungs because the temperature there is too high for replication.

replication
a process whereby viruses use the genetic material of host cells to produce new virus particles

Diseases are not evenly distributed around the country, nor are the diseases always caused by the same strain of a particular virus. It is a well-known fact that the "seasonal flu" outbreaks we have each year during the winter months are caused by a different influenza virus each year. Moreover, various strains of influenza viruses can be present at the same time. If you examine Figure 13-4, you will notice that CDC's tracking of influenza during the 2009–2010 season involved the tracking of five strains of Type A Influenza, including H1N1 and one strain of Type B Influenza. Note also the number of H1N1 cases indicating that the H1N1 outbreak was early in the flu season and was quite strong and it existed among many other Type A cases that were not subtyped. The Type B cases were comparatively small, thus they do not appear clearly on the bars.

Did You Know...?

Smoking increases the risk of a secondary lung infection as a complication of the common cold by 50 percent.

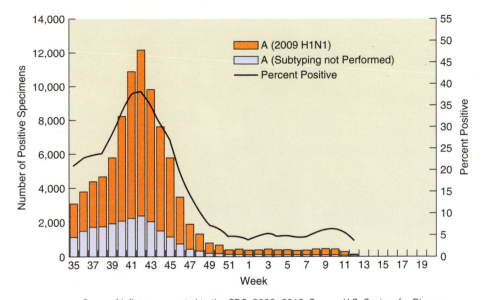

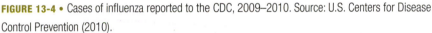

FIGURE 13-4 • Cases of influenza reported to the CDC, 2009–2010. Source: U.S. Centers for Disease Control Prevention (2010).

What's News

A virus usually found in the Middle East first appeared in New York City in 1999. Known as the West Nile virus, this organism is transmitted by mosquitoes that feed off infected birds. There were 62 human cases of West Nile infections in New York in 1999. In the years that followed, the disease moved from the New York area to the central United States, down the East Coast and west toward Texas. In 2009, the Centers for Disease Control (CDC) reported cases of West Nile infections in every state. The number of cases in New York was down to six in 2009, but Texas led the nation with 104 cases.

Bacteria

Bacteria are larger and more complex than viruses. They come in many forms. Figure 13-5 shows some of the common bacteria types. Most bacteria are harmless. In fact, at any given point in time, you have 10 times more bacteria in and on your body than you have body cells. Some bacteria are "friendly," living in your intestines, where they help digest food; other bacteria are used in baking, such as when putting the "sour" in sourdough bread. But some bacteria contribute to diseases in humans, causing conditions such as strep throat, food poisoning, wound infections, tuberculosis, gonorrhea, tetanus, and even toothache.

Bacteria produce illness to the body through one of two mechanisms. Some varieties of pathogenic bacteria produce **exotoxins**, which are poisons produced and released by the bacteria. These toxins are harmful to specific living body cells, producing such health effects as food poisoning, whooping cough, **botulism**, or diphtheria. Other bacteria may produce **endotoxins**, which are poisons contained within the cell wall of the bacteria and released as the bacteria die. Diseases such as **bacterial meningitis** and **tetanus** are caused by endotoxins. In other instances, the bacteria may transmit the toxin simply by coming into contact with the healthy cells.

exotoxins
poisons produced by and released from certain bacteria

botulism
a strong toxin that affects muscles in the body that can result in death if not treated quickly and properly; most often due to improperly canned foods

endotoxins
poisons that come from the cell wall of certain bacteria when they die

bacterial meningitis
inflammation of brain lining caused by various forms of bacteria

tetanus
a bacterial disease that affects the nervous system, commonly known as lockjaw; results in death about 10 percent of the time

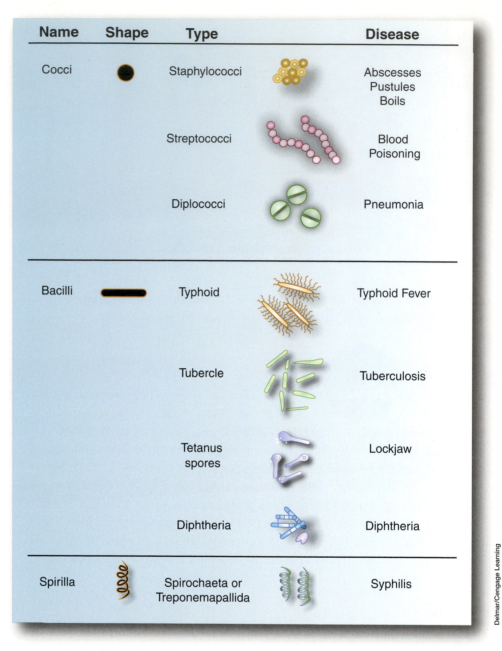

Name	Shape	Type		Disease
Cocci	●	Staphylococci		Abscesses Pustules Boils
		Streptococci		Blood Poisoning
		Diplococci		Pneumonia
Bacilli	▬	Typhoid		Typhoid Fever
		Tubercle		Tuberculosis
		Tetanus spores		Lockjaw
		Diphtheria		Diphtheria
Spirilla		Spirochaeta or Treponemapallida		Syphilis

Delmar/Cengage Learning

FIGURE 13-5 • Various forms of bacteria.

Bacteria are among the oldest life forms on the planet. They grow and reproduce under specific conditions, depending on the species of bacteria. The conditions required for bacterial growth are the following:

- *Suitable nutrients.* Each species of bacteria has specific nutritional requirements. Some bacteria use sulfur as a food source, while others may use living tissue.

- *Suitable atmosphere.* The atmosphere needed for bacteria survival isn't necessarily oxygen. For example, some bacteria *must* have oxygen for survival, some cannot survive in the presence of oxygen, and some will survive with very little oxygen.

- *Suitable temperature.* The most rapid bacterial growth occurs if the temperature is between 60 and 120 degrees Fahrenheit. In general, bacteria do not tolerate extreme heat or cold, yet there are bacteria that live and thrive only in hot sulfur springs and some species that can grow in the cold of outer space.

- *Suitable pH.* pH is a measure the acidity or alkalinity of a given solution. A pH of 1 is acidic, and a pH of 14 is alkaline. Hydrochloric acid has a pH of .5, healthy skin has a pH of 5, and household ammonia has a pH of 11.5. Bacteria thrive in species-specific pH ranges.

- *Suitable osmotic potential.* The ability of the bacteria to pull moisture into the cell as needed.

- *Suitable moisture.* Bacteria are 80–90 percent water, thus they must live in an aqueous environment. Some bacteria live in salty water such as the Dead Sea where the water contains 30 percent salt, other forms of bacteria will live in water that is only 2 percent salt.

If bacteria come in contact with an environment that is not specifically suitable for their growth and multiplication, they will die. For example, as concerned as many people are about their health, it is not likely that they would obtain a bacterial infection from a toilet seat, as the conditions for bacterial survival are not that good.

Bacterial diseases can be prevented with **immunization** and can be cured with the use of **antibiotics**. There are more than 150 antibiotics that can treat bacterial infections. Each disease has to be matched with the antibiotic that will destroy the pathogenic bacteria and cure that particular infection. Laboratory tests are needed to assess the particular bacterium causing a disease. One method to make this determination is to grow a culture of the bacteria in a laboratory (Figure 13-6) and examine the organism's characteristics. Only medical professionals know which antibiotic will work on which infection based on a test for the particular organism.

immunization
introduction of an agent that enables the body to become immune to effects of that agent

antibiotics
a class of medications that kill bacteria and clear up infection

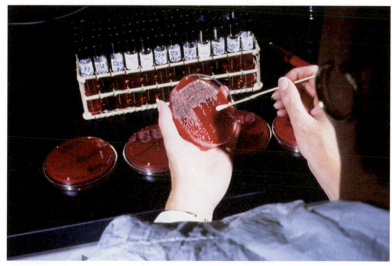

Courtesy of Photodisc

FIGURE 13-6 • Laboratory cultures are used to identify bacteria.

Fungi

Fungi are plantlike organisms such as molds, yeasts, and mushrooms. More than 70,000 forms of fungi have been identified. Fungi range from single-celled microscopic organisms to what might be one of the largest organisms on the earth. (In 1992, scientists in

What's News

Studies are showing that a strain of bacteria that causes tuberculosis is now resistant to the current treatment medications. This poses a serious threat to treating tuberculosis worldwide.

Michigan discovered an underground fungus that was almost 40 acres in size and an estimated weight of more than 100 tons.) Some fungi are pathogenic. Conditions such as ringworm, athlete's foot, nail fungus, bread mold, or vaginal yeast infections are troublesome but not life threatening. On the other hand, the pneumonia that is most likely to take the life of a person with acquired immune deficiency syndrome is a fungus, and the "death cap" mushroom kills the consumer after about six days of illness. Never pick and eat wild mushrooms unless you are able to clearly identify them as safe. Not all fungi are pathogens. For example, many forms of mushrooms are used as a food source; certain yeasts can be used to make bread, wine, and beer; and one form of mold, *Penicillium chrysogenum*, is used to make penicillin.

Protozoa

parasites
organisms that rely on a host organism for survival; usually the host organism is harmed in some way

scabies
infection caused by a small mite

Protozoa are one-celled, animal-like microscopic organisms. Some protozoa are harmful to humans because they are **parasites**, although there are fewer than a dozen such parasites in the United States. One of them is *Giardia intestinalis* (Figure 13-7), which can be picked up by drinking untreated water, particularly from mountain streams and lakes. The organism makes it way into water sources from infected wild animals (and, in some cases, humans), and hikers who drink the contaminated water can become very ill after a few days, with abdominal cramps, nausea, vomiting, and diarrhea. The condition is not life threatening, but it is very uncomfortable. Giardia can be avoided by boiling water or treating it with appropriate chemicals. If the source of drinking water is not a treatment plant, an approved well, or the site of a melting glacier, it must be treated before it is safe for drinking. Dysentery, a severe form of diarrhea, is caused by an amoeba.

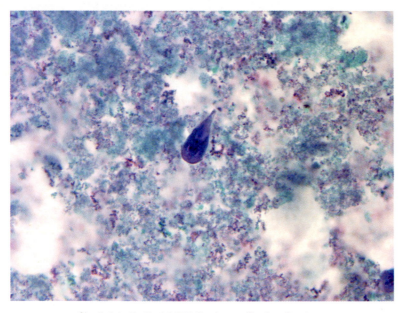

FIGURE 13-7 • *Giardia intestinalis* at 1,000-times magnification. Courtesy of CDC/Melanie Moser

Multicellular Parasites

The largest of the pathogenic organisms are the multicellular parasites. These organisms generally undergo a life cycle that includes stages of development that are outside the human host. There are very few multicellular parasites that affect humans in the United States, and those cases that do occur are confined to the southeastern United States. Some multicellular parasites are very small, such as small mites (0.3 to 0.5 millimeters), which cause **scabies** (Figure 13-8). The condition is cured with the correct type of prescription lotion. Other multicellular parasites can be up to 20 feet long, such as tapeworms that come from eating infected raw meat and cause severe intestinal illness.

Another example of a multicellular parasite is a roundworm known as *Ascaris lumbricoides*. This roundworm is the most common worm infection in humans and can be found in rural areas of the southeastern United States. It is transmitted as an egg through contaminated soil that may be accidentally swallowed. Once it enters the host's body, it lives in the small intestine, where it feeds off the host. The organism may live one or two years and generally produces no discomfort unless there are several worms present.

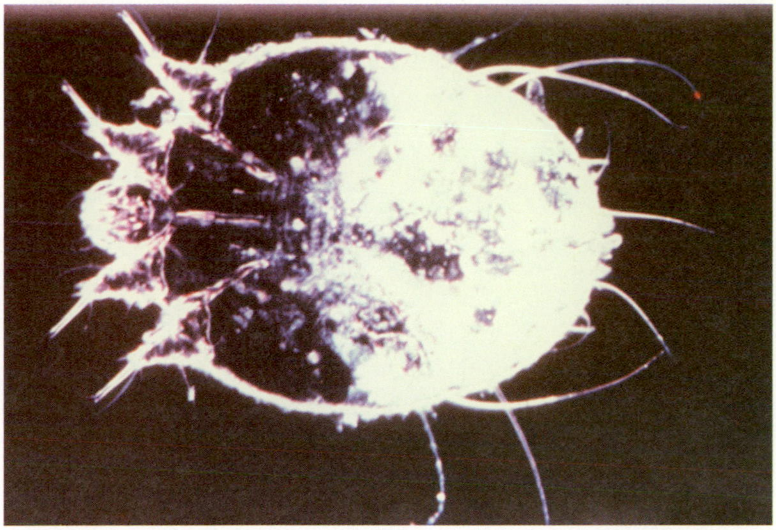

The Chain of Infection

Infectious diseases are spread in a variety of ways. Some diseases are communicable, which means they can be spread directly from one person to another. Some pathogens can be transmitted in the air or by touch, which is why it's important to cover your mouth when you sneeze and wash your hands before handling food. Other ways of transmitting infectious diseases include contact with infected soil, food, or animals. What we know about communicable disease has come from the development of the germ theory of disease. Although germ theory evolved during centuries of scientific growth, it was the works of Louis Pasteur and Robert Koch during the mid-1800s that confirmed the role of pathogens in causing diseases and how to prevent their spread.

An outcome of germ theory was a model that proposed an understanding of the infection process. The chain of infection, presented in Figure 13-9, illustrates each of the conditions or links in the model that must be present for infection to spread. If any of the elements in the chain are not available, transmission cannot continue. This is an extremely important concept. Infectious diseases are controlled by breaking one of the links through preventive practices, medications, changes in the environment such as ensuring clean water supplies, and/or careful hand washing.

FIGURE 13-8 • Scabies mite (microscopic view). Courtesy of CDC

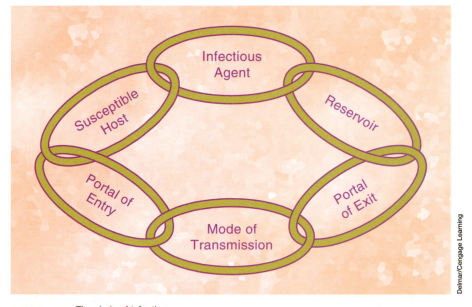

Delmar/Cengage Learning

FIGURE 13-9 • The chain of infection.

There are six "links" in the chain of infection. Let's look at the model as it pertains to the common cold:

1. *Infectious agent.* A pathogenic organism, such as a virus or a bacterium, is present. *The virus for the cold may be from a number of viruses, but a variation of the rhinovirus is the cause in most cases.*

2. *Reservoir.* A place where the organism can grow and reproduce. This may be inside a human or an animal or in a material such as water, soil, or food. *The reservoir for the cold virus is the back of the nose. Moisture and temperature are appropriate for the virus to multiply.*

3. *Portal of exit.* A specific way for the pathogenic organism to leave the reservoir. Portals of exit vary, depending on the organism. *The cold virus exits from the nose or mouth.*

4. *Mode of transmission.* A way for the organism to move from the reservoir via the portal of exit into another host. Modes of transmission may involve direct contact, such as kissing, sneezing, coughing, consuming or handling contaminated food or water, and insect or animal bites. Some organisms are transmitted by way of **fomites**. A desktop, doorknob, soda can, and cutting board are examples of fomites. *The cold virus may be transmitted via droplets in the air or from a fomite, but you are actually more likely to catch the cold virus from a desktop or doorknob than from breathing the same air as another person who has a cold.*

fomites
inanimate objects that transmit pathogenic organisms

5. *Portal of entry.* The location and means by which the pathogen is able to enter the body. The portal of entry is specific to the disease condition. Bacteria that produce food poisoning enter through the mouth and then move down the esophagus to the stomach. The portal of entry for human immunodeficiency virus infection is the bloodstream. The virus cannot get into the body through the skin unless there is an open sore. *Cold and flu viruses enter through the nose, mouth, or eyes.*

6. *Susceptible host.* An individual lacking immunity against the pathogen is vulnerable to developing the illness. This can be a person who is not immunized against the disease, who has a weak immune system, or whose behavior puts him or her at risk for a disease. Not everyone who is exposed to a pathogen becomes ill. Some people have very good immune systems that keep them healthy. Depending on the disease, a susceptible host can become a new reservoir.

Did You Know...?

Researchers at the University of Arizona analyzed samples from personal work spaces and found that the average desk held 400 times more bacteria than the average toilet seat. But the "germiest" place among all the work spaces examined was the telephone.

Preventing Infectious Diseases

Management of infectious diseases occurs when the chain of infection principles is applied. Information about the organisms, host characteristics, and the environment is helpful in controlling the spread of disease. Having this information allows us and health care workers to develop behaviors and regimens to prevent infections.

Breaking the Chain of Infection

It's only necessary to break one link in the chain of infection to stop infectious organisms in their tracks. Each of the links may have its own specific breaking point:

1. *Infectious agents.* Organisms can be killed with chemicals that destroy them or prevent their reproduction. Water in our local water supplies is chlorinated because chlorine kills harmful bacteria that have not been otherwise removed during the water treatment process. When you are camping, you can make your drinking water safe by boiling it for at least one minute, and you can add water treatment tablets as an additional precaution. Other things you can do to eliminate infectious agents include thoroughly cooking foods that require cooking and keeping your environment clean of waste materials and trash. Bacterial infections can be treated with antibiotic tablets, lotions, or ointments. If the doctor prescribes an antibiotic, be sure to use it according to directions and for the prescribed amount of time. Failure to do so may result in a recurrence of the infection, possibly with bacteria that have developed mutations that are resistant to the antibiotic. This makes follow-up treatment more difficult.

2. *Reservoir.* Prevent bacteria and other harmful pathogens from multiplying by taking away the reservoir where the pathogens may live. Bacteria can't grow on food if you refrigerate it or freeze it properly. If you cover food that sits on a counter, the bacteria in the air can't fall on the food and grow. Wash your hands before and after handling raw meat to reduce the possibility of contaminating the meat. Keep cold foods cold and hot foods hot. The West Nile virus is carried and transmitted by mosquitoes, and eliminating standing water on your property will eliminate mosquito breeding grounds. Stay home when you are ill; there is no need to take the "reservoir" to class or work.

3. *Portal of exit.* Cover your mouth when you cough or sneeze. Throw away infected tissues or bandages, disposing of them in a covered trash can. If you have a communicable disease, stay away from other people. This method is called **self-imposed quarantine**. A person with a sexually transmitted infection can use barrier protection to block transmission of the pathogens.

4. *Mode of transmission.* One of the most effective ways of stopping the mode of transmission, according to the CDC, is to wash your hands often. Sexually transmitted infections can be avoided by practicing abstinence or postponing sexual activity until you know your intended partner very well and are comfortable discussing these infections and ways to prevent them. Medical personnel never touch the body fluids of another person without protective gloves.

5. *Portal of entry.* Avoid touching your face, especially your nostrils and eyes, during the cold and flu season. *Stay away* from injected drug use unless prescribed by a doctor. Don't share eating utensils, straws, or drinks. Never share toothbrushes or razors.

6. *Susceptible host.* Keep your body healthy with plenty of rest, exercise, and a balanced diet. Don't put yourself at risk of getting diseases. Have regular checkups to detect signs of disease. Get all necessary immunizations and keep them up to date.

self-imposed quarantine
voluntarily staying away from other people when you are ill so as not to spread disease

Did You Know...?

One major study showed that children with asthma were more likely to have upper respiratory infections if they lived where there was a high cockroach population.

Immunizations

Immunity means being resistant to the pathogens causing certain diseases. In order to understand immunization, you need some knowledge of the body's antigen–antibody response to pathogenic agents. An antigen is a protein substance that is characteristic

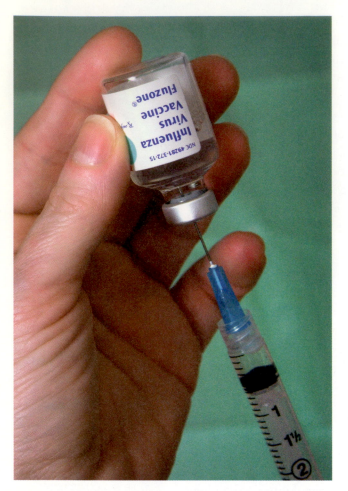

FIGURE 13-10 • Vaccines are given in specific dosages. Courtesy of CDC; photo by Jim Gathany

of the pathogen. When the antigen enters the body, it is "read" by the body's immune system which triggers the release of antibodies, structures that identify and neutralize pathogens. People can develop immunity in a number of ways:

1. *Active naturally acquired immunity* occurs when the person experiences a natural infection of a pathogen and becomes immune to that pathogen on recovery. This explains why the person may only get that particular disease once. Chicken pox is an example.

2. *Active artificially acquired immunity* happens when an individual is actively vaccinated with a protein of the pathogen that confers immunity (Figure 13-10). An example is the vaccination for diphtheria. Tetanus is another example, but, unlike diphtheria, tetanus requires booster immunizations every 10 years.

3. *Passive naturally acquired immunity* takes place when a baby receives antibodies from his or her mother by a natural process, such as in breast milk or through the transfer of antibodies from mother to fetus during pregnancy. This form of immunity does not protect one from a particular disease; rather, it helps strengthen the immune system in general.

4. *Passive artificially acquired immunity* occurs when someone is injected with pooled serum from immune individuals that contains antibodies.

Active artificially acquired immunization (also known as vaccination) is a procedure that encourages immunity to specific infectious diseases by developing and testing vaccines that contain various forms of the virus or bacteria that cause a disease. In some cases, the vaccines are designed to prevent a disease from occurring or to lessen the effects if the disease does occur. An example is immunization to prevent respiratory influenza. In other circumstances, a vaccine can be used to prevent a disease from progressing. Clinicians are currently testing a vaccine that would prevent people infected with the human immunodeficiency virus from developing acquired immune deficiency syndrome.

Most of the important immunizations we have today were developed at the beginning of the twentieth century. Since the process of immunizing began, billions of people have been protected from devastating diseases such as smallpox, diphtheria, whooping cough, tetanus, and yellow fever. Perhaps you never heard of some of those diseases. The fact that you have not heard about them demonstrates the miracle of immunizations because in the past, these diseases commonly affected every neighborhood. Smallpox, once a major life-threatening concern, is now virtually extinct, and polio and measles have been virtually eradicated from the United States. Polio and measles are still found in countries that do not have aggressive immunization programs.

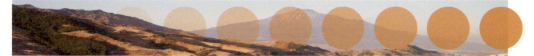

What's Your View?

A Position on Immunization

Although immunizations have saved countless lives, the procedure is not without controversy. States require children to have immunizations before starting school. In 2007, the state of Texas passed a law requiring all 12-year-old females to get immunized against human papillomavirus, a sexually transmitted infection that is a precursor to cervical cancer. There are arguments against requiring vaccines. Some people say, for example, that people should have a choice to receive the vaccine, that some people get sicker from the immunization, and that immunizations are costly. Those in favor, however, argue that everyone should get immunized to protect themselves and the public. Do you think schools should require this form of immunization?

- If your local health department announced it had a new vaccine that prevented human immunodeficiency virus infections, would you be willing to get the vaccine, or would you hold off and see how it affected other people?

- What would your reaction be if the immunization were required?

Disease Progression

Once a pathogen enters the body, the infected person's immune system goes into action and distributes antibodies to fight the infection. A person with a very strong immune system will destroy the invader before the organism has a chance to produce symptoms. This is an example of a *nonsusceptible* host. In the instances when the immune system cannot destroy the invader, the infected person gets ill. Infectious diseases progress through five separate stages (Figure 13-11):

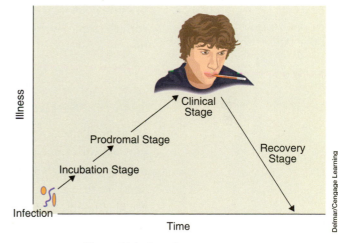

FIGURE 13-11 • Stages of infectious diseases.

1. *Infection.* Infectious diseases begin when a susceptible host becomes infected with a pathogenic organism. The organism enters the body through its specific portal of entry and "sets up housekeeping" where it can grow and multiply.

2. *Incubation stage.* During this stage, the pathogenic organism starts to multiply. The incubation period varies with each disease and ends when symptoms appear. Incubation may last hours (food poisoning), a couple of days (common cold), or even years (**human immunodeficiency virus [HIV]**). At the end of the incubation stage, a disease is usually highly contagious.

3. *Prodromal stage.* Infected people in this stage will begin to feel sick, although they won't have all the symptoms of the disease. With a common cold, the person may

human immunodeficiency virus (HIV)
a virus that can multiply and destroy a portion of the human immune system

feel a sore throat or feel achy and tired. Although the person is not really ill, he or she can still pass the disease on to someone else. Obviously, this is a very significant aspect of the communicable disease process because people who are prodromal don't feel sick enough to stay home or seek medical treatment.

4. *Clinical or illness stage.* It is during this stage that symptoms appear. For example, a person who is clinically ill with a cold will sneeze, cough, and have a runny nose. One of the reasons the common cold is so prevalent is because it is a disease that is uncomfortable but not so much so that it causes most people to avoid their daily activities, such as attending classes or going to work.

5. *Recovery stage.* Recovery begins when the body's immune system starts to overcome the pathogenic organisms and illness symptoms begin disappearing. This may take a few hours or a few weeks, depending on the disease and the treatment given. Many bacterial illnesses can be treated with antibiotics. Specific antibiotics cure specific diseases; there is no single antibiotic that treats all diseases and infections. An important fact about antibiotics is that they can't kill viruses, which is one reason why there isn't a cure for the common cold. It is important when taking antibiotics to take the entire prescription, even if you begin to feel better before you use all the medication. If you stop taking the antibiotic just because you think you are cured, the few bacteria that remain can reproduce, but they become capable of altering their genetic core to create a resistance to the antibiotic. One form of the bacterium causing gonorrhea has now mutated to the point where the bacteria use antibiotic penicillin as a food source. Thus, physicians now use tetracycline to treat gonorrhea.

During the recovery stage, disease-causing organisms are still in the body. It is possible in some instances for a person suffer a **relapse**, a condition in which someone gets sick with the same illness before fully recovering. It is important to take care of yourself during the recovery stage so that relapse does not occur.

relapse
a condition in which someone gets sick with the same illness before fully recovering

●●● Major Infectious Diseases

Many kinds of infectious diseases affect humans; however, we are more likely to be infected with some pathogens than with others. Knowing which diseases are most likely to infect adults, along with knowing the pathogens that cause them, how they are spread, and how they can be prevented, will help you develop wellness skills to prevent or reduce the likelihood of infecting you and others.

The Common Cold

The most frequently occurring infectious disease in America is the common cold. More than 200 rhinoviruses are known to cause colds. Contrary to popular belief, colds are *not* caused by cold temperatures or cool drafts. The "cold season," the time of year when the majority of colds occur, is usually between early September and late April. The reason colds are more frequent during that time period has to do with how colds are transmitted, which is from person to person. During the cooler months, people spend more time indoors together, thus increasing the chance of being exposed to cold viruses.

There are several mechanisms whereby colds can be spread from one person to another. The most common is by touching a fomite and then touching the eyes, nose, or mouth. You can see how effective frequent hand washing is for preventing illness during the cold season. Inhaling the virus when someone sneezes or coughs is another way of becoming infected. The least likely way a person can become infected with a cold is by inhaling virus particles that have been suspended in the air because the virus particles are widely dispersed in the air.

Colds are usually most contagious from the second to the fourth day of infection, when the greatest number of viruses is present in nasal fluids. It takes only one or more virus particles to cause the cold. Colds usually peak in a couple of days and run their course in 7 to 14 days. Symptoms include sneezing, nasal discharge, obstruction of nasal breathing, swelling of the sinus membranes, sore throat, cough, and headache.

Because most colds are caused by viruses and usually go away on their own, seeing a doctor for medications or antibiotics won't help. It's actually a waste of money. The only effective way to treat a cold is to get rest and drink lots of fluids. You can take a pain reliever to reduce aches and discomfort you might experience. You may need to see a doctor, however, if you develop a **secondary infection**, one of the harmful side effects of a cold. Secondary infections occur when the cold turns into another type of infection, such as bronchitis, ear infection, or pneumonia. This type of complication involves the presence of some other pathogen. Colds, on their own, cannot produce secondary infections, nor is the cold life threatening. If you have a cold that worsens rather than improves after a couple of weeks, you should see your doctor to find out if you have a secondary infection that is treatable.

Influenza

Another common infectious disease is influenza, or "flu." There are three main types of flu virus: A, B, and C. The A and B viruses are more likely to be the cause of flu in humans, and there many variant subtypes of the A and B viruses. Flu is caused by one of these virus subtypes and is spread when an infected person coughs and the virus is transmitted into the air where it can be breathed in by others. The flu, like the common cold, can also spread through fomites, so it's important to avoid touching your face and mouth, especially during the flu season.

The incubation period for the flu is one to four days, and a person is considered contagious the day before symptoms appear until three to five days after symptoms begin. These symptoms include headache, chills, dry cough, body aches, fever, stuffy nose, and sore throat and may last for one or two weeks before they start to improve. People are often confused between flu and cold symptoms. A comparison of the symptoms for both of these diseases is presented in Table 13-2. Even though the flu may cause you to feel miserable for a week or two, it can be deadly for elder adults and young children. Influenza kills approximately 20,000 to 30,000 people each year. Approximately 90 percent of these deaths are among adults over age 65. The reason is that the immune system changes as one ages. In elder adults, the immune system begins to decline at all levels. Essentially, the way the body communicates among its cells and structures is altered, and the antigen–antibody reaction is greatly compromised.

Did You Know...? The National Institute of Allergy and Infectious Diseases estimates that there are more than 1 billion common colds in the United States within a one-year time span.

secondary infection an infection that arises at a location other than the original site; usually caused by a second pathogen or irritant

TABLE 13-2 • Comparison of cold and flu symptoms.

Condition Symptom	Cold	Flu
Fever	Fever is rare with a cold.	Fever is usually present with the flu in up to 80 percent of all flu cases. A temperature of 100°F or higher for 3 to 4 days is associated with the flu.
Coughing	A hacking, mucus-producing cough is often present with a cold.	A non-mucus producing cough is usually present with the flu (sometimes referred to as dry cough).
Aches	*Slight* body aches and pains can be part of a cold.	Severe aches and pains are common with the flu.
Stuffy Nose	Stuffy nose is commonly present with a cold and typically goes away within a week.	Stuffy nose is not commonly present with the flu.
Chills	Chills are uncommon with a cold.	About 60 percent of people who have the flu experience chills.
Tiredness	Tiredness is fairly mild with a cold.	Tiredness is moderate to severe with the flu.
Sneezing	Sneezing is commonly present with a cold.	Sneezing is not common with the flu.
Sudden Symptoms	Cold symptoms tend to develop over a few days.	The flu has a rapid onset—within 3–6 hours. The flu hits hard and includes sudden symptoms like high fever, aches, and pains.

Delmar/Cengage Learning

Scientists recently developed medications to help treat the flu, not cure it. Most of these medication are effective for type A influenza strains. At the present time, only Tamiflu and Relenza are effective against type A and type B influenza strains. Known as antiviral medications, they must be started very soon after the symptoms begin in order to be effective. Even with these medication, your bout with the flu will be shortened by only a day or so.

Food Poisoning

Food poisoning is another type of infectious disease, usually caused by food that is contaminated with certain types of bacteria. Some foods, such as certain varieties of fungi (mushrooms), are toxic in their natural form.

Campylobacter is a bacterial pathogen that causes fever, diarrhea, and abdominal cramps. It is the most commonly identified bacterial cause of diarrheal illness in the world. These bacteria live in the intestines of healthy birds, and most raw poultry meat has *Campylobacter* on it. Eating undercooked chicken or other food that has been contaminated with juices dripping from raw chicken is the most frequent source of this infection. The disease appears about two to three days after consuming the infected food. The infected person will generally recover without any medical intervention.

Salmonellosis, probably the most common form of food poisoning, is caused by *Salmonella* bacteria. Most persons infected with salmonella develop diarrhea, fever, and abdominal cramps 12 to 72 hours after infection. The illness usually lasts four to seven days, and most persons recover without treatment. However, for some people the diarrhea may be so severe that the patient needs to be hospitalized. In these patients, the salmonella infection may spread from the intestines to the bloodstream and then to other body sites and possibly causing death unless the patient is treated promptly with antibiotics. Elderly adults, infants, and those with weak immune systems are more likely to develop severe cases. Poultry, meat, or fish can be contaminated with the bacteria,

Campylobacter
a species of bacteria that causes diarrheal illness in the United States

salmonellosis
food poisoning caused by *Salmonella* bacteria from contaminated food sources, especially chicken and other meat products

which can multiply if the food is allowed to sit at room temperature. In the United States, there are there are between 1 million and 2 million cases of salmonella poisoning each year. Mild cases of salmonella are often undiagnosed, so the exact number of actual cases is difficult to determine.

An estimated 55 percent of all food poisoning cases are caused by improper cooking and storage of foods; 24 percent are caused by poor personal hygiene, such as not washing the hands before handling food and using unclean preparation surfaces. Only 3 percent of food poisoning cases are caused by an unsafe food source. You can prevent food poisoning by practicing the following safe food-handling behaviors, which were also presented in chapter 9:

> ## Did You Know…?
>
> Scientists have isolated at least 250 diseases that are caused by spoiled and contaminated food.

- Keep your hands clean while working with or eating food. This is the single most important thing you can do to prevent food poisoning. If you are going to contaminate your food, it is most likely to come from some bacteria you picked up during your regular activities during the day.

- Refrigerate leftover food as soon as possible. As food sits in the open air, it is subject to the "rain of terror"—pathogens that are falling from the environment. Once food is refrigerated, always check it before you eat it. If food of any kind smells bad, do *not* attempt to eat it. It should be discarded.

- Never eat vegetables, such as beans, asparagus, or greens, coming from a can that has a bulge in it. The bulge is created by gases produced by *Clostridium botulinum*, a potentially deadly bacterium that produces a nerve toxin. This type of food poisoning is called botulism.

- Always cook ground meat thoroughly. Undercooking the meat increases the likelihood of food poisoning.

- Never defrost poultry at room temperature; thawing should be done in the refrigerator. Poultry is a perfect environment for cultivating food-borne pathogens. If it is thawed outside the refrigerator, it is likely that pathogens will begin to grow on the warm outer surfaces before the inner tissues defrost.

- Avoid cross contamination. This means not allowing raw meat, poultry, or fish or any surface touched by these raw foods to come into contact with other foods.

- Don't use a wooden cutting board because organisms breed in the grooves made by knives. It is safer to use a ceramic or acrylic cutting board if the board is cleaned after each use. If you do choose to use a wooden board, be sure to periodically disinfect it with bleach.

Escherichia coli, a strain of rod-shaped bacteria that are found in the intestinal tract of humans and mammals, is the leading cause of food-borne illness. *Escherichia coli* O157:H7 (Figure 13-12) is one of hundreds of strains of the bacterium. An estimated 73,000 cases of *E. coli* infections and approximately 61 deaths result from *E. coli* in the United States each year. The organism is contracted when food, swimming pools, lakes, and streams are contaminated with infected feces. It can also be spread via human to human contact by way of contaminated feces, which is why good health practices include thoroughly washing hands after using the bathroom.

Escherichia coli
a form of bacteria that inhabit the intestinal tracts of humans and other mammals

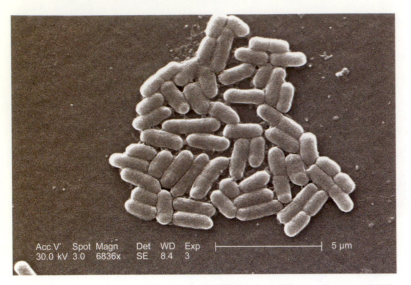

Food-borne spread of the disease can be prevented if beef and vegetables are cooked to at least 160 degrees Fahrenheit.

An infected, susceptible host will become ill two to three days after consuming the pathogen. Bloody diarrhea and intestinal pain are the obvious symptoms of infection. The patient is not likely to have a fever. There is no special treatment for this condition except drinking a lot of water and watching for complications. The patient should not take medicine to stop diarrhea unless approved by a doctor. Taking antidiarrheal medications prevents the intestines from getting rid of the *E. coli* germ.

FIGURE 13-12 • *Escherichia coli* O157:H7 at 6,836-times magnification. Courtesy of CDC

Acc.V Spot Magn   Det WD Exp
30.0 kV 3.0 6836x   SE 8.4 3
5 µm

Mononucleosis

Infectious mononucleosis is an extremely common disease among college students. It is caused by a common virus called the Epstein-Barr virus. Often referred to as "mono," infectious mononucleosis is nicknamed "the kissing disease" because it spreads primarily through intimate contact with infected saliva, but it can easily be spread by sharing drinking or eating utensils or via droplets if someone is sneezing or coughing. The incubation period for mono is from four to six weeks. Symptoms, which usually last about four weeks, include swollen glands in the neck, white patches in the back of the throat, fever, weakness, sore throat, headaches, tiredness, and lack of appetite. Although mono goes away without treatment, individuals with the disease should get plenty of rest and drink a lot of fluids. If symptoms don't go away in a couple of weeks, check with a physician. In some cases, the tonsils and adenoids become so enlarged that it is difficult to breathe. This more serious condition requires a doctor's care and may be treated with steroids to reduce the swelling.

What's News

In late September 2006, 199 people from 26 states were reported to the CDC with *E. coli* O157:H7 infections. Among the ill persons, 102 (51 percent) were hospitalized, and 31 (16 percent) developed a type of kidney failure called hemolytic-uremic syndrome. Three people died from their infections. It was soon discovered that the cases resulted from consumption of uncooked spinach from 13 packages. Further investigation revealed that the spinach was contaminated by cattle next to one of the growing fields. Water runoff carried the cattle waste and bacteria into the spinach field. The *E. coli* was absorbed into the spinach leaves; thus, washing could not remove the bacteria.

Conjunctivitis

Conjunctivitis, also known as pinkeye, is another common infectious disease. Conjunctivitis is caused by several types of viruses and bacteria and is spread by contact with either respiratory fluids or eye discharges from infected individuals. It can also be spread by sharing articles of clothing, towels, makeup, and grooming supplies that touch the face or eyes, so it's important that people not share these items.

Symptoms of conjunctivitis include a white or yellowish discharge from under the eyelid, matted eyelids during sleep, reddening and swelling of the eyelids, tearing, and pain. The incubation period is one to three days for bacterial conjunctivitis and 5 to 21 days for viral conjunctivitis. Most cases are mild and go away on their own. If you have conjunctivitis in which the symptoms are very painful or last for more than five days, you should see a doctor.

Strep Throat

Strep throat is a serious throat infection caused by a variety of round bacteria called *Streptococcus*. Strep throat is transmitted by sneezing and coughing or via fomites. The incubation period for strep throat is about five days. Some people, known as **carriers**, can be infected with strep throat and have no symptoms. Although they are not sick themselves, they can infect other people. Animals, including pets, can also be carriers of strep throat.

carriers
infected people who do not show symptoms of a disease but who can spread it to others

The symptoms of strep throat include fever, stomachache, headache, and a throat that hurts so badly that it is hard to swallow. Strep throat is usually easy to treat with antibiotics, but it is important to take the medicine exactly as it is prescribed. Not taking all the medicine or not taking it in the manner prescribed can result in a relapse. Strep throat that has relapsed can be harder to treat because the streptococci can develop resistance to the original antibiotic, rendering the antibiotic ineffective in killing the bacteria.

Strep throat can be very serious. If left untreated, it can even result in death. If you develop a sore throat and know you have been around someone who has been diagnosed with strep throat, you should see a doctor as soon as possible to be tested for the bacteria. The doctor will take a swab of your throat and have it tested for the presence of the bacteria. If the test comes back positive, your doctor will prescribe a 10-day antibiotic regimen, generally penicillin, unless you are allergic to penicillin, in which case erythromycin may be used.

Tuberculosis

Recall from chapter 1 that tuberculosis (TB) was the number one cause of death in the early 1900s. For many years, the number of cases declined, and in 2006 there were 13,779 cases of TB reported in the United States, the lowest rate since 1953. A number of those cases were reported among immigrant populations. This infection is caused by bacteria that travel through the air. It is spread when an infected person coughs or sneezes, propelling the bacteria into the air, where they can be inhaled by other people. Because the bacteria are inhaled, TB usually infects the lungs, but it can also infect other organs, such as the brain, kidneys, and liver. Left untreated, it can be fatal. Some types of TB are easily cured with antibiotics, but there is a new type of the bacteria that is resistant to many antibiotics and can be deadly.

Did You Know...?

In any given year, two-thirds of the world's population is infected with tuberculosis, and almost 2 million people die from tuberculosis-related illnesses.

TB is caused by a bacterium known as *Mycobacterium tuberculosis*. Symptoms of TB include weight loss, night sweats, feeling sick or weak, and fever. When the bacteria infect the lungs, the symptoms include coughing, chest pain, and coughing up blood. If you think you have been exposed to TB, you should see your doctor as soon as possible because exposure can be determined by a simple skin test. People who test positive for TB exposure may have medications prescribed to kill the bacteria before they develop the illness.

Sexually Transmitted Infections

Sexually transmitted infections (STIs; sometimes called sexually transmitted diseases [STDs]), as their name suggests, are infections spread by sexual contact. The United States has the highest rates of STDs in the industrialized world. The rates of STDs, accounting for more than 18 million *new* cases each year, are 50 to 100 times higher in the United States than in any other industrial nation. Most cases of STIs in America occur among people in the 15- to 24-year-old age-group, and African Americans are disproportionately represented among other racial groups. Each of the major STIs is discussed next and summarized in Table 13-3. For a variety of historical and political reasons, some STDs are reported from all 50 states to the CDC. At the present time, the reportable list includes gonorrhea, syphilis, and chlamydia.

Chlamydia

The most common STI in the United States is chlamydia, caused by a bacterium called *Chlamydia trachomatis*. Chlamydia is associated with almost 3 million cases a year in the United States. The number of cases has been steadily rising since 1984, when chlamydia reporting began. In 2008, there were 1,210,523 new cases of chlamydia reported to the CDC (2009a). Women are three times more likely to have a chlamydia infection than are men, and women aged 15–24 had a case rate of over 3,100 infections per 100,000 women in that age range (Figure 13-13). Women had infections rates three trime higher than men. Although the infection rates for all races increased in 2008, minorities had far more new cases than whites (Blacks, eight time higher, Native Americans, 4.7 times higher, and Hispanics 2.9 times higher). The greatest number of new cases is found in the South, the fewest in the Northeast.

Most people infected with chlamydia don't have symptoms. If symptoms do develop, they usually appear within one or two weeks after exposure. Symptoms of chlamydia include a burning sensation when urinating, eye inflammation, minor discharge from the vagina or pus discharge from the penis, and pain or swelling of the testicles. More advanced cases may cause lower back and abdominal pain and fever. If chlamydia is left untreated, it can result in many serious complications, such as sterility, in both men and women.

Gonorrhea

Gonorrhea is caused by *Neisseria gonorrhoeae*, a bacterium that grows easily in the warm, moist areas of the male and female reproductive tracts, though infections can occur in the anus,

WEB LINK

Sexually Transmitted Infections

http://www.engenderhealth.org

At this Web site, you will find a complete "minicourse" on sexually transmitted infections.

SEARCH TERMS: understanding STIs, guide to infectious disease, infectious disease information

TABLE 13-3 • Common sexually transmitted infections.

Pathogen	Description	Symptoms	How Spread	Comments	Treatment
Pubic lice (crabs)	Parasites that live in pubic or armpit hair. They do not enter the genitals.	Intense itching in the area where they are found	Contact with infected bedding, clothing, towels, and toilet seats. Intimate and sexual contact. No protection from condom.	Pathogen is highly contagious. The only protection is limiting the number of intimate and sexual contacts.	Over-the-counter and prescription medication
Chlamydia	A type of bacteria that can enter the internal sex structures and can lead to sterility if not treated	Discharge from the penis or vagina. Pain when urinating. Up to 85 percent of women and 40 percent of men do not show any symptoms.	Sexual contact with someone who is infected with Chlamydia. Correct condom use can prevent transmission.	The number one STI in the United States	Must be treated with antibiotics. Partner must also be treated.
Gonorrhea	Caused by a bacterium. There are more than 700,000 new cases of gonorrhea reported each year.	Burning when urinating. Females may not have any symptoms.	Sexual contact; not typically transmitted by clothing	It is possible for some people to be infected for months without showing symptoms.	Antibiotics. Left untreated, gonorrhea can lead to pelvic inflammatory disease and sterility in women.
Syphilis	Caused by a spiral-shaped bacterium, *Treponema pallidum*	Various symptoms for each of the three active stages	Through direct sexual contact with an infected person	Blood test needed to confirm diagnosis	High doses of penicillin; other antibiotics for those with penicillin allergy
Herpes	Herpes simplex virus. More than 45 million people have been diagnosed with the disease.	Itchy or painful blisters that may appear on the shaft of the penis, vulva, vagina, buttocks, or scrotum	Sexual contact. Herpes can be spread even if the blisters are not present. Correct condom use offers limited protection.	Infected person has a responsibility to notify any present or future sexual partners.	There is no cure. Medications are available to relieve symptoms of the blisters.
Genital warts/ human papillomavirus (HPV)	Three varieties of a virus that attaches to the skin in the genital area. More than 20 million Americans are already infected.	Small, white bumps that resemble cauliflower. No pain or itching. Some forms of these viruses contribute to cancer of the cervix.	Sexual contact. Correct condom use offers limited protection.	There are more than 70 different types of HPV. HPV infections predispose women to cervical cancer.	There is no cure. The small tumors can be surgically removed.
HIV infection	Human immunodeficiency virus	Generally no symptoms with HIV infection. Symptoms of acquired immune deficiency syndrome will begin to appear years later, such as certain infections, fever, and respiratory problems.	Sexual behaviors and sharing needles during drug use	More than 36 million cases worldwide	No cure. Medications can help relieve symptoms and reduce likelihood of infections.

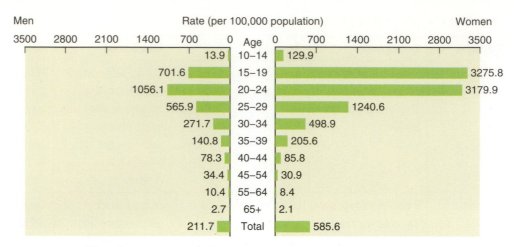

FIGURE 13-13 • Chlamydia age- and sex-specific rates, United States, 2008. Courtesy of CDC, 2009c

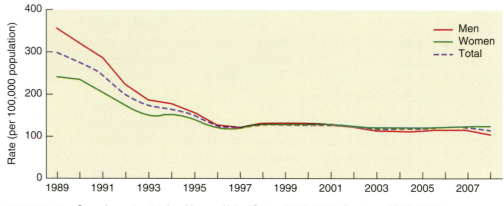

FIGURE 13-14 • Gonorrhea rates: total and by sex, United States, 1989–2008. Courtesy of CDC, 2009b

eyes, and throat. There are more than 300,000 new cases of gonorrhea in the United States each year; in 2008, this meant a rate of 111.6 cases per 100,000 people (Figure 13-14). The disease can be transmitted via oral, vaginal, or anal contact with an infected person. Any sexually active person is at risk for gonorrhea, but the disease is disproportionately prevalent among women, adolescents, young adults, and African Americans. Symptoms such as a burning sensation when urinating or yellow discharge from the penis or vagina may appear as soon as three to five days after exposure.

Because there are numerous strains of antibiotic-resistant gonorrhea in the United States and because many patients are showing chlamydia infections concurrently with gonorrhea, physicians presently prefer to treat patients with antibiotics such as Ofloxacin, tetracycline, Ciprofloxacin, or Cefixime.

Syphilis

Syphilis is an STI that is transmitted through direct sexual contact with a sore containing the causative pathogen, a bacterium called *Treponema pallidum*. The disease can also be transmitted from a woman to her baby during pregnancy. This condition is known as congenital syphilis. Because the symptoms of early syphilis resemble other illnesses, it has been called "the great imitator." Once infected, a person will exhibit the symptoms of *primary syphilis* in about three weeks. The first sign of primary syphilis is a raised, painless sore called a "chancre" that appears near the portal of entry. Other symptoms include swollen lymph glands. The chancre will go away without treatment after three to four weeks.

The disease will go into *secondary syphilis* after 2 to 10 weeks. During this stage, the infected person will experience a sore throat, fatigue, swollen glands, and a rash that is neither painful nor itchy. A person can get a second round of secondary syphilis. Again, the condition will go away without any treatment. After secondary syphilis passes, the infected individual enters *latent syphilis*. During this stage, there may be no symptoms, but the infected person is still able to transmit the pathogen to others. Once the disease progresses to the *tertiary syphilis*, the organism has gone deeper into the body tissues, affecting body organs and the nervous system. For this reason, a person with tertiary syphilis can no longer infect anyone else. This stage is not reached by all infected persons. It may take two to three years to reach tertiary syphilis. Once organs are damaged, they will not return to normal after treatment. The typically preferred treatment for syphilis is injection of penicillin G.

Herpes Simplex

Herpes simplex is a virus that causes genital herpes. There are two types of herpes simplex viruses (HSV). HSV-1 is the form that generally causes recurring sores (cold sores or fever blisters) on the lips, mouth, or face. HSV-2 is sexually transmitted herpes. Evidence indicates, however, that these two organisms can affect their alternate reservoirs. Symptoms include small blisterlike sores that heal themselves in one to two weeks. There are medications, such as acyclovir, that can hasten the recovery, but there are no cures for HSV infections. Once infected, the virus remains in the body, alternating between months or years of dormancy and active stages. A condom can reduce the probability of getting an HSV infection, but the condom offers no protection if the infection site of the carrier is on the pubic area where the condom does not provide a barrier. Not all HVS-2 sores are on or in the genitalia.

Human Papillomavirus

The human papillomavirus (HPV) is actually a collective title for approximately 100 viruses of this type. The virus precipitates a condition known as genital warts or condyloma. The warts appear at the site of the infection, someplace near the genitalia. The warts are not painful, nor are they cancerous, but they are unsightly. The greatest concern about HPV is its relationship to cervical cancer. In 2006, it was estimated that 10,000 women would be diagnosed with cervical cancer and that 4,000 would die from the cancer. The known relationship between HPV and cervical cancer is so strong that researchers have developed a vaccine that prevents two forms of HPV responsible for 70 percent of cervical cancers. The virus is transmitted from host to susceptible host via sexual contact. Approximately 20 million people are presently infected with HPV. Much like HSV infection, HPV cannot be destroyed or removed from the body; hence, genital

What's News?

A recent study confirms condom protection against HPV (Winer, et al., 2006). Young women whose partners used condoms every time they had intercourse were 70 percent less likely to contract HPV than were women whose partners used condoms less than 5 percent of the time.

cryosurgery
superfreezing tissue to destroy it

cauterization
using a small electrical probe to burn tissue to destroy it

acquired immunodeficiency syndrome (AIDS)
a condition caused by HIV infection whereby a portion of the immune system is destroyed, making it easy for the infected person to get life-threatening diseases

opportunistic infections
infections caused by organisms that would not be present in people with normal, healthy immune systems

warts will be a continual nuisance. The growths can be removed using surgery, **cryosurgery**, laser therapy, or **cauterization**.

HIV

HIV, as we now know it, was first identified in 1981, though it probably existed before that. It all began in June 1981, when the CDC received reports of five young men who died of complications of what we now know as **acquired immune deficiency syndrome (AIDS)**. Between 1981 and 1995, there were 551,515 reported cases of AIDS in the United States (85 percent male, 15 percent female). The fatality rate was almost 80 percent. Between 2001 and 2004, there were 163,809 new cases reported (71 percent male, 29 percent female) with a 7 percent fatality rate. Such is the changing face of the HIV/AIDS epidemic. The good news is that persons with AIDS are living longer; the bad news is that the disease is still a very significant public health problem. The CDC estimates there almost 1,000,000 people in the United States who are infected with HIV. The majority of cases are still among those in the 20- to 44-year-old age-group. Moreover, the condition is growing most rapidly among minority populations and is a leading cause of death among African American males ages 25 to 44 (Figure 13-15).

The portal of entry for HIV is any opening to the bloodstream; hence, open sores on the body or intravenous drug use are primary portals of entry. When HIV gets into the bloodstream, it seeks out T4 helper cells, a type of white blood cell that fights infection. The virus enters the T4 cell and then uses the material inside the cell to create more viruses that are then sent off to the bloodstream to find more T4 cells. At this point, a person is HIV positive, meaning that the virus is present and multiplying. Years later, the part of the immune system using the T4 cells for defense is weakened to the point where pathogens that would otherwise be fought off by the immune system appear. Infections with these specific pathogens are known as **opportunistic infections**. Once opportunistic infections are present, the patient fits the definition of having AIDS. These opportunistic infections become life-threatening conditions for a person with AIDS. Many people don't realize that no one has ever died from AIDS. Rather, people with AIDS generally die from complications associated with opportunistic infections, such as those listed in Table 13-4.

There is no cure for AIDS, but recent advances in antiretroviral therapy have minimized the effects of the opportunistic infections. Worldwide, there are more than 36 million people infected with HIV. Of these cases, only

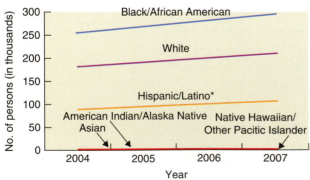

Estimated Number of Persons Living with HIV/AIDS, by Race/Ethnicity, 2004–2007—34 States

FIGURE 13-15 • Persons living with AIDS by race. Source: U.S. Center for Disease Control and Prevention (2009b).

TABLE 13-4 • Common opportunistic infections.

Affected Body System	Examples of Disease
Respiratory	Tuberculosis *Pneumocystis carinii* pneumonia
Gastrointestinal	Mycobacterium
Nervous	Toxoplasmosis
Skin	Kaposi's sarcoma Herpes simplex Varicella zoster
Urogential	Candidiasis Herpes simplex

Delmar/Cengage Learning

about 25 percent are receiving antiretroviral treatment for their condition. Currently, there are 26 antiretroviral drugs approved by the Food and Drug Administration to treat individuals infected with HIV. The recommended treatment for HIV is highly active antiretroviral therapy (HAART). Each HAART regimen is specific to the patient and contains a combination of three or more medications.

Preventing STIs

The research findings are clear. There are two ways to avoid transmission of STIs. The most reliable way to prevent the spread of these conditions is to abstain from sexual activity (oral, vaginal, and or anal sex) or be in a long-term monogamous relationship with an uninfected partner. Sexual behavior outside these two conditions poses a risk for contracting an STI. There are some practices that pose varying levels of protection, but none are 100 percent effective.

Male Condoms

Male condoms, if used correctly, can be effective in reducing the risk of contracting an STI during sex, but there are some STIs for which a condom may not provide complete protection. For example, HPV and herpes simplex can be transmitted by skin-to-skin contact. If one partner has an infection on his or her pubic area, the condom may not cover it, and the virus can be transmitted to the other person through skin-to-skin contact. Following are some precautions:

- Use a new condom with each sex act (e.g., oral, vaginal, and anal).

- Handle the condom carefully to avoid damaging it with fingernails, teeth, or other sharp objects.

- Put the condom on after the penis is erect and before any genital, oral, or anal contact with the partner.

- If a lubricant is needed, use only water-based lubricants (e.g., K-Y Jelly™, Astroglide™, AquaLube™, and glycerin) with latex condoms. Oil-based lubricants (e.g., petroleum jelly, shortening, mineral oil, massage oils, body lotions, and cooking oil) tend to destroy latex and will cause the condom to fail.

- Ensure adequate lubrication during vaginal and anal sex; this might require the use of water-based lubricants.

- To prevent the condom from slipping off the penis, hold the condom firmly against the base of the penis during withdrawal and withdraw while the penis is still erect.

- Use of animal membrane condoms is not recommended. The pores in the animal membrane can be 1,500 nanometers in diameter. While this size of a pore will block the penetration of sperm, a pore this size is about 10 times larger than the human immunodeficiency virus.

Female Condom

The female condom was approved for use by the U.S. Food and Drug Administration in 1993. It is a polyurethane sheath that is approximately six and a half inches long and is inserted into the vagina prior to any sexual intercourse. The inside of the female condom is lubricated with silicone, but additional lubricant can also be used, and the female condom can be used in addition to the male condom. One advantage of the female condom is that it can be inserted up to eight hours before intercourse. It also represents an alternative contraceptive device if the male partner refuses to use a condom. The pores in the female condom are sufficiently small to prevent transmission of sperm, bacteria, and viruses. Research indicates that the female condom is an effective barrier contraceptive device and offers protection against transmission of viruses and bacteria. It is a recommended option in the absence of the male condom. The failure rate for the female condom is related to human error. Used exactly as intended, the female condom is 95 percent effective but in actual usage is more like 80 percent effective.

Other Contraceptives

All other contraceptive methods, including the diaphragm, do not offer a high level of protection from STIs. Any contraceptive device that does not ensure adequate barrier protection will not protect against STIs. Some offer a higher degree of protection than others. Likewise, there are no sexual chemical lotions that prevent the spread of STIs. There is no clinical evidence, for example, that Nonoxynol-9 destroys the bacteria and viruses associated with STIs.

● ● ● Bioterrorism

bioterrorism
a form of terrorism in which biological agents (pathogens) are used to infect large segments of a population

You may be familiar with terrorism as a behavior used by some political groups to gain control, inflict damage on communities and terrorize the citizens, or raise awareness of their political causes. Terrorism can occur in many forms, such as suicide bombings. **Bioterrorism** is terrorism through the use of biological weapons, specifically the intentional release of pathogenic biological agents into the environment in an effort to cause death or injury to humans, animals, or plant life. For example, in 2001, anthrax was spread into the U.S. postal system and resulted in 22 deaths. In response to such events, the threat of bioterrorism is monitored by the U.S. Department of Homeland Security, created in response to terrorist attacks in New York City and Washington, D.C., in 2001. In addition to developing plans to address threats by all forms of terrorism, the department developed categories to classify biological weapons in order of their potential threat. Category A agents pose the greatest threat to the American public, are easily transmitted, and have high mortality rates. Anthrax and smallpox are examples of category A threats. The government is doing the most to address threats from this category. Category B and category C threats are not easily transmitted and are considered less life threatening.

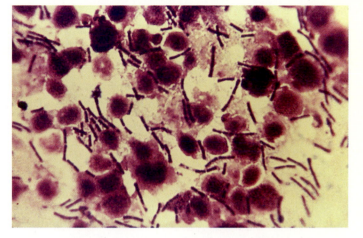

FIGURE 13-16 • Photomicrograph of *bacillus anthracis* (Anthrax Bacteria). Courtesy of CDC Public Health Image Library, 2005

Anthrax

Anthrax is a category A agent that was used in a biological attack in October 2001. Several citizens and government employees received letters in the mail containing a fine white powder that, when analyzed, turned out to be anthrax. Anthrax is a bacterial infection (Figure 13-16) that can be transmitted in a number of ways, but it cannot be spread from person to person:

1. *Inhalation.* This is the most serious form of anthrax and causes death in 99 percent of the cases if not treated quickly. This is what happened to some of the people who opened the contaminated mail in 2001. Inhaled anthrax infection usually starts with symptoms that are the same as severe colds and flu, but breathing soon becomes difficult. The general public does not come into contact with this form of anthrax unless it is introduced to the environment by criminals or terrorists. Farmworkers can be exposed to anthrax when they deal with materials from infected animals.

2. *Skin contact.* Anthrax can cause infections if it comes into contact with cuts or scratches. This is the least serious form, causing painless blisters that break and develop black scabs.

3. *Oral consumption.* This is the least common method of spreading anthrax to humans. It can be caused by eating undercooked meat from an infected animal.

Our bodies have some natural defenses to anthrax so that not everyone who is exposed to the bacteria will get the disease. All three types of anthrax are treatable with antibiotics, so it is important see a doctor quickly if exposure is suspected. Although there is a vaccine available for anthrax, the vaccine is in limited supply and not available to the general public at this time.

> **WEB LINK**
> ## Bioterrorism
> **http://www.bt.cdc.gov**
> At this Web site, you will find good, up-do-date information on bioterrorism and emergency preparedness. The site also has information in Spanish, but information on specific agents is available in many languages.
>
> **SEARCH TERMS:** bioterrorism, biological threats, biological agents

Smallpox

Another category A agent is smallpox. Smallpox is a serious, contagious, and sometimes fatal infectious disease that is caused by a virus. There is no treatment or cure for smallpox, but there is a vaccine. Because of this very effective vaccine, the last case of naturally occurring smallpox in the United States was in 1949, and the last case in the world was in Somalia in 1977. The symptoms of smallpox are high fever, headaches and body aches, nausea, and scabs that crust over and leave scars. Smallpox is usually spread by person-to-person contact, body fluids, or touching clothing or other contaminated items. Smallpox is rarely spread through the air because it is a fragile virus. There are smallpox vaccines available, but they are no longer given because the disease is considered eradicated, but if a bioterroristic attack were to occur, there would be enough vaccine to immunize the public.

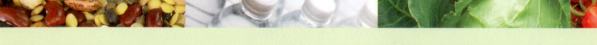

BUILDING YOUR LIFETIME WELLNESS PLAN

Infectious diseases continue to be significant health problems, but controlling infections and protecting your health is easy to do. Infections can be easily prevented by including certain behaviors discussed in this chapter in your wellness plan:

- Keep your hands clean, especially after using the toilet and before eating.

- Be sure that you and your family members are fully immunized according to medical recommendations.

- Understand the chain of infection and practice the behaviors that prevent transmission of infectious diseases.

- Understand that barrier contraception, such as a condom, is only partially effective in preventing the transmission of STIs. Abstinence from sexual behaviors and intravenous drug use is the only 100 percent effective strategy for preventing STIs.

- Learn all you can about infectious diseases and keep up to date with prevention practices and treatments.

●●● **End-of-Chapter Activities**

Opportunities for Application

1. Construct a table such as the one shown here for each of the major pathogenic agents, list three specific diseases, and fill in the empty columns for each disease.

Pathogen	Common Diseases	Prevention	Treatment
Viruses			
Bacteria			
Fungi			
Protozoa			
Multicellular parasites			

2. Select two of the infectious diseases you cited in item 1 previously and draw or describe the conditions of the chain of infection at each stage for the diseases. For each condition, describe the most efficient means of preventing transmission. Learners should list their chosen conditions and then research and describe the prevention measures for each element of the chain.

3. Summarize the best prevention strategy for reducing the probability that you would not contract an STI.

Key Concepts

1. Explain why even though the common cold is caused by a virus, there is no vaccine available and why we continually catch colds.

2. List the six conditions necessary for bacterial growth.

3. List at least five safe food-handling practices.

4. Explain the value and limitations of condom use in preventing STI transmission.

Answers to Personal Assessment: Personal Habits

This assessment is actually a checklist of good preventive health practices.

1. You want to make sure you have all the immunizations you need for your age-group. Some immunizations require booster injections at certain time periods.

2. The pathogens that make you sick, such as the common cold virus, are most likely to get into your body because of dirty hands.

3. Some diseases, such as head lice or ringworm, can be transmitted by hair care devices. Blood-borne diseases such as HIV can be transmitted by razors.

4. If you don't cover up to prevent spreading the virus, you may be contaminating surfaces and spreading disease to others.

5. If the person with whom you share with has cold or flu, you can become infected. And remember that you can't wipe the germs off the bottle, can, or straw.

6. Clean footwear can reduce the possibility of foot odor and athlete's foot.

7. The need for an examination becomes more important as you get older. A checkup can find disease problems before they get too advanced.

8. HIV infection is incurable. It is transmitted by blood-to-blood contact.

9. Everyone should know how to handle food products to reduce the possibility of food poisoning.

10. Each of these activities is a good wellness practice. They help maintain a healthy immune system.

References

Centers for Disease Control and Prevention. (2009a). *HIV/AIDS Surveillance by Race/Ethnicity (through 2007)*. Retrieved March 22, 2010 from http://www.cdc.gov/hiv/topics/surveillance/resources/slides/race-ethnicity/index.htm

Centers for Disease Control and Prevention. (2009b). *Sexually transmitted disease surveillance, 2008*. Atlanta: U.S. Department of Health and Human Services.

Centers for Disease Control and Prevention. (2009c). Table 11 B. Chlamydia—Rates per 100,000 population by race/ethnicity, age group and sex: United States, 2004–2008, *Sexually Transmitted Diseases Surveillance, 2008*. Retrieved April 1, 2010 from http://www.cdc.gov/std/stats08/tables/11b.htm

Centers for Disease Control and Prevention. (2009e). *West Nile Virus Activity in the United States*. Retrieved March 28, 2010 from http://www.cdc.gov/ncidod/dvbid/westnile/surv&controlCaseCount09_detailed.htm

Centers for Disease Control and Prevention. (2010). 2009–2010 Influenza Season Week 12 ending March 27, 2010. *Flu View*. Retrieved April 1, 2010 from: http://www.cdc.gov/flu/weekly/

Public Health Image Library. (2005). *Bacillus anthracis*. Retrieved January 20, 2008 from http://phil.cdc.gov/phil/home.asp

Winer R. L., et al. (2006). Condom use and the risk of genital human papillomavirus infection in young women. *The New England Journal of Medicine, 354,* 2645–2654.

CHAPTER 14

Chronic Diseases

●●● Introduction

For centuries, infectious diseases were the major killers of people of all ages. With the introduction of better personal health practices, advances in environmental conditions, and the development of antibiotics, infectious diseases are no longer the threat they once were. **Chronic diseases** are currently the leading causes of death and disability among Americans. Chronic diseases are conditions that are not caused by pathogens and tend to last for a long period of time. Presently, almost 70 percent of all deaths are attributable to three chronic conditions—heart disease, cancer, and diabetes (Figure 14-1). The medical care costs of people living with chronic diseases account for more than 75 percent of the nation's $1.4 trillion medical care costs. Diabetes alone is responsible for nearly $132 billion a year. With the control of infectious diseases, people live much longer, and, as they age, the risks increase for conditions such as heart disease and cancer. In addition,

chronic diseases
disease conditions that continue for a long time

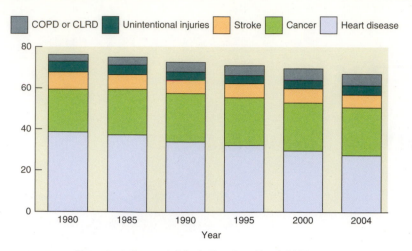

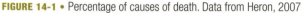

FIGURE 14-1 • Percentage of causes of death. Data from Heron, 2007

there are many chronic conditions that are not life threatening, but these conditions can reduce the quality of life for people who have them.

Many people don't worry too much about chronic diseases, especially young adults, believing chronic illnesses to be problems of older adults. The truth is that the conditions predisposing someone to chronic ailments develop over a lifetime. Chronic diseases are very much preventable because they are related to lifestyle factors and behaviors. The young adult years are the best time to develop the wellness skills and personal habits to help

PERSONAL ASSESSMENT
Heart Disease

Heart disease is the leading cause of death in the United States. What do you already know about heart disease? Read each of the statements below and whether you think each is true or false. You will learn about this condition as you read the chapter, but the answers appear at the end of the chapter.

1. High blood cholesterol is a risk factor for heart disease that you can control.

2. A blood cholesterol level up to 240 is okay for adults.

3. Fish oil supplements are good for lowering blood cholesterol.

4. Using margarine instead of butter is heart healthy.

5. Heart disease death rates are higher among African Americans than for whites.

6. All children should have their cholesterol levels checked.

7. All types of vegetable oils help lower blood cholesterol levels.

8. Being overweight is a risk factor for heart disease.

9. A person suffering a heart attack has a greater chance of survival if he or she gets treatment within five minutes.

10. Cocaine use is a risk factor for heart disease.

prevent chronic conditions from occurring later, but even in middle age, behavior changes can add years to life. This chapter contains information on many chronic diseases, what they are, and what you can do to reduce your risks of getting many of them.

The Nature of Chronic Diseases

Chronic diseases affect the majority of people in the United States at some point in their lives. To see just how widespread these conditions are, count the number of learners in your next class. Divide the total by four. Then multiply your answer by three. This number represents how many of the learners in that group are likely to die of a chronic disease later in life. That's right; about 70 percent of all deaths in this country are caused by some form of chronic illness. Given those figures, where do you see yourself in the years to come?

The chronic diseases to be discussed in this chapter are not caused by pathogenic organisms. They are not contagious, and they cannot be cured with antibiotics. Research is clear that virtually all the chronic conditions are related to lifestyle factors. To some degree, a person's genetic makeup also plays a role in his or her level of susceptibility to specific chronic conditions. The public health system was established to be the first line of defense against the leading causes of death, which at that time were infectious diseases. The system has yet to catch up with the shift to the morbidity and mortality of chronic conditions. In addition, the health care system, while it is developing procedures to address the increase in chronic disease conditions, is costly. Because chronic conditions last longer and the treatments are costly, chronic conditions have resulted in much higher costs associated with prevention and treatment.

The good news is that chronic conditions can be prevented or at least have their onset delayed by practicing health wellness behaviors. These behaviors result from choices you make, and the behaviors under your control are your best defense against chronic diseases. Prevention does not cost much. It is certainly less expensive than treatments. Applying what you learn in this chapter can reduce your health care costs while having a positive influence on how long you might live, but, more important, it can have a positive effect on how well you live.

The Cardiovascular System

The cardiovascular system is a closed circulation system, meaning that all the structures in the system are full of blood. The major components and structures of the cardiovascular system are illustrated in Figure 14-2. When one section of blood moves, all the blood moves. The heart is the muscular pump that pushes the blood through the system. Major blood vessels carrying blood away from the heart are known as arteries. Arteries branch off and become smaller and smaller as they infiltrate the body tissues, becoming **arterioles**. Eventually, the blood vessels become capillaries, vessels so small in some places that red blood cells have to pass through them in single file. It is at the capillary level that materials are exchanged through the cells of the body. The capillaries also pick up waste materials from the cells and carry them to body structures for processing, especially the lungs and kidneys. On the way back to the heart, the vessels get larger, forming veins. This causes a loss of pressure, so the veins have valves in them that keep the blood from moving backward between heart beats. The heart has four chambers because there are two loops of circulation. One loop circulates the blood around the body and back to the heart, and the other loop circulates the blood from the heart to the lungs and back.

arterioles
the smallest of the arteries leading to capillaries

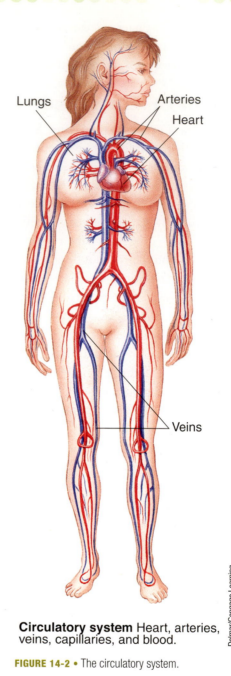

Delmar/Cengage Learning

Circulatory system Heart, arteries, veins, capillaries, and blood.

FIGURE 14-2 • The circulatory system.

whole blood
blood that contains all the major components of blood—red cells, white cells, and platelets

WEB LINK
The Cardiovascular System

http://www.innerbody.com/image/cardov.html

At this interactive Web site, you will find good information about the circulatory system. In fact, you can find information on any of the body systems.

SEARCH TERMS: cardiovascular system, heart and blood vessels

Blood

The blood that circulates through the circulatory system is known as **whole blood** because it contains all the blood components— red blood cells, white blood cells, and platelets suspended in a watery substance known as plasma. Red blood cells transport gases around the bloodstream, most notably oxygen and carbon dioxide. White blood cells are part of the body's immune system, and platelets assist in the blood-clotting process. The bloodstream is also a vehicle for transporting food nutrients and cell waste products. Among these materials are lipoproteins, also collectively known as cholesterol. Cholesterol is a waxy, fatlike substance that is found in all cells of the body. Your body makes all the cholesterol it needs, but cholesterol is also found in some of the foods you eat. The body uses cholesterol to make hormones, vitamin D, and substances that help you digest foods. There are essentially two forms of cholesterol comprised of lipoproteins:

- Low-density lipoprotein (LDL) cholesterol is sometimes called "bad cholesterol." High levels of LDL cholesterol can lead to a buildup of cholesterol in the arteries. The higher the LDL level in the blood, the greater the risk of getting heart disease (Table 14-1).

- High-density lipoprotein (HDL) cholesterol is sometimes called "good cholesterol." Think of HDL cholesterol as a being cholesterol "sponges." You can see in Table 14-2 that the higher your HDL cholesterol level, the lower your chance of getting heart disease.

During a physical examination, your physician may order a "lipid blood panel." The frequency of lipid testing will depend on your age and whether any other cardiovascular risk factors are present. Your physician will advise you accordingly, but by the time you reach age 40, you should have your lipid values checked at least every five years (more frequently if other risk factors are present). The lipid panel will test for your total cholesterol, LDL cholesterol, HDL cholesterol, and triglycerides. Although a high HDL level is good (60 and above) and low cholesterol (less than 200) level is good, the ratios of these values are more important indicators. You will find examples of these ratios in the following tables. Table 14-3 illustrates two examples of the ratio between total cholesterol and HDL, and Table 14-4 illustrates examples of LDL/HDL ratios.

TABLE 14-1 • Interpretation of total cholesterol values.

Total Cholesterol Levels	Relationship to Heart Disease
Less than 200 mg/dL	The "desirable" level that puts you at lower risk for heart disease. A cholesterol level of 200 mg/dL or higher increases your risk for heart disease.
200 to 239 mg/dL	Anything within this range is considered "borderline high."
240 mg/dL and above	"High" blood cholesterol. Someone with a cholesterol level in this range has more than twice the risk of developing heart disease compared to someone whose cholesterol level is below 200 mg/dL.

Source: National Heart, Lung, and Blood Institute (2005).

TABLE 14-2 • Relationship of HDL cholesterol levels to heart disease risk.

HDL Cholesterol Levels	Heart Disease Risk
Less than 40 mg/dL	A major risk factor for heart disease.
40 to 59 mg/dL	The higher your HDL, the better, but still may be a risk factor.
60 mg/dL and above	An HDL of 60 mg/dL and above is considered protective against heart disease.

Source: National Heart, Lung, and Blood Institute, 2005.

TABLE 14-3 • Examples of two total cholesterol and HDL cholesterol ratios.

Relationship of Total Cholesterol to HDL—determined by dividing the HDL level into the total cholesterol value. For example, two separate tests revealed:		
1. Cholesterol = 203	Divided by HDL = 21	Equals total cholesterol/HDL ratio of 9.6
2. Cholesterol = 220	Divided by HDL = 50	Equals total cholesterol/HDL ratio of 4.4

Delmar/Cengage Learning

TABLE 14-4 • Examples of two LDL and HDL cholesterol ratios.

Relationship of LDL to HDL—determined by dividing the HDL level into the LDL value. For example, two separate tests revealed:		
1. LDL = 130	Divided by HDL = 21	Equals total cholesterol/HDL ratio of 6.1
2. LDL = 160	Divided by HDL = 50	Equals total cholesterol/HDL ratio of 3.2

Delmar/Cengage Learning

In Table 14-3, notice that even though subject 2 has a higher cholesterol level than subject 1, he or she also has a higher HDL level; thus, the ratio is only 4.4. The lower this ratio, the lower the risk factor for heart disease.

In the example in Table 14-4, you can see once again that HDL provided a protective factor, offsetting the higher LDL level in subject 2.

There are things you can do to manage your cholesterol, such as increasing your HDLs and reducing your LDLs. Doing so creates a favorable HDL/LDL ratio. If you want to increase your HDLs, you can do the following:

- Engage in regular aerobic exercise for at least 20 to 30 minutes at a time two or three days per week.

- Keep your weight under control. Obesity encourages increased LDL. Losing weight will reduce the LDL levels while improving your HDL.

- Don't smoke. If you are a current smoker, quitting will increase HDL levels.

- A *little* alcohol, fewer than two drinks a day, can increase your HDL levels.

- Keep trans fats out of your diet.

- Consume as much low-fat foods as you can. Lipoproteins are manufactured from fats in the diet.

> **Did You Know...?**
>
> The average adult has about 10 pints of blood in his or her body.

Cardiovascular Disease

cardiovascular disease
Any number of medical conditions that affect the heart or blood vessels servicing the heart

The most common chronic disease, responsible for more than 40 percent of the deaths in the United States, is **cardiovascular disease**. The name of the disease is descriptive of the two conditions it describes:

- *Cardio* refers to the heart.

- *Vascular* describes the blood vessels.

Cardiovascular disease is not one particular disease; rather, it is a descriptive class of diseases. The most common cardiovascular diseases are **hypertension**, **coronary heart disease**, and **stroke**.

Hypertension

Hypertension is the term given to blood pressure that is higher than normal. Blood pressure is the force exerted by the blood on the walls of the arteries as it is pumped through the body. Normal blood pressure is about 120/80 mm Hg. Blood pressure is measured in millimeters of mercury (mm Hg) because mercury was used in the older **sphygmomanometer** (Figure 14-3). This is a special cuff that is put around the upper arm and inflated with air to cut off the blood flow through the arm. The air is then let out of the cuff to allow the blood flow to return to the arm. With a manual sphygmomanometer, a trained person listens to the sounds in the blood vessels with a stethoscope. With an electronic sphygmomanometer, the electrical activity in the blood vessels is detected with a small computer. The test is reported as a ratio, such as 123/81. The higher number in this ratio is the measure of pressure when the heart contracts and squeezes blood out into the arteries. This is known as **systolic pressure**. The lower number, **diastolic pressure**, is the pressure of blood in the arteries as the heart relaxes between beats. Hypertension is a consequence of the arteries losing their elasticity. This loss of elasticity can be caused by cholesterol buildup in the arteries that narrows the opening (Figure 14-4) or from the aging process whereby the linings of the arteries lose their elasticity as the person ages. The lack of elasticity results in blood vessels that don't expand to accommodate the blood as it is pumped through the arteries. The heart is trying to push the blood through a smaller-diameter opening. Hypertension can strain the heart, causing it to enlarge and weaken. It can also be a warning sign that blood vessels in the heart or brain can be narrowing—early signs of heart attack or stroke.

In the United States, one in four adults has hypertension, and most of these cases are among minority populations. About one-third of these people don't know they have it, which is why hypertension is often referred to as "the silent killer." Because there are no symptoms of hypertension, the only way to diagnose the condition is to have one's blood pressure checked periodically with a sphygmomanometer. You can purchase a sphygmomanometer at any drug store and check your blood pressure periodically at home.

Blood pressure readings above 140/90 are considered high. Individuals with high blood pressure may be advised to change one or more of their lifestyle behaviors. Left untreated, hypertension can lead to stroke or damage the heart, kidneys, and other organs. The cause of hypertension in 90 to 95 percent of cases is unknown, although the risk factors for cardiovascular disease, discussed later in this chapter, also contribute to hypertension.

Depending on the person, lifestyle changes to reduce hypertension might include increasing physical exercise, quitting smoking, reducing alcohol consumption,

hypertension
increased pressure in the arteries against which the heart must pump the blood

coronary heart disease
a condition whereby the arteries servicing the heart muscle get blocked

stroke
an event in the brain that cuts off the blood supply to a section of brain tissue

sphygmomanometer
a device used to measure blood pressure

systolic pressure
pressure measured in the arteries as the heart is pumping blood into the arteries

diastolic pressure
pressure measured in the arteries as the heart relaxes to fill with blood

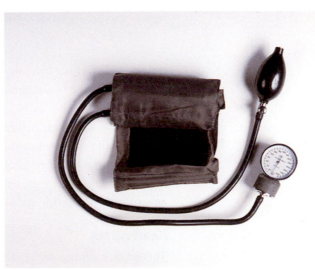

FIGURE 14-3 • A sphygmomanometer.

Delmar/Cengage Learning

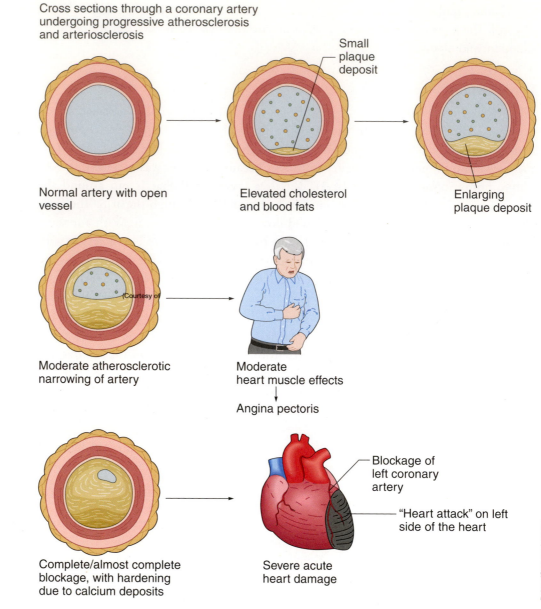

Cross sections through a coronary artery undergoing progressive atherosclerosis and arteriosclerosis

Normal artery with open vessel

Elevated cholesterol and blood fats

Small plaque deposit

Enlarging plaque deposit

Moderate atherosclerotic narrowing of artery

Moderate heart muscle effects

Angina pectoris

Complete/almost complete blockage, with hardening due to calcium deposits

Severe acute heart damage

Blockage of left coronary artery

"Heart attack" on left side of the heart

FIGURE 14-4 • Atherosclerosis: narrowing of the arteries.

Delmar/Cengage Learning

losing weight, using less salt, or managing diabetes. If following these recommendations doesn't lower the blood pressure to within normal range, your physician may prescribe medication.

There is a medical condition known as low blood pressure, but the condition is generally not life threatening the way high blood pressure is. Low blood pressure does not cause a strain on the heart; rather, it can produce feelings of light-headedness or dizziness. It is important to see your health care provider if you experience symptoms such as shortness of breath, fainting spells, headaches, or fever over 101 degrees Fahrenheit.

Heart Attack

The heart is a muscular organ that needs its own blood supply to function properly. Special arteries, different from those that supply blood to the rest of the body, ensure that the heart receives the nutrients it needs to continue pumping. Called coronary arteries, their interior linings are normally smooth, much like a nonstick cooking surface. This surface can become very uneven because of the gradual buildup and hardening of fatty material inside the artery known as plaque. This process is known as **atherosclerosis** and can be the result of both hereditary factors and lifestyle habits, but it is related to the level of cholesterol in the diet and bloodstream. If there is too much atherosclerotic plaque, the coronary arteries can become partially blocked and unable to supply the heart muscle with the blood and nutrients it needs (Figure 14-5). This condition is called **coronary artery disease**. As the arteries become more and more clogged, the heart labors as it tries to pump blood through smaller blood vessels that are not very elastic. The heart may actually start to hurt, a condition called angina. This is the heart's way of saying that it needs more oxygen. If the condition continues to worsen, it can result in a heart attack, known in medicine as a **myocardial infarction**. Heart attacks vary in the amount of damage to heart depending on the size of the coronary artery that becomes blocked. The blockage occurs when some of the plaque, built up inside the artery, breaks off and reaches a point in the artery where the material cannot pass though the small diameter of the artery. The blockage prevents the needed blood supply from reaching the heart muscle beyond the blockage. The cells in that area of the heart muscle not receiving oxygen die. In some cases, the heart continues to pump. In other cases, a coronary artery becomes so restricted that the heart stops working altogether. These differences explain why some people have heart attacks and don't even know it, whereas others die before they fall to the floor.

Did You Know...?

The average person's heart beats 72 times a minute, or 103,680 times a day. A good aerobic exercise program will make the heart muscle more efficient so that when the body is at rest, the heart can beat at a slower rate to move the same amount of blood.

atherosclerosis
a buildup of firm fatty deposits along the inner lining of the arteries that causes the opening inside the artery to narrow and lose elasticity

coronary artery disease
atherosclerosis in the coronary arteries

myocardial infarction
medical term for heart attack

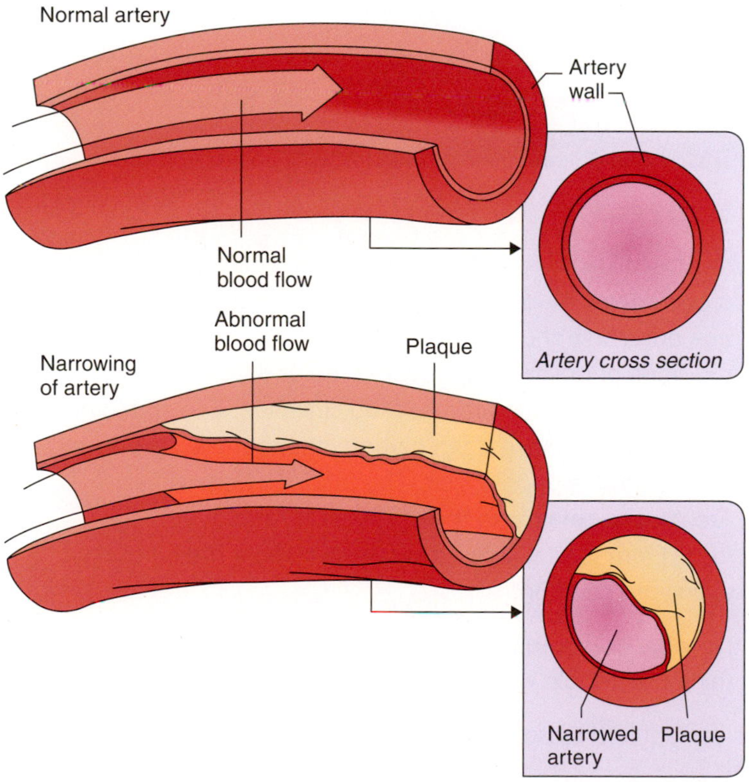

Normal artery

Artery wall

Normal blood flow

Abnormal blood flow

Plaque

Artery cross section

Narrowing of artery

Narrowed artery   Plaque

FIGURE 14-5 • Plaque buildup in the artery. Courtesy of National Heart Lung and Blood Institute, 2009

Symptoms of a heart attack vary from person to person, ranging from no symptoms at all to any of the following:

- *Chest pain.* The pain is not usually sharp. Victims of heart attacks describe it as a crushing, squeezing pain or a tight constriction across the top of the chest. This pain usually starts in the center of the chest and then spreads or moves around, going to either shoulder, down the arms, or into the jaw.

- *Heavy sweating.* Most heart attack victims sweat very heavily, even if they are not doing any physical activity.

- *Nausea.* Nausea is a common heart attack symptom, especially in women.

- *Shortness of breath.* Many heart attack victims report it is hard for them to "catch their breath."

- *Fainting.* Fainting may also occur.

What's News

Numerous research studies have now confirmed a possible link between gum disease and heart disease. It appears the bacteria that contribute to gum disease may also play a role in causing plaque buildup in coronary blood vessels. This is one more reason to take good care of your teeth and gums—one more personal wellness behavior to reduce heart disease risk.

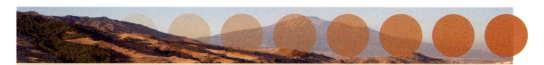

Should Tobacco Companies Pay?

Cigarette smoking has been linked to both heart disease and cancer. Believing that the tobacco companies have been responsible because they market a product known to be addicting and unhealthy, many states have sued the tobacco industry for billions of dollars to recover some of the money the states spent caring for people with tobacco-related illnesses. The states believe that the tobacco companies have been dishonest about their products and don't care if cigarettes make people sick. The tobacco companies, on the other hand, feel that people make the decision to smoke, and the companies do not force them to buy cigarettes. Gather some background information and explain your position:

- Do you believe the tobacco companies bear some responsibility for illness, or do you think the people who use tobacco products are at fault?

- Should smokers be required to pay more than nonsmokers for their own health care?

Most heart attack victims, when experiencing symptoms, deny the possibility they are having a heart attack. They know they don't feel well, but the symptoms may subside after a while, so they pass it off as some other ailment that has "gone away." This attitude prevents them from getting needed help. Most deaths from heart attacks occur within two hours after symptoms begin, without the victim ever reaching the hospital. Permanent damage to the heart and death can often be prevented if the victim gets help and treatment without delay. If you are with someone who is experiencing any of the symptoms of a heart attack, have the person stop whatever he or she is doing and rest. If the symptoms last for more than a couple of minutes, contact the emergency medical services. Heart attack is a true medical emergency.

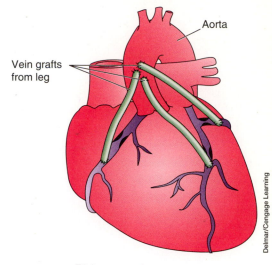

Aorta

Vein grafts from leg

Delmar/Cengage Learning

FIGURE 14-6 • Triple coronary bypass.

Treating Heart Disease

Medical advances have resulted in a variety of treatments for heart disease, ranging from cholesterol-lowering medications to heart transplants. One commonly used procedure to enlarge clogged arteries is called **angioplasty**, in which a small balloon is inserted into a clogged artery. The balloon is then inflated to press the plaque against the wall of the artery and increase the size of the opening allowing better blood flow. If the blockage is too great, coronary bypass surgery is performed. In this procedure, the surgeon removes a small section of vein from the patient's leg and attaches it to the heart to create a "bypass" around the damaged artery (Figure 14-6). Have you heard the term *triple bypass*? This is the procedure performed when three arteries are blocked and are replaced by three veins. The new blood vessels allow blood to pass safely through the heart muscle.

What if a person suffers a heart attack? Getting him or her to a medical facility is of the utmost importance. Medical treatment is most successful if begun within five minutes of the heart attack. Since the arrival of an ambulance is generally longer than that, it is important that cardiopulmonary resuscitation (CPR) be performed until help arrives. Do not attempt to drive the victim to the hospital—unless there is no other alternative. Performing CPR and waiting for the ambulance is the recommended course of action because when the ambulance arrives, the emergency management team can administer medication and oxygen to stabilize the patient before transport. More important, an ambulance can move more quickly and safely through traffic, and the emergency medical personnel can stay in communication with the hospital along the way.

When the patient arrives at the hospital, medical staff will evaluate the patient's condition and assess whether the individual is suffering from a myocardial infarction. In the meantime, the patient is given oxygen and placed on an **electrocardiograph (ECG)**. Heart tissue that has been damaged by a heart attack will show up on the ECG printout. Blood is also drawn and processed by the laboratory to test for specific enzymes that appear in the bloodstream following a heart attack. Medication will be administered to relieve the patient's anxiety and physical discomfort. The rest of the treatment will be specific for the seriousness of the patient's condition and the specific area of the heart muscle that was affected.

angioplasty
medical procedure in which a small balloon is inserted into a clogged coronary artery and inflated to reduce an obstruction

electrocardiograph (ECG)
a device that measures the electrical output of the heart muscle

WEB LINK
CPR Training
You can find out locations for CPR training programs at the Web sites of the American Heart Association at **http://www.americanheart.org/cpr** or the American Red Cross at **http://www.redcross.org**. Having this training may prepare you for saving a life some day.

SEARCH TERMS: CPR training, cardiopulmonary resuscitation

Stroke

A stroke occurs when the blood supply to brain tissue is cut off, much like the process leading to a heart attack. Stroke can be caused by a blockage in the arteries (atherosclerosis) that supply oxygen to the brain, known as **ischemic stroke**, the most common form, accounting for 80 to 85 percent of all strokes. A stroke can also be caused by a ruptured blood vessel in the brain, known as a **hemorrhagic stroke**. Although not as common as ischemic stroke, hemorrhagic stroke is more likely to be fatal. No matter the cause of the stroke, brain tissue in the area of the stroke will be deprived of oxygen, causing the tissues to die. Because a stroke usually happens on one side of the brain, symptoms usually occur on only one side of the body. There is no way of telling what effect the stroke will produce on the body. It all depends on the section of the brain that is afflicted and how much of the brain tissue dies. For example, a stroke in the frontal lobe may affect speech. Figure 14-7 illustrates the functions controlled by the various sections of the brain.

People should be aware of stroke symptoms. It is essential for anyone experiencing stroke to get medical attention immediately. This is especially true if a person has a "ministroke." Symptoms that last for less than 24 hours are characteristic of a ministroke. Even though a ministroke is not fatal and the patient recovers easily, about one-third of all major strokes are preceded by ministrokes. This is why everyone should have familiarity

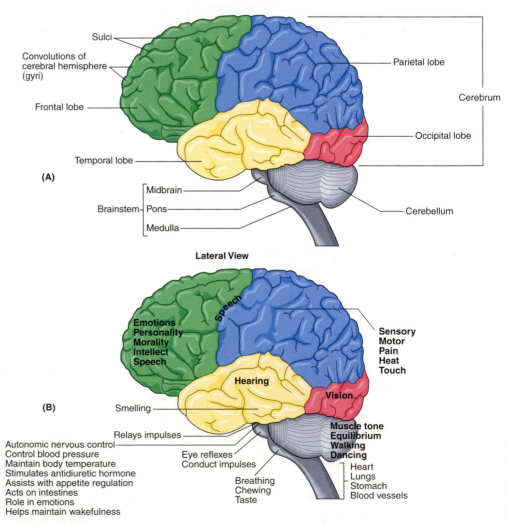

FIGURE 14-7 • Parts of the brain and areas of brain function.

Delmar/Cengage Learning

with stroke symptoms, and medical care should be sought for any stroke, no matter how small or if the symptoms go away. Possible symptoms of stroke include the following:

- Sudden weakness, numbness, or paralysis in an arm, a hand, a leg, a foot, or the face

- Sudden loss of speech, slurred speech, or incoherent speech and/or trouble understanding the speech of others

- Sudden loss of vision or experience of dimness (usually happens in only one eye)

- Sudden unexplained dizziness, unsteadiness, or falling

- Loss of consciousness

Because stroke affects the brain, it is important to contact emergency medical services immediately, even if symptoms are slight or only temporary. The sooner a stroke victim gets medical attention, the less brain damage will occur. Stroke is a true medical emergency.

> **WEB LINK**
> ## American Stroke Association
> **http://www.strokeassociation.org**
> This Web site provides information and current updates about stroke.
>
> **SEARCH TERMS:** stroke, cerebrovascular disease

Risk Factors for Cardiovascular Disease

The Framingham Heart Study began in 1948. The project was designed to study a cohort of 5,209 men and women between the ages of 30 and 62 from the town of Framingham, Massachusetts. The purpose of the study was to observe members of the cohort to determine the physical and lifestyle factors related to cardiovascular disease. After years of research, the Framingham Study presented a clear picture of the risk factors associated with heart disease. Two categories of risk factors have been identified:

1. Risk factors you cannot change or control (*nonmodifiable* risk factors)
   - *Heredity.* Having close family members who have heart disease is a significant risk factor for the disease. Certain racial groups are at a higher risk than others. For example, approximately 30 percent more African Americans will die from heart disease than will white Americans.
   - *Age.* The older a person is, the more likely he or she will develop heart disease. More than half of all those who have heart attacks are over age 65, and four out of five people who die from heart attacks are over age 65. One reason older people are prone to heart disease is that as a person ages, arteries lose some of their ability to expand and relax easily as the blood is pumped through them. It may be that the groundwork for heart disease begins when a person is younger. For example, deposits of plaque have been observed in the arteries of children and teenagers, so it is clear that preventive behaviors are important for young people.
   - *Gender.* During their childbearing years, women have less heart disease than men of the same age because of a protective effect from estrogen. This may explain why women develop heart disease about 10 to 15 years later than men. Once women go through menopause and their estrogen levels decrease, they are just as likely to develop heart disease as men.

> **WEB LINK**
> ## Women's Heart Health
> **http://www.hearthealthywomen.org**
> This Web site is a complete, well-documented source of information about heart health specifically intended for females. It contains information for women and health professionals.
>
> **SEARCH TERMS:** women's health, women and heart disease

What's News

Increased Heart Disease Risk for Hispanic Women

A study conducted at the University of Rochester indicates that Hispanic women are more likely to have heart attacks than Anglo women (Kreimer, 2007 Kreimer is from Rochester). The findings indicated that the cardiac risk for Hispanic subjects was equal to risk for Anglo women who were 10 years older.

- *Race*. African Americans, Native Americans, Mexican Americans, Native Hawaiians, and some Asian Americans are at higher risk for developing heart disease. This is due in part to higher occurrences of diabetes, high blood pressure, and obesity in these populations.

2. Risk factors you can change or control (*modifiable* risk factors)
   - *Smoking*. Smokers have a much higher risk of heart disease than nonsmokers because smoking raises the level of carbon monoxide in the blood, which can damage the walls of veins and arteries. Smoking also makes the heart beat faster, narrows the blood vessels, raises blood pressure, and causes the blood to become sticky so that it clings to the walls of arteries more easily. It is interesting to note that smoking is a greater cardiovascular risk factor for men under age 50 than those over age 50.
   - *Inactivity*. Lack of exercise is a major risk factor for cardiovascular disease. Exercise, especially aerobic exercise, makes the heart stronger and more efficient, helps the body manufacture the good kind of cholesterol known as HDL cholesterol, and improves circulation.
   - *High cholesterol*. Cholesterol is a type of fatty substance found in the body and circulates in the bloodstream. By now, you know there are different types of cholesterol, each with a different effect on the body. The "bad" cholesterols are LDLs and very low-density lipoproteins. Lipoproteins are protein molecules that carry fat. HDL is considered "good" cholesterol because HDL molecules act as "cholesterol sponges," picking up and carrying off large amounts of fat from the bloodstream. When large amounts of bad cholesterol are present in the bloodstream, the cholesterol can accumulate in the arteries and make them narrower. Therefore, as blood cholesterol rises, so does the risk of coronary artery disease.

     Whereas smoking and a high-fat diet cause the body to produce bad cholesterol, exercise helps it produce good cholesterol. Smoking and a high-fat diet are independent risk factors, but these two risk factors are not additive; that is, one risk factor + one risk factor does not equal two risk factors. What happens is that the two risk factors become multiplicative, meaning that one risk factor + one risk factor equals three risk factors.

     Cholesterol level is also affected by age, sex, and heredity. Have you heard the term *hardening of the arteries*? Atherosclerosis is the medical term for this condition, and it is one of the consequences of high cholesterol levels, especially LDLs. As fat deposits and calcium build up along the walls of the arteries, they form a substance called plaque. Atherosclerosis can start early in childhood. In

What's News

A new blood test is now available that detects heart attack risk. The test detects levels of C-reactive protein, an indicator of inflamed blood vessel walls, which are associated with heart attack risk.

fact, scientists have found evidence of the beginning of fat streaks in the arteries of children as young as three years old.

- *Obesity and overweight.* People who have excess body fat are more likely to develop cardiovascular disease even if they have no other risk factors. Excess weight raises blood pressure, which in turn causes a strain on the heart and also raises LDL cholesterol and triglycerides (fats that are converted from foods we eat). Excess body fat contributes to lower levels of HDLs.

Thirty years ago, according to the NHANES II survey, data indicated that 25 percent of the U.S. population was obese. Data from NHANES III in 1985 revealed that 33 percent of the population was obese. In chapter 9, you learned about weight management and the health problems associated with obesity. Cardiovascular health is affected by obesity because obesity does the following:

- Causes an increase in blood cholesterol
- Reduces HDL cholesterol
- Causes an increase in blood pressure levels
- Contributes to the development of diabetes

- *Hypertension.* It is normal for blood pressure to vary from moment to moment, and it is highly influenced by factors such as activity level, dietary patterns, and stress. But blood pressure that consistently measures over 140/90 is labeled as hypertension, or high blood pressure. Nearly one-third of Americans are diagnosed with high blood pressure. Many more people may have it and don't know it because they have not had it checked.

Understanding your risk factors not only helps you know if you are at risk for cardiovascular disease but also empowers you with information about the specific modifiable risk factors you can change. Knowing these risk factors is only part of the prevention strategy for reducing the chance of developing cardiovascular disease. The knowledge must be put into practice. More important, the earlier in your life you begin addressing risk factors, the better your cardiovascular health will be later in life.

Preventing Cardiovascular Disease

Armed with knowledge of the modifiable cardiovascular risk factors and having the motivation to practice wellness, one must apply his or her health literacy skills to develop a wellness plan that protects against development of modifiable risk factors. Some of the wellness behaviors already been discussed in previous

WEB LINK
The Framingham Study
http://www.framinghamheartstudy.org

This is the official Web site of the Framingham Heart Study. You can find a lot of historical and technical information about the study, but you can also link to "risk scores" and complete a table to determine your risk for heart disease.

SEARCH TERMS: Framingham Heart Study, Framingham study

chapters, but let's review and summarize some of the heart-protective behaviors we learned from cardiovascular studies, such as the Framingham Heart Study.

Exercise

More than 40 years of research confirms the health benefits of exercise. It appears that approximately 250,000 deaths each year are attributable to lack of regular physical activity. But, more important, long-term studies of active individuals have confirmed the protective value of exercise. Even exercise programs adopted during the middle years of life are associated with decreases in mortality. What are the benefits of regular exercise on cardiovascular health?

1. *Strengthens the heart muscle.* A healthy heart muscle can be made stronger and more efficient with exercise. Depending on the type of exercise program, the heart muscle responds to the demands placed on it by the exercise program. The heart not only becomes stronger, pumping more blood volume per stroke, but also performs more efficiently by contracting fewer times each minute. The resting heart rates of well-trained athletes like marathon runners may be 40 to 60 beats per minute. It is best if you get 30 to 60 minutes of vigorous activity most days of the week, but research shows that any exercise is better than none. The definition of vigorous activity will vary depending on your age. A 20-year-old can perform a 60-minute aerobic routine of high intensity or run six miles at a time. As a person ages, his or her exercise goals will change because of age-related physiological changes. A 50-year-old can still perform a 60-minute exercise routine, but the intensity is lower. Exercises can come in many forms and are adaptable to various age-groups and one's physical limitations (Figure 14-8).

2. *Lowers blood pressure.* The effect of exercise on blood pressure comes about in two ways. As mentioned previously, the heart muscle gets stronger and more efficient. The second effect occurs in the other parts of the circulatory system. The demands of exercise trigger the body to grow more capillaries in the exercised muscles of the body. With more blood vessels, the heart is pumping against less resistance.

3. *Creates a better HLH/LDL ratio.* Exercise tends to increase the production of HDL molecules and discourages the production of LDL cholesterol.

4. *Enhances blood flow.* Because of the changes in cholesterol levels induced by exercise, the increase in capillaries, and strengthening of the heart muscle, blood flows with less resistance to all areas of the body.

All these benefits reduce the risk of stroke, heart disease, and high blood pressure. Research suggests it is the *amount* of physical activity rather than the *intensity* that has the greatest effect on cholesterol levels. Not only that, it appears that *any exercise* is better than no exercise.

Cancer

Under normal conditions, almost all the cells in our bodies go through the process of cellular growth and reproduction. The exceptions would be cells such as bone cells, nerve cells, and muscle cells. Liver cells will reproduce only if the liver is damaged. The process of growth and reproduction is very systematic and controlled by the genetic codes within the cells. The four phases of cellular reproduction known as mitosis are illustrated in Figure 14-9.

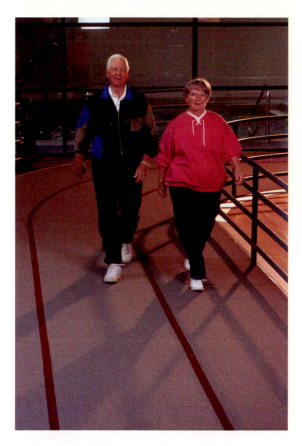

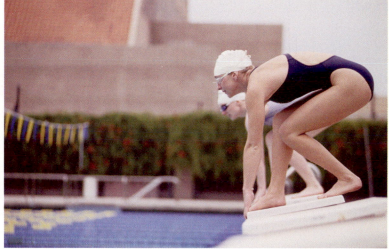

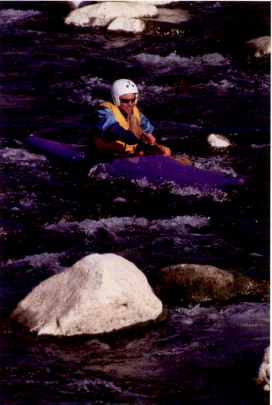

Courtesy of Photodisc

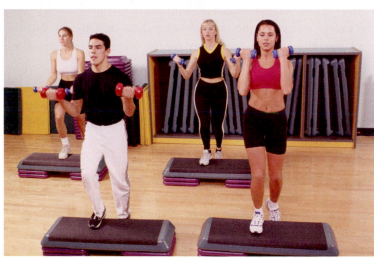

FIGURE 14-8 • Healthy exercise comes in many forms.

During the *prophase*, the 46 chromosomes within the cell are duplicated, and the **centrioles** move to opposite sides of the cell to pull the paired chromosomes into alignment for metaphase. The chromosomes are lined up at the cellular equator during the *metaphase* of mitosis. During the *anaphase*, the paired chromosomes separate from one another and move toward the respective cellular poles. The parent cell begins division during the *telophase*, and the new membranes begin to form for each of the two nuclei. The telophase is completed when the two new daughter cells are formed. This process averages about one hour, and it is consistent among the same type of tissue. More important, the new cells are identical in all respects from the original cells.

centrioles
two spindlelike structures within the cell that help align chromosomes during cell division

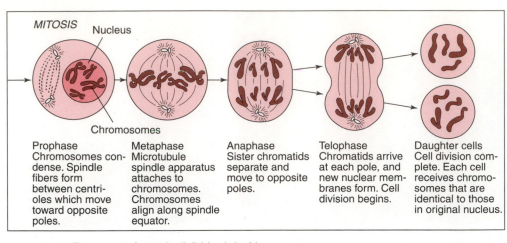

FIGURE 14-9 • The process of normal cell division (mitosis).

cancer
the uncontrolled growth and spread of abnormal cells in the body

Cancer, on the other hand is quite unlike normal mitotic divisions. Cancer is the uncontrolled growth and spread of abnormal body cells. All the mechanisms that govern mitosis no longer apply when cancer cells form. The growth is rapid and uncontrolled, and the duplication of genetic material entering prophase results in daughter cells that are unlike the parent cells. Moreover, the genetically altered cells continue to reproduce genetically altered cells and so forth. The result is the rapid formation of tissue that has lost its original function and purpose.

The American Cancer Society reports that one out of every two men and one out of every three women will have cancer sometime during their lifetime. Hardly anyone escapes either having cancer or having someone close to them develop the disease. Although 77 percent of all cancers occur in people over age 55, it can occur at any time during the life span.

Can you see the difference between the cancerous and normal cells in Figure 14-10? As a normal biological process, body cells reproduce and grow at a certain set, controlled rate. This rate is controlled by the genetic makeup of the person and the code programmed in the cells. For example, one cell divides into two cells, two cells become four, and so on. Cancer cells grow at a faster, abnormal rate. They develop into bundles of genetically altered cells called **malignant tumors**, which can interfere with the body's normal functions. In essence, the cancer cells displace normal cells from the organ's tissue. When cancer cells first begin to grow, they usually stay in one area of the body. If they are not treated, they can eventually detach from the original tumor and spread to other sites in the body. The cells will travel by just spreading, for example, in the case of smokeless tobacco, from the gum to the jaw to the brain, or cancer cells can spread through the lymph system, say, from the prostate to the lymph nodes to the spine. This process is called **metastasis** and often results in death. Lung cancer, for example, often spreads to the brain.

malignant tumors
abnormal growth of cells forming a cancerous tumor

metastasis
the spread of cancer from one site to another location in the body

benign tumors
abnormal growth of cells that form a noncancerous tumor

biopsy
the removal of a tiny piece of a tumor for examination under a microscope

Not all tumors are cancerous, however. Some tumors, such as cysts, moles, or fatty tumors, are known as **benign tumors** because they don't spread wildly or threaten life. If a doctor suspects that a person has cancer, a **biopsy** is performed. This is a surgical procedure that involves removing a tiny piece of the tumor and examining it under a microscope to see if the tissue is cancerous. Malignant tumor cells are irregular in shape, size, and growth patterns and usually invade the surrounding tissue (Table 14-5).

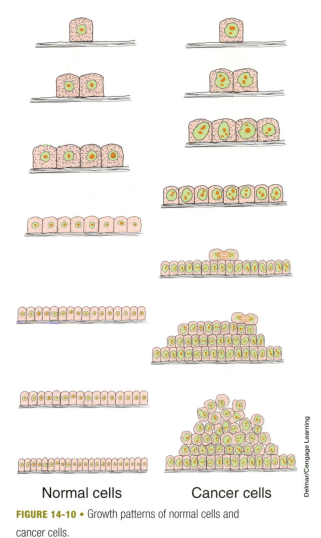

Delmar/Cengage Learning

Normal cells   Cancer cells

FIGURE 14-10 • Growth patterns of normal cells and cancer cells.

TABLE 14-5 • Comparisons of normal and cancerous cell growth.

Characteristic	Normal Cells	Cancer Cells
Genetic makeup	All cells genetically identical	Varied genetic makeup
Cell structure	Identical	Varied
Cell function	Serve a purpose	Loss of identity so they fail to function as normal cells do
Location	Stay where they originated	Loose; cells can easily spread to other areas of the body
Cell life	Fixed and finite	Longer than normal cells
Cell reproduction	Regulated	No regulation

Delmar/Cengage Learning

Factors That Contribute to Cancer

Certain types of cancer are related to personal behaviors. For example, smoking causes lung cancer and contributes to other types of cancer, such as cancer of the bladder, esophagus, and breast. In fact, one-third of all cancer deaths are caused by smoking. Smokeless tobacco causes oral cancers such as cancer of the tongue and mouth.

Many years of scientific research have disclosed a number of other factors, in addition to smoking, that are related to cancer formation. Notice how many of these are under your control. Think about how having this information gives you the power to effectively fight one of the top killers of our time. The behaviors may not prevent cancer from ever occurring, but they may well delay its onset.

1. *Diet.* There appears to be a strong relationship between diet and certain cancers. What we know about dietary influences are both positive and negative. Some foods, especially fruits and vegetables supply cancer-protective substances, such as fiber, antioxidants (e.g., beta-carotene, vitamin E, and lutein), and macronutrients. On the other hand, some foods, especially those that contain large amounts of sugar and dietary fat, can contribute to cancer formation. Excessive amounts of alcohol also contribute to the development of certain cancers.

2. *Occupational and environmental factors.* Exposure to certain chemicals may cause brain, lung, and other cancers. Asbestos, for example, is a fibrous mineral used in a number of industrial products including roofing shingles. Years ago it was used as a flame-resistant form of insulation. Asbestos is known to cause lung cancer. Often overlooked as a carcinogen but perhaps the most common environmental factor is sun exposure, which is strongly related to skin cancer. Most cancers from sun exposure develop years after the exposure takes place. Every year in the United States, there are about a million new cases of skin cancer, more than the number of all other cancers combined. Individuals exposed to the sun for more than half an hour are advised to use sun protection. Among other environmental carcinogens, there is some public concern about cellular phone use contributing to brain tumors. Medical researchers are conducting studies to determine the effects of cellular phone use on health (Figure 14-11).

3. *Infectious Agents.* Certain viruses are related to some types of cancer. For example, the same virus that causes mononucleosis is responsible for Burkitt lymphoma, a type of cancer found in African children. Many cases of liver cancer have been connected to hepatitis A and B viruses. And some cases of cervical cancer have been linked to the human papillomavirus, the same virus that causes genital warts and is transmitted through sexual contact. The human immunodeficiency virus (HIV) plays an indirect role in the causation of Kaposi's sarcoma, a cancer that is prominent among those with acquired immune deficiency syndrome. HIV weakens the immune system paving the way for infection of the *Kaposi sarcoma herpesvirus.*

4. *Obesity.* An obese individual is not assured of getting cancer, but evidence does suggest that obesity may be a risk factor making the person more cancer prone. For example, obesity and overweight have been clearly associated with an increased risk for kidney cancer in both men and women (i.e., a twofold risk compared to non-obese people).

5. *Inactivity.* Scientists believe that about one-third of all cancer deaths are related to diet and lack of exercise. The latest guidelines suggest that exercising for at least 30 minutes a day five times a week can protect against cancer. Forty-five minutes is recommended for preventing breast and colon cancers.

6. *Genetics.* Some types of cancer tend to run in families. These include breast cancer, colon cancer, ovarian cancer, and uterine cancer.

There are three main reasons why people are concerned that cellular telephones may cause certain types of cancer:

1. Cellular telephones emit radiofrequency (RF) energy (radio waves), which is a form of radiation and is under investigation for its effects on the human body.
2. Cellular telephone technology is relatively new and is still changing, so there are few long-term studies of the effects of RF energy from cellular telephones on the human body.
3. The number of cellular telephone users has increased rapidly. As of 2008, there were more than 270 million subscribers to cellular telephone service in the United States, according to the Cellular Telecommunications and Internet Association. This is an increase from 110 million users in 2000 and 208 million users in 2005.

One of the problems associated with the research on the effects of cellular phone use on humans is the fact that exposure to the RF varies with the amount of time one spends on the phone, that is, the number of minutes per call and the number of calls per day. To date, there is no causal relationship between cellular phone use and cancer, but the only studies have been on the short-term effects. The long-term effects have yet to be completed. The U.S. Food and Drug Administration has suggested some steps that cellular telephone users can take if they are concerned about potential health risks from cellular telephones:

- Use of cellular telephones for shorter conversations or for times when a conventional phone is not available.
- Switch to a type of cellular telephone with a hands-free device that will place more distance between the antenna and the head of the phone user.

FIGURE 14-11 • The effects of cellular phone use on brain cancer. Source: National Cancer Institute, 2009

Cancer Treatments

The sooner cancer is detected, the greater the likelihood the cancer can be cured. One of the best things you can do to protect yourself against this disease is to know and watch for the warning signs of cancer (Figure 14-12). If any of these conditions are present for more than a week, you should contact your health care provider. Having any of these symptoms does not mean a person has cancer. They may be symptoms of other noncancerous conditions, but they should be examined anyway. In most all medical conditions, the sooner you attend to adverse conditions, the greater the likelihood of a more rapid and less costly cure.

In addition, regular self-examinations are recommended for men and women. Breast self-examinations are *one* recommended detection regimen for women, but the American Cancer Society advocates that all women should receive an annual **mammogram** since it is a more accurate diagnostic tool. Men are advised to perform a regular testicular self-examination and self-refer to a physician if any suspicious masses are detected. Details for performing these examinations can be found at the American Cancer Society Web site.

mammogram
type of imaging that uses a low-dose X-ray system for early detection and diagnosis of breast diseases in women

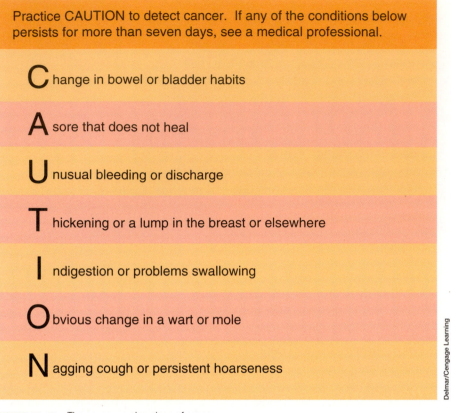

Practice CAUTION to detect cancer. If any of the conditions below persists for more than seven days, see a medical professional.

Change in bowel or bladder habits

A sore that does not heal

Unusual bleeding or discharge

Thickening or a lump in the breast or elsewhere

Indigestion or problems swallowing

Obvious change in a wart or mole

Nagging cough or persistent hoarseness

Delmar/Cengage Learning

FIGURE 14-12 • The seven warning signs of cancer.

There are several kinds of treatment for cancer; the specific type of treatment used depends on the type of cancer and the stage at which it is detected. The most common treatment is surgery, whereby the malignant tumor and a large area of normal tissue around it are removed. Nearby lymph nodes are often removed to ensure that cancer cells do not travel through the lymph system and metastasize. A patient is considered cured if the cancer has not metastasized into nearby lymph nodes or the bloodstream and if the surgeon is able to remove all the cancerous cells. Cancers that are treated with surgery include cancers of the head and neck, lung, breast, colon, ovaries, prostate, uterus, and thyroid.

The second most common type of treatment is radiation, received by almost half of all cancer patients. Radiation beams do not kill cancer cells but destroy their ability to reproduce. Radiation is used for treating Hodgkin's disease and cancers of the brain, throat, bone, testicles, and cervix. Unfortunately, radiation has some unpleasant side effects, which include diarrhea, fatigue, difficulty swallowing, intense itching, and lack of taste and smell.

Chemotherapy, another type of cancer treatment, involves giving drugs, hormones, or both to treat cancer that has spread from its original site. Essentially, the chemicals affect all fast-growing tissue. This explains why people are more likely to lose all their hair when they are taking chemotherapy treatments. As with radiation, chemotherapy often has unpleasant side effects, which can be quite uncomfortable and may include nausea, vomiting, diarrhea, anemia, hair loss, and lowered immunity.

Other treatments are gaining acceptance for various cancers:

• *Biological therapy.* Biological therapies are designed to stimulate the body's own immune system. As the immune system gets stronger, chemotherapy is used so that both modalities help fight cancer.

- *Cryosurgery.* **Cryosurgery** uses liquid nitrogen to freeze the cancer cells at the site of the tumor. It is currently gaining acceptance for cancers inside the body, such as prostate cancer, but it has been used for quite some time on basal cell cancer on the skin.

- *Laser surgery.* Lasers are most commonly used to treat superficial cancers (cancers on the surface of the body or the linings of internal organs) such as skin cancer and the very early stages of certain cancers like cervical, penile, or non–small-cell lung cancers.

cryosurgery
the use of liquid nitrogen to freeze cancerous tumors, thus destroying cancerous tissue

Other Chronic Conditions

In addition to the life-threatening chronic conditions such as cancer, heart disease, and stroke, there are less serious chronic ailments that are troublesome to good health and may require continual medical attention. These conditions can affect young adults and the elderly.

Osteoporosis

Your bones are living tissue. They are made primarily of calcium and **collagen**, a protein substance that gives structural flexibility in bones and other tissues such as your nose and ears. During your lifetime, calcium is constantly removed from bone and replaced. During your childhood and teen years, calcium was replaced faster than it was removed, causing the bones to become stronger. Through the adult years, the calcium tends to be removed faster than it is replaced.

Osteo means "bone," and *porosis* means "porous." Osteoporosis is a chronic condition that thins and weakens the bones to the point that the bones become fragile and porous and break easily. Women and men with osteoporosis most often break bones in the hip, spine, and wrist. Although the disease appears in elderly individuals, it appears to be a condition that begins in young adulthood. The condition can affect men and women, but of the approximately 44 million Americans at risk for this disease, 68 percent are women. Approximately 50 percent of the women and 25 percent of men over 50 years of age will break a bone because of osteoporosis.

Osteoporosis is considered a "silent disease" because a person is not aware that he or she has the condition until a bone breaks, but there are known risk factors, including the following:

- Getting older

- Being small and thin

- Consuming a diet low in calcium and vitamin D

- Lack of weight-bearing physical activity

- Having a family history of osteoporosis

- Taking certain medicines, such as steroids, thyroid hormone, and arthritis treatment drugs

- Smoking cigarettes

- Being a white or Asian woman, especially one who has completed menopause

- Having osteopenia (low bone mass)

WEB LINK

http://www.cancer.gov/cancertopics

Cancer treatment information can be found on the Web site for the National Cancer Institute, part of the National Institutes of Health. When you get to the site, click on "Cancer Treatments," and you can go to links with information on virtually any form of cancer.

SEARCH TERMS: cancer treatment, new cancer treatment, advances in cancer treatment

collagen
firm, flexible connective tissue in the body, made of protein

Knowledge of the risk factors is helpful because if you have some of these characteristics, you may suspect a propensity for osteoporosis. If you think you may be at risk, you can ask your physician to schedule a bone density test. It is a painless test that uses X-ray or ultrasound to measure the density of tissue in the bones. If the test indicates the possibility of osteoporosis, the doctor may prescribe a once-a-month medication to restore calcium retention. Osteoporosis can be prevented in most cases, beginning in young adulthood. The consumption of calcium-rich foods along with those that are rich in vitamin D is a very important preventive measure. Another preventive measure is to engage in weight-bearing exercises, such as walking, jogging, or tennis. Non–weight-bearing exercises, such as swimming, do not build bone density.

migraine
brain and nervous system disorder characterized by recurring attacks of severe headache

Migraine Headaches

Headaches are one of the most common reasons for doctors' office visits in the United States. There are many types of headaches, some more painful than others, but one of the most debilitating is the **migraine** headache. This is a brain and nervous system disorder that is characterized by recurrent attacks of severe headache accompanied by various combinations of symptoms that include nausea, vomiting, and sensitivity to light and sound. The headache lasts from 3 to 72 hours, with the pain usually occurring on only one side of the head. Some migraine sufferers see flashing lights and bright spots or experience other changes in their vision just before the onset of the headache.

There is no known cause of migraine. The most widely accepted theory is that migraines have a hereditary component. People prone to migraine seem to have a nervous system that is very sensitive to sudden changes in the body or the environment. Scientists believe that abnormal cells in the brain play a role in migraine and that certain factors, called migraine triggers, cause these abnormal cells to produce a headache. Here are some common triggers reported by migraine patients:

Did You Know …?

Women are three times more likely to suffer from migraine headaches than men. There is no clear reason why this is so, but scientists suspect that it is related to female hormones and the reproductive system.

- Lack of food
- Lack of rest or sleep
- Exposure to light
- Hormonal disturbance, especially in women
- Stress
- Alcoholic drinks
- Chocolate
- Foods, such as cheese, sour cream, and yogurt, that contain a chemical called tyramine
- Citrus fruit, such as oranges and grapefruits
- Certain food additives, such as nitrites, monosodium glutamate, and aspartame (NutraSweet and Equal sweetener)

What's News

Terrell Davis was an all-pro running back for the Denver Broncos when they won Super Bowl XXXII. His story is a good example of someone who lives successfully despite suffering migraine headaches. During the first quarter of the game, Terrell was hit hard and developed the symptoms of a migraine. The bright sunlight, for example, made him feel worse, so he left the field to take his medication. He was able to return to the game in the second half, scored the winning touchdown, and earned the Most Valuable Player Award for Super Bowl XXXII.

There are different types of treatments for migraines. In the past, doctors gave migraine sufferers pain medication and told them to go home and sleep. Now doctors can treat the migraine itself instead of just the pain because scientists have developed a family of prescription drugs, known as ergot alkaloids, which are effective in treating severe migraines. These drugs halt a migraine attack by preventing dilation of the blood vessels in the brain. Some migraine sufferers help themselves with relaxation exercises, stress management strategies, and biofeedback. These techniques can also be used to prevent migraine headaches from occurring in the first place.

Asthma

Asthma is a chronic disease in which the airways (bronchial tubes) swell, spasm, and produce larger-than-normal amounts of mucus. About 17 million Americans have asthma. Many people may have asthma as children and outgrow it by the time they reach adulthood. Nonetheless, each year, 5,000 people die from asthma. During an asthma flare, sometimes called an asthma attack, breathing is difficult. A flare may be brought on by a variety of triggers, such as allergens, tobacco smoke, exercise, changes in weather, viral infections, and smog. Because the triggers vary from person to person, treatment also varies. Some people can control their asthma by avoiding their triggers; others need medication.

Diabetes

Most of the food we eat is converted into sugar (glucose) to be used as energy by our body cells. The glucose circulates in the bloodstream and must be taken into the cells when needed. **Insulin**, a hormone produced by the pancreas, is necessary for the cells to get the glucose through their cell membrane. When the body either does not produce enough insulin or cannot correctly use the insulin that is produced, a condition known as diabetes develops. **Diabetes** is characterized by high levels of sugar in the bloodstream. Excessively high blood sugar levels can result in many serious complications, including death. In the United States, diabetes is the seventh-leading cause of death. There are two main types of diabetes, but a third form occurs in some women during pregnancy:

1. *Type 1 diabetes.* People with this form of diabetes have had the disease their entire lives. Their bodies don't manufacture insulin and must be controlled with a daily insulin injection. Type 1 diabetes is most often found in children and young adults.

asthma
a condition of the lungs characterized by periodic episodes of airway spasms, causing shortness of breath

insulin
a hormone produced in the pancreas that is used by the body to turn sugar into energy

diabetes
a disease characterized by high levels of sugar in the bloodstream caused by the body's either not producing enough insulin or not correctly using the insulin that is produced

2. *Type 2 diabetes.* People can develop type 2 diabetes at any age—even during childhood. This form of diabetes usually begins with insulin resistance, a condition in which fat, muscle, and liver cells do not use insulin properly. The pancreas loses the ability to secrete enough insulin in response to meals. Being overweight and inactive increases the chances of developing type 2 diabetes. Treatment includes using diabetes medicines, making wise food choices, being physically active, taking aspirin daily, and controlling blood pressure and cholesterol.

3. *Gestational diabetes.* Some women develop gestational diabetes during the late stages of pregnancy. Although this form of diabetes usually goes away after the baby is born, a woman who has had it is more likely to develop type 2 diabetes later in her life.

About 85 to 90 percent of American diabetics have type 2 diabetes, and most of these people are mature adults. Diabetes is becoming more prevalent, and, with the rising level of obesity in children, physicians are now seeing many teens with type 2 diabetes. Most type 2 diabetics can control their diabetes with diet, exercise, and weight control. In some cases, drugs are also used to bring the disease under control.

We don't know what causes diabetes, but heredity, obesity, and lack of exercise play an important role in the development of the disease. A diagnosis for diabetes is confirmed with blood tests, but a person may suspect that he or she has diabetes if all or some of the following symptoms are observed:

- Being very thirsty

- Urinating often

- Feeling very hungry or tired

- Losing weight without trying

- Having sores that heal slowly

- Having dry, itchy skin

- Losing the feeling in your feet or having tingling in your feet

- Having blurry eyesight

Diabetes can be very dangerous if it is not treated promptly. It can lead to cardiovascular disease, kidney disease, kidney failure, blindness, severe damage to the hands and feet that can require amputation, and damage to the nervous system. Diabetics must monitor their blood sugar to make sure it is under control. There now are simple test kits that require only one drop of blood, and the National Aeronautics and Space Administration is working on a painless technique that can monitor blood sugar through the skin.

BUILDING YOUR LIFETIME WELLNESS PLAN

The causes of many chronic diseases are under your control, and developing habits now to reduce your risks is a very important part of your wellness plan. The behaviors you practice now set the stage for preventing chronic conditions later in life. You may have noticed that all the chronic disease condition discussed in this chapter have behavioral risk factors associated with them. What can you do to practice wellness and reduce your risk factors? Complete your wellness plan and see.

●●● End-of-Chapter Activities

Opportunities for Application

1. Talk to as many of your family members as you can to find out if there is a history of heart disease among your relatives. If there is, collect information about family members who have heart disease, who had heart disease but did not die from the disease, or who had heart disease and died from it. What risk factors did they have? Prepare a short report of wellness behaviors (and wellness misbehaviors).

2. Perform an Internet search for a site related to various chronic diseases. Locate one reliable site for each disease and record the site name and URL. Make a list of the reasons under the URL explaining why you feel each particular site is a reliable and valid Web site.

3. Your doctor has just completed your annual examination. Your blood evaluation indicates that you have a total cholesterol value of 225 and an HDL value of 52. What does this tell you?

4. Imagine that you have a friend who complains about symptoms that you think relate to some of the chronic conditions discussed in this chapter. Explain what you could do to help your friend learn more about the condition and possibly seek treatment.

Key Concepts

1. Explain the difference between chronic and infectious diseases.

2. Explain the difference between systolic and diastolic blood pressure.

3. List and describe the symptoms of a heart attack.

4. List and describe at least four factors known to contribute to the formation of cancer.

5. Describe the difference between type 1 and type 2 diabetes.

Answers to Personal Assessment: Heart Disease

1. True

2. False. The desirable level is 200 or below.

3. False. Although fish oil supplements can have some beneficial effects, eating fish is the best way to receive the protective effect.

4. False. Remember from Chapter 9 that margarine contains trans fat.

5. True

6. False. Unless there is a medical condition that calls for it, children do not have to be tested.

7. False. Vegetable oils can help if they are in liquid form. But hydrogenated oils, such as margarine, contain trans fats, a risk for heart disease.

8. True

9. True

10. True

●●● References

Heron, M. P. (2007). Deaths: Leading causes for 2004. In *National Vital Statistics Reports* (Vol. 56, No. 5). Hyattsville, MD: National Center for Health Statistics.

Kreimer, S. (June 2007). Hispanic women face heart risks earlier. *DOC* News (American Diabetes Association), *4(6), 7.*

National Cancer Institute. (2009). Cellular Telephone Use and Cancer Risk. *National Cancer Institute: Fact Sheet.* Retrieved April 2, 2010 from http://www.cancer.gov/cancertopics/factsheet/Risk/cellphones

National Heart Lung Blood Institute. (2005). *High Blood Cholesterol: What You Need to Know.* National Institutes of Health, NIH Publication No. 05-3290. Retrieved April 2, 2010 from http://www.nhlbi.nih.gov/health/public/heart/chol/wyntk.pdf

National Heart Lung Blood Institute. (2009). *Atherosclerosis.* Retrieved April 2, 2010 from http://www.nhlbi.nih.gov/health/dci/Diseases/Atherosclerosis/Atherosclerosis_WhatIs.html

CHAPTER 15

Safety and Emergency Preparedness

CHAPTER OBJECTIVES

When you finish this chapter, you should be able to:

- Explain the difference between unintentional and intentional injuries.
- List the four major categories of unintentional injuries.
- Explain the major causes of motor vehicle injuries.
- Describe the relationship of age and gender to unintentional and intentional injuries.
- Describe key elements in being prepared for emergencies.
- Develop a personal and family safety plan.

KEY TERMS

bioterrorism

date rape or acquaintance rape

Heimlich maneuver

homicide

intentional injury

Rohypnol

sexual assault

sexual harassment

statutory rape

unintentional injuries

violence

violent victimization statistics

years of potential life lost

●●● Introduction

Living an interesting, healthy, and active life includes being aware of risks you may encounter, learning to recognize the potential for risky situations, and being able to avoid them. Some of these situations will be interpersonal in nature, such as circumstances where forethought about safety issues can protect you from harmful behaviors; others may be related to accidents beyond your control or disasters, such as hurricanes, tornadoes, ice storms, and so on. Although it is impossible to predict and avoid all types of risks, you can make some conscious choices that decrease the potential injuries and death. Moreover, it is helpful to think ahead for some of these events so that you have a plan of action in case they do occur. Many injuries, including those that are most

PERSONAL ASSESSMENT
Preventing Injury Quiz

Before reading this chapter, test how much you already know about keeping yourself and others safe from injuries. Read each statement and answer if you think the statement is true or false in the space provided. Then see the answers found at the end of the chapter.

1. Motor vehicle crashes are the leading cause of death in the United States for all age-groups.

2. It is estimated that 75 percent of all motor vehicle crashes occur on interstate highways.

3. Some studies show that talking on a cell phone while driving is as dangerous as driving while intoxicated.

4. The number of fatal crashes that are alcohol related has decreased over the past 20 years.

5. Most home injuries and deaths are caused by unintentional discharge of firearms.

6. Most deaths related to fires are due to smoke inhalation rather than to burn injuries.

7. The number of violent acts in the United States is at the lowest rate in almost 30 years.

8. Rates of violence are higher among persons over the age of 25 than among those younger than 25.

9. You are more likely to be killed or injured at home or in the community than at work.

10. Most cases of sexual assault involve an attack by a stranger.

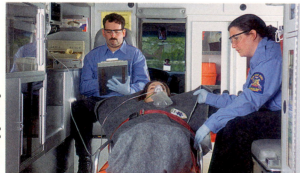

Delmar/Cengage Learning

FIGURE 15-1 • Many injuries can be prevented by learning their causes and practicing preventive behaviors.

serious, can be prevented by learning about their causes and practicing behaviors that are preventive (Figure 15-1). It is a well-known fact among safety experts that there really is no such thing as a person who is "accident prone." Rather, there are people who don't attend to safety practices. They move along performing unsafe behaviors, oblivious to the fact that foresight can be a form of prevention. This chapter presents information to help you develop strategies for safe living. You will also be challenged to determine what level of risk for injury or death you are willing to accept in order to live the kind of lifestyle you want.

●●● Choices and Consequences

As you were growing up, you probably felt that you didn't get to make as many of your own decisions as you would have liked. It probably seemed as if your parents or other adults made most of the important choices in your life. As an adult, you now have the responsibility for making your own decisions. It's wonderful to be in charge of your life, but it can also be a little intimidating. Every decision acted on results in a set of consequences. Needless to say, once you have chosen a pathway, you alone become responsible for the outcome. Furthermore, once acted on, it is nearly impossible to undo the behavior.

Deciding how much risk you are willing to accept is part of life. Think about how much risk you are willing to accept in exchange for the way you want to live and the probability of negative outcomes. For example, if you really enjoy bike riding but are unwilling to wear the necessary safety gear, are you willing to accept the risk of injury or death? What about other recreational activities, such as snowboarding, skiing, or rock climbing? Each of these activities comes with inherent risk of injury or possibly even death. Is this a risk that you are willing to accept in return for the pleasure you enjoy? Are there things that you can do to decrease your chance of injury while participating in these activities? Answers to these questions involve calculating risk and making decisions that correspond with the level of risk you determine to be right for you.

There is a difference between actual risk and perceived risk. While the actual risk of an activity may be relatively low, you may perceive it to be quite high. On the other hand, you may perceive that the risk for another activity is high when in fact risk may be low. Different individuals perceive risk differently, depending on their personalities and previous experiences. In addition to your own perceptions of risk, it is important to be aware of the objective facts concerning actual risk when you are making decisions about how much risk you are willing to accept. The information in this chapter will provide you with objective facts regarding various types of risk. You can then compare this with your subjective assessments of risk and make decisions about what levels of risk you are comfortable accepting.

●●● Unintentional Injuries

Unintentional injuries are injuries that happen when no harm was intended to occur. They are sometimes called accidents, but the word *accident* suggests that nothing can be done to prevent harm or injury. In fact, most unintentional injuries can be prevented.

The four major categories of unintentional injuries are the following:

1. Motor vehicle crashes

2. Injuries that occur in the home

3. Recreational or leisure-time injuries

4. On-the-job injuries

Unintentional injuries are the leading cause of death and disability among children, teens, and young adults (Figure 15-2). They are also the reason for more **years of potential life lost** than any other cause of death. When people are young, they have

unintentional injuries
injuries that happen when no harm was intended to occur; formerly called accidents

years of potential life lost
the difference in years between an individual's life expectancy and that individual's age at the time of death

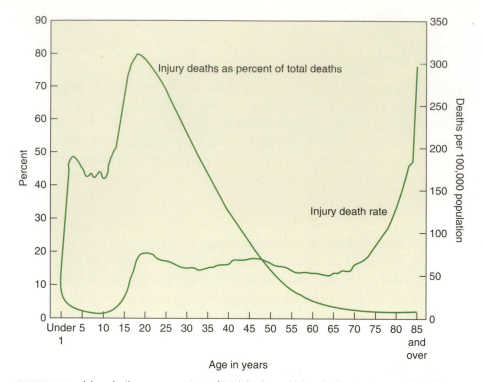

FIGURE 15-2 • Injury deaths as a percentage of total deaths and injury death rates by age: United States, 2003–2004. (Source: Centers for Disease Control and Prevention/National Center for Health Statistics, National Vital Statistics System; Bergen, Chen, Warner, & Fingerhut, 2008).

their whole lives ahead of them, up to 70 or 80 years and maybe more. Unintentional injuries accounted for 27.7 million emergency room visits in 2006. Preventing death from unintentional injury helps ensure that young people will live out their expected life span rather than having it cut short before they reach even middle age. Note in Figure 15-2 that unintentional injury contributes to a very high death rate among elder adults.

Motor Vehicle Injuries

Did You Know…?

According to the National Highway Transportation Safety Administration, on a per population basis, drivers who were under the age of 25 were more likely to be involved in a fatal motor vehicle crash than any other age-group.

According to the Centers for Disease Control and Prevention, in 2006, motor vehicle accidents represented the leading causes of death for individuals between the ages of 15 and 34 (2007). The National Highway Traffic Safety Administration (2008) reported 17,921 people in this age group were killed in motor vehicle accidents. Motor vehicle crashes are also the leading cause of traumatic brain injury death in the United States (CDC, 2010) as well as the cause of many cases of paralysis due to spinal injuries. Many of these deaths and injuries occur when the person is a passenger in a vehicle. It makes good sense to be concerned about safety whenever you are in an automobile, regardless of whether you are the driver or a passenger.

It has been estimated that 75 percent of motor vehicle crashes occur within 25 miles of home at speeds less than 40 miles per hour (Figure 15-3). This is exactly the type of driving we tend to do most often. As with any skill, driving takes attention, time, and practice to learn to drive well. Driving is a complex skill that requires attention to many factors at once. In fact, it is estimated that most motor vehicle crashes are a result of some type of human error. Five of the most common reasons for motor vehicle crashes are (1) excessive speed, (2) aggressive driving habits, (3) driver distraction, (4) alcohol and other drugs, and (5) improper use and nonuse of safety equipment. Driving at the posted speed limit based on road conditions, being courteous to others who share the road, and paying attention when driving can help minimize the likelihood that you will be involved in a motor vehicle crash.

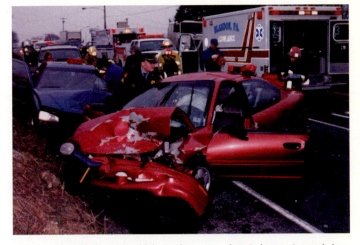

FIGURE 15-3 • Most motor vehicle crashes occur close to home at speeds less than 40 miles per hour. (Courtesy of David J. Reimer Sr.)

Excessive Speed

Excessive speed is cited as a contributing factor in many motor vehicle crashes. The faster you drive, the less time you have to react to an unexpected situation and the longer it takes to bring the vehicle to a stop. Think for a moment about speed limits in neighborhoods. Assume that the posted speed limit is 25 miles per hour. Your friend insists on obeying the speed limit and going only 25 miles per hour. You, on the other hand, always push it to at least 35 miles per hour. You may think that 25 miles per hour is "crawling" and that the police never monitor this street anyway. If a child suddenly runs into the roadway, will it be you or your friend who is most likely to stop to avoid hitting the child? Is this a risk that you are willing to take in order to drive faster (Figure 15-4)?

Aggressive Driving Habits

Reports of aggressive driving incidents have become more common over the past several years. Even so, most aggressive driving incidents still go unreported. As roadways become more crowded, drivers are more likely to find themselves in situations that are annoying or irritating. People also seem to be in more of a hurry these days. Some drivers deal with their frustrations by weaving in and out of traffic and making numerous lane changes in order to save a few seconds. Others try to make it through a yellow light that is sure to turn red before they completely cross the intersection. These are examples of aggressive driving behaviors that are, in fact, habits. The good thing about habits is that they can be changed. Becoming aware of your driving habits can be a good first step to changing them.

Driver Distraction

Driver distraction can be caused by fatigue and sleepiness as well as by the use of cellular phones, passengers in the vehicle, and performing other tasks at the same time as driving. Fatigue is also a major contributor to motor vehicle crashes. Fatigued drivers are not as alert to situations occurring on the roadway and have slower reaction times than well-rested, alert drivers. Some drivers even fall asleep while driving.

A study released in April 2006 conducted by the Virginia Tech Transportation Institute and the NHTSA found that almost 80 percent of crashes and 65 percent of near crashes

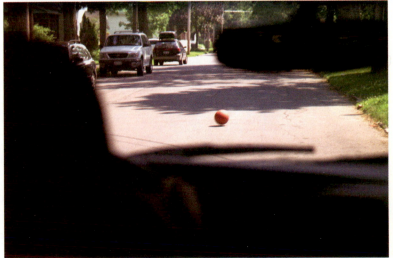

Delmar/Cengage Learning

FIGURE 15-4 • If a child runs in front of your car while you are speeding, will you be able to stop in time?

What's News

Road rage is an exaggerated form of aggressive driving that has received increased attention in the past few years. People who drive too aggressively may violate traffic laws, but those who exhibit road rage behaviors are guilty of criminal behavior. Road rage is demonstrated by uncontrolled anger that results in violence or threatened violence on the road. Road rage is often provoked by something trivial, such as someone driving too slowly or music that is too loud. Although road rage has many possible causes, it is commonly linked to personal attitudes about other drivers and a high stress level that the person lacks the skills to handle appropriately. Both males and females can exhibit road rage, but it is most common among teen and young adult male drivers.

WEB LINK

http://www.aaafoundation.org

Go to "Quizzes" and take a quiz that measures traits related to aggressive driving style. There are other driving quizzes at this Web site that you may find interesting.

SEARCH TERMS: aggressive driving, road rage

Did You Know…?

Almost half of all passenger vehicle occupant fatalities occur after dark, but only about 25 percent of travel occurs after dark. This makes the fatality rate per vehicle mile of travel about three times higher at night than during daylight hours.

involved some type of driver inattention in the seconds immediately preceding the event (Ranney, 2008). In crucial driving situations, response time is a critical factor for avoiding a collision. Driving safely is a skill that requires continual complex reactions. Any type of distraction can increase the likelihood of a crash. Unrestrained pets, changing the radio station, inserting a CD, or reaching for food or a drink are some of the many distractions that have led to motor vehicle crashes.

Traffic safety experts are becoming more and more concerned about the risks associated with the use of cellular phones by drivers. Talking on the phone is just one of the many possible distractions that drivers encounter each day. It seems, however, to be among the most potentially worrisome. The latest research shows that although using a cell phone while driving may not be the most dangerous distraction, it is by far the most common cause of distracted driving crashes and near crashes because there is such a high prevalence of cell phone use. Research indicates that a person using a cell phone while driving is four times more likely to be involved in a crash (Ranney, 2008). Although some people believe that hands-free cell phones are safer, a study published by the National Safety Council (2007) found no significant difference in response time between users of handheld and hands-free phones. A study conducted by researchers at the University of Utah concluded that talking on a cell phone while driving was as dangerous as driving drunk, even if the phone was a hands-free model (Strayer et al., 2006). It is important to know the laws in your state regarding the use of cellular phones. In some states, a driver can be ticketed for using a handheld phone while driving.

Alcohol and Other Drugs

According to the NHTSA, alcohol-related fatalities in 1982 represented about 60 percent of all traffic deaths. Alcohol-related traffic fatalities have declined since that time, and current statistics from the National Safety Council (2007) indicate that alcohol

What's News

A study conducted by Nationwide Mutual Insurance Company (2007) found that 73 percent of drivers used cell phones while driving. The percentage was highest among young drivers. Almost 20 percent of motorists said that they text messaged while driving. A study by the Polk Center for Automotive Studies (2006) reported that 92 percent of respondents agreed that talking on a cell phone while driving increased the risk of accidents. Despite this awareness, however, the same respondents admitted that they continued to engage in the behavior.

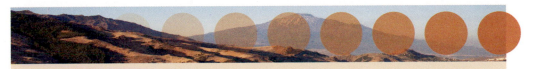

What's Your View?

Use of cell phones while driving is largely unrestricted by most states. No states totally ban the use of cell phones while driving, although a few states ban the use of handheld phones while driving. Some major cities also have restrictions on the use of handheld cell phones. Washington became the first state to ban the practice of text messaging on a cell phone while driving. As of January 2009, there were five other states that followed suit. Using a cell phone headset while driving is not something banned by any state or major city. Do you think there should be stricter laws in place regarding the use of cell phones while driving? Why or why not?

was a factor in approximately 40 percent of motor vehicle fatalities in 2005. Increasing the minimum legal drinking age to 21 and passing zero-tolerance-for-alcohol traffic laws are thought to have been partially responsible for this decrease.

Although we have seen a substantial drop in alcohol-related traffic deaths across time, there is still a lot of room for improvement. Even when the amount of alcohol in the bloodstream is below the legal limit, which varies by state, driving ability can be impaired. Reason, judgment, and response time are all affected by even small amounts of alcohol. Combining alcohol with driving is taking a big risk that may have life-or-death consequences—for yourself, your passengers, and others who share the road with you. Is this a risk that you are willing to take?

Improper Use and Nonuse of Safety Equipment

Over the past few decades, the safety equipment installed in motor vehicles has become more advanced. In addition to lap safety belts, new vehicles now have lap and shoulder belts, front air bags, and, in many cases, side air bags. Too many motorists, however, don't take advantage of all these protective devices. Recent reports by the NHTSA indicate that about 82 percent of Americans regularly wear their safety belts, although this figure decreases by about 10 percent at night. Although this is significant progress since the days of not even having safety belts in vehicles, many lives could be saved if safety belts were

What's News

Almost all 50 states have passed laws that permit or require ignition-interlock devices in the vehicles of all offenders convicted of driving under the influence of alcohol, even those who are convicted for the first time. In New Mexico, alcohol-related fatalities decreased 12 percent from 2004 to 2005, the first year after the law was passed. Ignition-interlock devices require a driver to blow into a machine that tests for alcohol in the breath before starting the car. Intermittent tests are also administered while the car is running. The devices cost the offender about $60 to $75 per month and may be installed for one year or more, depending on the state.

used more consistently. Every state except New Hampshire has some form of passenger restraint law. An individual is much more likely to be injured or killed in a motor vehicle crash if he or she is not wearing a safety belt. In fatal crashes in 2005, 55 percent of passenger vehicle occupants killed in motor vehicle crashes were unrestrained. The NHTSA reports that thousands of lives could be saved every year if drivers and passengers would just buckle up.

Air bags are a relatively recent innovation in safety equipment. It seems likely that air bags reduce the chance of injury and death. As air bags inflate, however, they can injure or even kill a child or small adult in the passenger seat. Children 12 years of age and under are always safest in the backseat. Infants and young children are required to be restrained in a safety seat. Following specific instructions for installation of an infant or child safety seat is critically important. Many inspections of safety seat installation have shown that the seats are installed incorrectly and are not providing proper protection. It is the driver's responsibility to make sure that all children and passengers in the vehicle are safely and properly restrained.

Motorcycles

Although less than 3 percent of passenger vehicles are motorcycles, motorcyclist fatalities represent about 9 percent of all traffic fatalities. Motorcycle fatalities have more than doubled in the past 10 years. This is partially due to the increased number of motorcyclists and to reduced helmet use. Motorcycles share the road with cars, trucks, recreational vehicles, and 18-wheelers that are much larger and heavier. A motorcyclist involved in a collision with one of these larger vehicles is almost always the loser. After an accident, a frequent comment from the driver of one of these larger vehicles is, "But I never even saw it." If you decide to operate a motorcycle, it is critically important that you make sure that you are easily visible to other drivers. Loss of control is another factor in many motorcycle accidents. This is often associated with excessive speed or skidding from improper braking.

Participating in a motorcycle safety training program can alert you to important safety precautions. Another way to increase your chance of survival in case of an accident is the consistent use of an approved motorcycle helmet at all times. Unfortunately, motorcycle helmet use is declining and is currently estimated to be about 58 percent.

At best, riding a motorcycle is a risky behavior. If this is a risk that someone wants to take, he or she should consider taking every available safety precaution. In nearly two-thirds of motorcycle accidents that involve another vehicle, it is the driver of the other vehicle who is at fault. As a motorcyclist, adopting a defensive approach to riding is critical to your safety. Automobile operators should recognize that motorcyclists are not easily seen because when drivers pull into an intersection or pull out to pass another car, they are looking for cars, not motorcycles.

Bicycles

Bicycles are usually included in statistics regarding motor vehicles because they are considered to be moving vehicles with all the rights and responsibilities of an automobile. Most serious injuries to bicyclists occur as a result of a collision with a motor vehicle. One of the major safety concerns for bicyclists is related to confusion regarding the manner in which bicycles share the road. Many motorists believe that bicyclists should get out of the way or stay on the sidewalk. On the other hand, cyclists are not legally able to use the sidewalk. Many bicyclists act as if they have a privileged status that allows them to cut through stopped traffic, run through stop signs and red lights, and switch from road to sidewalk depending on their mood. These attitudes and behaviors create dangerous situations in which neither motorists, bicyclists, nor pedestrians are at risk. Safety campaigns to help both bicyclists and motorists understand the rules of the road can make automobile–bicycle collisions less likely. Like motorcyclists, bicyclists are difficult to see. Wearing brightly colored, reflective clothing and riding defensively can reduce the risk of a collision.

The single most important factor in reducing deaths among bicyclists is wearing an approved safety helmet at all times. In 2008, there were 714 bicyclist deaths, of these, 622 (87 percent) of the victims were not wearing a helmet (Insurance Institute for Highway Safety, 2009). It is estimated that helmet use reduces the risk of death and brain injury by 85 percent, yet less than half of bicyclists consistently wear a helmet. From 1975 to 2005, deaths among bicyclists younger than 16 decreased by 79 percent, while deaths among bicyclists 16 and older increased by 96 percent. Since more than 80 percent of bicyclist deaths occur in those 16 and older, it is important for both adult and youth riders to wear helmets. Even just a short ride around the block can turn into tragedy if there is a fall or collision. A fall onto a concrete surface from only six feet can result in a fractured skull. Wearing a helmet *every single time you ride* might save you from serious brain injury or even save your life.

Injuries in the Home

According to the National Safety Council (2007), there is a fatal injury approximately every 18 minutes and a disabling injury every four seconds in homes across America. Yet most of us feel safer at home than anywhere else. We don't often think about the dangers that exist there. The leading causes of injury-related fatalities in American homes are falls, poisoning, falls, fire, choking, suffocation, and drowning. Many injuries in the home can be prevented by becoming aware of potential dangers and then taking simple safety precautions. The precautions may relate to the age of the home occupants. For example, if there are young children in the home, all toxic substances (cleaning materials, pest control materials, alcohol, and so on) should be stored out reach or under lock and key. If there are elder adults in the home, all throw rugs should have nonslippery backing, and there should be no carpeting on stairways to prevent falls.

Poisonings

According to National Safety Council statistics, 32 percent of deaths that occur at home or in the community are due to poisoning (2007). In fact, poisoning is the second-greatest risk of unintentional injury or death after motor vehicle accidents. Young children are particularly vulnerable to death by poisoning because of their curiosity and lack of knowledge about the harmfulness of common products. Even common, over-the-counter drugs such as aspirin can cause death if too many tablets are consumed. Cleaning agents, certain houseplants, and drugs should all be kept out of the reach of children.

Children, however, are not the only ones who are victims of poisonings. You may be surprised to learn that most poisoning fatalities occur in people over the age of 19, particularly in those aged 40 to 50. These poisonings are often related to ingesting nonlethal substances in toxic amounts or mixtures. Examples include the misuse or improper combination of legal prescription drugs, combining prescription drugs with alcohol, or illegal drug use, particularly narcotics. Exposure to household or home improvement toxins is also a factor.

In the event of a poisoning, the best action is to call the Poison Control Center. Keep your local Poison Control Center number next to the phone. Treatment for poisons will vary, depending on the type of poisoning, so it is important to call for advice. Inducing vomiting, for example, is recommended for some types of poisoning. For others, inducing vomiting can make the problem worse.

Falls

Falls are second only to poisonings as a cause of accidental death in the home. Although we usually think of a fall as something that occurs from a roof, tree, or ladder, many falls occur as a result of tripping or slipping at ground level. Tripping over a toy or other object left on the floor and slipping on icy or snowy sidewalks are common examples of falls that result in injuries and sometimes even death. It may be hard to imagine that a simple fall can cause death, but in 2000, falls caused or led to 15,400 deaths across the country (Bergen, 2008). About half these falls occurred in the home. Even slipping in the shower can lead to death if you strike your head against a hard or sharp object.

Falls are especially critical health threats for elder adults. Falls are the major cause of injuries, hospitalizations, and death among the elderly. Elders are especially vulnerable to injury from falls because their bones become more brittle with age. Every year, one out of three adults age 65 or older will take a fall. There are a number of reasons why elder adults are prone to falling. More important, there are the natural effects of aging. As people age, the changes in their nervous system will affect balance, and muscles lose tone, inhibiting elders from recovering their balance. Vision changes with age prevent elder adults from seeing well in dim light; thus, they will not see changes in terrain, carpeting, stairs, and so on. Elder adults are likely to be taking a number of medications, the effects of which can impair balance. There are also environmental conditions that contribute to falls among the elderly. They can trip on carpeted stairs or slip on small unfastened rugs on wooden or tile floors or icy sidewalks. To minimize the possibility of falls, home should be made "fall resistant" to the greatest extent possible (Figure 15-5). Elder adults can be encouraged to exercise. Research demonstrates that older adults who exercise on a regular basis are more fit and have better balance than those older adults who do not exercise.

When we talk about assessing risk and determining consequences, most of us could agree that even though there is a risk of death from falling in the shower, we would still choose to take regular showers. This is an example of a situation in which we assess the risk and the likelihood of negative consequences and decide that the benefits outweigh the risks. At the same time, we can take actions to reduce our risk of danger, such as using nonskid mats, or being careful to move carefully and in balance. Other actions that can lower the risk of falling in the home include making sure that stairs and living areas are well lighted, installing handrails in stairways and bathrooms, and keeping the floor and walkways clean and clear of clutter.

Fires

The most common cause of fatal fires in the home is the careless use of smoking materials. Most fire deaths are a result of smoke inhalation rather than burns. Maintaining working smoke detectors in key areas of the home is the best way to prevent smoke inhalation deaths. Too often, smoke detectors have been installed but do not function correctly. Batteries in smoke detectors should be tested at least once a month to make sure they are still able to sound an alarm in the event of a fire.

It's important to perform a home safety check to see if smoke detectors and fire extinguishers are present and working in key areas of your home, especially the kitchen and hallways. It's a good idea to set up a regular schedule for testing your smoke detectors, such as on the first day of each month, to make sure they are operating correctly. If the detectors are battery operated, the batteries should be changed once a year. Make sure all the members of your family know where the fire extinguishers are located and what to do in the event of a fire.

Another key aspect of home fire safety is having an established escape plan for every member of the family from every room in the house. Your local fire department can provide guidelines for establishing an escape plan. It is important to practice the plan, preferably at night, which is the time when most fires occur. Designate a prearranged meeting place for all members of the family once they have exited the house so that you will know that everyone is safe.

Suffocation and Choking

Many suffocation deaths involve children. Often these deaths occur when children are too young to recognize the dangers involved and adequate action has not been taken to protect them. Infants can suffocate if they become tangled up in bedding that obstructs their breathing. Other potential dangers for young children are plastic bags, which, when

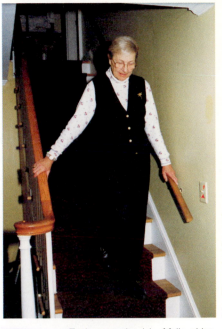

Delmar/Cengage Learning

FIGURE 15-5 • To decrease the risk of falls, elder adults homes should be made fall resistant, and they should be encouraged to use handrails when going up and down the stairs.

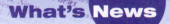

What's News

The Coalition for Fire-Safe Cigarettes is working for legislation to require cigarette manufacturers to only produce fire-safe cigarettes. Fire-safe cigarettes are a proven, practical, and effective way to reduce the risk of cigarette-ignited fires. Fire-safe cigarettes are manufactured in such a way that they have a reduced ability to burn when left unattended. The sale of these fire-safe cigarettes is legislated or already in place in all but three states.

placed over the face, can block the mouth and nostrils, and window-blind cords, which can strangle a child. Abandoned refrigerators and open car trunks can be particularly dangerous for inquisitive young children who are playing unsupervised.

Young children are also particularly susceptible to suffocation and choking deaths by airway obstruction. The airway can become obstructed when a child inhales food particles, pieces of a balloon, coins, or small toy pieces. Even adults often try to talk and eat at the same time, but doing so can put you at risk for food particles getting sucked into the windpipe.

Many lives have been saved by prompt use of the **Heimlich maneuver**, a relatively simple action that uses abdominal thrusts to dislodge items that are obstructing breathing. For information on how to use the Heimlich maneuver, see Figure 15-6.

Unintentional Discharge of Firearms

Although unintentional discharge of firearms is not one of the top four causes of death in the home, accidental discharge is a factor in many preventable deaths every year. This often occurs when young children find and play with guns without the knowledge of an adult. Some adults believe that the firearms they keep in the home are not loaded.

> **Heimlich maneuver**
> the use of abdominal thrusts to dislodge items that are causing choking; it is named after the physician who perfected the technique, Henry Heimlich

1. Ask the person if he or she is choking.
2. If the person starts to cough, wait.
3. If the person cannot speak, cough, or breathe, but is conscious:
   a. Stand behind the victim and wrap your arms around the victim's waist.
   b. Make a fist, keeping thumb straight (see A).
   c. Place the thumb side of your fist against the victim's upper abdomen, below the rib cage and above the navel (see B).
   d. Grasp your clenched fist with the other hand and press into the victim's upper abdomen with a quick upward thrust. Do not squeeze the rib cage or "hug" the victim (see C).
   e. Repeat the upward thrusting of your hands until the object is expelled.

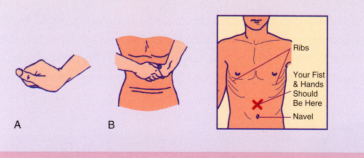

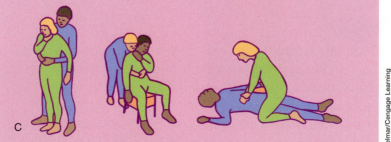

Delmar/Cengage Learning

FIGURE 15-6 • The Heimlich maneuver.

More often, however, adults know that the firearm is loaded but believe they have put it where the children can't find or reach it.

You can protect yourself and teach others to do the same by understanding the dangerous and unpredictable nature of guns. The careless use of a firearm, whether it is believed to be loaded or not, can result in tragedy. A good rule of thumb is to never point a gun at someone or something you don't intend to shoot. A firearm in the hands of someone who has no sense of how guns operate or knowledge of what a discharged bullet can do is very dangerous. If you are ever around someone who brings out a gun, especially if the gun does not belong to him or her, leave the area immediately.

Many states require people to attend gun safety classes before they can purchase a handgun. These classes teach people to respect the power of weapons and to use guns safely. This information helps reduce accidental shootings. Non–gun users can do some things to protect themselves:

- Never attempt to handle guns without proper training.

- Avoid situations where untrained people are handling guns.

- Never challenge or threaten someone who has a gun.

Young children should be educated about gun safety and trained to respect firearms and leave the area *anytime* someone they know produces a firearm. If they mistakenly think that they will leave if the gun happens to be fired, it may be too late.

Recreational Injuries

Numerous safety hazards are associated with recreational or leisure-time activities. Americans are spending more time engaging in recreational activities, so it is important to be aware of potential risks. Since most of these recreational activities occur outside the home, unintentional injuries are likely to occur at a place where assistance is not readily available in case of an injury. A basic level of first-aid training can be useful in case of an accident until help arrives. With all recreational activities, some of the keys to preventing unintentional injuries are the following:

- Learn proper skills and techniques for participation and using any devices needed for the activity.

- Use safety and protective gear properly.

- Avoid the use of alcohol and drugs before or during participation in activities.

- Be aware of your actions and the actions of others.

All water sports are potentially hazardous. Swimming and boating can result in drowning deaths, particularly for those who do not swim well. These deaths are often caused by a combination of carelessness and alcohol use. If you are not a strong swimmer, you should always wear a life jacket when boating. Household pools should always be fenced and locked to keep unattended young children from wandering into the pool. Children should not be permitted to use the pool facilities without adult supervision, even if the children have swimming skills (Figure 15-7).

Skateboards, in-line skating, and scooters are frequent causes of injuries to the head, wrist, arm, and hand. Proper and consistent use of safety equipment, including a helmet, knee pads, wrist braces, and so on, can help prevent many of these injuries

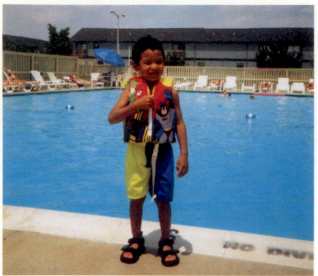

Delmar/Cengage Learning

FIGURE 15-7 • Even the proper use of life vests doesn't replace the need for adult supervision when children are swimming.

(see Figure 15-8). Many of these injuries occur as people go beyond the basic use of the equipment and attempt stunts they think they can perform. There are videos all over the Internet showing people performing stunts and seriously injuring themselves in the process. Would you put on a pair of in-line skates, roll down the metal roof of an office building, and attempt to land on the railing of the steps coming up from the parking lot? Can you imagine what happened to the young man who thought he could perform this stunt without safety equipment?

Work-Related Injuries

Remember the material you read earlier in this chapter about perceived risk versus actual risk? According to the National Safety Council's American Worker Safety Survey (2006), 31 percent of people in the survey indicated that they felt safest at home, and 62 percent said that they felt equally safe at home or work. Only 5 percent felt safer at work. Yet time spent at work is actually safer than time spent driving, being home, or engaging in recreational activities. Work-related injuries and deaths have declined as job safety procedures have become stricter.

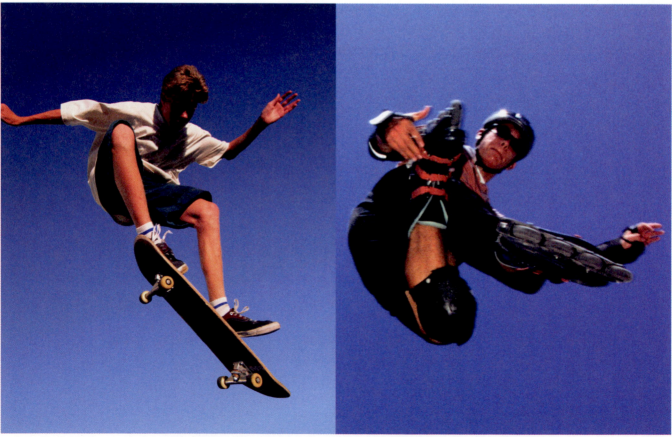

Courtesy of Photodisc

FIGURE 15-8 • Both of these men are skilled at doing skating tricks, but only one is demonstrating awareness of personal safety.

Employers want to protect their workers, and they also recognize that job-related injuries can cost the company money.

Motor vehicle crashes that occur while a person is on the job are the number one cause of work-related injuries. In 2005, motor vehicle crashes accounted for approximately 25 percent of all workplace fatalities, followed by falls, being struck by a flying or falling object, and workplace violence.

Employees sometimes feel as if on-the-job safety precautions are a waste of time. These attitudes must be addressed so that employees and employers can work together to create a safe workplace. Some employees lack the knowledge or skills to perform their jobs safely. In that regard, safety orientation programs for new employees should be put in place. Education and training techniques can prevent many work-related injuries. Back injuries, for example, account for about 20 percent of all injuries on the job. Teaching workers the safest and most efficient ways to lift heavy objects can lead to a decrease in back injuries and a reduction in workers' compensation claims.

> ### Did You Know...?
>
> In the largest study of its kind ever conducted, the National Institute for Occupational Safety and Health (Wassell, et al., 2000) found no evidence that back support belts were helpful in reducing back injury or back pain in retail workers. The study found no significant difference in back injury rate, incidence of self-reported back pain, or rate of back injury claims, even for workers in the most strenuous types of jobs. Instead of using back supports, experts recommend that employers focus on training employees to use good lifting techniques.

Stress and fatigue can contribute to carelessness and result in injuries. Environmental conditions in the workplace can also be a source of injuries or illness. Work-related deaths and injuries are particularly high for laborers and agricultural workers. Some keys to preventing work-related injuries and deaths are the following:

- Be sure you have received proper workplace safety training.
- Always follow safety guidelines for your workplace.
- Exercise caution when engaging in any potentially risky activities.

In addition to their on-the-job safety programs, many employers have instituted off-the-job safety programs for their employees. Employee injuries and deaths are costly to employers in terms of loss productivity, increased medical expenses, loss of valuable personnel, and the costs of hiring and retraining replacement employees. Since most unintentional injuries and deaths occur off the job, employers are recognizing the value of helping to keep their employees safe in all situations, whether at work, at home, or at play. Developing a "culture of safety" that transcends the workplace yields benefits for employers as well as employees and their families.

●●● Intentional Injuries and Violence

Intentional injury is any harm, injury, or death that is caused deliberately. **Violence** is the use of physical force with the intent to inflict harm, injury, or death. A variety of violent crime statistics are compiled by different organizations in the United States. The FBI Uniform Crime Reports Program collects information about crimes that are reported to the police for the following seven offenses: homicide, forcible rape, robbery, aggravated assault, burglary, larceny-theft, and motor vehicle theft. The U.S. Department of Justice, through its National Crime Victimization Survey (NCVS), collects statistics on all nonfatal violent crimes against persons 12 years of age and older.

intentional injury
any harm, injury, or death that is caused deliberately

violence
the use of physical force with the intent to inflict harm, injury, or death

violent victimization statistics
statistics for rape, sexual assault, robbery, aggravated assault (assault with a weapon), and simple assault; statistics do not include murder

Violent victimization statistics include rape, sexual assault, robbery, aggravated assault, and simple assault. Although the statistics gathered are not exact, they give a good estimation of violent crimes other than murder. According to the NCVS, the overall violent victimization rate has declined steadily since 1994 and in 2005 was the lowest ever recorded. The FBI Uniform Crime Reports showed that the overall rate of criminal violence decreased 26 percent between 1996 and 2005. This is great news, but many forms of violence still exist, and much work needs to be done to further reduce violence.

Homicide

homicide
the deliberate killing of one human being by another

At the national level, no crime is measured as carefully as is **homicide**. One obvious reason is the seriousness of the crime. An additional reason is that homicide can also be used as a relatively reliable indicator for all violent crime. Homicide is the second-leading cause of death among young people aged 16 to 24, second only to motor vehicle crashes, and is the third-leading cause of death (after motor vehicle crashes and suicide) for young adults 25 to 34 years of age. Males, teenagers, young adults, and persons of color are most likely to be victims of homicide. According to the Bureau of Justice Statistics (2006), older teens and young adults ages 18 to 24 years had the highest homicide victimization rates per age-group. Historically, this same age-group has the highest rates as homicide offenders. Once a person reaches the age of 25, his or her chances of being a victim of violent crime begin to decline significantly.

In most homicides, the perpetrators are male. Females do kill, but they do not initiate violence as often as males, and they kill for different reasons, often in self-defense. Homicides are frequently the result of an argument that gets more and more intense and leads to angry and aggressive behavior. If a person decides to use force and a firearm is available, all too often the argument ends in a homicide.

In 2005, about 70 percent of all homicides involved the use of a firearm, usually a handgun. Contrary to popular opinion, people are unlikely to be killed by a stranger. Only about 15 percent of homicide victims were murdered by strangers. Since you are much more likely to be at risk from someone you know than from a stranger, you should be aware of potentially violent behavior in people with whom you associate. For example, it might not be safe to be closely involved with a person who gets angry easily and threatens or seems capable of violence.

Gang-Related Violence

Gang-related violence was once thought to be a problem only in urban, inner-city neighborhoods. Today, however, gangs exist not only in urban areas but also in suburban and rural areas. Gangs tend to develop when teens and young adults perceive the need to "stick together" to protect themselves or establish dominance over another group. All humans need companionship, support, security, and a way to gain self-esteem. Gangs provide a way of belonging to a specific group. Conflicts over territory, the need to establish dominance, and the need to experience excitement and victory are some of the most common reasons for rival gangs to fight. Gang violence tends to spread beyond the gang itself, sometimes resulting in family members or innocent bystanders being injured or killed.

Hate Crimes

Hate crimes are acts of violence committed against an individual because of his or her race, ethnicity, national origin, religion, or sexual orientation. Hate crimes occur when people are unable to accept the many differences that exist between individuals and groups in our society. Sometimes persons who lack the knowledge and skills to deal effectively with those differences feel as if violence is the only way to express their dissatisfaction or frustration with people who are different.

Hate crimes can be directed at either individuals or groups. They can also be focused on the disfigurement or destruction of property, such as painting graffiti or burning a church or place of worship. According to a 2008 FBI report on hate crime, the motivation for just over half the hate crimes was the result of racial bias, about 18 percent associated with religious bias, 16 percent related to sexual orientation bias, and about 13 percent of hate crimes appeared motivated by ethnic origin. In approximately 30 percent of the cases, the perpetrator was known to the victim.

School/Campus Violence

School violence has received a lot of attention in the past few years because of several school shootings that resulted in the deaths of teachers and students. These shootings have occurred not only in K–12 schools but also on college campuses. Statistics consistently show, however, that learners are safer at school than they are at home, in the workplace, or on the road. Despite this fact, the possibility of violence in schools or on college campuses is real. Many schools and college campuses have now adopted school/campus safety plans to deal with both unintentional injuries and intentional violence.

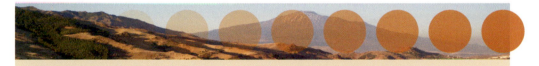

What's Your View?

The 2007 shootings on the Virginia Tech campus that left 32 people dead and many others injured raised many questions about the lengths to which campus officials should go to prevent campus violence. Some individuals believe that it is unreasonable to expect campus security plans to protect students, faculty, and staff from all incidents of this nature. They point out that there is no definitive way to know that an individual is capable of this type of violence and that there is no proven way to prevent this magnitude of violence before it happens. Other individuals believe that it is the responsibility of campus officials to have safety plans that address all possible scenarios for violence. What do you think? Is heightened security the answer? To what extent should freedom be restricted in order to increase security and safety?

Workplace Violence

Relatively few deaths occur in the workplace, and in 2005, only about 10 percent of workplace deaths were from homicides. In 1992, homicide was the second-leading cause of death on the job, second only to motor vehicle crashes that occur on the job. By 2005, however, workplace homicide dropped to fourth, behind falls and being struck by an object. Women account for a higher percentage (24 percent) of workplace fatalities from homicide than do men (9 percent). While women truly may be at higher risk for workplace homicide, it is also possible that women are simply at lower risk for other types of workplace fatalities, such as transportation-related deaths and falls.

In about 85 percent of workplace homicides, the perpetrator is committing a crime (often a robbery) in conjunction with the violence. In contrast to homicides in other situations, the majority of workplace homicides involve perpetrators and victims who don't know each other. Although the media give a lot of attention to violent acts by someone employed or previously employed in the workplace, the National Institute for Occupational Safety and Health (2006) found that only 7 percent of all work-related homicides involved a coworker or former coworker. Table 15-1 identifies the four main categories of workplace violence.

TABLE 15-1 • Typology of workplace violence.

Type	Description
I: Criminal intent	The perpetrator has no legitimate relationship to the business or its employees and is usually committing a crime in conjunction with the violence. These crimes can include robbery, shoplifting, trespassing, and terrorism. The vast majority of workplace homicides (85 percent) fall into this category.
II: Customer/client	The perpetrator has a legitimate relationship with the business and becomes violent while being served by the business. This category includes customers, clients, patients, students, inmates, and any other group for which the business provides services. It is believed that a large portion of customer/client incidents occur in the health care industry in settings such as nursing homes or psychiatric facilities; the victims are often patient caregivers. Police officers, prison staff, flight attendants, and teachers are some other examples of workers who may be exposed to this kind of workplace violence, which accounts for approximately 3 percent of all workplace homicides.
III: Worker on worker	The perpetrator is an employee or past employee of the business who attacks or threatens another employee(s) or past employee(s) in the workplace. Worker-on-worker fatalities account for approximately 7 percent of all workplace homicides.
IV: Personal relationship	The perpetrator usually does not have a relationship with the business but has a personal relationship with the intended victim. This category includes victims of domestic violence assaulted or threatened while at work and accounts for about 5 percent of all workplace homicides.

Source: National Institute of Occupational Safety and Health (2006).

Family and Intimate Violence

Women are most frequently the victims of violent acts committed by family or intimate partners, accounting for approximately 85 percent of cases of violence by intimate partners. According to the U.S. Department of Justice (2006), about 22 percent of women surveyed reported being physically assaulted by an intimate partner in their lifetime. In fact, about one-third of all female murder victims were killed by an intimate partner. In every age-group, female murder victims were four to five times more likely to have been killed by an intimate partner than were male victims.

The majority of perpetrators of family violence have two characteristics in common: they are male, and they witnessed family violence while they were growing up. Abusive partners have a need to control their partner and are unable to communicate, negotiate, and compromise to get their needs and desires met. Figure 15-9 presents the four-phase cycle of violence that most acts of family violence follow.

Abusive behaviors often develop early in the relationship, although they do not become recognized until much later. Abusers use many different mechanisms to isolate, intimidate, and control their partners. See Table 15-2 for some tips from the American Psychiatric Association for early signs of abuse and questions to ask yourself regarding your relationships.

Did You Know...?

Interacting with the public, exchanging money, delivering services or goods, working late-night or early morning shifts, and working alone are all factors that increase the risk of work-related homicide. If you have a job, consider the potential risks associated with the job responsibilities and take precautions to protect yourself to the greatest extent possible.

2. The tension explodes into some form of violent behavior.

1. Tension builds between the partners, often over a relatively minor problem.

3. The abuser begs for forgiveness and promises that the violence will never happen again.

4. If the victim forgives the abuser, a "honeymoon" period of calm follows, but chances are high that the cycle will soon be repeated.

Delmar/Cengage Learning

FIGURE 15-9 • The cycle of violence.

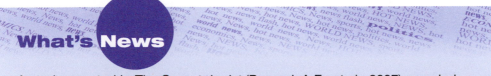

What's News

A study reported in *The Gerontologist* (Bonomi, A.E., et al., 2007) revealed that about 4 percent of women aged 65 and older said that they had been physically or mentally abused by an intimate partner within the previous five years. Once viewed as a problem only in younger women, this study indicates that intimate partner abuse can happen at any age.

TABLE 15-2 • Indicators of an abusive relationship.

Your Inner Thoughts and Feelings
Do you:
√ feel afraid of your partner much of the time?
√ avoid certain topics out of fear of angering your partner?
√ feel that you can't do anything right for your partner?
√ believe that you deserve to be hurt or mistreated?
√ wonder if you're the one who is crazy?
√ feel emotionally numb or helpless?
Your Partner's Belittling Behavior
Does your partner:
√ see you as property or a sex object rather than as a person?
√ force you to engage in sexual behaviors that make you uncomfortable?
√ ignore or put down your opinions or accomplishments?
√ treat you so badly that you're embarrassed for your friends or family to see the behavior?
√ humiliate, criticize, or yell at you?
Your Partner's Controlling Behavior
Does your partner:
√ attempt to control where you go or what you do?
√ constantly check up on you to see what you are doing and where you are?
√ act excessively jealous and possessive?
√ accuse you of having affairs?
√ try to keep you from seeing your friends or family?
√ limit your access to money, credit cards, or the car?
Your Partner's Violent Behavior
Does your partner:
√ hurt you or threaten to harm someone very close to you?
√ hurt you, or threaten to hurt or kill you?
√ threaten to take your children away or harm them?
√ threaten to commit suicide if you leave?
√ destroy your belongings?
Go through the checklist and count the number of "yes" responses. In a healthy relationship, there should be none. The more "yes" answers you give, the more serious is the risk for abuse.

Source: Adapted from: American Psychiatric Association (2010).

Many women stay with abusive partners because they lack the financial resources to leave, have low self-esteem, fear that they cannot find another partner, or don't believe that they can make it on their own. When children are involved, the situation is even more difficult. Children, as well as women, are at risk when family violence is present. In homes where there is partner abuse, children are significantly more likely to be abused than in families where partner violence is not present.

Violence against Children

Violence against children can take many forms: physical, emotional, sexual, or simply neglect. A violent act committed by a parent is one of the five leading causes of death among children ages 1 to 18. As difficult as it is to believe, approximately two-thirds of murders of children under the age of five are committed by a parent or other family member. Parenting is a difficult and demanding task, even under the best of circumstances. Parents who lack the knowledge and skills to cope effectively with the demands of parenthood may become angry and frustrated with their children. If they cannot express this anger and frustration appropriately, they may take it out on the children.

Sometimes one child is singled out as the target for the parent's frustration. Trying to work, taking care of children, and managing all the details of a household can put a big strain on all parents, but the strain can be especially severe for single parents. Single parents who don't have adequate support from others are at risk for acting violently toward their children.

If you are involved in a violent situation at home or are a witness to violence, confide in a trusted person who can assist you in finding the help you need. Getting help early before the situation gets completely out of hand can prevents more serious problems later.

Cyberviolence

As discussed in chapter 5, the rapid growth of the Internet has produced new concerns about "virtual" violent acts that are the result of Internet interactions. Concern has been raised about the violent content of some Web sites and electronic messages. There is more concern, however, about the possibility of a "real-life" violent act committed against someone after an Internet relationship has been established through e-mail or chat rooms.

The anonymity of the Internet allows people to pretend to be someone they are not. For example, a much older man might convincingly pretend to be someone near a younger person's age in order to establish an online friendship. He might then make arrangements to meet the younger person with intentions that are dishonorable or even dangerous. Some people like to make a game of posing as someone older, younger, or of a different gender on the Internet. While this can be an innocent pastime, it can be problematic if the people involved ever decide to meet in real life.

With the popularity of Web sites such as Facebook.com and MySpace.com and hundreds of other opportunities to meet new friends, romantic partners, or even potential roommates online, using the Internet for these purposes becomes a delicate balance. Because it is almost impossible to be absolutely sure about the identity of people you "meet" on the Internet, you should be especially careful revealing personal information about yourself that could allow the other person to identify and locate you. Many experts suggest that you never give out your last name, home address, school, or workplace until you have solid data about the other person that warrants your trust. It may seem harmless to talk to people on the Internet, but the risk for danger should always be considered. Never assume that the people you are "chatting" with are who they portray themselves to be. Even if you begin to trust them, by all means never agree to meet with them anywhere except a very public place, such as a restaurant, library, shopping mall, and so on.

If you decide to meet someone in person whom you have previously interacted with only on the Internet or over the telephone, experts recommend that you always meet for the first time in a public place, during the daytime. Common sense dictates that these relationships should be approached with some degree of caution until you are absolutely sure you can trust the other person. While you may be tempted to throw caution to the wind and quickly become closely involved with someone whom you have just met, this is not generally wise. Of course, that is true regardless of however you met the person.

Sexual Assault

sexual assault

a sexual act involving the use of force or threat of force to get the victim to cooperate

Sexual assault is a violent crime involving the use of force or threat of force to have sexual relations with someone without that person's voluntary consent. Acts of sexual violence can be directed toward both males and females, although it is more common for them to be directed toward females. Although many females fear sexual assault by a stranger, women are most at risk of being assaulted by men they know. About 70 percent of female rape or sexual assault victims report that the offender was an intimate, another relative, a friend, or an acquaintance.

In most cases of sexual assault, a weapon is not used. In 2000, only 6 percent of sexual assaults involved a weapon, such as a gun or knife. The lack of a weapon, however, does not mean that it is not sexual assault. Verbal threats and physical intimidation can be used to force the victim into submitting to a sexual act. Experts have different opinions about whether a victim should fight back when being sexually assaulted. If the perpetrator is a stranger rather than someone the victim knows, there is a greater likelihood that the victim will be physically injured or killed, especially if he or she tries to fight back. Victims of sexual assaults should never be criticized for their decision about how much to resist or the type of resistance they used. They are not at fault for being assaulted.

statutory rape

any sexual relations committed by an older individual (generally over the age of 18) with an individual who is under the legal age of consent (generally age 14 or younger)

date rape or acquaintance rape

any forced sexual activity in which the victim is acquainted with or is dating the rapist

If the victim is younger than the state's legally defined age of consent, a sexual relationship is considered "sexual assault on a minor," sometimes referred to as **statutory rape**, regardless of whether there was mutual consent. The laws in states vary, but generally it is a "victim," the youngest of the two, being seduced by the older perpetrator. For example, a college male of 19 who engages in a sexual relationship with a 14-year-old female, who would be under the legal age of consent, could be charged with sexual assault on a minor even if both parties agreed to the sexual relationship.

About 60 percent of all sexual assault victims report that a current or former spouse, boyfriend, or date was the perpetrator. This crime is known as **date rape or acquaintance rape**. Many of these incidents are never reported to legal authorities. The woman often feels that the incident may have been her fault because she was attracted to the man. There may have been no weapons, direct verbal threats, or strong use of force. Nevertheless, if a woman is coerced into having sexual relations without her consent, she is the victim of sexual assault.

Rohypnol

a drug used in countries outside the United States as treatment for insomnia but most commonly known in the United States as a date-rape drug

Date rapes are frequently alcohol related. Alcohol can affect the judgment and reasoning ability of both the perpetrator and the victim. The effects of alcohol may make it impossible to determine if there was consent. Sometimes drugs such as **Rohypnol** are used to produce temporary amnesia so that the victim will not remember the incident clearly. Use of these so-called date-rape drugs is a criminal act, whether or not sexual assault actually occurs.

Engaging in any type of sexual behavior without establishing clear and direct verbal consent is a risky behavior for both males and females. Males can later be accused of rape, even if they thought the sexual activity was consensual at the time it occurred. Sexual boundaries should be communicated clearly and directly early in the relationship. Once boundaries have been established, follow through by mutually enforcing those boundaries.

Sexual Harassment

Sexual harassment is a milder form of sexual violence than sexual assault, but it can still have many negative consequences for the parties involved. Unwelcome sexual advances, requests for sexual favors, sending unwanted sexually explicit e-mails, or any other conduct that is sexual in nature and creates an intimidating atmosphere can be considered sexual harassment.

Sexual harassment often occurs in situations where there is an imbalance of power, such as between a teacher and a learner, or a supervisor and an employee, or between two employees. Sometimes, sexual favors are demanded in exchange for a passing grade or maintaining employment. If you find yourself in a situation in which you feel that sexual harassment is occurring, tell the person clearly and directly that you find the sexual comments or behaviors inappropriate. Tell him or her to stop the objectionable behavior immediately. If the individual continues the behavior, file a formal complaint with the person's supervisor, employer, or the school administration. If it persists, you can file a complaint asking for a legal remedy with the state or federal Equal Employment Opportunity Commission.

sexual harassment
any unwelcome sexual advances, requests for sexual favors, or other conduct that is sexual in nature and creates an intimidating atmosphere in an academic or work environment

●●● Resolving Conflict Nonviolently

There are many life situations where conflict occurs. Conflict is an unavoidable part of life. Some people attempt to resolve conflict with violence, especially with the use of handguns. The best way to avoid violent conflict is to try to use calming words to reduce the tension and reach a solution or escape a potentially violent situation. If that fails, depending on the circumstances, it may be better to give in to your opponent. Standing your ground unnecessarily to someone with a weapon can lead to tragic consequences.

Factors That Contribute to Violence

Recent rates of violence and intentional injury in the United States have declined. However, they are still higher in the United States than in other similar countries, particularly for murder. Many factors contribute to this situation. Understanding those factors can help you avoid being a victim of violence.

Population Characteristics

Rates of violence are not consistently distributed across the United States. The geographic area of the country that you live in, your gender, your age, and your socioeconomic status all affect the amount of violence to which you are likely to be exposed. For example, rates of murder, especially those involving guns, are higher in southern states than in other states.

Most perpetrators of violent acts are male. Although females do commit violent acts, including murder, they do not do so nearly as often as males. In fact, males are nine times more likely to commit murder than

Did You Know...?
Between 1992 and 2001, Native Americans experienced violence at rates that were more than twice that of blacks, whites, and asians.

are females. Males are also more likely to be victims of violent acts. Three-fourths of all murder victims in the United States are males.

Rates of violence are higher among young people than among older adults. One-half of all persons arrested for violent crimes are under the age of 25. Teenagers and young adults are also victims as well as perpetrators of violence. People from the 12- to 24-year-old age-group have historically had the highest levels of violent victimization of any age-group.

Violence occurs in all racial and ethnic groups as well as at all socioeconomic levels, but it is highest among minority groups with low socioeconomic status. Living or working in an area in which the majority of residents lack status, power, and economic resources puts one at greater risk for experiencing some type of violence.

Interpersonal Relationships

Although we often hear warnings about being careful around strangers, the fact is that most victims of violence know their attacker. Victims and perpetrators are usually similar to each other in gender, ethnicity, educational level, and socioeconomic status. Women, especially, are often the victims of attack by someone who is known to them. In cases of murder, more than 60 percent of the women knew their attacker. The rates for sexual assault are even higher: approximately 70 percent of the women knew their attacker. Men are less likely to know their attacker: about 50 percent of male victims of violence identified a stranger as the perpetrator of the violence.

Use of Alcohol and Other Drugs

Use of alcohol and other drugs is closely related to violent behavior. Many individuals behave much more aggressively when they are under the influence of alcohol or other drugs than they normally would because chemical products release inhibitions. Judgment and reason are among the first things affected by alcohol. A simple argument, fueled by alcohol or drugs, can turn into an angry confrontation that leaves someone injured or dead.

Violence in the Mass Media

Graphic images of violent acts appear frequently in the mass media. Dozens of television programs and movies focus on various aspects of crime. News reports also contain detailed reports of crime and violence.

In most cases, violent incidents are shown in great detail. Research indicates that receiving a constant dose of violent images through the media makes real-life violence seem more common and acceptable. What are often left out from these images are the consequences of violent acts: the suffering of victims and the punishment faced by perpetrators. This unbalanced presentation may give the false impression that there are no real consequences of violence.

Availability of Firearms

In the United States, many different types of firearms are readily available. It is easier to obtain handguns in the United States than in any other industrialized country in the world. Many people believe that the easy accessibility of handguns is one of the reasons that the rate of homicide is so much higher in the United States than in other industrialized countries.

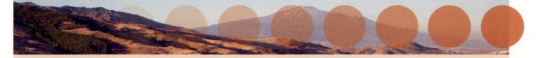

What's Your View?

Violence in the Mass Media

There is a great deal of debate about whether seeing frequent graphic images of violent acts in television programs, cartoons, video games, and movies makes people more likely to act violently themselves. What do you think?

- Would your opinion change depending on how old the person viewing the violent acts is?

- Would your opinion vary with the violent act shown (i.e., if it is a cartoon, a movie, or a video game)?

- Is the violence in "fantasy," such as in a cartoon or video game, different from "reality," such as in a news program or dramatic movie?

Perhaps the main reason that firearms increase the homicide rate is because firearms are so effective in causing death. Other weapons may cause serious injury, but the injuries are less likely to result in death. Approximately two-thirds of all homicides in America are committed using a firearm.

Easy availability of firearms is also a major contributor to suicide in the United States. Suicide is the third-leading cause of death in persons ages 10–14 and the fourth-leading cause of death in young adults ages 25 to 34 (CDC, 2007).

Emergency Preparedness

In the aftermath of the terrorist attacks of September 11, 2001, the subsequent anthrax scare that same year, and the natural disasters of Hurricanes Katrina and Rita, Americans have been bombarded with information about "emergency preparedness." Although the events of September 11 brought emergency preparedness to the forefront of our consciousness, being prepared in the event of an emergency is something that each of us should be mindful of. Unlike natural disasters, **bioterrorism** is a planned threat or release of biologic or chemical toxins released into the air, food systems, or water sources. Bioterrorism is an act that is intentional and criminal in nature, meaning that it requires additional prevention and response strategies that include law enforcement agencies. Since it poses a great threat to society by creating numerous health hazards, many resources are being allocated to ensure surveillance of reemerging infectious diseases along with a thorough public health response to bioterrorist threats.

While terrorist attacks are shocking and tragic, for Americans such attacks are the least likely causes of emergencies. The most common types of emergency situations are natural disasters and severe weather. Contagious disease, explosions, chemical emergencies, violent incidents, and bioterrorism are other examples of emergency situations. While different types of emergencies require different preparations, there are at least three elements that remain constant: having the necessary information about how to respond to an emergency, having a well-stocked emergency supply kit (including food and water),

bioterrorism
the threatened or intentional release of viruses, bacteria, or other toxins to intimidate or harm a civilian or government population

and having a plan about what you and your family will do in the event of an emergency. Most experts suggest that you should have enough food, water, and other supplies to allow you and your family to be self-sufficient for at least three days. In addition, depending on the nature of the emergency, you may be required to provide your own shelter, first aid, and sanitation.

Information on Emergency Preparedness

Several agencies have information, planning guides, and checklists regarding what you need for an emergency. The Department of Homeland Security, the Federal Emergency Management Agency, the Centers for Disease Control and Prevention, and the American Red Cross all provide extensive information about emergency preparedness. Keep in mind that once an emergency occurs, you will usually not have the time or the resources to locate this valuable information. Properly preparing for an emergency includes making the effort now to ensure that you already have the information that you will need in the case of an emergency.

Emergency Supply Kits

Imagine that there is some type of emergency in your community. You do not have any gas, water, or electric service. All the businesses are closed, and emergency personnel are unable to reach you. What will you do until help arrives? One of the most important

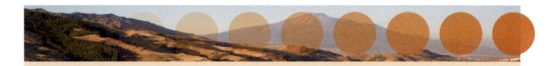

What's Your View?

Some people believe that all the talk about emergency preparedness is just simply encouraging people to be fearful. They feel that the likelihood of an emergency is rare and that the probability is high that emergency personnel will be able to handle any emergency that does occur. Therefore, they see no need to make individual preparations. Other people believe that every individual has the responsibility to be self-sufficient during an emergency. They believe that it is essential that individuals have emergency supply kits and emergency plans in place to provide for themselves and their families during an emergency. What's your view on the following questions?

Is it realistic to expect individuals to be prepared for widespread emergency situations, such as a weather or bioterrorism event? Why or why not?

What about people who are disabled or otherwise unable to care for themselves?

What percentage of resources (time, money, personnel, and supplies) should community and government agencies devote to emergency preparedness given the other pressing needs of our communities, such as education and health care?

things you can do to prepare for a possible emergency is to have a well-stocked emergency supply kit that can help sustain you and your family until help reaches you. Figure 15-10 provides a list of items recommended by the Department of Homeland Security for an emergency supply kit.

Recommended items to include in a basic emergency supply kit:

- Water, one gallon of water per person per day for at least three days, for drinking and sanitation
- Food, at least a three-day supply of nonperishable food
- Battery-powered or hand-crank radio and a NOAA weather radio with tone alert and extra batteries for both
- Flashlight and extra batteries
- First-aid kit
- Whistle to signal for help
- Dust mask to help filter contaminated air and plastic sheeting and duct tape to shelter-in-place
- Moist towelettes, garbage bags, and plastic ties for personal sanitation
- Wrench or pliers to turn off utilities
- Can opener for food (if kit contains canned food)
- Local maps

Additional items to consider adding to an emergency supply kit:

- Prescription medications and glasses
- Infant formula and diapers
- Pet food and extra water for your pet
- Important family documents, such as copies of insurance policies, identification, and bank account records in a waterproof, portable container
- Cash or traveler's checks and change
- Emergency reference material such as a first-aid book or information from http://www.ready.gov
- Sleeping bag or warm blanket for each person (consider additional bedding if you live in a cold-weather climate)
- Complete change of clothing including a long-sleeved shirt, long pants, and sturdy shoes (consider additional clothing if you live in a cold-weather climate)
- Household chlorine bleach and medicine dropper. When diluted nine parts water to one part bleach, bleach can be used as a disinfectant. Or, in an emergency, you can use it to treat water by using 16 drops of regular household liquid bleach per gallon of water.
- Fire extinguisher
- Matches in a waterproof container
- Feminine supplies and personal hygiene items
- Mess kits, paper cups and plates, plastic utensils, and paper towels
- Paper and pencil
- Books, games, puzzles, or other activities for children if necessary

FIGURE 15-10 • Emergency preparedness kit checklist. (Source: Adapted from U.S. Department of Homeland Security, http://www.ready.gov/america/getakit).

Creating an Emergency Plan

You and your family should have an emergency plan in place that you can follow in the event of an emergency. One of the most confusing things about an emergency is that everyone is in a heightened emotional state. As a result, many people are not able to think calmly and logically about the best action to take. Planning ahead can help you avoid this chaotic confusion at the beginning of an emergency. Emergency preparedness should not be an "after-the-fact activity." If you want the necessary provisions for survival after a disaster, you should get them before the event. After the disaster, you will be competing for same resources as the many other people who did not prepare.

Your first decision will probably be whether to stay where you are or to evacuate from the source of the emergency. Depending on the nature of the event, you may not have the option to evacuate, and you may have to stay where you are. In practical circumstances, this may mean that one adult member of the family is at work, another is at home, and any children may be at school or at another location in the community. It is frightening to be separated from those you love in an emergency, but it may be more dangerous to try to get everyone in one place. Each situation requires a determination of whether it is best to stay wherever you are or to try to move to a different location. You should have an emergency plan that considers the likelihood that family members may be separated and unable to communicate. This plan should include a known meeting place in the community, if not your home. Don't count on a cell phone; everyone else will be trying to use their phone, and even if there is working service, the lines will be overcrowded with everyone trying to call. Knowing in advance what you have agreed to do in specific situations can make the uncertainty more tolerable. Advance planning is even more important when you are responsible for young children, the elderly, disabled individuals, or animals.

> **WEB LINK**
>
> **http://www.ready.gov**
>
> At this Web site, you can obtain information from the Department of Homeland Security about staying put or evacuating in an emergency. When you get to the Web site, follow the link to "Make a Plan."
>
> **SEARCH TERMS:** evacuation, shelter-in-place

It is important that you are prepared in the event of an emergency. Having an out-of-town contact person, someone who is unlikely to be affected by a local emergency, a neighborhood and regional meeting place, and an evacuation location can help ensure that family members who are separated in an emergency can be reunited as quickly as possible.

Emergencies Away from Home

If you find yourself in an emergency situation at work, at school, in the community, or while traveling in a vehicle, it is important to have a plan for how to respond. Knowing that you have an emergency plan regardless of where you and your family members are located when the emergency occurs provides a sense of control and safety in a frightening situation. By talking with your workplace and, if applicable, your children's school(s) ahead of time, you can determine whether you are comfortable with the existing emergency plans that are in place or whether you need to take further action. Thinking ahead as to what you would do if you were not at home in the event of an emergency is an important part of an overall emergency preparedness plan.

BUILDING YOUR LIFETIME WELLNESS PLAN

Although it is impossible to guarantee that you can always stay safe, certain actions can help you increase the likelihood. After reading this chapter, consider the importance of the following safety and emergency preparation elements and decide whether to incorporate them into your personal wellness plan:

- Become a skilled driver and take all possible safety precautions in driving situations.

- Create an emergency plan for your home and make sure the smoke detectors are working and your family has a first-aid kit.

- Learn the facts about the causes of unintentional and intentional injury so that you can make informed decisions about the level of risk you are willing to accept.

- If you participate in high-risk activities, make sure that you have and use the proper safety equipment every time.

- Identify actions that you can take to decrease the likelihood of being the victim of an unintentional or intentional injury.

●●● End-of-Chapter Activities

Opportunities for Application

1. Research homicide rates in the United States and in three other industrialized countries. Use visual graphics to report your findings. Do the same for suicide rates. What differences did you discover? What do you think the reasons are for any differences you find?

2. Research and discuss how social environment affects attitudes toward violent behavior. For example, if it is socially acceptable for television programs and video games to have graphic acts of violence, how does that affect attitudes toward real-life violence? Consider how income level might affect a person's attitudes toward violence. What other sociological factors might influence attitudes toward violence?

3. Research a recent disaster in the United States (due to either natural causes or terrorism). Be sure to identify the state and community where it occurred. Research the response efforts in that community. Write a paper that describes if an emergency plan was planned, if it was implemented, and how effective it was. Identify specific ways that it was handled well in addition to identifying areas where it could have been better handled.

Key Concepts

1. Describe your personal attitude regarding risk and how you make decisions about what risks to take.

2. List the four major categories of unintentional injuries and give an example of each.

3. Explain how age and gender are related to violence and intentional injury.

4. Describe the ways in which firearms contribute to violence.

5. Identify the resources you can use to develop safety and emergency preparedness plans.

Answers to Personal Assessment: Preventing Injury Quiz

1. False. Motor vehicle accidents are the number one cause of death for ages 4 to 34.

2. False. Most motor vehicle accidents occur within 25 miles of the home, and the driver is usually traveling at less than 40 miles per hour.

3. True

4. True

5. False. The leading cause of injuries at home is poisoning.

6. True

7. True

8. False. Rates of violence are highest for persons between the ages of 18 and 24.

9. True

10. False. In most cases of sexual assault, the attacker is often someone known by the victim.

●●● References

American Psychiatric Association. (2010). *Domestic Violence*. Retrieved from http://www.healthyminds.org/Main-Topic/Domestic-Violence.aspx?css=print [April 5, 2010]

Bergen, G., Chen, L. H., Warner, M., & Fingerhut, L. A. (2008). *Injury in the United States: 2007 chartbook*. Hyattsville, MD: National Center for Health Statistics.

Bonomi, A. E., et al. (2007). Intimate partner violence in older women. *Gerontologist*, 47(1), 34–41.

Bureau of Justice Statistics. (2006). *Criminal Victimization-2008*. Retrieved May 12, 2010 from http://bjs.ojp.usdoj.gov/index.cfm?ty=pbdetail&iid=1975

Centers for Disease Control and Prevention. (March 2010). *Traumatic Brain Injury in the United States*. Retrieved May 16, 2010 from http://www.cdc.gov/traumaticbraininjury/pdf/blue_book.pdf

Centers for Disease Control and Prevention. (2007). *10 leading causes of death by age group highlighting unintentional injury deaths, United States 2006*. Retrieved May 18, 2010 from:http://www.cdc.gov/injury/Images/LC-Charts/10lc%20-Unintentional%20Injury%202006-7_6_09-a.pdf

Federal Bureau of Investigation. (2008). *Hate Crime Statistics, 2007*. U.S. Department of Justice. Retrieved April 5 from: http://www.fbi.gov/ucr/hc2007/summary.htm

Insurance Institute for Highway Safety. (2009). *Fatality Facts 2008*: Bicycles. Retrieved May 18, 2010 from http://www.iihs.org/research/fatality_facts_2008/bicycles.html

National Highway Traffic Safety Administration. (2009). *Traffic safety facts: Bicyclists and other cyclists*. Retrieved May 17, 2010 from: http://www-nrd.nhtsa.dot.gov/pubs/811156.pdf

National Highway Traffic Safety Administration. *Persons killed, by age–state : USA, year: 2008*. Retrieved May 18, 2010 from http://www-fars.nhtsa.dot.gov/People/PeopleAllVictims.aspx

National Institute for Occupational Safety and Health. (2006). *Workplace violence prevention strategies and research*. Retrieved May 15, 2010 from http://www.cdc.gov/niosh/docs/2006-144

National Safety Council. (2007). *National Safety Month 07*. Retrieved June 16, 2007 from http://www.nsc.org/resources

National Safety Council. (2006). *American Worker Safety Survey, 2006*. Retrieved April 4, 2010 from: http://www.hreonline.com/pdfs/NSCExecSummary.pdf

Nationwide Mutual Insurance Company. (2010). *Driving while distracted: Statistics you need to know*. Retrieved May 17, 2010 from http://www.nationwide.com/newsroom/dwd-facts-figures.jsp

Polk Center for Automotive Studies. (2006). *Consumers admit phones cause careless driving*. Retrieved November 11, 2006 from http://usa.polk.com/News/LatestNews/2006_0517_phones.htm

Ranney, T. A. (2008). *Driver Distraction: A Review of the Current State-of-Knowledge*. Washington, D.C.: National Highway Traffic Safety Administration.

Strayer, D. L., Drews, F. A., Crouch, D. J. (2006). A comparison of the cell phone driver and the drunk driver. *Human Factors: The Journal of the Human Factors and Ergonomics Society*, 48, (2), 381–391.

Wassell, J. T., Gardner, L. I., Landsittel, D. P., Johnston, J. J., & Johnston, J. M. (2000). A prospective study of back belts for prevention of back pain and injury. *JAMA*, 284, 21, 2727–2732.

CHAPTER 16

Environmental Wellness

●●● Introduction

The planet we live on seems very large, but by astronomical measurements, it is not that big; in fact we are much like a speck of dust in the universe. We may not realize it, but the planet we call home is getting smaller every day, not because the physical size of the planet is shrinking but rather because the world's population is rapidly increasing. This population increase requires more environmental resources in order to thrive. Thus far, people have taken this consumption of resources very lightly, maintaining an "out-of-sight, out-of-mind" attitude. People don't realize the amount of the Earth's resources that are needed to support all the people on the planet. In the United States alone, we need materials from

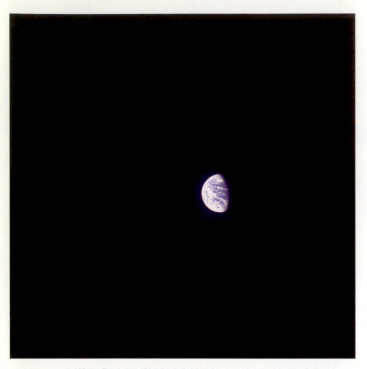

FIGURE 16-1 • While Earth itself isn't shrinking in size, the rapid population growth we are experiencing is consuming our planet's resources and producing waste at an alarming rate. Photo courtesy of NASA.

the Earth to heat our homes, operate our cars, produce our books and papers, grow our food, and build our homes and office buildings. As all these materials serve their purpose, they either produce waste by-products or become waste in and of themselves. We are using the Earth's resources at an alarming rate and producing waste that somehow must be dealt with (Figure 16-1). If we do not effectively deal with these concerns, we will eventually be living in a highly polluted environment.

●●● Human Population and the Environment

Hippocrates, the fifth-century Greek, known as the father of medicine, said it best: "If you want to learn about the health of a population, look at the air they breathe, the water they drink, and the places where they live." Have you ever taken the time to examine the environment where you live? To find out what the environmental health of your community is, read your local newspaper and see how often the paper carries news articles related to environmental issues, such

---

PERSONAL ASSESSMENT

Environmental Health Behaviors

Read each of the statements below and answer whether you think the statement is true or false. Think about why you chose the response you chose. Answers to this assessment can be found at the end of the chapter.

1. When mowing your lawn, it is best to collect your grass clippings, bag them, and send them to the landfill.

2. Most of the solid waste in landfills is made of paper.

3. What we know as "acid rain" does not pose a threat to human health.

4. Hazardous household wastes can safely be poured into a drain because contaminants will be removed at the water purification plant.

5. Natural gas is a good fuel source because is does not pollute the environment.

6. You can dissolve more materials with water than you can with sulfuric acid.

7. Rainwater is the purest form of water.

8. Water treatment facilities are regulated by law.

9. Federal regulations require that the water quality of every town in the United States is the same.

10. Noise pollution can damage hearing.

as air pollution, waste management, toxic materials in the environment, and/or flooding. You may be surprised to learn how many of these subjects appear.

Over many centuries, human beings have developed numerous ways of using environmental materials to enhance their lives. Wood has been used for constructing dwellings, furniture, and other household items (Figure 16-2). Stone has been used for building and paving; plants have been consumed for food, fabric, and medicines; and fossil fuels have been used for heating, cooking, and transportation. Using these materials resulted in two things: the consumption and reduction of the products and an accumulation of waste. Of critical importance is the fact that more and more of these resources became necessary as the population increased, and the Earth's population has indeed increased in unprecedented numbers. The world's population has grown significantly in the past 2010 years. The population grew slowly for the first 1800 of those years, but it grew very rapidly over the last 200-plus years as you can see in Figure 16-3. The world's population has mushroomed to more than 6.5 billion people, and it is still growing at a rapid rate. This means that more people will consume additional materials from the environment while creating more waste. One can only guess what the future holds as the world's population continues to grow at an incredible rate. One thing is for sure. Our environmental health issues are intimately related to the increasing numbers of people on the planet.

Human population has a profound impact on the environment. To illustrate this point, let's examine the impact urban growth has on groundwater. In order to develop the community, land has to be cleared to make room for buildings and roads. Trees and shrubs are removed and burned (which may add to air pollution), and sewers are installed. Each of these actions results in less vegetation to slow runoff of rainwater. Instead, much of the rainwater runs into the sewer and doesn't stay in the ground.

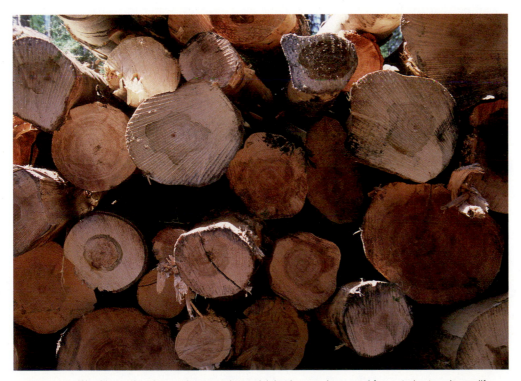

FIGURE 16-2 • Wood is an abundant environmental material that humans have used for centuries to enhance life, for everything from creating fire to building homes and constructing furniture and household items. Photo by Jeff Vanuga, U.S. Department of Agriculture, Natural Resources Conservation Service.

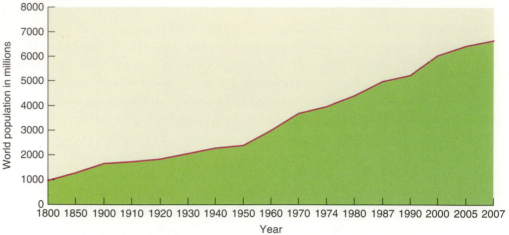

FIGURE 16-3 • World Population Curve 1800 through 2007.

Flooding occurs because the natural landscape pattern of water runoff has been altered. As urban growth continues, bulldozers clear the land to make way for the construction of houses and subdivisions. To make more use of the land, developers may fill ponds. More roads are built, contributing further to an increase in runoff. Streams may be diverted from their natural locations to increase the water supply. Unless it is carefully controlled, these changes are likely to produce discharged sewage into streambeds. Urbanization is completed by the addition of more roads, houses, and commercial and industrial buildings. More pavement and concrete means less soil to absorb water, meaning that the underground water table may have less water to recharge it, causing the water table to drop. Some existing wells will not be deep enough to get water and might run dry.

The runoff from the increased pavement goes into storm sewers and then into streams. This runoff, which used to soak into the ground, now goes into streams, increasing the likelihood of flooding. When the environment gets distorted to this degree, municipalities eventually take action to address the runoff problems. Currently, environmental engineers assume the task of redeveloping the land to return some of it to a state where the water is not lost and to prevent homes and neighborhoods from flooding.

Paul Ehrlich (1971) was a well-known biologist and researcher in the 1960s and 1970s whose interests included the effects of overpopulation on world hunger. His premise was that in the years to come, population growth was going to outpace the ability of countries to produce enough food for population survival, especially among underdeveloped countries. He was a strong advocate for "zero population growth," a proposal calling for each couple to have no more than two children, meaning that if all couples worldwide produced offspring to replace themselves, exponential population growth would level off. The reality is, however, that developed countries like the United States were more likely to practice birth control in this fashion, and less developed countries would not subscribe to this philosophy. Ehrlich's work was controversial at the time, and his predictions of widespread famine never occurred, but the implications for addressing uncontrolled population are relevant to environmental health concerns.

Did You Know...?

Forty percent of all energy and resources worldwide is associated with building construction.

Health and the Environment

The condition of the environment can produce significant health effects among the population. About 18 months after Michael's family moved back to their old neighborhood, Michael started doing poorly in school. Michael's teacher said that he was often tired and did not feel well. Michael's parents took him to the doctor, who did some blood tests. They learned that he had higher-than-normal levels of lead in his body. Tests revealed that he got it from the paint in the house where he lived.

John was usually a very healthy man who had 20 years of experience as a construction worker. He worked long, hard hours and usually had an abundance of energy. Lately, he felt tired and had difficulty breathing. John went to see his doctor and submitted to a series of diagnostic tests. He soon learned he developed lung cancer even though he was a nonsmoker—probably from being exposed to asbestos in and around his construction sites.

Something was definitely wrong with many children in this town. It appears that they developed rare cancers or blood conditions. Moreover, many babies were born with birth defects or were stillborn. When citizens and medical personnel expressed concern, a complete investigation of the town's environmental conditions was undertaken. Research revealed that somehow there was illegal dumping of radioactive waste products in the old public landfill that was closed six years ago.

Mary moved her business into a larger but older office building. Shortly thereafter, about 80 percent of the workers reported numerous episodes of flulike symptoms, memory loss, and/or muscle aches. Mary recalled reading something about this kind of condition, so she ordered an environmental assessment of the building's ventilation system. The investigation revealed the offices into which they moved had evidence of *Stachybotrys chartarum*, a toxic mold.

What do these situations have in common? All the people experienced effects of an unhealthy environment. Of the four previously described scenarios, only one of the four resulted from a naturally occurring environment threat: the toxic mold. People in the other instances suffered the consequences of some type of human effect on the environment:

- *Lead exposure*. Paint before 1978 often contained lead, a highly toxic substance. Many houses were painted with lead-based paint, and the lead could get into the house dust, making airborne exposure possible. Lead exposure can cause several problems, such as reduced IQ, learning disabilities, attention deficit disorders, behavioral problems, stunted growth, impaired hearing, and kidney damage. At high levels of exposure, a child may become mentally retarded, fall into a coma, and even die from lead poisoning.

- *Asbestos exposure*. Asbestos is a group of minerals that occur naturally in the environment. Many years ago, the material was used often in construction for insulation, soundproofing, fireproofing, roofing, floor and ceiling tiles, and brake shoes for cars. It was first regulated in the late 1970s by the U.S. Consumer Product Safety Commission and was banned from use in wallboard patching products and gas fireplaces. This was because using it could release it into the environment for inhalation. By 1989, scientists discovered that asbestos was even more dangerous than originally believed, so the U.S. Environmental Protection Agency (EPA) banned it from all new construction projects. Asbestos can cause scarring and

mesothelioma
a form of cancer almost always caused by exposure to asbestos

asbestosis
chronic inflammation of the lung tissue caused by exposure to asbestos

mycotoxins
a class of toxins produced by certain types of fungi

WEB LINK
Radiation

http://www.epa.gov/radiation

At this Web site, you will find a great deal of information about radiation, but click on the link "Becoming Aware of Radiation Sources," and it will take you to "Rad Town," an interactive city where you can scan the town and learn about many sources of radiation that may be in your environment.

SEARCH TERMS: environmental radiation, radiation, health effects of radiation

ecosystem
a complete, self-sustaining community of living organisms and the nonliving materials that support them

inflammation in the lungs and airway, **mesothelioma** (a type of lung cancer), and **asbestosis**. Exposure also elevates the risk for cancers of the gastrointestinal tract, throat, kidney, esophagus, and gallbladder.

- *Radiation.* Radiation sickness can occur when people are exposed to a large dose of radiation (acute exposure) or small doses over time (chronic exposure). Chronic exposure can result in delayed diseases such as cancer. The severity of the symptoms depends on the type of radiation and the amount of exposure.

- *Toxic mold.* Black mold grows easily on walls or any type of porous surface. The health effect of the mold depends on the type of mold, the concentration of the mold, the length of exposure, and the susceptibility of the exposed person. This type of mold produces **mycotoxins** that may compromise one's health. Sometimes people do not know that they are breathing in these mycotoxins until they become sick because the molds can be tolerated in small doses. Those people who leave the affected area will usually recover with few serious side effects. However, if the condition persists, infected individuals can suffer from a plethora of serious medical conditions, including chronic bronchitis, chronic fatigue, lupus, fibromyalgia, rheumatoid arthritis, multiple chemical sensitivity, and more.

Understanding the Environment

In order to understand environmental health issues, you must first have an understanding of an **ecosystem**. An ecosystem is a community composed of living organisms that is self-sustaining because of the relationship of the organisms to each other (Figure 16-4). When you were younger, did you ever create a terrarium as a science project? A terrarium is a glass bowl that contains a number of living and nonliving things that create an environment that is self-sustaining. For example, the glass bowl might contain some moss from the forest, some small plants that grow in the same type of habitat as the moss, a plastic container to hold water, soil around the container where the moss can grow, some small worms or insects that feed off the moss, and perhaps a salamander or newt to live in the habitat. The ecosystem becomes self-sustaining because water provides an energy source for the plants, small insects may feed off the plants, and the salamander may feed off the insects. The salamander provides waste that contains nutrients to help the plants grow. Plants give off oxygen and moisture to the ecosystem for the animals; the animals give up carbon dioxide for the plants. The essence of the ecosystem is that under ideal circumstances, it is a balanced system. All organisms flourish because they take products from one organism and give up products that they consider waste for the other organisms to use for their own good.

The entire Earth is an ecosystem (Figure 16-5). It has been a well-balanced global ecosystem for millions of years. Animal life and plant life coexisted in a mutually supportive manner. Over time, there were occasions where plant and animal species disappeared, evolved, or appeared, but those changes occurred within the natural changes of the ecosystem. When humans became part of the ecosystem millions of years ago, the Earth's ecosystem was still well balanced. Over the centuries, however, humans have taken control of the ecosystem by using more resources than they returned to the ecosystem. Moreover, humans have done some things in the name of progress that specifically harm the Earth's ecosystem. This is illustrated with the earlier example of urbanization's effect on groundwater. All these changes in the name of progress are convenient for the people, but as the ground and vegetation are torn up and replaced with nonliving physical structures, the ecosystem is affected. The animals that occupied part of the ecosystem must move or die. In essence, the balance of nature is destroyed. A "new nature" appears that may be deficient in some of the organisms that were present before humankind. Some organisms adapt to the ways of the human ecosystem. You may see news reports, for example, of bears that roam the streets of northern communities looking for food in trash containers. The townspeople don't want the bears around, but they forget that the bears were members the original ecosystem before humans arrived.

The ecosystem of the planet has always varied because of natural disasters, but the population explosion on the planet is producing a serious effect on the Earth's global ecosystem. Up until now, little has been done to consider the implications and consequences of "population pollution." At some point in time, humans will need to address population growth. If not, there will be consequences. In one of the science classes you may have taken, you probably cultivated bacteria in a Petri dish. The Petri dish contains a medium that supports bacterial growth (Figure 16-6). It seems that the bacteria could be sustained by the food in the Petri dish for quite some time, but this is not the case. The bacteria will use the food and reproduce easily. As time passes, an interesting thing happens. Before the entire food source is gone, the bacteria will die.

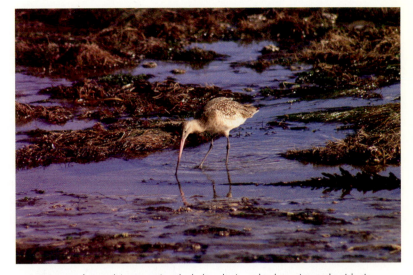

FIGURE 16-4 • A complete ecosystem includes plants, animals, water, and nutrients. Photo courtesy of Steve Lonhart/SIMON NOAA.

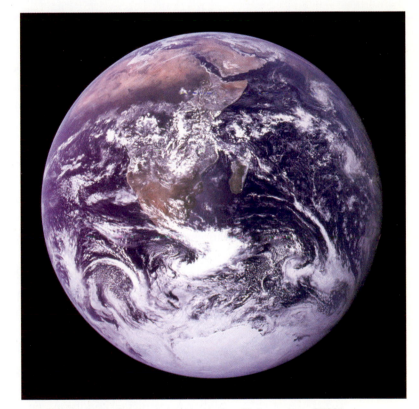

FIGURE 16-5 • The earth is a very large ecosystem. Photo courtesy of NASA.

The effect of environmental conditions on health has long been a factor on human existence. In the years between 1347 and 1354, approximately 20 million people died from the Black Death, also known as the bubonic plague: that was about one-third of the European population. The plague was an enormous environmental health disaster. The disease, as you may know, was caused by bacteria transmitted from fleas that lived on infected rats. The disease came from Southeast Asia when rats were unknowingly transported by ships and travelers. Medical science was not advanced enough to

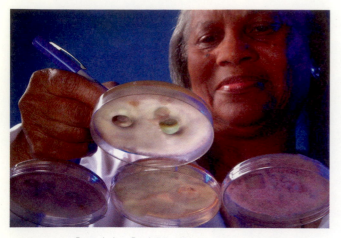

FIGURE 16-6 • Bacteria in a Petri dish will eat, reproduce, and then die before their entire food source has been consumed. Courtesy of the Centers for Disease Control and Prevention; photo by James Gathany.

cholera
an acute infectious diarrheal disease caused by a bacterium

determine the causes of death. Bodies were burned and buried in mass graves (that sometimes were not even covered over), and some people, ill from the disease, were boarded up in their own homes and left to die. The rats lived and multiplied on garbage left out in the open because no one knew about the importance of sanitation procedures; thus, there wasn't any real science to support a way of controlling the plague.

One of the earliest examples of an environmental health practice to protect the public occurred in 1854 in London, England. Dr. John Snow, an anesthesiologist, noted that numerous people who came to the hospital ill with **cholera** and died were from addresses in the same part of town. He investigated further and found that people took their drinking water from public pumps located in different parts of London. (Remember, the homes back then had no running water because treatment facilities had not been invented, nor did medicine have any working knowledge of how "germs" were transmitted.) Snow noted that almost 500 people within the area of one city block died from cholera, and all of them lived near the Broad Street pump. Snow convinced the city government to remove the pump handle to prevent people from drinking the contaminated water. It was later discovered that water from the pump was contaminated with sewage containing the cause of the cholera. Cholera outbreaks still pose problems to underdeveloped countries, but the illness is more treatable. In Snow's time, most people who contracted cholera died from it in less than a day.

As the scientific community learned more about pathogens and the chain of infection, the growth of the environmental health field followed close behind. Largely grounded in science to determine environmental threats and establish the best ways for protecting human life, environmental health experts work hand in hand with lawmakers. The population enjoys a better quality of life because of laws and policies created with the help of environmental scientists.

The World Health Organization (2007) describes environmental health as "those aspects of human health, including qualities of life that are determined by physical, chemical, biological, social, and psychosocial factors in the environment. It also refers to the theory and practice of assessing, correcting, controlling, and preventing those factors in the environment that can potentially affect adversely the health of present and future generations."

There are currently numerous programs evolving within academic institutions around the country to train environmental professionals. For example, researchers are needed to study environmental conditions; engineers are needed to help construct environmentally

What's News

The *British Medical Journal*, in a worldwide poll of 11,000 people, reported that the greatest medical advancement since 1840 was sanitation, ranking above antibiotics, anesthesia, and vaccines.

friendly landscapes, buildings, and automobiles; and scientists and mechanical engineers are needed to develop alternative fuel sources for turbines and vehicles. There are also courses within academic programs, such as this course you are now taking, to help the general public understand the importance of protecting the ecosystem by living in an environmentally friendly manner. It is hoped that by the time you complete this unit of study and your wellness plan, you will incorporate ecologically friendly behaviors into your wellness lifestyle.

Fossil Fuels and the Environment

Fossil fuels are closely linked to the environmental and political interests of the United States and the entire world. Oil-based fuels are either used directly by every adult in the United States or are part of the production and distribution of commodities we use on a daily basis. There are three major forms of fossil fuels: coal, oil, and gas. These products were formed millions of years ago before dinosaurs lived on the Earth—that is why they are called fossil fuels. As animals and plants died, they began to fall to the bottom of lakes and rivers, and their remains turned into peat. Over millions of years, rocks and dirt piled up on the peat, and eventually the rocks and dirt pressed down on the peat and pressed out all the water. Over time, the mass of peat was transformed into coal, oil, or natural gas. These three products account for about 88 percent of all energy worldwide.

Coal is a hard, black, solid substance that is made up of carbon, hydrogen, oxygen, nitrogen, and varying amounts of sulfur. It comes in a variety of forms, some of which contains more energy than others. Coal is found in many states throughout the United States and is generally found in deep coal mines, though some coal is taken from strip mines near the surface of the Earth. The United States has more coal than the rest of the world has oil, and scientists estimate that the country has enough coal to last another 200 to 300 years. Some people burn coal in their homes as a source of heat in the winter, but most coal is burned to make steam that drives powerful turbines to generate electricity. In fact, 87 percent of all coal mined in the United States is used to generate electrical power.

One of the downsides of using coal as fuel is that it does not burn very cleanly. Of all the fossil fuels, coal is the most polluting. This is significant because most electrical power plants currently use coal as the primary energy source to power turbines that generate electricity. As the coal burns, impurities and by-products of combustion can go into the atmosphere and mix with water to produce acid rain. The good news is that current technology is demonstrating that it is possible to remove up to 90 percent of the impurities before they reach the atmosphere (Figure 16-7).

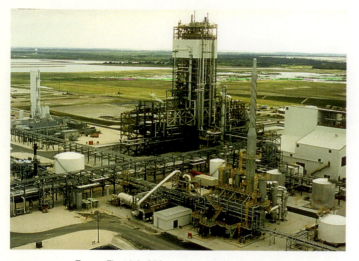

FIGURE 16-7 • Tampa Electric's 250-megawatt power facility near Lakewood, Florida, is one of the cleanest coal-fueled power stations in the world. It first turns coal into a gas and then filters out acid rain and smog, causing impurities and achieving emission levels much closer to a natural gas plant than a traditional coal-burning facility. Courtesy of the U.S. Department of Energy.

Oil, also referred to as petroleum, is another type of fossil fuel. Oil has been used for more than 5,000 years. The early civilizations of the Middle East used liquid oil as a medicine for wounds, and oil was used in lamps to produce light. Native Americans used oil for medicine and for waterproofing canoes. Oil became an important commodity as Europe and the United States entered the age of the industrial revolution. With industry came the need for power, and eventually oil became a significant energy source not only for powering the production plants but also as a fuel source for vehicles distributing products. Continued population growth created a need for more manufacturing, the growth of cities, and the emergence of motorized transportation, all requiring more energy sources. More important, research to use petroleum in more creative ways resulted in many scientific discoveries. Look at Figure 16-8 and see the products that are produced from a typical barrel of oil. There are many common products that are manufactured using petroleum chemicals—things like medications, crayons, dinnerware, lipstick, shampoo, and toothpaste. Oil is useful for manufacturing many products in addition to gasoline.

Oil is found in porous rock layers under the Earth's crust. It is a mistaken belief that oil lies in large pools underground. The oil is trapped between the porous rock layers, but it is under pressure, and that's why it may shoot out of the ground when the layer is first penetrated. Through normal drilling techniques, companies are able to extract only

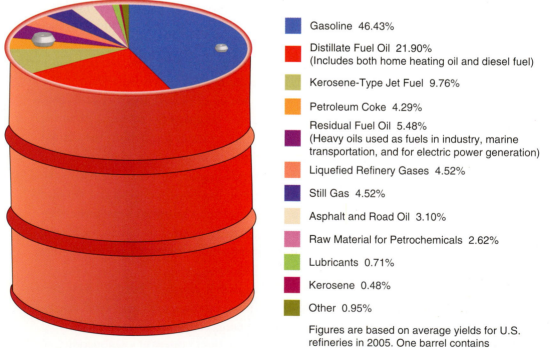

Gasoline 46.43%

Distillate Fuel Oil 21.90%
(Includes both home heating oil and diesel fuel)

Kerosene-Type Jet Fuel 9.76%

Petroleum Coke 4.29%

Residual Fuel Oil 5.48%
(Heavy oils used as fuels in industry, marine transportation, and for electric power generation)

Liquefied Refinery Gases 4.52%

Still Gas 4.52%

Asphalt and Road Oil 3.10%

Raw Material for Petrochemicals 2.62%

Lubricants 0.71%

Kerosene 0.48%

Other 0.95%

Figures are based on average yields for U.S. refineries in 2005. One barrel contains 42 gallons of crude oil. The total volume of products is 2.7 gallons more than the original barrel of oil.

FIGURE 16-8 • What comes from a barrel of oil? Source: California Energy Commission, 2002.

about 30 percent of the oil. Other methods are utilized to obtain about another 20 percent. A barrel of oil is equal to 42 U.S. gallons, and not all the oil is used to produce gasoline.

Natural gas is a nonrenewable fossil fuel formed by the decomposition of small plants and animals more than 100 million years ago. The remains of these organisms were trapped under many layers of rock. The pressure and the heat of the Earth's core caused the production of gases. There are numerous gases associated with natural gas, but the main component of natural gas is **methane**, an odorless, colorless, tasteless, flammable gas. Natural gas is used in our homes for heating and cooking, but during the manufacturing process, a chemical odorant that smells like rotten eggs is added to the gas. This is so that gas leaks can be detected by their distinctive odor before there is an ignition problem.

Natural gas supplies about 25 percent of the energy we use, and it is the most environmentally friendly of the fossil fuels. It burns cleaner than coal or petroleum because it contains less carbon than its fossil fuel cousins. Natural gas also has less sulfur and nitrogen compounds, and it emits less ash particulates into the air when it is burned than coal or petroleum fuels. Using natural gas to heat your home is an economical choice. Natural gas is the least expensive of all home heating sources. Moreover, the United States has the largest natural gas deposits in the world.

methane
an odorless, colorless, tasteless, flammable gas created by decomposition of organic material

●●● Environmental Pollution

Environmental pollution begins and ends with human population. Human beings and some of the products they use contribute greatly to the transformation of the Earth's ecosystem. At the same time, solutions for addressing the change in the ecosystem are within the power of people's ingenuities. Just as humans have created pollution, they are capable of preventing it and cleaning up the environment. As you read through the following sections, give some thought to the things you personally could do to address pollution in your environment.

Solid Waste

Call it garbage, trash, refuse, or solid waste, but by whatever name we use to describe it, it represents the "stuff we want to throw away," the things we don't want cluttering or fouling our immediate environment. As long as it leaves our immediate environment (e.g., our home) and we don't have to look at it anymore, we are pleased. But where does all this material end up, and what effect does it have on our towns and communities?

Solid waste is generally called *municipal solid waste* (MSW) by people who study it. Not surprisingly, solid waste has been around for thousands of years, and each year we produce more of it. Athens, the ancient Greek city-state, opened the first municipal garbage dump more than 2,500 years ago. From then until the present, people generally view waste disposal with an out-of-sight, out-of-mind philosophy. Historically, the waste was cast into places that hid it or took it away from the population. The improper disposal of solid waste became such a problem for England that in 1388 the British Parliament banned waste disposal from the local waterways.

To find the most abundant material in MSW, you need to look no further than the printed page you are reading right now. Yes, it is paper; we recycle only about 50 percent of the paper we use.

The most environmentally sound management of MSW is achieved when these approaches are implemented according to the EPA's preferred order of generating less waste. Think of the three Rs: source reduction first, followed by reusing and then recycling. After these measures are used, we can think about composting and then disposal in landfills or waste combustors.

According to the EPA, over the past 35 years, the amount of waste each person creates has almost doubled, from 2.7 to 4.5 pounds *per day*. Needless to say, the United States leads the world in the amount of waste per day per person; Australia ranks number two. Of interest is the news that much of the country's waste is now being recycled, composted, or used to create usable energy (Table 16-1). The most effective way to stop the trend toward more waste per person is practicing **source reduction** by preventing waste in the first place. Examples of waste reduction include the reduced weight of plastic used in one-liter soft drink bottles. Since 1977, the weight has been reduced from 68 to 51 grams. Seemingly insignificant in individual units, the change has resulted in the reduction of 250 million pounds of plastic in the environment. In another example, a licorice company in California decided to stop sending unacceptable products and scraps from their production line to the landfill. Instead, these materials were sold to cattle ranchers as a food source for the cattle. In addition to reducing waste to the landfill, the company saved $26,000 in hauling costs to the landfill and earned more than $8,000 from the sales to cattle ranchers.

source reduction

change in the design, manufacture, purchase, or use of materials or products (including packaging) to reduce their amount or toxicity before they become municipal solid waste

TABLE 16-1 • Generation, materials recovery, composting, combustion with energy recovery, and discards of municipal solid waste, selected years 1960–2008 (in pounds per person per day).

Activity	1960	1970	1980	1990	2000	2005	2008
Generation	2.68	3.25	3.66	4.50	4.63	4.54	4.50
Recovery for recycling	0.17	0.22	0.35	0.64	1.03	1.08	1.10
Recovery for composting*	Negligible	Negligible	Negligible	0.09	0.32	0.38	.40
Total materials recovery	0.17	0.22	0.35	0.73	1.35	1.46	1.50
Combustion with energy recovery†	0.00	0.01	0.07	0.65	0.66	0.62	.58
Discards to landfill, other disposal‡	2.51	3.02	3.24	3.12	2.62	2.46	2.43
Population (millions)	179.97	203.98	227.25	249.90	281.42	296.41	304.06

Source: Office of Solid Waste (2009).

*Composting of yard trimmings, food scraps, and other MSW organic material. Does not include backyard composting.
†Includes combustion of MSW in mass burn or refuse-derived fuel form and combustion with energy recovery of source-separated materials in MSW (e.g., wood pallets and tire-derived fuel).
‡Discards after recovery minus combustion with energy recovery. Discards include combustion without energy recovery. Details may not add to totals because of rounding.

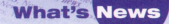

Another way of preventing materials from ending up in the landfill is to reuse the material. Old tires used to end up in the landfill, and some people reuse them in different ways. An old tire can be made into a backyard swing. Some people take old tires, fill them with dirt, and use them as planters. A retiree, known to one of the authors, uses some of his spare time to search for lost golf balls on the local golf course. He takes all the balls he finds and places them in empty egg cartons that his neighbors donate to him. The "packaged" balls then become gifts for his friends. Country farmers who sell eggs encourage their customers to bring their empty egg cartons with them when they buy their eggs. Empty milk cartons can be trimmed down to be used as planters to start vegetable seedlings early in the spring.

Recycling is another method of reducing waste in the landfill. The current rate of municipal recycling reported by the U.S. General Accounting Office is 32 percent. The 2008 goal was 35 percent. Americans are looking for ways to recycle materials and protect the environment. Old tires can be ground into granules, added to asphalt, and used as a highway covering or in the construction of running tracks at schools and universities. Tires are also shredded and used as garden mulch. Perhaps the most recycled product in the United States is aluminum. When aluminum cans are recycled, they can be reprocessed and back on the store shelves in as little as 60 days. According to the Aluminum Association, two-thirds of all the aluminum ever produced is still in use. In 2008, there were 1.557 billion pounds of aluminum collected for recycling (The Aluminum Association, 2009). Not only is recycling beneficial to the solid waste environment, but it also saves money and energy needed for production costs. For example, remanufacturing 20 aluminum cans from recycled material uses the same amount of energy needed to produce *one new can*. You would be amazed at the number of products we use that can be recycled. Use your health literacy skills to find out more.

Landfill

The modern landfill, sometimes still referred to as the "dump," is a carefully planned site for disposing of waste material. Landfills may vary depending on the type of waste being disposed. Virtually all large communities have landfills for handling MSW. The location of a landfill is carefully selected because the purpose of the landfill is not just to "hide" trash. The site is designed to manage the waste carefully in order to protect the ecosystem.

The location of the landfill is of prime importance. Landfills located near large cities are located in huge pits or ravines. The area must be easily accessible, and consideration must be given to ensure that constructing the landfill to meet government requirements is cost effective. The landfill must allow for the decomposition of waste without attracting rodents and scavengers, allow for the recovery of certain usable by-products, and prevent any toxic material from entering the surrounding area or groundwater. The geology is carefully studied to ensure that the land on which the landfill is constructed is stable and away from faults, wetlands, floodplains, or other restricted areas. The landfill is lined with a landfill liner, an impermeable membrane that prevents leakage of toxic **leachate** into the ground. Leachate is the liquid produced when water seeps through the landfill material. As the water percolates through the waste, it picks up particles and chemicals that could be harmful to the environment if it is not contained. Landfills generally have a containment and pumping system that permits the collection of leachate so that it can be disposed safely. The site is also engineered to capture **biogas**, such as methane, for use as a fuel for a nearby power generation plant.

Landfill Management

When waste arrives at the landfill, the material is weighed and inspected to ensure that there are no toxic materials entering the landfill. The truck is directed to the working area of the landfill, and the contents are added to the landfill. After the loads are dumped, they are spread out and compacted using heavy equipment. At the end of each day, the compacted material is covered by a layer of soil, and periodically a chemical additive is used to eliminate odors and discourage rodents, scavengers, and birds. Biogas is collected on an ongoing basis. In 2003, 440 trillion **British Thermal Units (BTUs)** of biogas were produced from U.S. landfills. At some point in time, the landfill will reach capacity. When this happens, the landfill is covered by a heavy layer of soil and earth, and the land is reclaimed as a park or a wildlife refuge.

Household Hazardous Wastes

There are some activities around the house for which materials that are used contain products that are potentially hazardous to the ecosystem. These products may include such materials as paints, cleaners, stains and varnishes, batteries, motor oil, and pesticides. These materials are referred to as *household hazardous waste*. Household hazardous wastes are sometimes disposed of improperly by individuals pouring wastes down the drain, on the ground, or into storm sewers. Unknowingly, people will also put them out with the trash. The dangers of such disposal methods may not be immediately obvious, but certain types of household hazardous wastes have the potential to cause physical injury to sanitation workers, contaminate septic systems or wastewater treatment systems if poured down drains or toilets, and present hazards to children and pets if left around the house. This is especially important if your household is dependent on a well as your source of drinking water.

In order to safely handle hazardous material, be sure that you can identify what constitutes hazardous waste. The best way to know is to read the warning label on the container. Hazardous materials have at least one the following features:

- *Ignitable*. The product is capable of burning or causing a fire.

- *Corrosive*. The material is capable of eating away materials and destroying living tissue when contact occurs between the hazardous material and the skin, mouth, or eyes.

---

leachate
liquid produced when water passes through landfill materials

biogas
gas, such as methane, produced from the decomposition of natural material

British Thermal Units (BTUs)
a unit of energy used worldwide in the power, steam generation, and heating and air-conditioning industries (one BTU = about .25 calories)

Did You Know…?

Americans generate 1.6 million tons of household hazardous waste per year. The average home accumulates as much as 100 pounds of household hazardous waste in the basement or garage and in storage closets.

- *Explosive.* The substance can cause an explosion or release poisonous fumes when exposed to air, water, or other chemicals.

- *Toxic.* The material is poisonous or harmful, either immediately (acutely toxic) or over a long period of time (chronically toxic).

One way to reduce potential hazards is to use products that are harmless or at least less harmful to people or the environment to start with. One way to do this is to purchase cleaning products, weed killers, insecticides, and so on that can accomplish the same objective without including hazardous chemicals and to use the minimal amount of the product to do the job. A second way of protecting the environment is to handle your hazardous material correctly by doing the following:

- Use and store products containing hazardous substances carefully to prevent any accidents at home, such as inhalation of toxic vapors, accidental poisoning, and so on. Never store hazardous products in food containers. Keep products containing hazardous materials in their original containers and never remove the labels. Read the labels and be sure to use and store products according to instructions. Corroding containers should be repackaged and clearly labeled. This will prevent accidental ingestion and can also help protect sanitation workers once the product is discarded.

- Never mix household hazardous waste with other products. Chemicals may react, ignite, or explode; contaminated household hazardous waste may become unrecyclable if it is contaminated. Mixing chlorine bleach and ammonia will create toxic fumes.

- Try to purchase water-based products or products labeled as environmentally friendly.

- Wear protective clothing/gloves when handling toxic materials like insecticide or pest removal products.

Another way to keep the environment safe is to look for creative ways to dispose of leftover products. Leftover materials can be shared with neighbors or donated to charity for use elsewhere. Your community or state may also have a hazardous waste disposal program where you can drop off hazardous materials on certain collection dates. Car batteries can be recycled to service stations or auto parts stores. The EPA estimates that about 80 percent of all batteries collected in this manner can be recycled. While federal law does not require households to separate household hazardous waste from MSW, some states have special requirements. Call your local or state solid waste officials to learn what requirements apply to household hazardous wastes.

The Precautionary Principle

During a 1998 landmark meeting of scientists, government officials, lawyers, labor activists, and grassroots environmental leaders, the Precautionary Principle was crafted. The Precautionary Principle was not proposed in response to any particular environmental issue. Rather, it was proposed as a universal answer to the

WEB LINK
Tox Town

http://toxtown.nlm.nih.gov

If you want to obtain more information on some environmental issues, go to Tox town, an interactive Web site produced by the National Institutes of Health. The site is intended for use by public school learners, but as you navigate the site, you will obtain links to numerous sites with advanced scientific information about many environmental concerns. It may also be a useful site to share with your children.

SEARCH TERMS: environmental pollution, environmental education

prevailing public mind-set that perpetuates many environmental problems. In part, the Precautionary Principle reads, "When an activity raises threats of harm to human health or the environment, precautionary measures should be taken even if some cause and effect relationships are not fully established scientifically. In this context the proponent of an activity, rather than the public, should bear the burden of proof." (Wingspread Conference on the Precautionary Principle, 1998).

Air Pollution

There are many causes of air pollution. In that regard, the elements of air pollution can vary from location to location and from time to time. Some of the most common causes of air pollution are factories, wildfires, automobiles, dry cleaners, and electric plants. Air pollution can be unsightly and hazardous to one's health. Air pollution can cause damage to the health of human beings, animals, plants, forests, and vegetation. In some instances, the pollution can even destroy building material. Air pollution is also an indirect cause of skin cancer.

The EPA (2009a) indicates that the United States is doing a better of job of cleaning up air quality. According to measures of the six major pollutants (carbon monoxide, lead, nitrogen monoxide, volatile organic compounds, particulates, and sulfur dioxide), the quality of the air for all measures is better than it was in 1980. For example, measured carbon monoxide (178 million tons in 1980 was 78 million tons in 2008). It is important to remember, however, that the data reflect the entire country. While some communities experience better air quality, there are some that have not. Despite air quality improvements, in 2008 over 126 million people nationwide still lived in counties with pollution levels above the EPA's national air quality standards.

The Atmosphere

Air pollution is better understood if one is able to comprehend the role of the Earth's atmosphere on our air quality. The Earth is surrounded by a blanket of air called the atmosphere. It extends approximately 348 miles from the surface of the Earth. Without the atmosphere, there would be no life on Earth. Our atmosphere is responsible for protecting the Earth's surface from dangerous solar radiation and for the weather that circulates moisture around the planet. The atmosphere has been divided into four levels (Figure 16-9). The *troposphere* starts at the Earth's surface and extends upward for five to nine miles. This is the region that is most dense and where all weather patterns are formed. The *stratosphere* starts just above the troposphere and extends to 31 miles high. This is where the ozone layer is located. The ozone layer absorbs and disperses the solar radiation as it arrives from the sun. These two layers contain 99 percent of our air. The *mesosphere* starts just above the stratosphere and extends to 53 miles high. The *thermosphere* starts just above the mesosphere and extends to 372 miles high.

Causes of Air Pollution

Air pollution can be caused by many different things. The most likely cause of pollution is the internal combustion engine (like the one in your car) because they are designed to burn fossil fuel, there are so many automobiles, and they are driven so frequently—often with only one occupant. The automobile is *most* polluting when it is coasting or idling while at a standstill. Imagine what this means to the air quality in cities with rush-hour traffic. Other principal sources of air pollution are factories, wildfires, dry cleaners, and electric plants. Air pollution can damage the health of human beings, animals, plants, forests, and crops; it can also interact with construction materials and damage the facing of buildings. Some of the chemicals in air pollution can contribute to itchy eyes, asthma, cancer, birth defects, and nervous system injury. At the height of the industrial revolution, there was so much industrial smoke polluting the air, especially during days of high humidity and fog, that the term *smog* was coined (smoke + fog). Now, our air pollution contains many chemicals that are not visible, so we speak of air pollution instead of smog.

After many years of rampant, visible pollutants in the air, the U.S. government formed the EPA in 1970. The first EPA administrator was Donald Ruckelshaus, and one of his first duties was to address the National Press Club. It was there that he described not the importance of the EPA but the importance of the environment: "An environmental ethic is needed. Each of us must begin to realize our own relationship to the environment. Each of us must begin to measure the impact of our own decisions and actions on the quality of air, water, and soil of this nation. (Wisman, 1985, p. 2)" That same year, Congress passed the Clean Air Act, which did the following:

- Set standards for industrial emissions

- Set standards for automobile emissions

- Classified other pollutants

- Gave the EPA the power to enforce policies

- Gave economic incentives for those complying with EPA standards

- Made each state responsible for its own plan

The Clean Air Act, with amendments added in 1990, has done much to advance the quality of our air, but there is still much to be done given that we still rely so heavily on fossil fuels.

Temperature Inversion

There are communities in the United States that are more prone to air pollution than other communities. It has a lot to do with the geological and temperature conditions that exist around the community. If the conditions are right, the city ends up with an atmospheric "lid" over the city that traps pollution at the surface. Los Angeles, California, is located in a basin near the coast of California. The basin is formed by the small mountains and foothills that are north and east of the city. During the summer months, cool air from the Pacific Ocean settles into the basin during the nighttime hours. When the sun comes up in the morning, it heats the atmosphere above the basin. The warm air above and the still cold air at the surface create a **temperature inversion** that traps all pollution close to the surface of the land. During a peak pollution event in

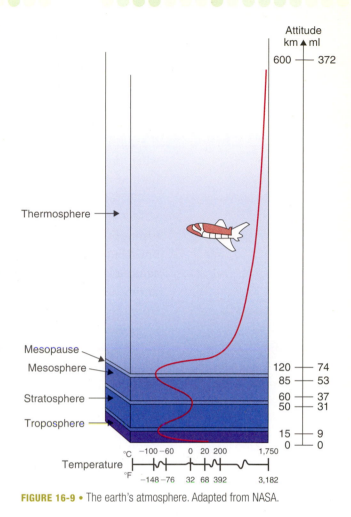

FIGURE 16-9 • The earth's atmosphere. Adapted from NASA.

temperature inversion

an atmospheric condition when cold air at the Earth's surface is trapped by warm air above it

the late morning hours in the summer, a person can fly from Los Angeles International Airport and observe a gray or brownish haze over the city, and there will be a breaking point where the air will be clear above the cloud of pollution. In contrast, Denver, Colorado, has peak pollution episodes during the winter months. Denver also sits in a type of basin with the foothills of the Rocky Mountains to the west of the city. Overnight, during the winter months the air becomes cold and settles over the city. When the sun rises east of the city, the air above the city heats up and creates the inversion when the air is still. Morning commuter traffic is the major source of air pollution in both of these cities.

Ozone

Ozone is a highly reactive gas molecule composed of three oxygen atoms (O_3). On the one hand, ozone is protective when it resides in the stratosphere because it prevents damaging solar radiation from getting to the Earth. On the other hand, tropospheric ozone during air pollution events is damaging to human health. Tropospheric ozone is formed from the chemical reaction when **nitrogen oxides** and **volatile organic compounds** enter into a chemical reaction in the presence of heat and sunlight.

Ozone is a powerful oxidant. In cities where the ozone levels are high, people find that rubber products and certain plastics around their homes will deteriorate because of the effects of ozone. If ozone can do this to manufactured material, imagine what it can do to the human body. Ozone attacks lung tissue by reacting chemically with it in a process called "oxidizing." At levels often found in many of the cities across the country, ozone becomes a strong lung irritant. Some compare this to getting a "sunburn" on the lungs. People exposed to high ozone levels may experience symptoms such as shortness of breath, chest pain when inhaling deeply, wheezing, and coughing. The EPA has identified three groups of people who are at risk; people with preexisting lung disease, people who exercise during ozone alerts who respond with decreased lung function (about 15 percent of that group), and vulnerable population subgroups, such as children and the elderly. Major cities where inversions occur often issue "ozone alerts" advising children and elder adults to stay indoors during ozone episodes.

But in a different way, ozone can be good for humans. Stratospheric ozone is a naturally occurring gas that filters the sun's ultraviolet (UV) radiation. A diminished ozone layer allows more radiation to reach the Earth's surface. Studies during the 1980s indicated that the level of ozone in the stratosphere was deteriorating, largely because of the release of **chlorofluorocarbons (CFCs)** into the atmosphere. CFCs were developed in the 1930s as a safe alternative to ammonia as a refrigerant. More recently, CFCs were used as propellant in aerosol spray cans. Chlorine is a main ingredient in CFCs. When CFCs are released into the atmosphere, they rise into the stratosphere, where the chlorine destroys the ozone molecules. Loss of ozone in the stratosphere allows harmful solar radiation to enter the Earth's atmosphere.

Between September 21 and September 30, 2006, the average area of the ozone hole over Antarctica was the largest ever observed, at 10.6 million square miles. As shown in Figure 16-10, on September 24 of that year, the Antarctic ozone had the record single-day largest area of 11.4 million square miles. This discovery is disturbing because with all the data we had from earlier findings, there was a worldwide effort to control the use of CFCs. Without

nitrogen oxides
nitrogen-based compounds formed from burning fossil fuels

volatile organic compounds
chemical compounds formed largely from the combustion of fossil fuels

chlorofluorocarbons (CFCs)
highly stable compounds used as components of aerosol propellants and refrigerants

WEB LINK
Ozone Hole
http://www.theozonehole.com
This is a very interesting Web site where you will find numerous links to all the current information about ozone and the effects of its loss in the stratosphere.
SEARCH TERMS: ozone hole, ozone depletion

the protection of the ozone layer, there is potential for great harm to life on Earth. For humans, overexposure to UV rays can lead to skin cancer, cataracts, and weakened immune systems. Increased UV can also lead to reduced crop yields and disruptions in the marine food chain.

Health effects of a diminished ozone layer include the following:

- *Skin cancer.* Melanoma is a deadly form of skin cancer. It is believed that there is a relationship between sunburn during childhood and melanoma. The recent increase in melanoma-related deaths in the United States has followed the depletion of the Earth's ozone layer discovered in the 1980s.

- *Cataracts.* Cataracts are a form of eye damage in which one or both lenses of the eyes lose transparency, resulting in clouded vision (Figure 16-11). Left untreated, cataracts can lead to blindness. Research has shown that UV radiation increases the likelihood of certain cataracts. Modern medical practices can treat cataracts, but the treatment is costly and not available to those people who cannot afford it. This is one reason why there has been a great deal of interest in having people wear appropriate eyewear that provides protection against both UVA and UVB radiation.

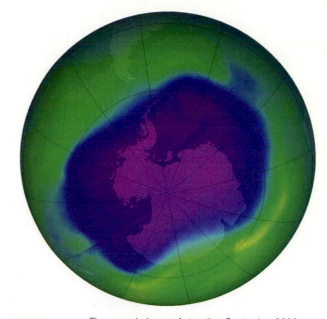

FIGURE 16-10 • The ozone hole over Antarctica, September 2006. Courtesy of NASA.

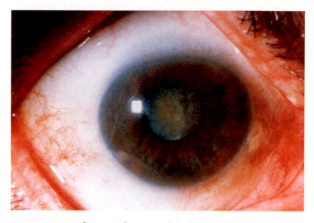

FIGURE 16-11 • Cataract. Courtesy of the National Eye Institute, Bethesda, Maryland.

Health Effects of Air Pollution

Determining the relationship between air pollution and health continues. Many circumstances, such as the features of the pollutants, the density of pollution, the length exposure, and the susceptibility of the host, vary greatly.

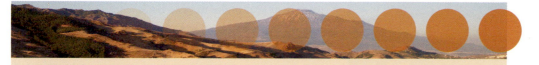

What's Your View?

The federal government has taken measures to mandate less polluting modes of transportation because of the effects of burning fossil fuels on air pollution. There are laws and standards that mandate reduction of emissions that pollute the environment. But what about other personal machines and devices that are dependent on fossil fuels? Motorcycles, lawn mowers, and charcoal grills are all dependent on fossil fuels that, when used, emit pollutants into the atmosphere. Should these items be subject to government and scientific standards, or should we depend on people to take appropriate action to protect the environment?

point contamination
pollutants that are added directly at the site of the aquatic source

nonpoint contamination
pollutants that make their way to a body of water through runoff from rain or irrigation

Data thus far seem to point to the fact that people with preexisting respiratory problems are most likely to be affected by air pollution, especially if they are exercising. More research is needed to confirm the health effects of pollution, but because research is less definitive than that done on cigarette smoking, all of us should still do what we can to reduce or eliminate pollution. Rest assured that there are no benefits to chemically polluted air.

Water Pollution

Water covers three-fourths of the Earth's surface. As you know, one water molecule is comprised of two atoms of hydrogen and one atom of oxygen. The way these atoms are arranged makes a drop of water a perfect sphere. The only reason that "drops" are teardrop shaped is because the water molecules are affected by outside forces such as gravity (Figure 16-12). Water possesses unique physical properties. It is the only material on Earth that can exist as a solid, liquid, and gas at temperatures normally found in the Earth's environment. Water is also known as the "universal solvent" because it dissolves more materials than any other liquid. It also has a high surface tension that keeps the molecules clumped together. The latter characteristic is very important because it is this property that allows a plant to absorb water through its root system and transport it throughout the plant. Water is necessary for all life on the planet and is very important to the world's ecosystems.

Did You Know…?

The overall amount of water on Earth has remained the same for 2 billion years.

A person can live about a month without food but only about a week without water. If a human does not absorb enough water, dehydration may occur, eventually leading to death.

Water pollution can damage all forms of life. Pollution can negatively affect drinking water, lakes and aquatic life, recreation, fishing, transportation, and commerce. Water pollution can damage aquatic ecosystems such as coral reefs, estuaries, freshwater ecosystems, lakes, marine ecosystems, oceans, rivers and streams, watersheds, and wetlands. Some of the pollutants getting into the waterways may also make its way back to humans when they consume fish or other aquatic animals that are contaminated with unsafe chemicals in the water. Water pollutants are often materials such as arsenic, contaminated sediment, disinfection by-products, dredged material, lead, mercury, and microbial pathogens such as bacteria.

Water pollution occurs when a body of water in contaminated with large amounts of materials from outside the ecosystem to the point that the water becomes unfit for its intended use. Pollution in waterways occurs in one of two ways: either **point contamination** or **nonpoint contamination**. The addition of polluting materials directly to a body of water is known as point contamination. An example of point contamination occurred in 1989 when an oil tanker, *Exxon Valdez*, struck a reef in

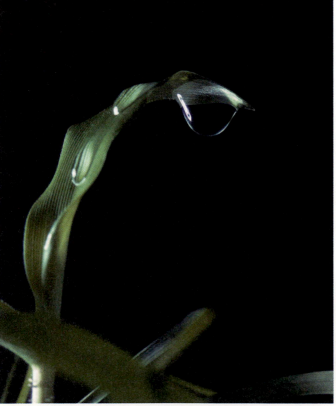

FIGURE 16-12 • Water, made up simply of hydrogen and oxygen, is vital to all life on our planet. Photo by Tim McCabe, U.S. Department of Agriculture, Natural Resources Conservation Service.

TABLE 16-2 • Eating tuna safely.

| If You Weigh | Don't Eat More Than One Can Every | |
	White Albacore	Chunk Light
50 pounds	4 weeks	9 days
100 pounds	2 weeks	5 days
130 pounds	10 days	4 days
150+ pounds	9 days	3 days

Source: Adapted from Natural Resources Defense Council, (n.d.)

Alaska's Prince William Sound. The hole in the tanker resulted in dumping approximately 11 million gallons of oil into the sound. Thousands of animals died immediately; the best estimates include 250,000 to 500,000 seabirds, 2,800 to 5,000 sea otters, approximately 12 river otters, 300 harbor seals, 250 bald eagles, and 22 orcas as well as the destruction of billions of salmon and herring eggs. Nonpoint contamination occurs when environmental contaminants are deposited on the land and carried to the waterway by water from rain or irrigation runoff. Fish become contaminated with mercury because of nonpoint contamination. Mercury is not a normal toxin in fish, so you may wonder how the mercury gets there. It appears that the chain of events toward contamination begins on land. Industrial activities such as garbage incineration, automobile recycling, and power generation from coal produce airborne mercury molecules that fall on land and water. The mercury is converted by microorganisms into a more biologically active form of mercury. This active mercury is carried by rainwater into waterways, where it eventually ends up in the ocean. Once the mercury arrrives in the ocean, it enters the food chain—contaminated small organisms are eaten by larger organisms and so on. Eventually, fish contaminated by mercury, such as tuna, are consumed by humans. Given all this information, perhaps you are concerned about how much tuna is safe to eat. Mercury poses the greatest threat to the health of children and women who are pregnant or planning to become pregnant, but you may wish to use the information in Table 16-2 as a guide.

Causes of Water Pollution

In general, all causes of water pollution are man-made (Figure 16-13). Although pathogenic organisms are deposited into waterways by animals, the presence of the organisms represents a natural consequence of activities within the ecosystem. These microorganisms are not harmful to other animals within the ecosystem. Much of the pollution in the water comes from agricultural runoff, particularly in the form of fertilizer residue. Another source is sewage from human waste. When these

WEB LINK
Mercury Action
http://www.mercuryaction.org
This Web site contains information regarding the health effects of mercury, and what you can do to protect yourself and your family from contamination.
SEARCH TERMS: health effects of mercury, mercury poisoning, mercury contamination

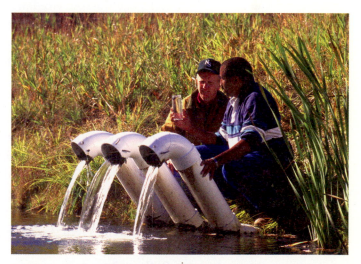

FIGURE 16-13 • Two Natural Resource Conservation Service workers survey the water quality in a mine water filtration pond in Somerset County, Pennsylvania. Photo by Bob Nichols, U.S. Department of Agriculture, Natural Resources Conservation Service.

materials get into the waterway, the natural balance of the ecosystem is affected. In excess levels, nutrients such as these are so strong that they overstimulate the growth of aquatic plants and algae. Excessive growth of these types of organisms eventually clogs our waterways. These organisms use up dissolved oxygen as they decompose, causing harm to animal life in the water, and block light to deeper waters, preventing organisms within the ecosystem from flourishing. All these changes to the ecosystem prove harmful to aquatic organisms, as they affect the respiration of fish and other invertebrates that reside in water.

Arsenic

Arsenic occurs naturally in rocks and soil, water, air, plants, and animals. It can be released into the environment through natural activities such as volcanic action, erosion, and forest fires or through human actions by the mishandling of materials. Approximately 90 percent of industrial arsenic in the United States is currently used as a wood preservative, but arsenic is also used in paints, dyes, metals, drugs, soaps and semiconductors. High arsenic levels can result from certain fertilizers and animal feeding operations. Industrial practices such as copper smelting, mining, and coal burning may contribute to arsenic in our environment.

Long-term exposure to arsenic has been linked to cancer of the bladder, lungs, skin, kidneys, nasal passages, liver, and prostate. There are short-term effects of arsenic exposure, but the dosage necessary to create those effects would be much higher than the amount encountered in the water supply. To protect the public, the EPA set standards for arsenic levels in municipal water supplies. Beginning in 2006, all municipal water systems were prohibited from allowing treated water to exceed arsenic levels of 10 parts per billion. Families who get their water from private wells are not protected by this policy unless they have their water voluntarily tested periodically since arsenic is tasteless and odorless.

Lead

Lead, a metal found in natural deposits, is common in household plumbing materials and some water service lines. Exposure to lead is most likely to occur through swallowing or breathing lead paint chips and/or dust containing lead. However, lead can also found in drinking water. Contaminated drinking water does not come from the water treatment facility; it is most likely to be present in homes built prior to 1986 when building contractors installed pipes containing lead and used lead-containing solder during construction.

Lead is a toxic metal that is harmful to human health; it has no known value to the human body. The human body cannot tell the difference between lead and calcium. Thus, like calcium, lead remains in the bloodstream and body organs for months before it is excreted. The unexcreted lead is absorbed into the bones, where it can collect for a lifetime. To help block the storage of lead in your body or the tissues of your family members, prepare meals that are low in fat and high in calcium and iron, including dairy products and green vegetables.

Pathogens

The disinfection of drinking water is one of the major public health advances of the twentieth century. One hundred years ago, typhoid and cholera epidemics were common throughout European and American cities because the drinking water was not treated to remove pathogens. Disinfection was a major factor in reducing these epidemics, and it is an essential part of drinking water treatment today. However, the disinfectants themselves can react with naturally occurring materials in the water to form unintended organic and inorganic by-products, posing health risks. Over the past 10 years, we have also learned that there are specific microbial pathogens, such as *Cryptosporidium*, that are highly resistant to traditional disinfection practices. *Cryptosporidium* is a parasite commonly found in lakes and rivers, especially when sewage and animal wastes contaminate the water. *Cryptosporidium* has caused several large waterborne disease outbreaks of gastrointestinal illness with symptoms such as diarrhea, nausea, and/or stomach cramps. People with severely weakened immune systems are likely to have more severe and more persistent symptoms than people with healthy immune systems. Moreover, *Cryptosporidium* has been a contributing cause of death in some people infected with HIV/AIDS and cancer as well as transplant patients taking immunosuppressive drugs and people born with a weakened immune system. Personal contact with this organism is more likely to come from swimming in lakes and streams than from municipal drinking water. There is little chance of *Cryptosporidium* infections via today's water supplies. The EPA has established new water treatment rules to make certain that municipal water supplies are free from this parasite.

Private Wells

The public water supply in the United States is carefully monitored and controlled by federal and local regulations. These regulations do not apply to private wells. People who get their drinking water from a private well must remember that the underground water supply, though generally clean, does not reside specifically under the well owner's property, meaning that the water comes from an underground source that is vulnerable to chemical runoff and contamination miles from the owner's property. For this reason, it is best to follow some basic rules for well safety:

- Check the well every spring to make sure there are no mechanical problems; test it once each year for pathogens and once every two to three years for harmful chemicals.

- The well should also be tested if the following occur:
  - There are known problems with well water in the surrounding area
  - There are observed problems near the well (e.g., flooding, land disturbances, and nearby waste disposal sites)
  - Any part of the well system, such as pipes or motors, are replaced periodically

Protecting the Waterways

The contamination of freshwater sources can result from organic sources such as bacteria, one-celled pathogens, and decayed material. Contamination can also come from chemical pollutants dumped into the water source. The former problem is easily treated by municipal water treatment facilities; the latter is a much more serious concern because treatment facilities are set up to handle only organics materials. The best way to prevent chemical pollution is for community members to be very careful about any chemical dumping into waterways or down the drain. Storage of toxic material is a concern as well. If left out in the open, the chemicals can be washed into the drainage system by rain or irrigation runoff. Just because waste goes down the drain or sent to a landfill does not mean that it has been disposed of safely.

How can you be sure that you are disposing of materials properly? Don't pour unused household products, such as cleansers, beauty products, medicine, auto fluids, paint, pesticides and lawn care products, down the drain. Properly dispose of them at your local household hazardous waste facility. If you don't know where the facility is, contact your local government office. Dispose of excess household grease (meat fats, lard, cooking oil, shortening, butter and margarine, and so on), diapers, condoms, and personal hygiene products in the solid waste collection. Pouring them down the drain can clog pipes and could cause raw sewage to overflow in your home or yard or in public areas. Overflows often occur during periods of high rainfall or snowmelt and can result in basement backups, overflows at manholes, or discharges directly into rivers, lakes, and coastal waters. Don't pour used motor oil down the drain. Used motor oil can diminish the effectiveness of the treatment process and might allow contaminants to be discharged. The contaminants could pollute local waterways or harm aquatic life. Motor oil can be recycled through oil change shops. If you're a darkroom hobbyist, dispose of spent fixer, developer, and other photographic chemicals in separate containers and transport them to a hazardous waste facility.

Healthy Community Environment

What do you think about when you hear individuals talk about *our environment*? Many people immediately think about the problems of pollution because of what they hear in the media. The quality of our air and water may be important, but there are many other aspects of our physical and natural environment that affect health. The climate of the region where you live is one example. Extreme temperatures encourage people to stay inside rather than engaging in exercise and outdoor activities. The natural vegetation in an area can either relieve or aggravate allergies. And the natural landscape can affect the flow of the wind, resulting in either a reduction or an increase in air pollution. Los Angeles is a clear example. Air quality is affected not only by artificial pollutants but also by natural phenomena, such as radioactive radon gas, which can be found all over the United States. Sometimes the environment is in our favor. Did you know that a high level of natural salts, such as fluoride in drinking water, tends to prevent tooth decay by hardening the teeth?

> ### Did You Know...?
>
> Each year, of disposed materials, approximately 50 percent of all paper, 34 percent of all plastic soda bottles, 45 percent of all aluminum beverage cans, 63 percent of all steel packaging, and 67 percent of all major appliances are sent to recycling.

Of great importance is the fact that each of us is a member of the ecosystem in which we live. Unlike natural ecosystems, humans have the ability to create a disruption of the ecosystem where they reside. To the contrary, people have the ability to protect and clean up the environment. The problem is that so many people do not know enough about environmental issues, or perhaps they do not care enough to protect the environment. They may be too busy trying to earn a living and raise a family to worry about environmental health. Some folks think that "it's someone else's problem," but the bottom line is that humans will have to pay attention to the condition of the environment or eventually suffer the consequences of pollution and hazardous materials in the environment. We are part of the community ecosystem; thus, we can participate in the destruction of our ecosystem, or we can clean it up or protect it. There is too much at stake for the task to be left with one person, but every one of those persons can contribute to the movement to preserve the ecosystem. If everyone helps, everyone can be protected. If each of us fails to do our part, we are leaving a legacy for our ancestors that will eventually need to be addressed, or life on this planet may disappear. If not *us* now, then *who* later?

Noise Pollution

Sounds are with us all the time. Because hearing is one of our senses, we depend on our hearing to bring us important information from the outside world. In our modern world of machines, motors, technology, and personal behavior patterns, much of the sound in our world has become noise. Simply put, noise is unwanted sound. A person's loud rock music being played in the room next door may be music to them, but it can be noise to you if you are trying sleep or study. Our communities are now dealing more and more with noise pollution. In fact, may municipalities now have noise ordinances that prevent loud sounds during certain hours of the day.

Because sound cannot be produced in a vacuum, an explosion in outer space would not be heard. Sound travels in waves and has two characteristics that are important to the hearing process:

1. *Frequency.* The **frequency** of a sound wave refers to how often the material through which the wave passes vibrates in response to the wave. The frequency of sound is measured in **hertz (Hz)**: 1 Hz is one cycle per second, and 100 Hz is 100 cycles per second. The higher the number, the higher the pitch of the sound. The human ear can hear frequencies between about 10 and 20,000 Hz. Dolphins can hear frequencies up to 120,000 Hz.

2. *Intensity.* Simply put, the intensity of sound is how loud it is. This loudness is measured in units called **decibels (dB)**. The higher the decibel number, the louder the sound. You can learn about the decibel level of common sounds in Table 16-3.

Decibels are damaging, but given two sounds of equal decibels, the sound with the highest pitch is more harmful to hearing.

frequency
how often the material in a medium vibrates when a wave passes through the medium

hertz (Hz)
unit used to measure the frequency of sound

decibel
a measure of the intensity, or loudness, of a sound

TABLE 16-3 • Decibel levels of common sounds.

Sound	Decibel Level	Likelihood of Ear Damage
Whispers	40 dB	None
Everyday conversation	60 dB	None
Restaurant	70 dB	None
Heavy city traffic, vacuum cleaner, factory noise	80 dB	Minimal
Workshop tools, lawn mower	90 dB	Damage at exposure for eight hours per day
Jet takeoff	100 dB	Damage at exposure for two hours per day
Amplified rock music, shotgun blast	110 to 130 dB	Damage at exposure for 10 to 30 minutes per day
Air-raid siren, military jet	130 dB	Damage at five minutes per day
Pistol shot	140 dB	Danger level

Delmar/Cengage Learning

Caring for Your Ears

The sounds we hear can range from very pleasing (soft music) to annoying (loud traffic or road noise) to painful (an explosion). In fact, sound can be so loud that it permanently destroys hearing. Figure 16-14 lists the noises that people feel are the most annoying. Many young people prefer their music loud rather than soft. The most damaging sounds are probably from loud music delivered through the head phones of a personal disk player or listening to loud music in a very confined space. They may not worry much about loud sounds because their hearing quickly recovers, but this changes as one gets older. There are two reasons for concern. The first is that habits established during young adulthood tend to be kept for a lifetime. The second is that every loud assault on the hearing mechanism during one's lifetime can leave the hearing mechanism slightly damaged. The damage may not be noticeable at first, but an accumulation of assaults over

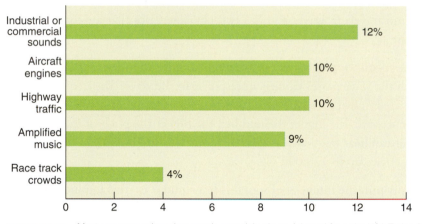

FIGURE 16-14 • Most common noises that people complain about. Adapted from the USA Today 2000.

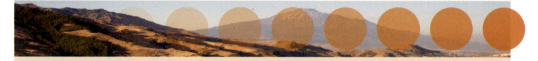

What's Your View?

Modern sound systems have been engineered to produce an accurate reproduction of sound. But these same systems have also been manufactured to allow the sound to be delivered loudly. These conditions present two problems—one personal and one social. The personal problem is the possible harm to hearing from playing the music too loudly. The social problem is one of playing music so loudly that it can be heard by someone outside the listener's location (house, car, and so on).

- Just how loudly should people be allowed to play music?

- While the listeners have the right to enjoy themselves, others outside the location have the right to listen or *not* to listen. Whose rights should be respected?

- Should there be a limit to how loudly people can play music in their home or car?

the years is likely to rob older adults of their hearing. Do you ever feel your ears buzzing after listening to loud music? Your ears buzz because your hearing mechanism has been challenged by varied frequencies at high decibels.

Look back at Table 16-3 for examples of damaging sounds. People working in occupations where they are exposed to loud noises are required by law to wear ear protection. Companies must provide ear protection for employees who are exposed to sounds of 90 decibels or higher during an eight-hour period. Many rock stars actually wear earplugs to protect their hearing when they play in concerts.

Noise pollution seems to be more tolerated than any of the other forms of pollution presented in this section. The effects are not immediately noticeable, and noise doesn't look or smell bad like other forms of pollution. That does not mean that noise is safe. It is part of the environment and needs to be attended to.

Doing Your Part

The quality of our environment is in our hands. We can destroy it, or we can protect it. We can allow others to negatively impact the ecosystem in which we live, or we can ignore them. We can teach our children to value and protect the world where we live, or we can allow them to use and abuse resources and "let some-one else" take care of the environment. The choice is ours. The choice is yours. You have to define what you want the world to be like and, it is hoped, take your turn at helping make it better than you found it. For example, if every coffee-drinking American used a refillable mug instead of a disposable cup, we would spare the environment about 7 million pounds of car-bon dioxide emissions every day, or we could plant about 140,000 trees to neutralize the effects of carbon dioxide. When you complete your wellness plan for this chapter, give serious thought to what you can do to practice environmental wellness.

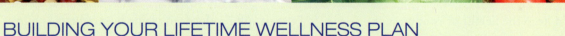

BUILDING YOUR LIFETIME WELLNESS PLAN

Environmental wellness is a very interesting part of wellness. In one sense practicing environment wellness is something you can do for yourself by doing your part to maintain the ecosystem where you live. But in another sense you are caring for and shaping the environment for your family, friends, and community members perhaps for decades to come. If everyone on the planet did all they could to make the environment a better place, the task of preserving the planet for future generations would be an easy one. The only thing we can do is do our best to maintain the ecosystem. As you develop your wellness plan for this topic, consider the following:

- Don't litter, even if "everyone else does". Encourage others to dispose of their trash appropriately. If we all do our part, the environment can change. If we DON'T do our part, the environment WILL change.

- Look for opportunities to help with environmental issues, such as highway cleanup, neighborhood recycling programs; help take school children on environmental field trips like to the city dump.

- Create ways to have a positive effect on the environment. Earlier we suggested using the stairs to help with caloric expenditure, but by NOT using the elevator, think of the energy that is being saved by not using the machine.

●●● **End-of-Chapter Activities**

Opportunities for Application

1. Contact your local water supplier and ask for information on the water quality in your area. Suppliers are required by law to provide the information to the public "in an understandable fashion." You may be able to find the information on the town's Web site, or you can call the treatment facility and ask that they send it to you. Summarize what you find.

2. Use your health literacy skills to prepare a letter to the editor of your local newspaper. Choose an environmental health concern that interests you and develop a three- to four-paragraph letter explaining why that particular issue should concern the citizens of your town. Be sure to include the latest data on the topic you can find and make it as relevant to your city as possible, such as information from the closest city if it is not yours or data from your state rather than the nation.

3. Look in your garage or the storage area under your kitchen sink and choose three cleaning products, fertilizers, or pest control products. Construct a chart that includes the type of product, the main chemicals or cleaning agents for each product, and the possible health effects of each product.

Key Concepts

1. Learn more about the polluting effect of tropospheric ozone. Search the Web to obtain two key pieces of information: the chemical reaction that produces tropospheric ozone and the effects of ozone on people and property.

   Explain the chemical process for ozone production in the troposphere.

   Make a list of ozone's destructive properties.

2. Chlorine is added to municipal water supplies. Explain why and describe the protective effect it has.

3. We know that using fossil fuels is harmful to the environment. There is a great deal of interest about finding new sources of energy. Some of these new energy sources are "renewable sources" of energy. Explain what is meant by renewable energy and list and describe some examples of renewable energy sources.

Answers to Personal Assessment: Environmental Health Behaviors

1. False. You should keep the height of your grass at three inches and allow all your clippings to stay on the lawn. They will provide nutrients to your lawn as they decompose.

2. False. Most of the health effects are cases of asthma and bronchitis caused by sulfur dioxide and nitrogen oxides.

3. False. It disrupts the ecosystem and can cause harm to humans.

4. False. Water treatment plants cannot remove toxic chemical.

5. False. It still produces the same by-products as burning gasoline.

6. True

7. False. Rainwater actually has a lot minerals in it. Distilled water is pure.

8. True

9. False. Remember that there are some chemicals that water treatment cannot remove.

10. True. High-decibel sounds are especially harmful.

●●● References

The Aluminum Association. (2009). *Industry Statistics.* Retrieved May 18, 2010 from http://www.aluminum.org/Content/NavigationMenu/NewsStatistics/StatisticsReports/default.htm

California Energy Commission. (2002). *Energy Quest (Chapter 8: Fossil Fuels - Coal, Oil and Natural Gas).* Retrieved April 2010 from http://energyquest.ca.gov/story/chapter08.html.

Duke, J.S. (2003). Burning buried sunshine: Human consumption of ancient solar energy. *Climatic Change* 61, 31–44.

Ehrlich, P. R. (1971). *The population bomb.* Cutchogue, NY: Buccaneer Books.

Natural Resources Defense Council. (n.d.). *Eating Tuna Safely.* Retrieved April 5, 2010 from http://www.nrdc.org/health/effects/mercury/tuna.asp.

New Scientist. (April 4, 2010) *Which is the greenest US city of all?.* Retrieved April 5, 2010 from http://www.newscientist.com/article/mg20627543.800-which-is-the-greenest-us-city-of-all.html.

Office of Solid Waste. (2009). *Municipal solid wastes in the United States: 2008 facts and figures* (Report No. EPA530-S-06-001). Washington, DC: U.S. Environmental Protection Agency.

USA Today. (December 15, 2000). Worst Noise Pollution Offenders. *USA Today,* p.1.

U.S. Environmental Protection Agency. (2009a). *Air Quality Trends, 1980–2008.* Retrieved April 5, 2010 from http://www.epa.gov/airtrends/aqtrends.html.

U.S. Environmental Protection Agency. (2009b). *Municipal Solid Waste Generation, Recycling, and Disposal in the United States: Facts and Figures for 2008.* Document no. EPA-530-F-009-021. Retrieved April 5, 2010 from http://www.epa.gov/osw/nonhaz/municipal/pubs/msw2008rpt.pdf.

Wingspread Conference on the Precautionary Principle. The Science and Environmental Health Network. January 26, 1998. http://www.sehn.org/wing.html. Retrieved April 5, 2010.

Wisman, P. (November 1985). EPA History (1970-1985): William D. Ruckelshaus, (December 4, 1970 to April 30, 1973). The Environmental Protection Agency. Retrieved April 4, 2010 from http://www.epa.gov/history/topics/epa/15b.htm.

World Health Organization. (2007). *Public health and environment.* Retrieved 2010, April from http://www.euro.who.int/envhealth/20060609_1.

CHAPTER 17

Health and Wellness through the Life Span

●●● Introduction

As you begin the last chapter in this book, you should have a good understanding about health and wellness, the health risks you might face during your lifetime, and how to use health literacy skills to obtain valid information. You know many risk factors can be controlled by making good decisions and practicing health-enhancing behaviors. It is hoped that during this course, you obtained information that will act as a wellness road map driven by your health literacy skills to optimize your health and that of your family and friends. Travel well!

This final chapter contains material to enhance your wellness goals through the rest of your life span. As a mature adult, you may already have encountered stressors specific to

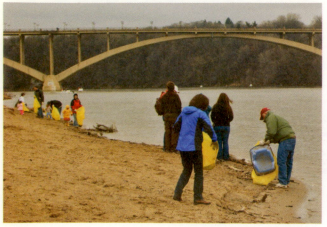

Courtesy of Shutterstock

FIGURE 17-1 • Health and wellness across the life span include contributing to the health of your family and your community, as demonstrated by these volunteers celebrating Earth Day by cleaning up the banks of the Mississippi River.

adulthood. Perhaps some of this stress was associated with helping to enhance the well-being of others, be they your parents, family members, relatives, or friends. Parenthood may be part of your life, now or in the future; consequently, a need will arise for you to contribute to developing the wellness skills of your family members. As a member of your community, you will have the occasion to contribute to the health of your community (Figure 17-1). Information and activities in this chapter will help you understand your role as an adult and provide you with information for developing a wellness plan that will serve you well as a caring member of your family and community.

●●● Challenges of Adulthood

At any stage of life we are faced with stressful events that cause us to worry, problem solve, and cope in order to address the challenge of responding to the events. Adulthood is no different. While stressful events are still a part of life, the nature and magnitude of the events may be more demanding. It is one thing to feel stressed because you

PERSONAL ASSESSMENT
Being an Adult

Before reading this chapter, take this personal assessment to discover more about your thoughts and feelings concerning adulthood and aging. Read the questions below and answer them according to what you believe at the present time. Formulate your answers, using the following scale, on the way you feel most of the time: 1 = definitely true, 2 = mostly true, 3 = mostly false, and 4 = definitely false. An interpretation of your results is located at the end of the chapter.

1. I will still like to do the same activities no matter how old I am.

2. The type of stressors that I experience will not change as I grow older.

3. There's really nothing I can do now to help me be happier when I am older.

4. Thinking about getting old is depressing to me.

5. There is no need to think about retirement until I am much older.

6. I believe I could be happy in more than one occupation.

7. Even when I am old, I expect to be healthy and active.

8. I believe you are only as old as you think you are.

9. Age has its privileges and benefits.

10. Parenting adolescents is a very difficult task.

had a homework assignment due when you were a fifth grader and another thing to suddenly have to deal with some acne when you were getting ready for an important social occasion as a senior in high school. Those kinds of things pale if, as an adult, you have to make a life-changing decision, such as deciding to marry or having to deal with medical and home care for an aging parent with Alzheimer's disease. The point is that with maturity comes a whole set of challenges demanding more intellectual and financial resources than were necessary to respond to the challenges experienced during one's youth. Some of the major life events that result from maturation are shown in Figure 17-2.

Medical psychiatric researchers Thomas Holmes and Richard Rahe (1967) researched the effects of life events on health. As a result, they devised a survey that measured the relative impact of stressful life events on health. The instrument, known as the Holmes-Rahe Social Readjustment Scale, gained popular acceptance in the health field because it was a way of looking at the health effects of stressful life events. The findings from the data that Holmes and Rahe collected on almost 400 subjects and compared to health effects that the subjects encountered two years after taking the survey indicated that the higher a respondent's measure of stressful events, the greater the likelihood of serious illness within the next two years. While the work of Holmes and Rahe indicates a strong relationship between stressful life events and health, it should not be taken as an absolute. Examination of the life events scale will quickly reveal that not all stressful life events are included on the questionnaire. In chapter 3, you learned about the concept of stress hardiness. Someone scoring high on the Holmes-Rahe Scale may also exhibit the characteristics of stress hardiness, thus reducing the likelihood of illness. Refer to Figure 17-3 and determine your Holmes-Rahe score and see if you agree with the assessment while giving consideration to your personal assessment of stress hardiness.

When you were younger, many of your psychological and physical needs were probably attended to by parents or other family members. Currently, you are held to a higher standard of self-care. By now, you should have mastered the skills in life to be an independent self-directed, lifelong learner. The older you become, the more self-care you will develop. It is possible that you may be in position to care for others—children, elderly parents, sick spouse, and so on. If you enter into a committed relationship and possibly have children, you will be responsible for another whole set of circumstances to which you must attend. It's possible that you are not the typical 18- to 20-year-old college student. If you are what colleges refer to as the "nontraditional student," you may want to use the information in this chapter that is directed toward the typical college student to help children of your own or those of other family members.

Challenges of Adulthood

Between the ages of 20 and 35, you will experience many life changes because this is a time when young adults must adapt to new roles and responsibilities. Young people entering adulthood typically experience more role changes during this period than during any other stage of life. Let's consider a young man named Mike. Mike graduated from college at 22 and got his first full-time job. Not too long after that, the relationship with his girlfriend, whom he dated throughout college, ended. When he was 24, he met Lisa, and they fell in love. At 25, he was offered a new job in a neighboring state, so he and Lisa married and moved to the new state. Mike had never lived so far away from

- Leaving home
- Making educational choices
- Developing adult relationships
- Choosing an occupation
- Progressing at work
- Developing a financial plan
- Making decisions about marriage and a family
- Caring for aging parents
- Planning for retirement
- Confronting health issues
- Growing older
- Facing death

FIGURE 17-2 • Major life events associated with maturation.

Delmar/Cengage Learning

Rank	Life Events	Life Change Units	Rank	Life Events	Life Change Units
1	Death of a child	123	24	Mortgage or loan greater than $10,000	44
2	Death of spouse	119	25	Change in responsibilities at work	43
3	Divorce	98	26	Change in living conditions	42
4	Death of close family member	92	27	Change in residence	41
5	Marital separation	79	28	Begin or end school	38
6	Fired from work	79	29	Trouble with in-laws	38
7	Major personal injury or illness	77	30	Outstanding personal achievement	37
8	Marriage Jail term	75	31	Change in work hours or conditions	36
9	Death of close friend	70	32	Change in schools	35
10	Pregnancy or birth of a child	66	33	Christmas	30
11	Major business readjustment	62	34	Trouble with boss	29
12	Foreclosure on mortgage or loan	61	35	Change in recreation	29
13	Gain of new family member	57	36	Mortgage or loan less than $10,000	28
14	Marital reconciliation	57	37	Change in personal habits	27
15	Change in health or behavior of family member	56	38	Change in eating habits	27
16	Change in financial status	56	39	Change in social activities	27
17	Retirement	54	40	Change in the number of family get-togethers	26
18	Change to a different line of work	51	41	Change in sleeping habits	26
19	Change in number of arguments with spouse	51	42	Vacation	25
20	Marriage	50	43	Change in church activities	22
21	Spouse begins or ends work	46			
22	Sexual difficulties	45			
23	Child leaving home	44			

FIGURE 17-3 • Social readjustment rating scale. Miller, M.A. and Rahe, R.H. (1997) Life changes scaling for the 1990's. *Journal of Psychosomatic Research, 43,* (3), 279–292. (Used with Permission)

his childhood home, but he found himself becoming more and more independent from his parents. When he was 28, he received a promotion at work about the same time that he and Lisa had their first child (Figure 17-4). The next year, at age 29, Mike and Lisa bought their first house. Just two years later, Mike's father had a heart attack. Mike and Lisa had to decide if they should move their family to live closer to Mike's parents. In just a few short years, Mike experienced all these life events: being a college learner, becoming a full-time employee, breaking up with a girlfriend, dating, marrying, getting a job promotion, moving far away from home, having children, and coping with the serious illness of a parent.

By this point in this course, you understand the importance of the wellness lifestyle and the behaviors and strategies needed to develop and maintain high-level wellness. Without question, such a preparation will help you meet the challenges and role changes of adulthood. No matter what your age, as an adult, you will continue developing your knowledge, skills, and personal values to guide your decision making. You will be setting goals for the completion of your education and your transition to a career. At the same time, you will cultivate the self-discipline needed to work and achieve those goals. As time goes by, you will be tested to acquire new knowledge, make many decisions, and develop new behaviors to address the obstacles and challenges that arise.

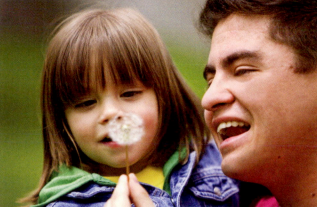

FIGURE 17-4 • During early adulthood, people undergo many life changes.

Career Stressors

One of the biggest decisions you will ever make is choosing your career path because this choice will affect many other aspects of your life. Your career choice will determine the type and amount of education you pursue, the knowledge and skills you need to find employment, and how much money you will earn. Even arriving at a career choice can be stressful. Many people go to college not really knowing what they want to do in life. Moreover, in today's business world, there are many more specialty areas than there were decades ago. For example, people don't just go into computing. Computer science positions include programmers, technical supporters, systems analysts, system administrators, software developers, and numerous engineering positions specializing in hardware development. It sometimes takes students a few years of schooling to finally determine what they really want to do professionally. Choose carefully, as your life is likely to be much more satisfying if you select a career or vocation that you really enjoy. To choose a career that is right for you, step back and consider your personality and interests as well as your job options. Here are several points to consider when choosing a career:

1. Choosing a career can be a way of expressing your personality. Many social scientists agree that personal traits such as aptitudes, abilities, and interests play a strong role in which career you are likely to choose. For example, some individuals are "people oriented"; they are well suited for occupations where they interact with people, such as teaching, sales, nursing, marketing, counseling, or management. Those who are not people oriented may be more comfortable in accounting, software development, drafting, engineering, or veterinary medicine.

2. Look for success in more than one type of job. The U.S. Department of Labor produces a book called the *Dictionary of Occupational Titles*, which lists more than 20,000 occupations. Depending on your interests, you can probably find dozens of jobs that interest you and in which you can be very successful.

3. Your level of education will affect your career options. Education past high school can help any person be more gainfully employed. According to the U.S. Department of

WEB LINK
Career Choices

http://www.bls.gov

If you are undecided about your career or want more information about the career you are seeking, go to this Web site. At the home page, go to the bottom left of the page and click "occupations," then click "occupational outlook handbook." You can then search for almost any occupation. When you get to the occupation, you will find the potential of that profession, training needed for the position, and salary information.

SEARCH TERMS: occupations, job prospects, job market

TABLE 17-1 • Education and earning power of persons age 25 and over, 2009.

Education Level	Average Income Male	Average Income Female
Some high school—no completion	$23,830	$14,710
High school diploma (includes GED)	$33,930	$22,300
Some college no degree	$40,260	$26,440
Associate degree (2-year)	$45,080	$30,870
Bachelor's degree	$47,240	$60,290
Master's degree	$56,710	$40,230
Doctorate degree	$95,880	$64,080

Source: National Center for Education Statistics, *Outcomes of Education Report* (2009).

Labor, people who drop out of high school are 72 percent more likely to be unemployed than are those who finish high school. Education also plays a big role in how much money you earn. On average, people with a college degree earn more than twice what a person earns who never finished high school. So the more education one has, the more earning potential one is likely to achieve. Table 17-1 give you some idea of the differences between education levels and the earning power differences between men and women.

4. Career choices can be made throughout life. In the distant past, many people followed their parent(s) into their job and worked their entire lives in the same type job that their parent(s) had. Today, people usually choose occupations different from those of their parents. They are also more likely to switch jobs and even pursue an entirely new career area as they get older.

Finding the right job and getting the necessary training to prepare you for that occupation is a challenging task. But there are certain things you can do to increase the likelihood of choosing a career that you find satisfying:

- *Research job characteristics.* Talk to people working in occupations that interest you, conduct research in the library, or go online to get more information. Find out which jobs appeal to you the most. Learn about the working conditions, responsibilities, duties, and qualifications involved in the job. You should also consider the earning potential, opportunities for advancement, and personal satisfaction you can expect to obtain.

- *Visit the career center on your campus.* Colleges and universities have offices to help find their professional niche and even support with job placement. You might ask a counselor in the career center if they have an **occupational interest inventory** you could take. An occupational interest inventory is a test that measures a person's interests as they are related to various jobs and careers. These tests can help you discover what types of careers might be the best fit for you based on your interests and personality.

occupational interest inventory
a test that measures a person's interests as they are related to various jobs and careers

Did You Know…?

That each year, the U.S. Department of Education provides more than $83 billion in financial aid to nearly 14 million postsecondary students. About 50 percent of college graduates leave school owing student loans. The average student loan debt is $10,000.

- *Set your goals early to obtain the job you choose.* Once you have decided on the job you would like to have, you can research information about that professional area. You can find out what courses you can expect to take to prepare for that field. If you have little skill or interest in math and physics, engineering would not be a good choice for you. Determine how to best train for the job you want. If special courses or education are required, begin working to acquire those qualifications.

- *Do the things in school that will lead toward the job you want.* While you are working on your degree, you can volunteer to work for a company that hires people to do the job you would like to have. For example, if you would like to become a court reporter or legal assistant, see if you can volunteer to work in a law office. If you want to become a veterinarian, volunteer to help in an animal clinic. You may be able to set up your volunteer program as an internship experience and get school credit for the work you do.

- *Don't get stuck in a job you dislike.* If you find that the first job you choose doesn't result in the job satisfaction you expected, find one that does. With more than 20,000 types of occupations available, surely you can find the job that is right for you.

Financial Stressors

As an adult, you are more responsible for your own living expenses than you were when you lived at home. If you have been living on your own for a while, you may have adjusted to the necessity of generating a steady and rewarding income and establishing a budget you can live with. No matter what your situation, you probably realize that your educational experiences are an investment in the future, preparing you with the knowledge and skills necessary for employment that holds financial security. After you complete the necessary education, it is up to you to secure the right job and do all the personal and professional things necessary to achieve financial success. The journey to get there, however, will still be fraught with financial challenges.

Common Financial Problems

Many people believe that if they just had more money, they would have fewer problems. But this is not necessarily true. Both the rich and the poor can have financial problems (as well as other kinds of problems). Have you heard the phrase "living from paycheck to paycheck"? Some people save little or nothing from what they earn. Perhaps they earn only enough to cover their necessary living expenses, with little or no money left for personal spending or savings (Figure 17-5). Or they may spend a lot of money on things that aren't necessities. If unexpected emergencies arise, people who haven't saved may find themselves with serious financial problems.

Another common problem is depending too heavily on borrowing. Buying a lot of things on credit can be an indication that people are living beyond their financial abilities. You can begin learning good money management skills at

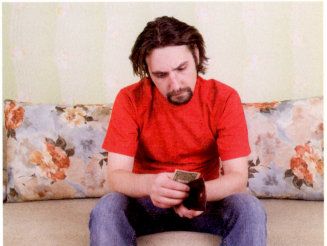

FIGURE 17-5 • Living paycheck to paycheck with no money for personal spending or savings is a common financial problem and a huge stressor.

Courtesy of Shutterstock

any point in your life. Developing and practicing good money management skills now will help you manage your money well in the years to come and help reduce some of the financial stressors of life.

Money Management

Good money management means balancing your expenses with your income. By acquiring the skills needed to make wise choices about spending and saving your money, you can begin to prepare for the future. Consider the following strategies for practicing wise money management.

Determine Your Priorities. You have goals in life and some may include financial comfort. Being clear about your priorities helps you decide where you want to invest your time, energy, and money. For example, is $180 spent on a tattoo a wise investment if you have to borrow money to get the tattoo in the first place? What about having to borrow money for the books you need this semester because you purchased the tattoo. Worse yet, think about the decision to borrow money so that you can do both. Unless you obtain a loan that offers terms like 0 percent interest for 12 months and you are positive that you can pay the loan off before the deadline, you are *always* going to pay more for that item than you planned to. Credit card and loan companies use their money to make money. Imagine charging the $180 for the tattoo to a credit card that has 15 percent interest. Table 17-2 illustrates what the payout would look like if it were paid off monthly for one year and **amortized** at 15 percent. You can see that the $180 tattoo has an additional cost of almost $15 because of the loan. Imagine what happens to the cost of the tattoo if you make nothing more than the minimum payment each month.

Set Goals for Your Future. Once you have decided what is most important to you, you can choose what you want to accomplish in the future and what it will take to get there. For example, you may want to purchase a car, you may want to travel with friends, or you may want to finish college with no student loans. Once you have set your goals, you can determine how much money you will need to achieve those goals and set a plan for success.

Make Saving a Priority. It is wise to always be mindful of your financial future, especially in terms of saving money and preparing for retirement. Although it may seem to you that retirement is a long way off, when it comes, you want to be ready. Saving along the way can help a great deal, and if you get a job with a retirement program, that is even better. If you were to begin saving $100 a month and continue to do so while keeping

amortized
the provision of paying off a borrowed amount of money over a predetermined time period

TABLE 17-2 • Amortization schedule for a $180 loan.

Month Year	2 2010	3 2010	4 2010	5 2010	6 2010	7 2010	8 2010	9 2010	10 2010	11 2010	12 2010	1 2011
Payment ($)	16.25	16.25	16.25	16.25	16.25	16.25	16.25	16.25	16.25	16.25	16.25	16.25
Principal paid ($)	14.00	14.17	14.35	14.53	14.71	14.89	15.08	15.27	15.46	15.65	15.85	16.05
Interest paid ($)	2.25	2.08	1.90	1.72	1.54	1.35	1.17	0.98	0.79	0.59	0.40	0.20
Total interest ($)	2.25	4.33	6.22	7.94	9.48	10.83	12.00	12.98	13.76	14.36	14.76	14.96
Balance ($)	166.00	151.83	137.48	122.96	108.25	93.35	78.27	63.00	47.55	31.89	16.05	0.00

Calculated with Amortization Calculator, http://www.bretwhissel.net/cgi-bin/amortize

the money in a savings account that would pay 4 percent interest, at the end of 40 years you would have $118,590.12. In fact, you would earn more than $70,000 in *interest* from the bank.

Consider How and Where You Spend Your Money. Keep a record of all your purchases and expenses. You may discover that you spend a lot of your money on things that are not high priorities. If this is the case, you may need to reevaluate where you are spending your money in order to have enough money for those things that are most important or necessary to you. There is another reason for keeping track of your spending, and that is having receipts for the things you paid for. It is not uncommon for a business to bill you twice for the same purchase. Without receipts, you have little chance of recovering the loss.

Make a Commitment to Spend Money Wisely. Before making a purchase, ask yourself, "Will this purchase help me reach my financial goals and take care of my priorities? Is this purchase necessary? Can I wait to buy this?" If you decide to buy something, then do some comparison shopping for the best bargain. Take your time to make sure that you are getting the best deal. For example, one of the authors was interested in purchasing a headset for a cellular phone. The headset in question was $99.99 at the cellular phone store. The author found the same headset, new and in the factory box, on e-Bay for $29.90, including shipping.

Create a Budget. First, list all your anticipated expenses, *including savings*. Next, write down how much money you expect to earn or receive. Do you have enough to cover your expenses? If you don't, look for expenses you can eliminate or for a way to increase income. Try to eliminate expenses other than savings. Plan what to do with the money you have left, if any. You can spend it now, save it, or invest it. Learn to say no to purchases that don't fit your priorities and budget. Think about saving for unexpected future expenditures, such as car repairs, home repairs, and tuition increases.

Use Credit Wisely. Credit cards get many people into trouble. People apply for credit cards and begin purchasing items without a plan for paying off the debt. They don't think about what might happen if they get sick or lose their job. Moreover, they don't even understand how credit cards work. When you buy something on credit, someone (usually a bank or a credit card company) lends you the money to make the purchase. They will charge you interest for the privilege of using their money to purchase an item, usually because the item is an expense for which you don't have the ability to pay outright at that time. Interest rates vary from company to company and perhaps within the same company depending on a person's credit history. A person with no credit may get a card at 17 percent interest, while the same company will give a 10 percent interest rate to someone with a good credit history. Some credit card companies also charge an annual fee of $25 to $75 for the privilege of having the credit card, whether you use it or not. Many credit card companies charge a high interest rate; remember that the company or bank wants to make money by lending money. On cards with high interest rates, it is impossible to pay off the debt by making only the minimum payment each month. If you use a credit card to make purchases, it is wise to pay off what you owe as soon as you can. Doing so minimizes the amount of interest you pay, but, more important, it benefits your credit rating. You can reduce financial stress by managing your money well. Use your health literacy skills to learn all you can about credit card

Did You Know . . . ?

If you purchase a $1,800 flat-screen television with a credit card or store financial plan that has an 18 percent interest rate and pay for it over 24 months, the final cost of the television will be $2,157.

1. In 2009, the amount of outstanding consumer debt in the United States was $2.5 trillion. This translates into over $8,100 for every man, woman and child in the country.[1] Credit card debt alone averaged $16,007 per household that had credit card debt in July 2009. Compare this to working class people in the 1920s who had *NO* debt. In fact, banks would not sell homes to them; the banks rented the properties to families. If anyone wanted to own their own home, they paid for the work while the house was being built.

2. Typically, the American family today pays more than $1,200 a year in credit card interest. Twenty-three percent of American Families admit to "maxing out" their credit cards.[1]

3. A typical credit card purchase, paid off over time with minimal payments ends up costing 112 percent *more* than if the customer paid cash.[2]

4. Approximately 40% of American families spend more than they earn.[3]

5. With all this information, it is still surprising that nine out 10 people say credit card debt has never been a source of worry for them.[3]

Sources: [1]Money-zine.com (2009); [2]Woolsey, B., Shulz, M. (2010); [3]Bannister, P. (2004)

Delmar/Cengage Learning

FIGURE 17-6 • Facts about personal debt.

use before you get into financial difficulty. You can start by reviewing some interesting facts in Figure 17-6.

Relationship and Family Stressors

Adults, especially young adults, face many changes in their relationships. For some, such as those who have just started college, friendships and romantic relationships from high school may end and new relationships begin. As a college learner, you form new relationships from among those people who go to classes with you or whom you may meet at social functions or campus organizations. When you finish your current degree, you may continue your education, perhaps in another state. If you move, you will be geographically distant from the family and friends you grew up with. Some people find it difficult to leave all that is familiar to them. If you have the opportunity to move, you may have to engage in some serious decision making. You'll have to cope with the changes and challenges of ending some relationships and beginning others.

Even when relationships are going well, adults are often faced with important decisions. For example, consider Dwayne and Kerri, who have been dating for about four years. They just seemed to hit it off from the start. They love being together, but soon they will be graduating from college and looking for jobs. Dwayne is agonizing over whether to ask Kerri to marry him. "How do I know for sure this is really love?" he wonders. "Is there any test I can take to determine whether or not this is a 'forever relationship'?" He thinks about the things that he likes about Kerri. She has all the characteristics he wants in a partner: she's intelligent, kind, trustworthy, loving, emotionally stable, dependable, ambitious, honest, and fun to be with. Dwayne examines their relationship. They have many things in common, they enjoy being together, and each of them cares about what happens to the other person. Still, Dwayne wonders how he can know for sure whether he and Kerri will be happy together for the rest of their lives, especially given that each of them will have career interests.

Successful Relationships

There are no guarantees that two people will find love and happiness that lasts forever. But there are some characteristics for determining compatibility in relationships. In the United States, people tend to marry people who have a similar social standing. People also tend to marry individuals who have characteristics that are comparable to their own. These characteristics are called **similarity factors**. The most important similarity factors that lead to successful long-term relationships in our culture include social class, educational level, geographic location, age, race, ethnic group, religion, and values.

Relationships can cause stress, but not having relationships can cause stress, too. The lack of a romantic relationship is not necessarily a problem (unless the person wants to be in such a relationship), but everyone needs friends and acquaintances with whom they feel comfortable. As a mature adult, it's easy to become disconnected from the people who have been important in your life. You may have heard the old saying, "Make new friends, but keep the old—one is silver, the other gold." As you become an adult, you will see that there is a great deal of value in both old and new friendships.

similarity factors
those characteristics, values, and goals, shared by two people in a relationship

●●● Marriage and Family

The decision to marry someone should not be taken lightly. Marriage is intended to be a lifetime commitment and should be entered into only when both partners are certain that they want to enter into this "social contract." There are two sides of a marital relationship. The first is the love and excitement that comes from the nonmarital dating phase that leads up to the decision to marry, including the wedding ceremony. Take the marriage quiz in Figure 17-7 and see what you already know about marriage.

The wedding ceremony is a joyous time, and some people go to the limits of extravagance to make it a memorable time. The real part of the marriage comes after

---

Let's see what you already know about marriage. Read each of the statements below and mark down whether you think each statement is true or false and why you chose the answer you did. The correct answers and comments appear at the end of the chapter.

1. The secrets to long-term marital success are good communication and commitment.
2. Marriage offers more benefits to men that it does to women.
3. People today are getting married at a younger age than they did 10 years ago.
4. The more education a woman has, the greater her chance of getting married.
5. Married couples tend to be happier after they have children.
6. Marriage puts a woman at greater risk for physical abuse than if she stays single.
7. Couples who live together before marriage are more likely to have successful marriages than those couples who don't.
8. Couples can't be expected to stay married for life because people today live much longer than they used to.
9. Married people have more satisfying sex lives than single people.

Delmar/Cengage Learning

FIGURE 17-7 • Marriage quiz.

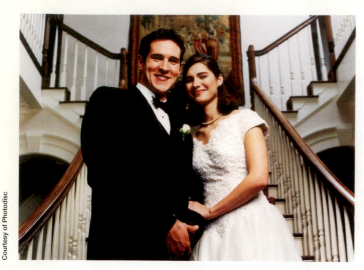

Courtesy of Photodisc

FIGURE 17-8 • The real task of marriage begins once the ceremony and honeymoon are over and the couple begins their life together.

the honeymoon is over and the couple returns to face reality. There is the *task* of being married that awaits the couple (Figure 17-8). In the ideal, marriage should forever be like the honeymoon, but that is not the case. The couple is faced with building the marital relationship so that it endures all the challenges to come. There will always be decisions to be shared and made, some of which will present immense challenges to the couple, but with patience, understanding, and good communication, the stress can be minimal, and the challenges will become opportunities to strengthen the bond.

Entering the Family Life Cycle

Many young couples decide to start a family of their own. A child can bring great joy, but he or she can also bring many new stressors. Parents must adjust to a lifestyle that is totally different from the one they previously experienced as a couple. Social scientists describe a **family life cycle** that illustrates the developmental stages of most families. There are six stages, and each stage has its own characteristics:

family life cycle
an orderly sequence of developmental stages that most families experience

1. *Between families.* This is the single young adult who has left his or her parents and has not married. Stressors during this stage can include learning to depend on peers for support, developing relationships, and establishing new living, study, and work habits. Some people use this time to look for a steady partner; others may use it to live the "single life."

2. *Marriage—newly married couple.* The newly married couple tends to be very happy, but the husband and wife must each learn to live with another person,

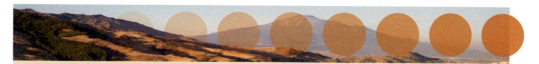

What's Your View?

What Is a Successful Marriage?

"A successful marriage requires falling in love many times, always with the same person" (anonymous). There is no instruction book for a successful marriage. When two people feel right about each other and decide to commit to a lifetime relationship, they may forget that there *are* things each person can do and say to strengthen the relationship as the years pass.

Think about the previous quote. What do you think it means? Do you agree with its message? Explain. Share the quote with your friends and see what they think about its meaning. Or you might want to share it with someone you are in a close relationship with if you have talked about marriage. Is his or her view similar to yours?

and new types of relationships must be formed with both sets of parents. The relationships become expanded—not only does the view of self change for each spouse, but there are complexities of the relationships with the blended family units as well.

3. *Family with young children.* This can be one of the most stressful of the family life cycle stages. New parents must take on greater responsibility. Relationships with other family members change. What was once a couple is now a family. The couple's parents expand their roles, too, as they become grandparents.

4. *Family with adolescents.* Parents often rate this period as the most difficult time in child rearing. Even families who had little conflict earlier in their marriage often experience family conflict during this time of transition. The manner in which children pass through adolescence is dependent on the relationships the parents established with the teens when the teens were children. Families with adolescents are tasked with preparing their children to leave home. They must also deal with their own midlife issues and possibly those of their aging parents.

5. *Beginning the empty nest.* An **empty nest** is a family whose children have grown up and left home. The parents may need to learn to be a couple once again. With children who are now adults, family relationships change. And when adult children marry, the family must accept outside members. The parents may also be dealing with the old age, disability, or death of their parents.

6. *Family in old age.* The original couple must face issues related to their advancing age. In some cases, these include retirement, financial concerns, and serious health challenges. One spouse may die and leave the other widowed.

empty nest
a family whose children have grown up and left home

Having Children

Aside from getting married, a couple's decision to start a family is probably the most significant decision the two of them will make. If they prepared well for their marriage, they will have shared their views about having a family with each other. Have you ever thought about how much children change the lives of parents? In fact, every aspect of marriage and life changes when there are children. And, although children are a source of great joy, they also bring many challenges. Mature partners who are considering becoming parents should ask the following questions of themselves and each other:

- Do I want to have a child? Why or why not?

- What kind of parent will I be?

- What are my views on child rearing?

- Am I willing to make the sacrifices necessary to be a good parent?

- How will a new baby affect the relationship with my spouse?

- If there are other children in the family, how will having another baby affect them?

Pregnancy and Delivery

In chapter 7, you read about the male and female reproductive systems, the process of conception, and the development of the fetus. Now let's take a closer look at pregnancy and childbirth. A full-term pregnancy is divided into three three-month time segments called trimesters.

The First Trimester

The first trimester lasts for 14 weeks. For both the mother and the baby, this is probably the most important period of a pregnancy because this is when the vital structures and organs are forming in the **embryo**, and it is a time of dramatic changes in the mother. Good prenatal care, as discussed in chapter 7, is extremely important early in the pregnancy to ensure both the health of the mother and the proper development of the child.

The Mother. Beginning in the fourth to sixth week of the first trimester, approximately 75 percent of pregnant women experience a condition known as **morning sickness**, which is characterized by an upset stomach and possibly vomiting. This condition is the result of the significant changes taking place in the mother's body, particularly changes in her hormone levels. Morning sickness is a misnomer since it does not always happen in the morning, nor is it really an "illness"; rather, it is a normal part of pregnancy. In some cases, morning sickness may persist all day. The accurate medical term for the condition is known as "nausea and vomiting of pregnancy." The symptoms of morning sickness can be reduced by eating four or five small meals a day instead of three large ones, eating a couple of crackers when first waking up in the morning, and avoiding spicy foods. If morning sickness is serious enough, the mother may require bed rest and will need extra help from her partner to take care of daily activities. By the time a woman reaches the second trimester, morning sickness usually has disappeared.

In addition to morning sickness, it is not uncommon for a woman to feel less romantic during the first trimester because of the discomfort of hormonal and physical changes. She needs patience and understanding from her partner during this time.

The Baby. During the first trimester, the embryo develops all its body organs and grows to a length of about one and a half inches. In addition to its organs, the embryo also develops an **umbilical cord**, which connects it to the placenta. The **placenta** is a structure that grows in the mother's uterus that allows the passage of nutrients from the mother's blood into the fetus's blood and the passage of waste materials from the fetus's blood to the mother's blood. This exchange takes place throughout the pregnancy.

The Second Trimester

The second trimester lasts from week 14 through week 28. The baby is now referred to as a fetus because it has developed all of its organs.

The Mother. As a woman enters the second trimester, several changes are likely to take place: her morning sickness goes away, her appetite improves, and her energy level increases. She now has to be careful not to eat *too* much. Some women think they need to consume a lot of food because they are "eating for two." But this is not exactly the case. The mother needs to eat for herself and for a

---

embryo
animal organism in the early stages of development; in humans, this stage begins with conception and lasts for 14 weeks

morning sickness
a feeling of nausea experienced by some women during the first trimester of pregnancy

umbilical cord
flexible structure that contains the arteries and veins that connect the embryo or fetus to the placenta

placenta
an organ that forms in the uterus during pregnancy to aid in the exchange of nutrients and waste products between mother and embryo or fetus

---

WEB LINK
Pregnancy

http://www.americanpregnancy.org/index.htm

If you want to learn more about pregnancy, go to this Web site, which contains a great deal of information related to pregnancy and childbirth, from ovulation calculation to paternity testing.

SEARCH TERMS: pregnancy, childbirth, birthing

"very little person" no more than 300 extra calories per day. Because of the growing fetus, she does have special nutritional needs: protein, calcium, iron, and **folate**. The woman will probably have to supplement her diet with calcium, iron, and folate because eating a normal diet does not provide the recommended levels of these nutrients. During this trimester, fetal growth causes the mother's abdomen to swell, so she now finds it more comfortable to wear loose clothing.

folate
a water-soluble B vitamin that occurs naturally in food

The Baby. All the fetus's organs have formed by the time the second trimester begins, and its heartbeat can be heard. Early in the trimester, the heartbeat makes a swishing noise, but as the trimester progresses, the sound begins to resemble a regular heartbeat. Sometime around the middle of this trimester, the fetus begins to move around. This is an exciting time for the family because it is a clear sign that the fetus is doing well. By the time the second trimester is over, the fetus is about 14 or 15 inches long and weighs approximately two pounds.

The Third Trimester

The third trimester is the home stretch—the most exciting part of the pregnancy. The parents become anxious to deliver the baby and will decide, with input from the doctor, how the baby will be delivered. Approximately two-thirds of all deliveries in the United States are vaginal deliveries, and most of them use a **prepared childbirth** technique. Prepared childbirth is often referred to as "Lamaze." Although the Lamaze method, developed by Dr. Ferdinand Lamaze, was popularized as birth without anesthesia in the 1960s, the current practice of prepared childbirth is collection of practices that help women give birth in a comfortable manner without the necessity of anesthesia. During the third trimester, the mother and her husband, partner, or friend may attend childbirth classes. Birthing classes are available to give couples information about labor and delivery. These classes usually teach the couple about prepared childbirth practices and explain the procedures of other birthing methods, such as a **cesarean-section delivery** where the baby is removed through an incision in the uterus. The classes give expectant fathers the opportunity to be actively involved with pregnancy and the birth process.

Did You Know...?

Loud or persistent noise is more than a nuisance—it is an environmental hazard! Rock concerts, loud boom boxes or radios, and street and airport jet traffic are all examples of environmental sources of noise. For pregnant mothers, it is very important to protect the developing fetus from environmental noise. Some studies have shown that pregnant women who are exposed to high levels of noise may deliver prematurely and have low-birth-weight babies and that their babies may have a higher risk for some hearing loss.

prepared childbirth
a birthing method that uses relaxation techniques and procedures to deliver the fetus without surgery

cesarean-section delivery
birthing procedure in which the fetus is surgically removed from the uterus

The Mother. Visits to the health care provider generally become more frequent as the physician monitors the last weeks of the pregnancy. The mother notices that the fetus is moving less as the trimester progresses because the fetus has grown so large that there isn't space for him or her to move freely. Near the end of the trimester, the mother feels somewhat uncomfortable as the baby continues to grow and starts to settle down in her pelvis in preparation for birth. At this time, it may be difficult for the mother to sleep comfortably because her abdomen is so large. The best sleeping position is on her side with a pillow between her legs.

The Baby. Although the fetus is completely formed by the beginning of the third trimester, there are significant events that take place in preparation for birth. The fetus gets a little fatter to make the transition from the comfortable warm space inside the mother to the colder air in the birthing area. During the latter part of this trimester, the fetus turns upside down and gets positioned at the bottom of the uterus to prepare for birth.

Childbirth

The birthing process normally takes place around the fortieth week of pregnancy, though 10 days before or after the due date is not unusual. Delivery usually begins when the fetus is completely ready to be born. Even though the mother is expecting the birth, the actual start may be a surprise, usually beginning with contractions of the uterus. The birthing process is broken down into three stages of labor (Figure 17-9):

Stage 1. The uterus is a muscular organ, and during the birthing process, the uterus pushes the baby out of the uterus and into the vagina. To do this, the uterus alternates between episodes of contractions and periods of relaxation. While the uterus is contracting, the cervix is dilating to allow for passage of the fetus. Uterine contractions will be about 20 minutes apart at the start of stage one but occur at one- to two-minute intervals by the end of the stage. During this time, the baby is moving headfirst downward from the uterus.

Stage 2. The baby emerges from the uterus headfirst. The head is the largest part of the baby, so after the head has emerged, the rest of the baby slips out easily. The pressure of the birthing process on the baby's chest causes the heart and lungs to become fully functional for its first breaths. The birthing cry is a sure sign that the baby is breathing.

Stage 3. The placenta detaches from the uterus and leaves the uterus through the vagina.

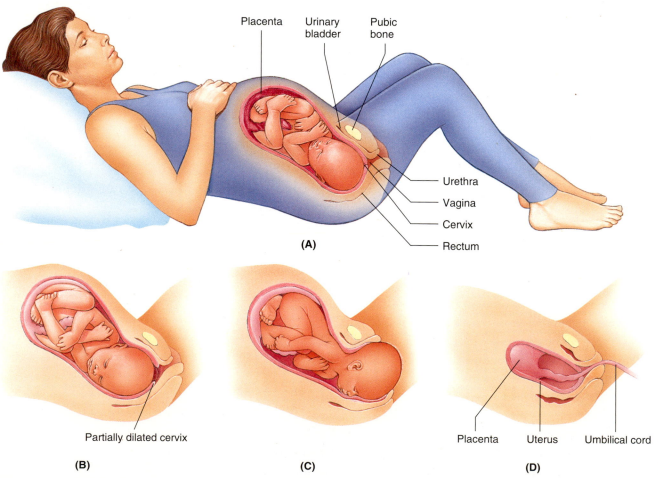

FIGURE 17-9 • Delivery of the fetus: (A) pre-labor, (B) first stage, (C) second stage, (D) third stage.

Middle Adulthood

Middle adulthood begins during the late thirties or early forties. When people enter middle adulthood, they may begin to ask themselves, "How am I doing for my age? Am I where I'm supposed to be?" Many people judge themselves by what is known as a **social clock**, a schedule of accomplishments they believe must be achieved by a certain age. When individuals don't accomplish one or more of the events or milestones of their social clock, they may become frustrated and disillusioned. This feeling is frequently referred to as a midlife crisis.

Middle adulthood is a transitional time. The excitement of being a young adult begins to diminish, and middle-aged adults are often faced with increased responsibilities for children and aging parents. At the same time, they are coping with the reality of their own aging and preparing for their retirement (Figure 17-10).

Career and Financial Stressors

In middle adulthood, individuals face many career and financial stressors. If one's chosen career has been successful and financially rewarding, these stressors may be minimal. When people are unhappy with their work, however, middle adulthood can be a time for career reevaluation. Individuals may decide to change jobs or return to school for additional training.

Financial stressors during this stage of life can be the result of trying to care for both children and aging parents as well as planning for one's own advancing age. The retirement age in our culture varies from person to person but has steadily decreased. People are retiring at younger ages than ever before, with many leaving work between ages 60 and 65. They hope to have plenty of time to enjoy things they didn't have time to do when they were employed. If they are financially secure, the prospect of retirement can be something to look forward to. If retirement means a substantial decrease in financial security, however, it may be viewed with a great deal of anxiety.

Relationship and Family Stressors

It would be nice if everyone who married lived happily ever after, but this ideal is not always the case. When two people marry, they face many problems and challenges together. Sometimes these troubles become overwhelming to one or both of the spouses, and the relationship may end in divorce. Although marital challenges can occur early in a marriage, they may also appear in a different form when the couple reaches middle adulthood. Any relationship with children that ends in divorce can be traumatic for any children. Parents would do well to read material to help prepare children for divorce.

Child Rearing

Child rearing can be a major family stressor during middle adulthood because this is often the time when the children are adolescents. Perhaps you remember how challenging it was for both you and your family when you were establishing your own separate

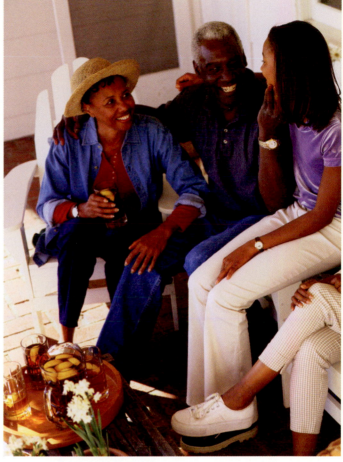

Courtesy of Photodisc

FIGURE 17-10 • Middle adulthood is often a transitional time, with couples raising a family, dealing with their own aging, and often taking care of their parents, who may be facing health problems.

social clock
a schedule of accomplishments a person believes he or she can or should achieve by a certain age

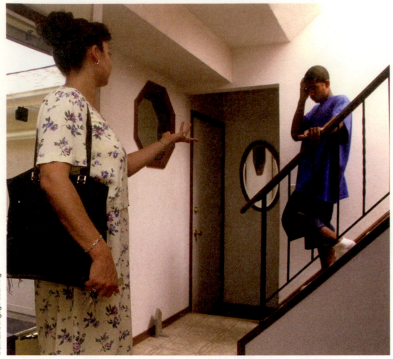

Delmar/Cengage Learning

FIGURE 17-11 • Families with adolescents often go through significant stress.

identity. Shifting hormone levels during adolescence contribute to unpredictable emotions and mood swings. It can be difficult for parents to watch their teenage children deal with the challenges of adolescence (Figure 17-11).

Parents must prepare their adolescent emotionally and intellectually for life as an adult. They want their teens well positioned to live independently, but, at the same time, they may still think of the teenagers as children. Some parents expect to help their children financially so that they can attend college or technical school. On top of all this, parents today are concerned about their children growing up in a world threatened by violence in schools, threats of bioterrorism, and the threat of nuclear weapons. In the midst of these concerns, parents may also be confronting their own personal challenges of middle adulthood and thinking about preparing for their upcoming retirement. The next time you say or think, "I'll never treat my kids like my parents treated me!" remember how much pressure there is on parents of teens today.

Common Marital Challenges

Many of the relationships we have in life are fraught with challenges. It does not matter if the relationship is a friendship, business relationship, social club, or marriage, when two or more people get together, there may be varying points of view. The disagreements or conflicts are not bad, and they cannot be avoided. The secret is to be able to recognize the effect on the relationship and work through the issues. In some instances, marital challenges do not end well. There are known factors that threaten a marriage. Here are some of the most common marital challenges that may lead to divorce:

- *Unrealistic expectations.* When one of the spouses has expectations of the other partner that are unrealistic, frustration and disappointment can occur. Unrealistic expectations can include role expectations. For example, a husband may expect his wife to do all the housework and cooking. She, on the other hand, may expect him to share those duties. Their conflicting expectations can result in a power struggle that leads to marital discontent.

- *Poor communication skills.* Poor communication is another common reason for divorce. To have a satisfying marriage, couples must recognize and resolve conflict in a positive manner in which both people feel like winners. Recall that there is a difference between poor communication and no communication, but both conditions are unproductive to a relationship.

- *Work and career issues.* If one or both spouses are unhappy in their job, this unhappiness often shows up at home. Spouses may disagree about the amount of time that should be allocated to work or career and the amount of time that should be devoted to the needs of the family, particularly if there are children. The home should be a place where these issues can be discussed safely.

- *Financial difficulties*. Disagreement about how to spend money is one of the most common reasons for marital conflict. Couples who work together to make joint decisions about spending have fewer divorces than those who don't.

- *Problems with in-laws*. In-laws sometimes interfere in a marriage. Even if this interference is unintentional, it can create a lot of pressure for a couple. The spouse of the person whose parent is interfering may become resentful if he or she is confronted about the level of interference. The person whose parent is interfering may not know how to handle the situation without creating stress in his or her relationship with the parents.

- *Infidelity*. One or both partners' being unfaithful to the marriage commitment can create a great deal of emotional pain. This pain and the resulting lack of trust often cause marriages to dissolve.

Deciding to seek a divorce is usually very difficult for both spouses. In fact, it is common for the decision to divorce to be postponed repeatedly. Separation usually results not from one incident but from a long chain of events. Adjusting to a divorce can be difficult for both spouses and for the children involved. It often causes frustration, conflict, pressure, and changes in the living situation. Most people who divorce eventually remarry. Unfortunately, divorce rates are even higher for second marriages than for first marriages. Some positive things about remarriages, however, are that partners often demonstrate better skills in conflict resolution and communication, and they share more of the housework and child-rearing duties.

Older Adulthood

The process of aging affects individuals physically, mentally, emotionally, and socially. Some people accept the effects of aging gracefully and learn to make the most of their later years (Figure 17-12). Others try to fight the aging process and end up depressed and frustrated. Much of how one handles being elderly is related to how one responds to his or her life cycle in general. The personality you have now can be the one you carry into your later years. Elder adults do not always become crabby, miserable people.

The effects of aging are more difficult for some people than for others. For example, serious health issues or financial difficulties can make older adulthood especially

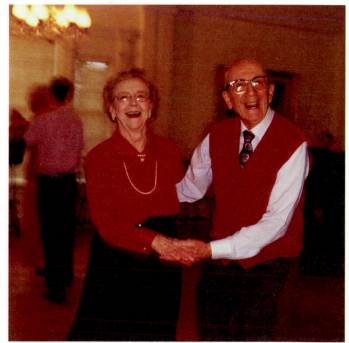

Courtesy of Photodisc

FIGURE 17-12 • Getting older can be a time of rejuvenation.

challenging. Learning now about the aging process and understanding upcoming life changes can influence your health and well-being as you become an older adult. The study of aging is called **gerontology**, and a researcher who studies aging is called a gerontologist. This is an important field of study because in the United States, the elderly population is growing larger every year. In 2000, people over age 65 represented about 13 percent of the total population. By 2050, about 20 percent of the population is expected to be over the age of 65.

In our culture, elderly people face many stressors, but perhaps none is more profound than that of ageism. **Ageism** is discrimination based on age and takes many forms. An example of ageism is the custom of requiring older Americans to retire at a certain age because of false beliefs about the competency of older people. For the same reason, businesses may not want to hire a "senior citizen" because the business world has the idea that old people can't perform well.

One of the best-known organizations formed by elder people to address ageism is the Gray Panthers, a political action group formed in the 1970s that now has more than 15,000 members across the United States. Other organizations that provide information and/or service for the elderly and conduct research on aging are the National Institute on Aging, the Administration on Aging, the National Council on Aging, and the American Association of Retired Persons.

Career and Financial Stressors

Historically, people in the United States retired from their jobs around age 65. This was an arbitrary age defined by Social Security. At the present time, retirement occurs in many forms. Some people still depend on Social Security, but they retire later than age 65 because their benefits are higher if they wait a few more years. Some people have individual retirement accounts that they set up earlier in life by contributing a certain amount of their salary each month. There are some people who plan well enough for retirement that they can retire at any age they desire. It all depends on one's goals in life. For those people who retire and planned ahead for their retirement, they will have the financial resources to enjoy their free time. A good retirement plan includes financial planning and goal setting.

Financial planning means saving and investing regularly during the years you work in order to ensure a steady and reasonable income during the retirement years. Many companies have a retirement plan that allows workers to invest while they are employed. Government workers and state public employees, such as teachers, may be covered by a retirement plan. Some people must rely only on the money they receive from Social Security. The nature of the plan and the age of retirement determine the retirement wage expected from these various kinds of plans.

Before people retire, they should decide what they want to accomplish during their retirement years. These goals usually involve activities that keep the retiree occupied in a productive life. People who retire without anything to do often end up bored and depressed.

---

gerontology
the study of aging

ageism
discrimination based on age

WEB LINK
Healthy Aging

http://www.healthyaging.net

At this Web site, you will find a number of links related to many aspects of healthy aging. There are tips for maintaining a healthy lifestyle into old age and information on mental health with tips from actual seniors.

SEARCH TERMS: healthy aging, health promotion for the elderly

---

Did You Know...?

Financial planning is especially important for women because they are much less likely to have retirement pensions or other investment savings than are men. At the same time, women generally live longer than men, so they have income needs for a longer period of time. As a result, older women are almost two times more likely to retire in poverty than are older men.

What's News

Scientists have discovered that a hormone called tumor necrosis factor (TNF) plays a role in aging. Healthy, active elderly people have a very low level of TNF, whereas people who are invalids have high levels of TNF. More research is needed to learn what causes the body to make this hormone.

Relationship and Family Stressors

As adults grow older, their children become grown adults and have families of their own. The parents now become grandparents and may eventually need extra help in performing their daily activities. When aging parents need extra help, the previous roles of the parents and children are reversed. The children become caregivers, and the older adults are the recipients of their care. These new roles can create stress for both the parents and the adult children. The children are challenged with balancing their job and their family needs with the needs of the parents. One or more of the adult children may have to assume a great deal of responsibility for their parents. In some cases, elderly parents move into the same house with their children. Some adult children decide to quit their job to care for their parents. For those adult children who work outside the home, elder adult day care centers provide assistance. These centers are much like child day care centers, providing a safe environment, activities, and meals during the day. Adult children drop their elderly parents off at the centers in the morning on their way to work and pick them up in the afternoon on their way home.

Older couples who don't have children lack this potential support structure. They may have to rely on friends or other family members if they need assistance. One of the major challenges of being an elder adult is accepting the fact that you are no longer able to be as independent as you once were.

WEB LINK
National Council on Aging
http://www.ncoa.org
This Web site contains a lot of information related to aging in America. From there, you can navigate the site and get health tips, Medicare information, and health newsletters.

SEARCH TERMS: healthy aging, elder health

Health Stressors

Elder adults find themselves coping with getting older. There are numerous **aging markers** that begin to appear as the years go by. Aging markers are those characteristics of aged people that characterize old age, such as wrinkled skin. As people grow toward being senior citizens, their bodies begin to change in many ways:

- *Changes in appearance.* Some older adults shrink in height. Their skin wrinkles and sags, yet some of their facial features will get heavier. They may begin balding, or their hair may turn gray become thinner and brittle.

- *Changes in physical senses.* All the senses change to some degree with aging. About a third of the elderly suffer hearing loss that requires corrective treatment. Vision often develops into a condition known as **presbyopia**. This condition does not allow the old person's eyes to focus on near objects, such as book print. Their visual acuity also diminishes with age. They do not see well in dim light. The sense of smell and taste diminish as well, presenting their specific effects on health. For example, old people who can't smell well may be prone to eating spoiled food, and

aging markers
physical changes that characterize old age

presbyopia
change in the eyesight of elder adults characterized by the inability to see close-up objects

the elderly are prone to overuse salt on their food because the taste receptors on their tongue don't register the salty taste they are used to.

- *Diseases.* Older adults may begin to experience age-related diseases such as osteoporosis, arthritis, and high blood pressure. These conditions may have been present when the individuals were younger, but the aging process makes the conditions worse. Of particular concern are conditions like Parkinson's and Alzheimer's diseases.

- *Changes in health status.* Organs of the body don't function as well as people age, and the immune system is not as strong as it was when they were younger. Illnesses can affect older people more severely than younger people. This is why influenza becomes a life-threatening condition among aged people.

- *Cognitive changes.* Memory can decline as the aging process advances. The elderly may not remember things as easily as they did in the past. Memory losses occur simply because nerve tissue among elder adults is not able to transmit impulses as well as it did when they were younger. Learning and problem solving may become more difficult.

Although many of these changes occur naturally as part of the aging process, staying active both physically and mentally can help slow the changes (Figure 17-13). Keeping active and practicing wellness behaviors throughout life have been shown to prevent many of the chronic diseases that affect older adults. It's never too early to start building the foundation for a healthy adulthood that extends into a happy old age.

Dealing with Death

One of the inevitable consequences of growing old is the fact that all human beings eventually die. Death is not a pleasant subject for most people, but it is something that has to be dealt with by family and caregivers. Developing an understanding of death and the grieving process that goes with it is a healthy addition to any wellness plan.

Psychologists have studied death and dying for many years. The pioneering work on the dying process was conducted by Dr. Elisabeth Kübler-Ross (1969). She studied

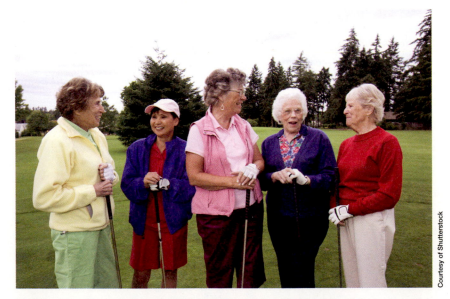

FIGURE 17-13 • Staying active and retaining social ties is important for older adults.

people with terminal illnesses and found that there appeared to be five specific stages that most of them passed through as they were dying:

1. *Denial.* The person doesn't accept the news that death is predicted by medical tests. Many people believe that the diagnosis is wrong or that the tests belong to someone else.

2. *Anger.* The person lashes out because he or she does not want to face the inevitable. The anger may be directed toward hospital personnel, family members, or friends.

3. *Bargaining.* The person may turn to prayer for help to find a cure for the condition. In essence, the person seeks a cure in exchange for promising to lead a better life.

4. *Depression.* The person may withdraw to a very personal space and refuse visitors. During this time, he or she needs the time to accept the reality that he or she will die.

5. *Acceptance.* The person finally accepts the impending outcome and reaches a peaceful state of readiness.

It is important to note that not every dying person passes through all these stages and that some people may float back and forth among the stages. Not every person exhibits the same behaviors during the stages, but all terminally ill people exhibit characteristics of some of these stages. Understanding the process can help you better respond to someone who needs support and understanding during a difficult time.

Grieving

Everyone responds to someone's death in their own way. Generally, we respond to death in a manner that reflects the values and personality of our family, and we may express our grief by participating in rituals and ceremonies defined by cultural and religious customs. These activities are designed to celebrate the deceased and help family and friends overcome the loss.

Adults exhibit their grief much differently than do young children. Children generally do not understand the permanence of death until they become teenagers. A four-year-old, for example, may believe that death is reversible and that the deceased person will return later. The grief response becomes deeper as a person gets older, largely because of the years of connection to the deceased and a mature understanding of the grieving process.

In Closing

The course you are now completing and this textbook have provided you with essential knowledge and skills to develop your personal wellness lifestyle. We hope you will consider this the start of your journey to lifetime wellness. The information you have and the health literacy skills that you have developed will serve you well for the rest of your life. Apply them wisely. Use your knowledge and skills to keep yourself well, and advocate for the wellness philosophy to your friends and family.

BUILDING YOUR LIFETIME WELLNESS PLAN

As you age and mature, you will have stressors that correspond to the various stages of your life cycle. Throughout your life, you will face numerous challenges and decision-making opportunities that will affect your career, financial condition, relationships, and family. You may face health challenges as well, especially in later life. Knowing what life events lie ahead and how to recognize the challenges they represent will help you develop behaviors and strategies to lead a healthy, happy life. Here are some things to consider for your wellness plan:

- Consider which stressors you are most likely to face in each stage of adulthood.

- List some ways you might work through those stressors.

- Think about what you can do *now* to prepare for future life events.

- Give some thought to how you might help your parents or grandparents with their life cycle challenges now or in the future.

●●● End-of-Chapter Activities

Opportunities for Application

1. Go to the Internet and find some quotations about the life cycle. Find two quotes for each of the following topics. Write down the quotes and comment on what each of them means to you.

Topic	Quote	Reaction
Love		
Marriage		

Topic	Quote	Reaction
Family		
Responsibility		

2. List what you consider to be the three most significant stressors of adulthood and describe the contributing factors.

3. Discuss the things couples should talk about before they marry.

Key Concepts

1. Describe how learning about aging contributes to a person's maturation process.

2. Explain why ageism is harmful to our society.

3. List and describe the six stages of the family life cycle.

Answers to Personal Assessment: Being an Adult

Answers will vary. A higher proportion of "definitely true" or "mostly true" responses to the first five questions indicates that you have negative or unrealistic views of adulthood and aging. A higher proportion of "definitely true" or "mostly true" responses to the last five questions suggest that you have more positive or realistic views of adulthood and aging.

Scoring for the Miller-Rahe Life Change Assessment

The higher the score, the more likely you are to experience an adverse health change within two years:

Score of 300 and higher = 90 percent chance of getting sick within two years.

Score of 150 to 299 = 50 percent chance of getting sick within two years.

Score below 150 = 30 percent chance of getting sick within two years.

Marriage Quiz

The following answers are based on research conducted over many years:

1. True. Good marriages don't just happen; they develop over time with good communication and commitment.

2. False. Studies now indicate that men and women benefit equally from being married.

3. False. The age at first marriage has risen to the mid-twenties. In the early 1960s, it was about 20 years.

4. True. Currently, college-educated women are more likely to be married than are non–college-educated women even though they marry later than non–college-educated women do.

5. False. It appears that the first child in a marriage tends to bring stress into the marriage.

6. False. Reported research indicates that being *unmarried*—especially living with a man outside of marriage—increases a woman's chances of being physically abused.

7. False. Their marriages are less satisfying and are more likely to end in divorce.

8. False. Longevity is not a factor. In fact, 50 percent of all divorces take place in the first seven years.

9. True. Research data support this conclusion.

●●● References

Bannister, P. (2004). *25 fascinating facts about personal debt*. Retrieved January, 2010 from http://bankrate.com/brm/news/debt/debtguide2004/debt-trivial.asp.

Holmes, T., & Rahe, R. (1967). Social Readjustment Scale. *Journal of Psychosomatic Research, 11,* 213–218.

Kubler-Ross, E. (1969). *On Death and Dying*. New York, NY: Scribner.

Miller, M. A. and Rahe, R. H. (1997) Life changes scaling for the 1990's. *Journal of Psychosomatic Research, 43,* (3), 279–292.

Money-zine.com. (2009). *Consumer Debt Statistics*. Money-zine.com. Retrieved April 2010 from http://www.money-zine.com/Financial-Planning/Debt-Consolidation/Consumer-Debt-Statistics/

National Center for Education Statistics. (2009). *Distribution of earnings and median earnings of persons 25 years old and over, by highest level of education and sex:2008*. Retrieved March 15, 2010 from http://nces.ed.gov/programs/digest/d08/tables/dt08_385.asp

U.S. Census Bureau. (January 15, 2010). Census Bureau reports families with children increasingly face unemployment. *U.S. Census Bureau News*. Retrieved April 2010 from http://www.census.gov/Press-Release/www/releases/archives/families_households/014540.html

Woolsey, B., & Shulz, M. (2010). *Credit card statistics, industry facts, debt statistics*. CreditCards.com. Retrieved April 6, 2010 from http://www.creditcards.com/credit-card-news/credit-card-industry-facts-personal-debt-statistics-1276.php

GLOSSARY

Abusive relationship Relationship in which one of the partners uses power and control over the other in order to get what he or she wants.

Acquired immunodeficiency syndrome (AIDS) A condition caused by HIV infection whereby a portion of the immune system is destroyed, making it easy for the infected person to get life-threatening diseases.

Acute bronchitis Inflammation of the bronchi (airways) by microorganisms.

Addictive relationship Relationship in which the object of your affection is the center around which your world revolves or your "drug of choice."

Adrenal glands A set of glands on top of each kidney that produce two types of hormones that regulate the stress response and sexual development.

Adrenaline and noradrenalin Hormones produced in the adrenal medulla that regulate blood pressure and blood flow under conditions of stress.

Aerobic activities Activities that require a continual supply of oxygen during the activity.

Aerobic capacity The maximum amount of oxygen that can be delivered to and used by the cells of the body during vigorous workouts.

Ageism Discrimination based on age.

Aging markers Physical changes that characterize old age.

Alcohol dehydrogenase (ADH) An enzyme in the liver responsible for alcohol metabolism.

Alimentary canal The tubular passage from the mouth to the rectum that functions in digestion, the absorption of food and water, and the elimination of waste.

Alkaloid An organic compound containing carbon, hydrogen, and nitrogen.

Alveoli Structures at the ends of the bronchioles that inflate with air when we breathe.

Amino acids Organic compounds that are the building blocks of protein.

Amortized The provision of paying off a borrowed amount of money over a predetermined time period.

Anaerobic activities Activities that require short bursts of energy that cannot be sustained for long periods of time because the body cannot supply enough oxygen quickly enough to keep up with the demand.

Androgens Male sex hormones produced in the adrenal cortex.

Android fat Fat that has accumulated in the region of the trunk.

Android fat pattern Accumulation of excess fat around the abdominal area, characteristic of male weight gain pattern.

Angioplasty Medical procedure in which a small balloon is inserted into a clogged coronary artery and inflated to reduce an obstruction.

Anorexia athletica A disorder that is most often common in competitive athletes and that occurs when someone starts compulsive exercising and does so in an amount of time or at an intensity that is beyond normal.

Anorexia nervosa An eating disorder in which a person does not eat enough food for the body to function at a healthy level or to maintain a healthy weight (can result in death by starvation).

Antibiotics A class of medications that kill bacteria and clear up infection.

Antioxidant Compound that interferes with the damaging effects of certain compounds in the body; may help lower LDL in the blood and prevent certain cancers.

Arterioles The smallest of the arteries leading to capillaries.

Asbestosis Chronic inflammation of the lung tissue caused by exposure to asbestos.

Asthma A condition of the lungs characterized by periodic episodes of airway spasms, causing shortness of breath.

Atherosclerosis A buildup of firm fatty deposits along the inner lining of the arteries that causes the opening inside the artery to narrow and lose elasticity.

Attempted suicide A deliberate, intentional, self-inflicted act that is intended to cause death but does not.

Autonomic nervous system The division of the nervous system that controls basic body processes that are largely involuntary, such as breathing, heartbeat, blood pressure, and digestion.

Bacterial meningitis Inflammation of brain lining caused by various forms of bacteria.

Bariatric Surgical interventions specific to obesity treatment.

Basal body temperature (BBT) The temperature of the body at complete rest.

Basal metabolism The amount of energy needed to maintain body functions at rest.

Benign tumors Abnormal growth of cells that form a noncancerous tumor.

Binge drinking Drinking consisting of five or more alcoholic drinks on a single drinking occasion for males and four or more drinks for females.

Binge-eating disorder A condition in which a person eats large amounts of food frequently and repeatedly.

Biogas Gas, such as methane, produced from the decomposition of natural material.

Biopsy The removal of a tiny piece of a tumor for examination under a microscope.

Bioterrorism The threatened or intentional release of viruses, bacteria, or other toxins to intimidate or harm a civilian or government population.

Birth control Any behavior or method designed to prevent conception or childbirth.

Bisexual Sexual attraction for both genders.

Blastocyst A mass of cells that implants in the uterus after fertilization of the ovum.

Blended family A family created when one or both of the partners who remarry bring children from a previous marriage into the new family unit.

Blood alcohol concentration (BAC) The percent of ethyl alcohol present in the bloodstream after drinking alcoholic beverages.

Body composition The relationship between fat-free mass (muscle, bone, and water) and fat tissue within the body.

Body image The way you see yourself when you look in the mirror or when you picture yourself in your mind.

Body mass index (BMI) A commonly used measure of the relationship (or ratio) of weight to height expressed in a mathematical formula.

Botulism A strong toxin that affects muscles in the body that can result in death if not treated quickly and properly; most often due to improperly canned foods.

Boundaries Imaginary lines that indicate a limit beyond which you will not go.

British Thermal Units (BTUs) A unit of energy used worldwide in the power, steam generation, and heating and air-conditioning industries (one BTU 5 = about .25 calories).

Bronchi The branches of the airway that enter the lungs.

Bronchiectasis A condition in which the airways of the lungs become scarred, swollen, and filled with mucus.

Bronchioles The very ends of the bronchial tree.

Bronchitis Inflammation of the major airways in the lungs (bronchi).

Bulbourethral gland Small gland near the base of the urethra that produces a fluid that conditions the urethra for the movement of sperm.

Bulimia nervosa An eating disorder in which a person eats a great deal of food and then vomits or uses other methods, such as laxatives or overexercising, to avoid gaining weight from the overeating.

Bullying The use of threats or force by one person or group to intimidate another person or group.

Calorie A measure of the amount of energy needed to raise the temperature of one kilogram of water one degree Celsius; scientists burn foods to measure the number of calories they contain.

Campylobacter A species of bacteria that causes diarrheal illness in the United States.

Cancer The uncontrolled growth and spread of abnormal cells in the body.

Capillaries The smallest of blood vessels, where oxygen and nutrients are exchanged for carbon dioxide and waste at the cell level.

Carbohydrates Food substances that provide energy for the body.

Carbon monoxide A colorless, odorless, poisonous gas.

Carcinogen A substance that causes cancer.

Cardiomyopathy An enlarged but weak heart muscle.

Cardiorespiratory fitness The ability of the respiratory and circulatory systems to deliver enough oxygen to sustain moderate levels of activity for long periods of time.

Cardiovascular disease Any number of medical conditions that affect the heart or blood vessels servicing the heart.

Carriers Infected people who do not show symptoms of a disease but who can spread it to others.

Cartilage A firm but elastic material that keeps the trachea open for the passage of air.

Cauterization Using a small electrical probe to burn tissue to destroy it.

Centrioles Two spindlelike structures within the cell that help align chromosomes during cell division.

Cervix Opening to the uterus.

Cesarean-section delivery Birthing procedure in which the fetus is surgically removed from the uterus.

Chlorofluorocarbons (CFCs) Highly stable compounds used as components of aerosol propellants and refrigerants.

Cholera An acute infectious diarrheal disease caused by a bacterium.

Cholesterol A waxy, fatlike substance in the body an excess of which may contribute to heart disease.

Chronic bronchitis Bronchitis characterized by a productive cough that continues for at least three months.

Chronic diseases Disease conditions that continue for a long time.

Cilia Microscopic hairlike projections on certain cells that line the airways and sweep mucus and debris up the airway to the throat.

Circumcision Surgical removal of the foreskin.

Clitoris A small mass of erectile tissue above the vagina which, when stimulated, is the source of sexual pleasure for a woman.

Coercion The use of physical or psychological threat or force to obtain a desired outcome.

Cognitive-behavioral therapy Used by a trained mental health professional to help a patient alter his or her response to a stimulus.

Collagen Firm, flexible connective tissue in the body, made of protein.

Complete protein Protein source containing all nine essential amino acids.

Completed suicide A term used to describe a suicide attempt that results in death.

Compromise A conflict resolution in which both parties give up something.

Compulsions Repetitive behaviors that are performed in response to obsessive thoughts.

Concentric A muscle shortens as a result of moving a resistance.

Conflict A struggle caused by incompatible or opposing interests, values, needs, or desires.

Conflict resolution A structured problem-solving process that uses reflective awareness, communication skills, problem-solving skills, and decision-making skills to prevent, manage, and peacefully resolve conflicts.

Contraception A method of preventing the union of sperm and ovum following an act of sexual intercourse.

Coronary artery disease Atherosclerosis in the coronary arteries.

Coronary heart disease A condition whereby the arteries servicing the heart muscle get blocked.

Corpus luteum Structure formed in the ovary where the ovum was released (produces progesterone).

Cortisol A significant hormone produced by the adrenal glands and involved in a number of body functions such as regulation of sugar metabolism and blood pressure.

Credentials Titles, education, or training that verify a person's intellectual or professional ability.

Critical thinking Evaluating the worth, accuracy, or authenticity of issues and information, leading to a level of conclusion that can direct thoughts or actions.

Cross training Participating in two or more different physical activities to achieve cardiorespiratory fitness.

Cryosurgery The use of liquid nitrogen to freeze cancerous tumors, thus destroying cancerous tissue.

Cyberbullying The use of electronic information and communication technologies, such as the Internet or text messaging, to harass and intimidate.

Daily Reference Values (DRVs) Reference values of eight selected nutrients for a 2,000-calorie diet; the basis of nutrition labels.

Date rape or acquaintance rape Any forced sexual activity in which the victim is acquainted with or is dating the rapist.

Dating Going out with another person in whom you have a romantic interest.

Decibel A measure of the intensity, or loudness, of a sound.

Deductive reasoning Reasoning that begins with the general and ends with the specific (arguments are based on laws, rules, and established principles, and conclusions are based on two or more premises).

Defense mechanisms Mental strategies and behaviors used to protect ourselves from situations that cause conflict or anxiety.

Deterrence The use of threats by one party to intimidate another party from exercising a particular behavior.

Diabetes Disease in which the pancreas does not produce enough insulin, a hormone needed to properly convert sugar to energy.

Diabetes A disease characterized by high levels of sugar in the bloodstream caused by the body's either not producing enough insulin or not correctly using the insulin that is produced.

Diaphragm A muscle just above the abdomen that supports breathing.

Diastolic pressure Pressure measured in the arteries as the heart relaxes to fill with blood.

Dieting Temporary patterns of eating that restrict calories for the purpose of losing weight.

Disaccharides Double sugar molecules that must be broken down to monosaccharides during digestion.

Disordered eating patterns Occasions when dieting, food restriction, fear of becoming overweight, and body image dissatisfaction interfere with normal daily life.

Distress A negative form of stress that occurs in reaction to something we perceive as bad.

Dopamine A neurotransmitter in the brain.

Dose related Drug effects increase as the frequency and quantity of a drug increases.

Drug abuse The intentional use of chemical substances to achieve an altered mental state.

Drug dependence A need for a drug that results in a continuous use of the drug.

Drug tolerance Physical change in the body that causes one to adapt to the effects of a drug, causing the person to use more of the drug to get the same effect.

Ductus deferens Duct that transports sperm from the epididymis to the penis.

Dynamic stretching Slow and controlled movement through a range of motion.

Dysfunctional family A family in which family interactions negatively affect the physical, emotional, and social development and well-being of the individuals in the family.

Eating disorders Problems related to food, weight, and body image that are harmful to physical or psychological health.

Eccentric A muscle lengthens in response to the release of weight held by a concentric contraction.

Ecosystem A complex collection of living things that share a specific environment.

Ecosystem A complete, self-sustaining community of living organisms and the nonliving materials that support them.

Electrocardiograph (ECG) A device that measures the electrical output of the heart muscle.

Embryo Animal organism in the early stages of development; in humans, this stage begins with conception and lasts for 14 weeks.

Emotionally healthy Refers to a person who is in touch with his or her entire range of feelings and can express those feelings in an appropriate way.

Emphysema A condition in which the alveoli tear because of overinflation.

Empty nest A family whose children have grown up and left home.

Endocrine system A system of glands, tissues, and cells that produce hormones to help regulate bodily processes.

Endometrium The innermost lining of the uterus where a fertilized ovum becomes implanted and nourished during pregnancy.

Endotoxins Poisons that come from the cell wall of certain bacteria when they die.

Environmental tobacco smoke Smoke that people breathe when they are in a smoky environment; also called secondhand smoke.

Epididymis Structure adjacent to the testes where sperm are stored.

Ergogenic aids Nutritional or pharmacological agents used by exercisers to help provide fuel and/or to gain a performance advantage.

Escherichia coli A form of bacteria that inhabit the intestinal tracts of humans and other mammals.

Essential amino acids The amino acids humans must get in their diet and that cannot be manufactured by the body.

Essential body fat The amount of fat necessary for use by the body to provide insulation, cushion body organs, and maintain normal bodily functions.

Essential fatty acids (EFAs) Fats needed by the body that must be consumed in the diet because the human body cannot manufacture them.

Estrogen The female hormone produced by the ovaries to repair the uterine lining after menstruation and to enhance feminine characteristics.

Eustress A form of stress that occurs in reaction to something we perceive as good but exciting.

Exhaled mainstream smoke Smoke that is exhaled by the smoker.

Exotoxins Poisons produced by and released from certain bacteria.

Extended family Sharing a home with numerous relatives.

Fad diet An eating regimen that overemphasizes one particular food or type of food and contradicts the guidelines of good nutrition.

Failure rate The number of pregnancies per 100 women using a particular birth control method during a one-year period.

Family household A householder and persons who live in the same household who are related to the householder by birth, marriage, or adoption.

Family life cycle An orderly sequence of developmental stages that most families experience.

Feedback A way to check if you understand what someone has said (a common method is to restate in your own words what you heard and to ask the speaker if this is what he or she meant).

Fermentation The process of converting sugars into ethyl alcohol and carbon dioxide.

Fetal alcohol syndrome (FAS) A characteristic set of birth defects that can occur among babies whose mothers drank alcohol during their pregnancies.

Fight-or-flight response The response of the nervous and endocrine systems to supply the body with energy to fight back or escape from a stressor.

Flexibility The ability to easily move the joints of the body through a full range of motion.

Folate A water-soluble B vitamin that occurs naturally in food.

Fomites Inanimate objects that transmit pathogenic organisms.

Frequency How often the material in a medium vibrates when a wave passes through the medium.

General adaptation syndrome (GAS) The body's physiological response to continuous stress; it includes three phases: alarm, resistance, and exhaustion.

Genes The small units of hereditary material found inside the nucleus of a cell.

Genitalia The external reproductive sex organs.

Gerontology The study of aging.

Glans The rounded head of the penis.

Gynoid fat Fat that tends to accumulate in the hips and thighs.

Gynoid fat pattern Accumulation of excess fat in the hips and thighs, characteristic of female weight gain.

Health literacy The ability to obtain, interpret, understand, and apply basic health information and services.

Health promotion Policies and activities designed to encourage wellness.

Health-related fitness Exercise activities that are specifically designed to provide health benefits to the participant.

Health risk appraisal A computerized assessment of an individual's health age in relation to his or her actual age.

Heimlich maneuver The use of abdominal thrusts to dislodge items that are causing choking; it is named after the physician who perfected the technique, Henry Heimlich.

Hemoglobin An iron-rich compound in the red blood cell that carries oxygen.

Hemorrhagic stroke A blood vessel in the brain bursts, flooding the surrounding area with blood.

Hertz (Hz) Unit used to measure the frequency of sound.

Heterosexual Sexual attraction for someone of the opposite gender.

Homeostasis A condition of the body's internal harmony as regulated by interaction of many body systems.

Homicide The deliberate killing of one human being by another.

Homosexual Sexual attraction for someone of the same gender.

Hormones Chemical messengers produced by the endocrine system to help regulate bodily processes.

Human immunodeficiency virus (HIV) A virus that can multiply and destroy a portion of the human immune system.

Hydrogenation The addition of hydrogen molecules to liquid fats to make them firm at room temperature.

Hypertension Increased pressure in the arteries against which the heart must pump the blood.

Hypokinetic diseases Diseases that are associated with prolonged periods of inactivity.

Hyponatremia A result of a chemical imbalance of too much water and not enough electrolytes in the body.

Hypothalamus An area in the center of the brain that exerts nervous system control over the pituitary gland and the rest of the endocrine system.

Hypothermia Loss of body heat due to exposure to extreme cold.

Ideal body weight The weight at which you feel strong and energetic and lead a healthy life.

Identity The recognition and expression of your uniqueness as a person, including your attitudes, beliefs, and behaviors.

Immunization Introduction of an agent that enables the body to become immune to effects of that agent.

Incomplete proteins Protein sources that do not contain all nine of the essential amino acids.

Inductive reasoning Reasoning that moves from the specific to the general; reasoning in which arguments are based on experience or observations rather than on laws or proven facts.

Infectious diseases Diseases caused by organisms that can spread through water, food, air, or human contact.

Infectious diseases Diseases that are caused by some form of pathogenic organism.

Inpatient Referring to treatment programs that take place while the patient stays in a hospital or other health care setting.

Insulin A hormone produced in the pancreas that is used by the body to turn sugar into energy.

Insulin and glucagon Two hormones produced in the pancreas that regulate the level of blood sugar.

Intentional injury Any harm, injury, or death that is caused deliberately.

Interpersonal conflict Disagreement or argument between persons or groups.

Intimacy A close personal knowledge of another person, characterized by feelings of warmth and closeness.

Intimate partner violence (IPV) Abuse that occurs between two people in a close relationship.

Intrapersonal conflict Confusion or struggle within yourself.

Ischemic stroke When a blood clot forms and blocks blood flow in an artery bringing blood to part of the brain.

Isometric Muscle contraction without movement through a range of motion.

Isotonic exercises Exercises where the muscles move heavy weight through their range of motion.

Job stress The harmful physical and emotional responses that occur when the requirements of the job do not match the capabilities, resources, or needs of the worker.

Ketosis Buildup of ketone bodies, potentially poisonous by-products of fat metabolism.

Labia Folds of skin at the entrance to the vagina.

Laparoscope A slender tube containing a small camera and/or a surgical instrument that can be inserted into the abdomen.

Leachate Liquid produced when water passes through landfill materials.

Leukoplakia A precancerous sore that develops after prolonged exposure to tobacco.

Life expectancy A measure of how long a person has left to live based on data related to current causes of death.

Lipids Fatty compounds in foods that provide energy and transport certain vitamins.

Longevity The length of a person's life.

Love A feeling of strong affection and devotion, characterized by unselfish and loyal concern for the well-being of another.

Mainstream smoke Smoke that comes directly to the smoker from the cigarette.

Malignant tumors Abnormal growth of cells forming a cancerous tumor.

Mammogram Type of imaging that uses a low-dose X-ray system for early detection and diagnosis of breast diseases in women.

Manic Referring to mania, excessive mental and physical energy often associated with mood disorders.

Maslow's hierarchy of needs A well-known representation of human needs progressing from most to least urgent; these needs include physical needs, safety and security, love and belonging, self-esteem, and self-actualization.

Media Methods of mass communication, such as radio, television, movies, magazines, and newspapers.

Mediation A process in which two disputing parties work out their problems by talking through them with an outside person who facilitates the discussion.

Medicine A chemical substance used to treat an ailment or illness.

Megadoses Doses that are much larger than what is recommended, approximately 5 to 10 times the RDI.

Meiosis The process of reducing chromosome numbers in reproductive cells to one-half the original number.

Melatonin A hormone produced by the pineal gland to help regulate sleep cycles.

Menopause A time period in a woman's life when she no longer experiences a menstrual cycle.

Menstruation A cyclical shedding of the uterine lining in response to changes in hormone levels.

Mentally healthy Refers to a person who has the ability to perceive reality in terms of facts and can respond appropriately to the challenges that life presents.

Mesothelioma A form of cancer almost always caused by exposure to asbestos.

Metabolic rate The rate at which your body uses food and oxygen to carry out various body processes.

Metabolism The process of converting food into energy for the body; also includes converting body fat to energy if other energy sources are not available.

Metastasis The spread of cancer from one site to another location in the body.

Methane An odorless, colorless, tasteless, flammable gas created by decomposition of organic material.

Migraine Brain and nervous system disorder characterized by recurring attacks of severe headache.

Milligram A unit of metric weight that is one one-thousandth of a gram; 100 milligrams is equal to 0.0035 ounces—about the same weight as a pinch of salt.

Mind mapping A technique that enables you to organize and illustrate your thoughts using both sides of your brain.

Mindful eating Paying attention to the food you are eating and enjoying its tastes, smells, and textures.

Mitosis The process of duplicating living cells.

Monosaccharides The simplest form of sugar that can be immediately absorbed into the bloodstream.

Monounsaturated fats Types of oils containing fats that contribute very little to the development of heart disease.

Morning sickness A feeling of nausea experienced by some women during the first trimester of pregnancy.

Muscle dysmorphia A male's excessive preoccupation with a very muscular body image.

Muscular endurance The ability of a muscle to contract repeatedly without becoming fatigued.

Muscular strength The amount of force a muscle is capable of exerting against a resistance with a single maximum effort.

Mycotoxins A class of toxins produced by certain types of fungi.

Myocardial infarction Medical term for heart attack.

Myotonia Involuntary muscle tension that occurs in males and females in response to sexual excitement.

Negotiation A process in which two disputing parties work out their problems by talking through them without the assistance of an outside party.

Neuron A specialized body cell that is the basic unit of nerve tissue.

Neurotransmitter A chemical in the body that regulates the movement of impulses among nerve cells.

Neurotransmitters Chemicals produced in the brain that allow transmission of impulses between nerve cells.

Nicotine An addictive chemical stimulant found in tobacco.

Nitrogen oxides Nitrogen-based compounds formed from burning fossil fuels.

Nonpoint contamination Pollutants that make their way to a body of water through runoff from rain or irrigation.

Nutrient density How many nutritional elements are present in a given amount of food.

Obese A term used to describe an excessively high amount of body fat in relation to lean body mass.

Obsessions Unwanted and distressing thoughts or impulses that occur repeatedly.

Occupational interest inventory A test that measures a person's interests as they are related to various jobs and careers.

Opinion A belief based on what seems to be true rather than on tested knowledge.

Opportunistic infections Infections caused by organisms that would not be present in people with normal, healthy immune systems.

Optimal health The condition in which a person is the healthiest that he or she can possibly be.

Orgasm A burst of nervous stimulation and muscular contractions that follows the sexual tension of the plateau phase.

Osteoporosis A condition where the bones get weak and brittle because of a lack of calcium.

Outpatient Refers to treatment given to a patient during periodic visits to a health care facility or physician's office.

Ovary Structure responsible for producing reproductive cells and female sex hormones.

Over-the-counter (OTC) medications Medicines that do not require a doctor's prescription.

Overweight A term to describe body weight that is too high in relation to height.

Ovulation The release of an ovum from one of the ovaries.

Ovum The female reproductive cell (the plural is ova).

Parasites Organisms that rely on a host organism for survival; usually the host organism is harmed in some way.

Parasympathetic nervous system The branch of the autonomic nervous system that slows down body processes and returns the body to homeostasis after a stressful situation has passed.

Parathyroid glands Four very small glands located on the thyroid gland that help regulate calcium.

Passion A strong liking for, desire for, or romantic attraction to another person.

Pathogenic organisms Also called pathogens, living organisms that can cause disease by invading the body's tissues and multiplying; commonly referred to as germs.

Pedometer A personal calculator worn by someone to measure the steps taken during a given time period.

Periodontal tissue Supporting tissue around the tooth root.

Personal identity A unified sense of self, expressing attitudes, beliefs, and actions that are uniquely characteristic of you.

Pheromones Substances produced by animals that serve to attract a partner for reproductive purposes.

Phobias Overwhelming, illogical fears of an event or object.

Pituitary gland Pea-sized gland in the center of the brain that regulates most of the endocrine glands in the body.

Placenta An organ that forms in the uterus during pregnancy to aid in the exchange of nutrients and waste products between mother and embryo or fetus.

Point contamination Pollutants that are added directly at the site of the aquatic source.

Polysaccharides Also known as "complex carbohydrates" because they are compounds of many monosaccharides.

Polyunsaturated fats Fats that come from plant sources that are better for heart health than saturated fats.

Posttraumatic stress disorder A mental disturbance that results from experiencing or witnessing a traumatic event that is replayed over and over in the mind after the event is over.

Prenatal care All the things done to safeguard the health of the mother and fetus throughout pregnancy.

Prepared childbirth A birthing method that uses relaxation techniques and procedures to deliver the fetus without surgery.

Presbyopia Change in the eyesight of elder adults characterized by the inability to see close-up objects.

Prescription drug abuse The use of a medical drug product for nonmedical reasons.

Prescription medicines Medicines that must be prescribed by a trained physician to ensure that they fit the medical condition for which they are being taken.

Progesterone The female hormone responsible for developing the uterine lining during pregnancy.

Proof The measure of the amount of alcohol in a liquor; a 90-proof liquor is 45 percent alcohol.

Prostate gland Accessory structure of the male reproductive system that supports movement of sperm.

Protein Nutrient used by the body to build and repair tissue and to manufacture enzymes.

Psychiatrists Medical doctors who specialize in treating mental illnesses.

Psychoneuroimmunology (PNI) The study of the interrelationships among the emotions, brain, nervous system, and immune system.

Psychotherapists Mental health professionals who are trained to treat mental disorders using psychological counseling techniques.

Psychotic Referring to a mental disorder in which the patient loses touch with reality by way of hallucinations, paranoid behavior, and fantasy thoughts.

Public health Sum of federal, state, and local health agencies and organizations working together to promote health and prevent disease for the community as a whole.

Purging Removing undesirable substances; in the case of bulimia nervosa, refers to vomiting or using laxatives or exercise to remove excessive amounts of food consumed.

Receptors Nerve endings that receive stimuli, as from the sense organs.

Reciprocity The "give-and-take" of a relationship; the evenness of exchange between the people involved.

Reference Daily Intakes (RDIs) The levels of a vitamin or mineral recommended to be included in the diet each day.

Reflective awareness The ability to identify to yourself what you are thinking or feeling at any given moment in time.

Relapse A condition in which someone gets sick with the same illness before fully recovering.

Replication A process whereby viruses use the genetic material of host cells to produce new virus particles.

Resiliency The ability to bounce back after experiencing distressing or traumatic events.

Respiration The exchange of oxygen and carbon dioxide in the lungs.

Risk factors Identifiable conditions or behaviors that increase one's risk of getting ill or injured.

Rohypnol A drug used in countries outside the United States as treatment for insomnia but most commonly known in the United States as a date-rape drug.

Romantic love A type of love that includes an attraction to another person based on affection and sexual interest.

Salmonellosis Food poisoning caused by Salmonella bacteria from contaminated food sources, especially chicken and other meat products.

Saturated fats Fats from animal sources that are firm at room temperature.

Scabies Infection caused by a small mite.

Schizophrenia A brain disease that is perhaps the most severe of the mental illnesses.

Secondary infection An infection that arises at a location other than the original site; usually caused by a second pathogen or irritant.

Self-actualization The highest level in Maslow's hierarchy of needs, representing an optimal level of mental and emotional function.

Self-disclosure Revealing personal information to others.

Self-imposed quarantine Voluntarily staying away from other people when you are ill so as not to spread disease.

Semen A translucent solution containing sperm and nourishing fluids from the seminal vesicles and the prostate.

Seminal vesicles Structures that produce a component of semen that nourishes and protects sperm.

Serotonin A hormone produced by the pineal gland to help regulate nerve impulses.

Sexual assault A sexual act involving the use of force or threat of force to get the victim to cooperate.

Sexual harassment Any unwelcome sexual advances, requests for sexual favors, or other conduct that is sexual in nature and creates an intimidating atmosphere in an academic or work environment.

Sexual identity The inner sense that individuals have about their own sexual identity.

Sexual orientation A lasting emotional, romantic, or sexual attraction for another person.

Sidestream smoke Smoke that comes from the burning end of a cigarette.

Similarity factors Those characteristics, values, and goals, shared by two people in a relationship.

Skill-related fitness The type of fitness required for participating in sports or other skill-related activities; includes such components as power, agility, coordination, speed, balance, and reaction time.

Smokeless tobacco Tobacco that is not smoked but is used orally, such as snuff or chewing tobacco.

Social clock A schedule of accomplishments a person believes he or she can or should achieve by a certain age.

Social network A person-centered web of social relationships.

Social psychology The study of how people's thoughts, emotions, and behaviors are influenced by the actual, imagined, or implied presence of others.

Social support Real or perceived emotional and physical support received by family, friends, neighbors, and coworkers.

Social support network People who are willing and able to provide emotional and physical resources to help you in time of need.

Source reduction Change in the design, manufacture, purchase, or use of materials or products (including packaging) to reduce their amount or toxicity before they become municipal solid waste.

Spermicide A chemical that is harmful to sperm.

Sphygmomanometer A device used to measure blood pressure.

Static stretching Stretching a muscle to the end of its range of motion and holding that position for an extended period of time.

Statutory rape Any sexual relations committed by an older individual (generally over the age of 18) with an individual who is under the legal age of consent (generally age 14 or younger).

Stepsiblings Brothers and/or sisters who joined your family when one or both of your parents remarry.

Stigma A belief that most people will devalue and discriminate against individuals who have a mental illness or seek treatment.

Storage fat Body fat as a result of excess calories stored by the body.

Stress The physical and emotional states experienced as a result of changes and challenges in our lives.

Stress hardiness Resilience when confronted with stressors, as identified by the characteristics of challenge, control, and commitment.

Stress response The physiological reactions that occur in the body when a stressor is experienced.

Stressors Situations that trigger physical and emotional reactions in our bodies.

Stroke An event in the brain that cuts off the blood supply to a section of brain tissue.

Suicide A deliberate, intentional, self-inflicted act that results in one's own death.

Surgeon general Highest-ranking medical officer in the United States.

Sympathetic nervous system The branch of the autonomic nervous system that responds to a stressor by accelerating body processes.

Systolic pressure Pressure measured in the arteries as the heart is pumping blood into the arteries.

Target heart rate range The percentage of the predicted maximum heart rate that must be reached to obtain improvements in aerobic capacity.

Temperature inversion An atmospheric condition when cold air at the Earth's surface is trapped by warm air above it.

Tendons Dense connective tissues that attach muscle to bone.

Testes Male sex glands that are located in the scrotum and are responsible for male sexual development and sperm production.

Testimony A firsthand declaration of fact.

Testosterone The male hormone that is produced in the testes.

Tetanus A bacterial disease that affects the nervous system, commonly known as lockjaw; results in death about 10 percent of the time.

Thymus Endocrine gland that helps with the development of a child's immune system.

Thyroid gland Gland that produces hormones that influence growth and development by regulating metabolism.

Tolerance Respect for people whose beliefs and practices differ from yours.

Toxic relationship Romantic involvement that results in negative consequences for one or both partners.

Trachea The airway that extends from the throat to the lungs.

Traditional family A family that consists of two parents and their biological or adopted children.

Trans fats Liquid fats that have been intentionally enhanced with hydrogen to make them firm at room temperature or more suitable for frying.

Type 2 diabetes A condition in which the body cannot transport enough glucose (sugar) to the cells to be converted into energy.

Umbilical cord Flexible structure that contains the arteries and veins that connect the embryo or fetus to the placenta.

Unintentional injuries Injuries that happen when no harm was intended to occur; formerly called accidents.

Unsaturated fats Fats that come from vegetable oil sources.

Urethra Passageway from the bladder to the outside of the body.

Uterine tubes Passageways that transport the ova from the ovaries to the uterus.

Uterus A pear-shaped, muscular organ that provides the proper environment where the fertilized ovum develops into a fetus and assists with childbirth.

Vagina A muscular, flexible passageway between the labia and the uterus.

Valid Based on evidence or supported by scientifically accurate data.

Vasongestion increased vascular blood flow in localized body tissue

Vegetarian The practice of consuming foods only from plant sources, except eggs or dairy products in some instances.

Violence The use of physical force with the intent to inflict harm, injury, or death.

Violent victimization statistics Statistics for rape, sexual assault, robbery, aggravated assault (assault with a weapon), and simple assault; statistics do not include murder.

Volatile organic compounds Chemical compounds formed largely from the combustion of fossil fuels.

Weight bias Negative attitudes and stereotypes that have a detrimental effect on interpersonal relationships.

Wellness Behaviors and habits that have a positive influence on health.

Wellness motives The sum of knowledge, beliefs, attitudes, and values that contribute to forming reasons for practicing wellness behaviors.

Whole blood Blood that contains all the major components blood—red cells, white cells, and platelets.

Withdrawal Feelings of discomfort that occur when the body is deprived of a drug to which it is addicted.

Years of potential life lost The difference in years between an individual's life expectancy and that individual's age at the time of death.

Personal Wellness Plan

1. Think about your responses to the health assessment at the beginning of the chapter. Record the behaviors that did not apply to you. List them in rank order starting with the behavior you feel is most important to you at this time.

_____

_____

_____

_____

2. Look at the behavior you designated for the first position on the list above. Check your ability to locate reliable information on the Web related to that behavior or topic. Fill in the table below.

Topic	URL	Search Terms Used:

3. List five new things you learned from any of the Web sites listed in your table.

_____

_____

_____

_____

Do you feel the information you obtained from the Web was reliable and credible? Explain.

_____

_____

_____

_____

4. Draw the four dimensions of health as they pertain to you at this time; that is, draw each of the dimensions to signify the strength and importance of that particular dimension as it relates to your health status at this time.

5. Using the drawing of the four dimensions of health as a starting point, draw a mind map of what you perceive the future of your health status to be in the next year. What changes would you like to make? What resources do you need to create a healthy life?

Personal Wellness Plan

1. A carefully developed wellness plan will help you easily meet the health and wellness goals you select for yourself. This chapter covered the components of wellness, personal attributes to wellness, and information on setting your wellness goals. Now would be a good time to assess your health condition. Go to the Real Age Web site (see chapter 2, p. 33) or some other site where you can take a free online health risk assessment. Evaluate your medical age as verified by the assessment and determine if you have any threats to your health. The object of this activity is to recognize any health risks you might face while you also identify the wellness behaviors that contribute to your "health age."

_____

_____

_____

_____

_____

2. Here are some things you may want to consider:

- Identify one or two ways you are practicing wellness for relevant behaviors you want to address.

_____

_____

_____

_____

_____

- Think about your current attitudes and motives toward wellness. List at least three attitudes you might develop to help you achieve your wellness goals.

_____

_____

_____

_____

_____

- Use the suggestions for goal setting to set a wellness goal that you could work toward this week. Try some of the strategies that were described in the chapter to increase your success rate and discover which strategies tend to work well for you.

_____

_____

_____

_____

_____

3. Visit the National Institutes of Health Web site and read about *Healthy People 2010*. Choose one of the *Healthy People 2010* objectives and list the personal wellness goals you would like to achieve that are related to that objective.

Objective: _____

_____

_____

_____

_____

4. Think about some things you could do to increase your health literacy skills. Use the Internet to obtain health information for yourself and your family. Practice evaluating the content of some health-related Web sites.

_____

_____

_____

_____

_____

Personal Wellness Plan

1. Start by identifying your major stressors at the current time.

   _____

   _____

   _____

   _____

   _____

2. Consider your stressors listed above. Are they temporary or long lasting? Will they resolve themselves relatively soon, or do you need to create an action plan to manage them?

   _____

   _____

   _____

   _____

   _____

3. Think about how you perceive life's problems and challenges. How can you approach these stressors more positively?

   _____

   _____

   _____

   _____

4. What coping resources do you have to manage these stressors (emotional support, tangible assistance, and so on)?

   _____

   _____

   _____

   _____

5. What steps can you take this week to manage these stressors?

_____

_____

_____

_____

_____

6. What steps can you take over the next week, month, or year to manage these stressors?

_____

_____

_____

_____

_____

7. Identify the specific strategies that you will use to manage these stressors.

_____

_____

_____

_____

_____

8. What benefits will you receive from taking action to manage your stressors?

_____

_____

_____

_____

_____

Personal Wellness Plan

1. Begin your mental health wellness plan by conducting a personal assessment of your mental health status at the present time. Go back through the chapter and review each of the mental/emotional health topics presented and prepare a checklist. For each concept, indicate on your checklist for each of the topic/concepts whether your condition is "fine," "could be better," or "really needs improvement." If you are not sure about your status, use your health literacy skills to locate assessments on the Internet that may help you.

_____

_____

_____

_____

_____

2. Take your assessment results and prioritize each of the items on your assessment that you labeled as "could be better" or "really needs improvement."

_____

_____

_____

_____

_____

3. From your prioritized list, choose the *one* condition that you would like to improve at this time. Do not try to change more than one condition at a time, as this will make your ability to accomplish anything much more difficult.

_____

_____

_____

_____

_____

4. Conduct an Internet search to learn all that you can about the condition you chose. List the sites and the URL addresses. You may want to print copies and make a notebook of the significant information you found at each site.

_____

_____

_____

_____

_____

5. Prepare a one- to two-page report summarizing what you learned and describing, in order, the first three things you intend to do to help you improve your mental health condition.

_____

_____

_____

_____

_____

Personal Wellness Plan

1. Use your health literacy skills to search the Internet for personal assessments that assess one's personal and psychological qualities related to conflict. List the sites you found and their URL addresses in the table. You may want to enter some notes about the sites in the second row. One site you may want to visit is http://www.nvcc.edu/home/npeck/conflicthome/index.htm. Go to "Personal Conflict."

Site Name	URL
1.	
Comments	
2.	
Comments	
3.	
Comments	

2. Write a summary of what you learned about yourself.

_____

_____

_____

_____

_____

3. Given what you learned about yourself, what would you say are the three most useful characteristics you possess for addressing conflict?

_____

_____

_____

_____

_____

4. What cues would you feel that would let you know that you are in a situation that contains conflict?

_____

_____

_____

_____

_____

5. Go back to the chapter and review the skills and qualities that will help you manage conflict in your life. What skills would you like to develop further? What are steps you can take to develop these skills?

_____

_____

_____

_____

_____

Personal Wellness Plan

1. Consider family relationships, friendships, and romantic relationships. What positive qualities do you have to contribute to these relationships?

   _____

   _____

   _____

   _____

   _____

2. What qualities would you like to develop more fully?

   _____

   _____

   _____

   _____

   _____

3. What can you do *this week* to begin working toward improvement in these areas?

   _____

   _____

   _____

   _____

   _____

4. What qualities would be important to you in making new friends or finding a new romantic partner?

   _____

   _____

   _____

   _____

   _____

5. What action steps would you take if you noticed that you were having repeated difficulties in your relationships with family, friends, or romantic partners?

_____

_____

_____

_____

_____

6. Where would you go for help if you or someone you knew were involved in a toxic or an abusive relationship?

_____

_____

_____

_____

_____

Personal Wellness Plan

1. There is much to learn about sexual health and wellness. It is impossible to cover all the information in one chapter. In this regard, using your health literacy skills can help you keep up with current information. You may even uncover information that would be useful for your family or friends. Test your knowledge of human sexuality. Enter the term "sex quiz" into your search engine. Take at least two of the quizzes, see how you score, and answer each of the following:

   • How did you perform on the quizzes? Did you score as well as you thought you would?

   _____

   _____

   _____

   _____

   _____

   • What were the five most significant things you learned from taking the quizzes?

   _____

   _____

   _____

   _____

   _____

   • List three quiz topics that interest you enough that you would like more information.

   _____

   _____

   _____

   _____

   _____

Search for information:

Topic	Search Term Used	URL/Notes

Imagine that you are a parent (if you are not one already). Develop a plan for communicating information on sexuality with your child. Search the Internet for information if you need it.

- At what point in your child's life do you think you should begin sexual education?

_____

_____

_____

_____

_____

- Make a list of the topics you would feel comfortable discussing with your child.

_____

_____

_____

_____

_____

- Make a list of the topics for which you think you need more information.

_____

_____

_____

_____

_____

- What advice would you give your child about having nonmarital sex as a teenager?

_____

_____

_____

_____

_____

2. Give some thought to the opposite sex. What is it about the opposite sex that most intrigues you but that you know the least about? Record your top three issues and fill in this table.

Topic	Information Learned

Personal Wellness Plan

1. The first step in developing a fitness program is to decide what fitness goals you want to pursue. Take the time to consider what dimension of fitness you need to develop the most. Make a list, in priority order, of the top three things you would like to address.

   _____

   _____

   _____

   _____

   _____

2. Decide which of those dimensions of fitness you wish to address as your goal for the next three months.

   _____

   _____

   _____

   _____

   _____

3. Use your health literacy skills to locate valid resources to help you with your goals and list them here.

Resource	Location/Citation	Notes

4. Create a personal activity plan similar to the one in this chapter for just that one fitness goal. Fill in the table with the necessary material.

_____

_____

_____

_____

_____

5. Develop a contract with yourself describing the activities you intend to pursue and the mechanism you will use to ensure that you can achieve your objectives (e.g., exercise partner, motivational strategies, rewards anticipated, exercise appointments, and so on). Include a calendar to help you stick to a schedule. Sign the contract and keep it with your fitness journal.

_____

_____

_____

_____

_____

6. Maintain a fitness journal where you can log your expectations, successes, challenges, and so on. If you can fulfill your contract and stay on target to meet your goal for three months, you are on your way. Then you can repeat the process with the two remaining dimensions you chose in item 2.

_____

_____

_____

_____

_____

7. Do you know someone in your family, at school, or at work who would be a good activity partner? Look for something that you and that other person might enjoy doing together. Strike up a conversation with him or her about physical activity. You might find that the two of you have something in common, and you may even find that he or she is also looking for someone to exercise with.

_____

_____

_____

_____

_____

Personal Wellness Plan

Go to http://www.mypyramid.gov and continue to the My Pyramid Tracker. It is necessary to register for this Web site by giving your user name, age, and gender. This is for privacy purposes and to allow the database to calculate your personal nutrition profile. After you sign up, you will be able to enter the Web site and search for the foods and portion sizes you ate during a 24-hour period. After you enter the foods, portion sizes, and quantity, select "Save and Analyze." After your information is analyzed, you will see a screen that offers a number of options. Select "Meeting Dietary Guidelines." The next screen will give you a comparison of your food intake compared to the recommended guidelines. (Note that if you enter data for alcohol consumption, it will not be reflected in the analysis, as there are no dietary guidelines for alcohol.)

1. How did your intake compare to the recommended guidelines?

_____

_____

_____

_____

_____

2. List the nutrients for which you exceeded the recommended guidelines.

_____

_____

_____

_____

_____

3. List the nutrients for which you fell below the recommended guidelines.

_____

_____

_____

_____

_____

4. Do you feel that this assessment was a reflection of a typical day for you?

_____

_____

_____

_____

_____

5. Given the information you received from the assessment, describe what changes you need to make in your dietary intake.

_____

_____

_____

_____

_____

6. List three dietary goals you expect to achieve in the next four weeks.

_____

_____

_____

_____

_____

7. List at least four resources that will help you reach your nutrition goals.

_____

_____

_____

_____

_____

Personal Wellness Plan

1. Make an effort to determine your percent body fat. You can check your weight on a scale or via a BMI chart, but to get a good body fat assessment, you will need to seek out some more precise methods. If you contact a health promotion, nursing, or physiology program on your campus, you may be able to get your body composition assessed for free by way of skinfold calipers, hydrostatic weighing, or electrical impedance. These programs often need volunteers as subjects to train learners on using the devices or as subjects for faculty/student research. If you are given the opportunity to get one of these assessments, ask if you can come back in six to nine months after you start an exercise program. You might find the results interesting.

_____

_____

_____

_____

_____

2. Do the weight management math and look into the future. Using the skills you learned in chapter 9, calculate the calories you get from foods you eat, each day for a three-day period. Calculate the average for the three days. Project that value to age 50. Then determine the caloric needs for someone of your gender and activity level at age 50. If eating habits stay the same, how many extra calories will you generate per day, per week, and so on? Determine what the weight gain will be between now and then. Explain what you think you could do to protect yourself.

_____

_____

_____

_____

_____

3. Use your health literacy skills and research information about weight loss drug regimens. Create a table of drug products, how they are designed to work, and their advantages, disadvantages, and costs. Summarize what you find and compare the use of drug regimens to a no- or low-cost program of sensible eating and exercise.

_____

_____

_____

_____

_____

4. Search the Internet for weight management Web sites that may be useful to your weight management program or one you may want to recommend to a family member or friend. Be sure that the sites are reliable and valid and that they present information from reliable professional sources. Make a list of the sites and their URLs.

_____

_____

_____

_____

_____

5. Use the Internet to find creative suggestions for weight management or create some of your own that may be helpful in your own program or recommendations you can give to others. An example might be the following: as a convenience, prepare healthy low-fat or low-calorie snacks ahead of time and keep them readily available.

_____

_____

_____

_____

_____

Personal Wellness Plan

In order to clarify your position on smoking, you may want to prepare yourself with information related to many aspects of tobacco use. Some of this information may help you solidify your attitudes or help you assist others to develop wellness patterns to prevent tobacco use.

1. If you have or plan to have children, describe what you would do to inoculate them from taking up tobacco use and justify at what age you would begin this process.

_____

_____

_____

_____

_____

2. In your opinion, what is the worst thing about tobacco use? Use your writing skills to prepare a personal statement describing social, physical, and psychological reasons why you choose to be tobacco free.

_____

_____

_____

_____

_____

3. Imagine you have a close friend or family member who smokes cigarettes. Write them a letter telling them what you have learned about the personal, medical, and social problems associated with smoking. Conclude the letter with a personal statement telling them how you feel about their smoking behavior.

_____

_____

_____

_____

_____

4. List and describe all the things you personally gain from not smoking. Categorize those things according to immediate, short-term, and long-term gains.

_____

_____

_____

_____

_____

Personal Wellness Plan

Alcohol consumption is viewed as an acceptable adult behavior by most people in our society. Yet not everyone needs to consume alcohol. Perhaps you already made your decision about alcohol's role in your life, but if you have not, now is a good time to do so. Consider the following suggestions as you develop your wellness plan.

1. Explore the significance of alcohol use (or future use) in your life. See if you can place yourself on the following continuum and explain how you feel about your position.

Nondrinker	Light drinker	Moderate drinker	Heavy drinker	Alcohol abuser

_____

_____

_____

_____

2. Respond to the following prompts if you have or plan on having a family, or you can respond as recommendations to a family member or close friend who has young children.

- Think about the role that alcohol might play in your family activities and describe how you might communicate expectations to your children and/or role model the behavior.

_____

_____

_____

_____

_____

- What education would you provide children to help them develop healthy attitudes and behaviors regarding alcohol use?

_____

_____

_____

_____

_____

- At what age do you think parents should begin conversations with young children to dissuade them from the use of illicit drugs?

_____

_____

_____

_____

_____

3. Make a list of what you perceive as the five most troublesome illicit drugs that people might use. Construct a table for each drug, like the one shown here, and describe the effects of each drug on the body and the personal and social problems associated with using each drug. Conclude with your personal view of the drug and your perception of personal risk if you were to use it.

Drug name	
Physical effects	
Personal effects	
Social problems	
Personal view of the drug	

Personal Wellness Plan

1. Conduct an Internet search for "adult immunizations." Use the information to construct a table of all the immunizations you already have, the dates of the immunizations, and the years of expected booster immunizations. In the "Comments" column, note any immunizations you need as an adult.

Vaccine	Year of Immunization	Booster Years	Comments

2. Create your own "Top 10 List" of things you can do to protect yourself from infectious diseases.

_____

_____

_____

_____

_____

3. Choose an infectious disease that currently has importance to you, a friend, or a family member and use your health literacy skills to gather information about the disease and develop a "chain of infection model."

Personal Wellness Plan

1. Consider the chronic diseases presented in this chapter and recall that all of them contained various behavioral risk factors known to predispose an individual to those particular conditions. Select at least three chronic diseases that are of interest to you. Create a table that includes each disease, the known behavioral risk factors associated with each disease, a list of the things you currently do to reduce any of the risk factors, and a list of things you want to change in your lifestyle to reduce or eliminate other risk factors.

2. List the seven warning signs of cancer. Do some additional research and under each warning sign describe the type of cancer(s) that may be associated with that warning sign.

_____

_____

_____

_____

_____

3. Research the various cures and treatments for heart disease. Then put your health literacy skills to work and find the medical care cost for each of the treatments. Consider the cost of treatment versus the cost of prevention.

_____

_____

_____

_____

_____

4. Examine each of the chronic diseases discussed in this chapter and note those that have a genetic component to them. Then review your family history and determine if you have a family history for any of these diseases or conditions. Write down what those diseases are and what you can do to reduce your risks of getting them.

_____

_____

_____

_____

_____

Personal Wellness Plan

1. Reflect on your level of comfort with various types of risks. Write your philosophy about taking risks with your health and safety here.

   _____

   _____

   _____

   _____

   _____

2. Consider the information that you have learned in this chapter regarding the objective risk levels associated with various activities. Which risky behaviors related to your safety concern you the most? Write them in the space here.

   _____

   _____

   _____

   _____

   _____

3. What can you do *this week* to begin working toward improvement in these areas?

   _____

   _____

   _____

   _____

   _____

4. What types of safety and emergency preparedness plans do you need to develop? Write them in the space here.

   _____

   _____

   _____

   _____

   _____

5. What action steps will you take to begin development of these plans? Write a "to be completed by" date along with your action steps.

_____

_____

_____

_____

6. Determine when you will need to review your safety and emergency preparedness plans. Write the date in the space here. Are there other people you need to communicate with about your plans? List these people in the space here as well.

_____

_____

_____

_____

Personal Wellness Plan

1. The topic of global warming will be an issue of debate between politicians and scientists for years to come. Research the topic on your own and see if you can develop an accurate summary of the scientific merit of global warming.

   _____

   _____

   _____

   _____

   _____

2. Given what you learned about global warming, what does the information mean to you? Describe the things that you and/or your family could do to prevent global warming.

   _____

   _____

   _____

   _____

   _____

3. Among the environmental issues you studied in this chapter, which do you think is the greatest threat to you personally? Explain why.

   _____

   _____

   _____

   _____

   _____

4. List and describe the three most important things you intend to do to help protect the ecosystem in which you live.

   _____

   _____

   _____

   _____

   _____

5. Solid waste is a major public health concern. Think about the ways you can reduce the amount of solid waste you produce and make a list of 10 behaviors you could adopt to reduce the amount. As an example, use the minimum amount of paper towel to dry your hands.

_____

_____

_____

_____

_____

Personal Wellness Plan

1. Give some thought to where you see yourself five years from today. Describe your goals and where you expect be with respect to the following:

   Education _____

   Work setting _____

   Financial condition _____

   Health status _____

   Relationship _____

   Family _____

   Living arrangements _____

2. For each of the previously mentioned themes, describe what you need to do in order to meet each of the goals you wrote down.

   Education _____

   Work setting _____

   Financial condition _____

   Health status _____

   Relationship _____

   Family _____

   Living arrangements _____

3. Perhaps there will be a time when you intend to have a family. Go to the Internet and search for sites to help you with aspects of family development. Be sure to verify the validity of the site and the information presented.

Topic	Site	URL
Pregnancy and childbirth		
Raising children		
Adolescent development		

4. Find out more about your family history, specifically the chronic disease conditions you might expect to experience as you get older. Research at least one of the conditions. Describe each condition and at what age you might expect to see symptoms and write a plan for what you could do to prevent or lessen the impact of the condition.
References to help you:

_____

_____

_____

_____

_____

5. Imagine that you don't engage in preventive behaviors but that you get the condition named in #4 sometime in the future. How much might it cost per year to treat it? Search the Internet or make calls to insurance companies or hospitals to get this information.
How do you think you will pay for the medical costs?

_____

_____

_____

_____

_____

INDEX